The

I C U

Book

Second Edition

PAUL L. MARINO, MD, PhD, FCCM

Clinical Associate Professor
Departments of Medicine and Emergency Medicine
University of Pennsylvania School of Medicine
Philadelphia, Pennsylvania

Illustrations by Paul Contino
and Graphic World Illustration Studio

The

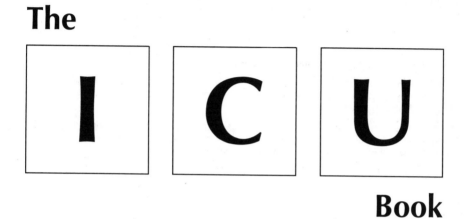

I C U

Book

Second Edition

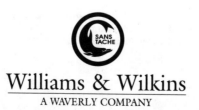

Williams & Wilkins
A WAVERLY COMPANY

BALTIMORE • PHILADELPHIA • LONDON • PARIS • BANGKOK
BUENOS AIRES • HONG KONG • MUNICH • SYDNEY • TOKYO • WROCLAW

Editor: Sharon R. Zinner
Managing Editor: Tanya Lazar
Production Coordinator: Felecia R. Weber
Project Editor: Robert D. Magee
Illustration Planner: Felecia R. Weber
Cover Designer: Cathy Cotter Visual Communications
Typesetter: Maryland Composition Co., Inc.
Printer: Victor Graphics, Inc.
Digitized Illustrations: Paul Contino and Graphic World, Inc.
Binder: Victor Graphics, Inc

Copyright © 1998 Williams & Wilkins

351 West Camden Street
Baltimore, Maryland 21201-2436 USA

Rose Tree Corporate Center
1400 North Providence Road
Building II, Suite 5025
Media, Pennsylvania 19063-2043 USA

Accurate indications, adverse reactions and dosage schedules for drugs are provided in
this book, but it is possible that they may change. The reader is urged to review the package
information data of the manufacturers of the medications mentioned.

Printed in the United States of America

First Edition, 1990

Library of Congress Cataloging-in-Publication Data
Marino, Paul L.
     The ICU book / Paul L. Marino.—2nd ed.
        p.   cm.
     Includes bibliographical references and index.
     ISBN 0-683-05565-8
     1. Critical care medication.   I. Title.
     [DNLM: 1. Intensive Care Units.   2. Critical Care.   WX 218 M3395i
1997]
     RC86.7.M369   1997
     616'.028—dc21
     DNLM/DLC
     for Library of Congress   96-48756
                                                                                     CIP

*The publishers have made every effort to trace the copyright holders for borrowed material.
If they have inadvertently overlooked any, they will be pleased to make the necessary
arrangements at the first opportunity.*

To purchase additional copies of this book, call our customer service department at **(800)
638-0672** or fax orders to **(800) 447-8438.** For other book services, including chapter reprints
and large quantity sales, ask for the Special Sales department.

Canadian customers should call **(800) 665-1148,** or fax **(800) 665-0103.** For all other calls
originating outside of the United States, please call **(410) 528-4223** or fax us at **(410) 528-
8550.**

Visit Williams & Wilkins on the Internet: http://www.wwilkins.com or contact our customer service department at **custserv@wwilkins.com.** Williams & Wilkins customer service
representatives are available from 8:30 am to 6:00 pm, EST, Monday through Friday, for
telephone access.

                                                                        98 99 00
                                                    2 3 4 5 6 7 8 9 10

dedication

To the memory of Mrs. Jean Marino,
my mother . . .
who was so much.

And to Daniel Joseph Marino,
my 9-year-old son . . .
who is even more.

I would especially commend the physician who,
in acute diseases, by which the bulk of mankind
are cutoff, conducts the treatment better than others.

Hippocrates

preface to the second edition

This second edition of THE ICU BOOK retains the purpose of the original text: to create a generic text for all (adult) intensive care units, regardless of the specialty ownership of any individual ICU. In addition, the emphasis on fundamental principles in the text should prove useful for patient care outside the ICU as well. As in the original text, this edition does not cover the highly specialized areas of critical care such as burns, trauma management, and obstetric emergencies because each of these areas has its own experts and comprehensive texts.

This edition represents a completely rewritten version of the original text, with updated references and new illustrations. The list of references at the end of each chapter has an added feature: each of the review articles in the list is accompanied by the number of citations in the review to give the reader an indication of the depth of the review. Ten new chapters have been added on topics that include oxidation injury (Chapter 3), analgesia and sedation (Chapter 8), assessment of tissue oxygenation (Chapter 13), inflammation and multiorgan injury (Chapter 31), the immunocompromised patient (Chapter 34), neurologic disorders (Chapters 50, 51, and 52), pharmaceutical toxins and antidotes (Chapter 53), and drug dosing adjustments for renal dysfunction, liver failure, and drug interactions (Chapter 54). The Appendix has also been completely revised, with new sections on units of measurements and conversions, and selected vital statistics.

Finally, this edition retains a single author, and thus personal preference is inevitably weaved into the fabric of the text. The hope is that this is not a shortcoming, or at least not an intolerable one.

preface to first edition

In recent years, the trend has been away from a unified approach to critical illness, as the specialty of critical care becomes a hyphenated attachment for other specialties to use as a territorial signpost. The landlord system has created a disorganized array of intensive care units (10 different varieties at last count), each acting with little communion. However, the daily concerns in each intensive care unit are remarkably similar because serious illness has no landlord. The purpose of THE ICU BOOK is to present this common ground in critical care and to focus on the fundamental principles of critical illness rather than the specific interests for each intensive care unit. As the title indicates, this is a 'generic' text for all intensive care units, regardless of the name on the door.

The present text differs from others in the field in that it is neither panoramic in scope nor overly indulgent in any one area. Much of the information originates from a decade of practice in intensive care units, the last three years in both a Medical ICU and a Surgical ICU. Daily rounds with both surgical and medical housestaff have provided the foundation for the concept of generic critical care that is the theme of this book.

As indicated in the chapter headings, this text is problem-oriented rather than disease-oriented, and each problem is presented through the eyes of the ICU physician. Instead of a chapter on GI bleeding, there is a chapter of the principles of volume resuscitation and two others on resuscitation fluids. This mimics the actual role of the ICU physician in GI bleeding, which is to manage the hemorrhage. The other features of the problem such as locating the bleeding site, are the tasks of other specialists. This is how the ICU operates and this is the specialty of critical care. Highly specialized topics such as burns, head trauma, and obstetric emergencies are not covered in this text. These are distinct subspecialties with their own texts and their own experts, and devoting a few pages to each would merely complete and outline rather than instruct.

The emphasis on fundamentals in THE ICU BOOK is meant not only as a foundation for patient care but also to develop a strong base in clinical problem solving for any area of medicine. There is a tendency to rush past the basics in the stampede to finish formal training, and this leads to empiricism and irrational practice habits. Why a fever should or should not be treated, or whether a blood pressure cuff provides accurate readings, are questions that must be dissected carefully in the early stages of training, to develop the reasoning skills needed to be effective in clinical problem solving. This inquisitive stare must replace the knee-jerk approach to clinical problems if medicine is to advance. THE ICU BOOK helps to develop this stare.

Wisely or not, the use of a single author was guided by the desire to present a uniform view. Much of the information is accompanied by published works listed at the end of each chapter and anecdotal tales are held to a minimum. Within an endeavor such as this, several shortcomings are inevitable, some omissions are likely and bias may occasionally replace sound judgment. The hope is that these deficiencies are few.

acknowledgments

This book owes its existence to the following individuals. First to Sharon Zinner and Tanya Lazar at Williams & Wilkins, who coordinated the effort with the patience and understanding that is so valuable to an author, particularly during the "dog days" of the writing effort. And to Carroll Cann at Williams & Wilkins, for his faith, guidance, and friendship over the past 15 years. Also to Paul Contino, a remarkable combination of scientist and artist who created most of the illustrations in this text, and added to the content of many as well. And finally to Phyllis Cassidy, for the *billions* of things she has done for this book and its author over the past 2½ years.

contents

section I
BASIC SCIENCE REVIEW

The first step in applying the scientific method consists in being curious about the world.
Linus Pauling

c h a p t e r

1

CIRCULATORY BLOOD FLOW

When is a piece of matter said to be alive? When it goes on "doing something,"
moving, exchanging material with its environment.

Erwin Schrodinger

The adult human being has an estimated 100 trillion cells that must go on exchanging material with the external environment to stay alive. To accomplish this, the circulatory system includes a vascular network that stretches more than 60,000 miles (more than twice the circumference of the Earth), and an average of 8000 liters of blood is pumped through this vascular network every day (1). This chapter describes the flow of blood through the circulatory system, and includes a description of flow through the heart (cardiac output) and flow through distant regions of the vascular circuit (peripheral blood flow). Most of these concepts are old friends from the physiology classroom, but this chapter applies them to actual practice at the bedside.

CARDIAC OUTPUT

Circulatory flow originates in the muscular contractions of the heart. Because blood is an incompressible fluid that flows through a closed hydraulic loop, the volume of blood ejected by the left side of the heart (in a given time period) must equal the volume of blood returning to the right side of the heart (over the same period of time). This reflection of the conservation of mass (volume) in a closed hydraulic system is known as the **principle of continuity** (2). It predicts that the volume flow of blood (volumetric flow rate), which is determined by the stroke output of the heart, will be the same at all points along the circulatory system. Therefore, the forces that determine cardiac stroke output also determine volumetric blood flow. The determinants of cardiac stroke output that can be measured or derived in a clinical setting are shown

3

TABLE 1.1. REFERENCE RANGES FOR HEMODYNAMIC PARAMETERS IN ADULTS	
Parameter	Normal Range
Ventricular end-diastolic pressure (EDP)	R 1–6 mm Hg
	L 6–12 mm Hg
*Ventricular end-diastolic volume (EDV)	R 80–150 mL/m²
	L 70–100 mL/m²
*Stroke volume (SV)	40–70 mL/m²
*Cardiac output (Q)	2.4–4.0 L/minute/m²
Pulmonary vascular resistance (PVR)	20–120 dynes·second/cm⁵
Systemic vascular resistance (SVR)	700–1600 dynes·second/cm⁵

* Indicates a parameter that is expressed in relation to body surface area.
R = right, L = left.

in Table 1.1. Each of these is described briefly in the paragraphs that follow.

PRELOAD

When a weight is attached to one end of a resting muscle, the muscle stretches to a new length. The weight in this situation represents a force called the **preload,** that is, the load imposed on a muscle before the onset of contraction. The preload force acts indirectly to augment the force of muscle contraction. That is, the preload force stretches the muscle to a new resting length and (according to the length–tension relationship of muscle) the increase in muscle length then leads to a more forceful muscle contraction.

Pressure–Volume Curves

In the intact heart, the stretch imposed on the cardiac muscle at rest is a function of the volume in the ventricles at the end of diastole. Therefore, ventricular end-diastolic volume (EDV) is used as a reflection of the preload force for the intact heart (3). The pressure–volume curves in Figure 1.1 describe the influence of preload on the mechanical performance of the left ventricle during diastole (*lower curves*) and systole (*upper curves*). The solid curves represent the normal pressure–volume relationships for diastole and systole. Note that the uppermost curve in the figure has a rapid ascent, indicating that small changes in diastolic volume are associated with large changes in systolic pressure. The normal relationship between diastolic volume (preload) and the strength of ventricular contraction was described independently by Otto Frank and Ernest Starling, and is commonly known as the Frank–Starling phenomenon (3). This relationship can be restated as follows:

In the normal heart, the diastolic volume (preload) is the principal force that governs the strength of ventricular contraction.

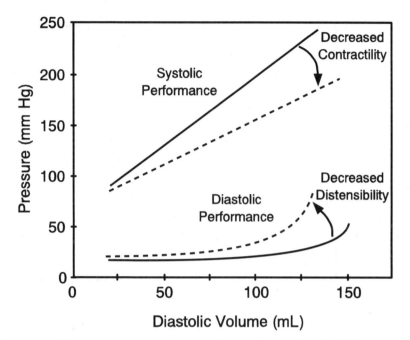

Figure 1.1. Pressure–volume curves for the intact ventricle. Solid lines represent normal pressure–volume relationships.

This indicates that the stroke output of the normal heart is primarily a reflection of the diastolic volume. Therefore, the most effective measure for preserving the cardiac output is to maintain an adequate diastolic volume. This emphasizes the value of avoiding hypovolemia and correcting volume deficits when they exist.

Ventricular Function Curves

Ventricular end-diastolic volume is not easily measured at the bedside, and the ventricular end-diastolic pressure (EDP) is more commonly used as a reflection of ventricular preload in clinical practice (see Chapter 11 for more information on end-diastolic pressure). The relationship between end-diastolic pressure (preload) and stroke volume (systolic performance) is used to monitor the Frank–Starling relationship in the clinical setting. The curves that define this relationship, known as *ventricular function curves* (4), are shown in Figure 1.2. Unfortunately, the interpretation of ventricular function curves can be misleading, as is demonstrated in the sections that follow.

Ventricular Compliance

The stretch imposed on cardiac muscle is determined not only by the volume of blood in the ventricular chambers, but also by the tendency of the ventricular wall to distend or stretch at any given chamber

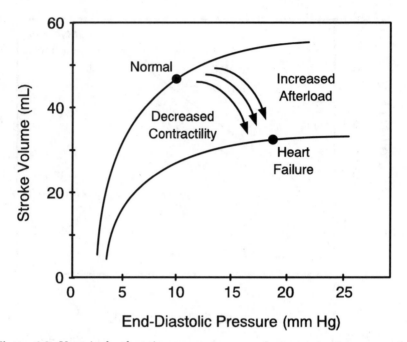

Figure 1.2. Ventricular function curves.

volume. This latter property is described as the **compliance** (distensibility) of the ventricle. Compliance is defined by the following relationship between changes in EDP and volume (EDV) (5):

$$\text{Compliance} = \Delta\text{EDV}/\Delta\text{EDP} \qquad (1.1)$$

The lower curves in Figure 1.1 show the end-diastolic pressure–volume relationships for the normal ventricle and a noncompliant (stiff) ventricle. As the ventricle becomes less compliant (e.g., when the ventricle hypertrophies), there is less of a change in diastolic volume relative to the change in diastolic pressure. Early in this process, the EDV remains normal, but the EDP increases above normal. As the compliance decreases further, the increase in EDP eventually reduces venous inflow into the heart, thereby causing a reduction in EDV. The decrease in EDV then leads to a decrease in the force of ventricular contraction. This illustrates how changes in ventricular compliance can lead to changes in cardiac stroke output, and how changes in cardiac stroke output can be independent of changes in systolic function.

The decrease in stroke output that accompanies a decrease in ventricular compliance is known as diastolic heart failure (6). The difference between heart failure caused by systolic and diastolic dysfunction is presented in Chapter 16.

The Preload Measurement

Changes in ventricular compliance also influence the reliability of EDP as a reflection of EDV. For example, a decrease in ventricular compliance results in a higher-than-expected EDP at any given EDV. Therefore, the EDP overestimates the actual preload (EDV) when the ventricle is noncompliant. The following points are important to remember when EDP is used as an index of ventricular preload:

> EDP provides an accurate reflection of preload only when ventricular compliance is normal. Changes in EDP provide an accurate reflection of changes in preload only when ventricular compliance is constant.

The influence of ventricular compliance on the assessment of preload surfaces again in Chapter 11. Chapter 16 describes the importance of an accurate preload measurement in distinguishing systolic from diastolic forms of heart failure.

AFTERLOAD

When a weight is attached to one end of a contracting muscle, the force of muscle contraction must overcome the opposing force of the weight before the muscle begins to shorten its length. The weight in this situation represents a force called the **afterload,** the load imposed on the muscle after the onset of contraction. The afterload is an opposing force that determines the force of muscle contraction needed to initiate muscle shortening (i.e., isotonic muscle contraction). In the intact heart, the afterload force is equivalent to the tension developed across the wall of the ventricles during systole (3).

The determinants of ventricular wall tension are derived from observations on soap bubbles made by the Marquis de Laplace in 1820. These observations were the basis for the law of Laplace, which states that the tension across a thin-walled sphere is directly related to the internal pressure and radius of the sphere: $T = Pr$. Because the ventricles are not thin-walled spheres, the Laplace relationship for the intact heart incorporates a factor that reflects the average thickness of the ventricular wall (5). The law of Laplace applied to the intact heart is then expressed as $T = Pr/t$, where T represents the tension across the wall of the ventricle during systole, P represents the transmural pressure across the ventricle at the end of systole, r represents the chamber radius at the end of diastole, and t represents the average thickness of the ventricular wall. The forces that contribute to ventricular wall tension are shown in Figure 1.3.

Pleural Pressures

Because afterload is a transmural force, it is influenced by the pleural pressures at the outer surface of heart. Negative pleural pressures increase transmural pressure and increase ventricular afterload, whereas positive pleural pressures have the opposite effect. Negative pressures surrounding the heart can impede ventricular emptying by opposing the inward displacement of the ventricular wall during systole (7).

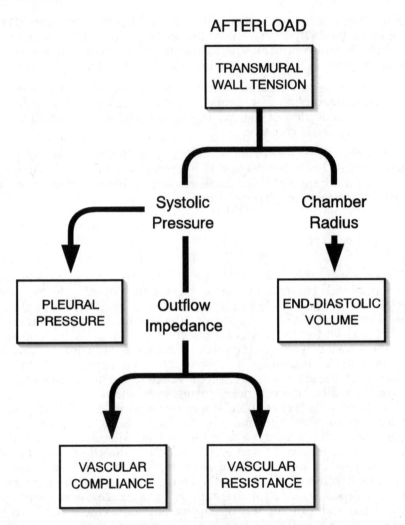

Figure 1.3. The forces that contribute to ventricular afterload. Forces enclosed in rectangles are readily defined or measured.

This action is responsible for the decrease in systolic blood pressure (reflecting a decrease in stroke volume) that occurs during the inspiratory phase of spontaneous breathing. When this inspiratory-related drop in pressure is greater than 15 mm Hg, the condition is called *pulsus paradoxus* (which is a misnomer, because the response is not paradoxical, but is an exaggerated version of the normal response).

Positive pleural pressures can promote ventricular emptying by facilitating the inward displacement of the ventricular wall during systole (7). Rapid and forceful rises in positive pressure surrounding the heart might also produce a massagelike action to expel blood from the heart and great vessels in the thorax. This is the proposed explanation for the success of cough CPR, which uses forceful coughing to maintain circulatory flow in patients with ventricular tachycardia (8). In fact, positive pleural pressure swings may be responsible for the hemodynamic effects of closed chest cardiac massage, as discussed in Chapter 18 (8).

Impedance versus Resistance

A major component of afterload is the resistance to ventricular out-flow in the aorta and large, proximal arteries. The total hydraulic force that opposes pulsatile flow is known as **impedance** (9). This force is a combination of two forces: (*a*) a force that opposes the rate of change in flow, known as **compliance,** and (*b*) a force that opposes mean or volumetric flow, known as **resistance.** Vascular compliance is not eas-ily measured at the bedside (10). On the other hand, vascular resistance is derived by assuming that hydraulic resistance is analogous to electri-cal resistance. That is, Ohm's law predicts that resistance to flow of an electric current (R) is directly proportional to the voltage drop across a circuit (E) and inversely proportional to the flow of current (I); $R = E/I$. The hydraulic analogy then states that resistance to the flow of fluid through a tube is directly proportional to the pressure drop along a tube ($P_{in} - P_{out}$), and inversely proportional to the flow of volume (Q):

$$R = P_{in} - P_{out}/Q \qquad (1.2)$$

This relationship is applied to the systemic and pulmonary circula-tions, creating the following derivations:

Systemic vascular resistance (SVR) = MABP − CVP/CO (1.3)

Pulmonary vascular resistance (PVR) = MPAP − LAP/CO (1.4)

where MABP is mean arterial blood pressure, CVP is central venous pressure, MPAP is mean pulmonary artery pressure, LAP is left-atrial pressure, and CO is the cardiac output. Vascular resistance is ex-pressed in units of pressure and flow. Because the pressures are mea-sured in mm Hg, the units would be mm Hg per mL/second. How-ever, the dislike for expressing pressures in mm Hg has led to the common practice of expressing vascular resistance in CGS (centimeter-gram-second) units, or dynes $\times$ second/cm^5. The conversion is dynes second/cm^5 = 1333 $\times$ mm Hg/mL/second.

Clinical Monitoring

Although afterload is a combination of several forces that oppose ventricular emptying, most of the component forces of afterload can-not be measured easily or reliably at the bedside. As a result, the vascu-lar resistance, derived as shown above, is often used as the sole mea-sure of ventricular afterload. However, as might be expected, vascular resistance is not an accurate measure of total ventricular afterload (11).

A shift in the height and slope of the ventricular function curve could be an indirect marker of changes in afterload, as shown in Figure 1.2. However, shifts in the ventricular function curve can also be caused by changes in the contractile state of the myocardium, and because it is not possible to determine whether myocardial contractility is constant using bedside measurements, a shift in the position of ventricular function curves cannot be used as a marker of changes in afterload.

CONTRACTILITY

The contraction of striated muscle is attributed to interactions between contractile proteins arranged in parallel rows in the sarcomere. The number of bridges formed between adjacent rows of contractile elements determines the contractile state or **contractility** of the muscle fiber. The contractile state of a muscle is reflected by the force and velocity of muscle contraction (3).

The contractile state of cardiac muscle in the intact heart is reflected in the systolic performance of the ventricles. This is demonstrated in the upper curves in Figure 1.1. The systolic pressures in this figure reflect isovolumetric contraction (i.e., the pressures are generated before the aortic valve opens), which eliminates the influence of outflow impedance (afterload) on systolic pressure. Therefore, the changes in systolic pressure at any given diastolic volume (preload constant) reflect changes in the contractile state of the myocardium.

Clinical Monitoring

Changes in myocardial contractility alter the height and slope of the ventricular function curve, as demonstrated in Figure 1.2. However, as just mentioned, changes in the position of ventricular function curves can also be the result of changes in ventricular afterload. Therefore, because it is not possible to monitor afterload to determine whether it is constant, a shift in the ventricular functions curve is not a reliable method for detecting changes in myocardial contractility (4).

PERIPHERAL BLOOD FLOW

The cardiac stroke output travels through a vast array of vascular channels that can differ markedly in size. The focus of the remainder of the chapter is the factors that govern flow through these vascular channels.

Caution: The determinants of flow through vascular conduits are derived from idealized hydraulic models that differ considerably from the conditions that exist in the intact circulatory system. For example, the flow in small tubes usually is steady or nonpulsatile flow, and does not represent the continually changing pulsatile pattern of flow that occurs in many regions of the native circulation. Because of discrepancies like this, the description of blood flow that follows should be used more as a qualitative than quantitative description of the hydraulics of vascular flow.

FLOW IN RIGID TUBES

The hydraulic analogy of Ohm's law, as mentioned previously, states that steady volumetric flow (Q) through a rigid tube is proportional to the pressure gradient between the inlet and outlet of the tube ($P_{in} - P_{out}$), and the constant of proportionality is the hydraulic resistance to flow (R):

$$Q = (P_{in} - P_{out}) \times 1/R \qquad (1.5)$$

The flow of fluids through small tubes was described independently by a German engineer (G. Hagen) and a French physician (J. Poiseuille), and their observations are combined in the equation shown below, called the Hagen–Poiseuille equation (12,13).

$$Q = (P_{in} - P_{out}) \times (\pi r^4/8\mu L) \qquad (1.6)$$

This equation identifies the components of hydraulic resistance as the inner radius (r) and length of the tube (L), and the viscosity of the fluid (μ). Because the final term in the Hagen–Poiseuille equation is the reciprocal of resistance (i.e., $1/R$), the hydraulic resistance to steady, volumetric flow is expressed as

$$R = 8\mu L/\pi r^4 \qquad (1.7)$$

The components of the Hagen–Poisseuille equation are shown in the diagram in Figure 1.4. Note that flow varies according to the fourth power of the inner radius of the tube.

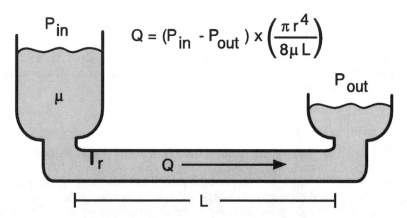

Figure 1.4. The forces that govern steady flow in rigid tubes. P_{in} = inlet pressure, P_{out} = outlet pressure, Q = flow, μ = viscosity, r = radius, L = length.

Thus, a twofold increase in the inner radius of the tube will result in a sixteenfold increase in flow: $(2r)^4 = 16\ r$. Flow varies much less with the other determinants of resistance; that is, a twofold increase in the length of the tube or the viscosity of the fluid results in a 50% decrease in flow rate. The influence of tube dimensions on flow rate has more practical applications as determinants of flow through vascular catheters, as presented in Chapter 4.

FLOW IN TUBES OF VARYING DIAMETER

The Hagen–Poisseuille equation predicts that as blood moves away from the heart and encounters vessels of decreasing diameter, the resistance to flow should increase and flow rate should decrease. However, the principle of continuity described earlier predicts that blood flow will be the same at all points along the vascular circuit. This apparent dilemma can be resolved by considering the relationship between flow velocity and cross-sectional area of a tube. For a rigid tube of varying diameter, the velocity of flow (v) at any point along the tube is directly proportional to the volumetric flow rate (Q) and inversely proportional to the cross-sectional area of the tube (A). These relationships are described below (2).

$$v = Q/A \qquad (1.8)$$

If flow is constant, a decrease in the cross-sectional area of a tube results in an increase in the velocity of flow. This is how the nozzle on a garden hose works, and is the rationale for jet ventilation.

Equation 1.8 can be rearranged to yield the relationship $Q = v \times A$. This relationship indicates that proportional changes in velocity and cross-sectional area in opposite directions result in a constant volume flow rate. This means that blood flow can remain unchanged in blood vessels of diminishing diameter if there are equal and opposite changes in the velocity of flow and the cross-sectional area of the vessels. The trick here is to use the total cross-sectional area of the vessels in a region rather than the cross-sectional area of individual vessels. This resolves the discrepancy between the principle of continuity and the Hagen–Poiseuille relationships.

Circulatory Design

The graph in Figure 1.5 shows the changes in flow velocity and cross-sectional area in different regions of the circulation (13). As expected, when blood moves toward the periphery, there are proportionate and reciprocal changes in cross-sectional area and velocity of flow. The high velocity of flow in the proximal arteries seems well suited for delivering blood quickly to the microcirculation, to allow more time for diffusional exchange with the tissues. The low velocity and large cross-sectional area in the capillaries are also well-suited for dif-

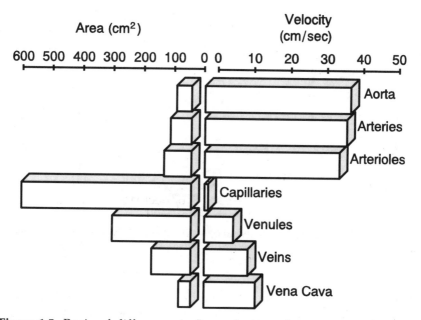

Figure 1.5. Regional differences in flow velocity and cross-sectional area in the human circulatory system. (Adapted from Little RC, Little WC. Physiology of the heart and circulation. 4th ed. Chicago: Year Book, 1989.)

fusional exchange. These features show a rational design in the circulatory system.

FLOW IN COLLAPSIBLE TUBES

The hydraulic relationships described above apply to flow through rigid tubes, but blood vessels are not rigid tubes. The determinants of flow in collapsible tubes are explained with the aid of the apparatus shown in Figure 1.6 (14). The apparatus shows a tube with collapsible walls passing through a fluid reservoir. The height of the fluid in the reservoir can be adjusted to vary the external pressure on the tube. As mentioned earlier, flow in a rigid tube is proportional to the pressure difference between the inlet and outlet of the tube ($P_{in} - P_{out}$). This is also the case in collapsible tubes as long as the external pressure is not high enough to compress the tube. However, as shown in Figure 1.6, when the external pressure exceeds the outlet pressure ($P_{ext} > P_{out}$) and compresses the tube, the driving force for flow is pressure difference between the inlet pressure and the external pressure ($P_{in} - P_{ext}$). In this situation, the driving pressure for flow is independent of the pressure gradient along the tube.

The Pulmonary Circulation

Vascular compression has been demonstrated in the cerebral, pulmonary, and systemic circulations. Extravascular compression is a par-

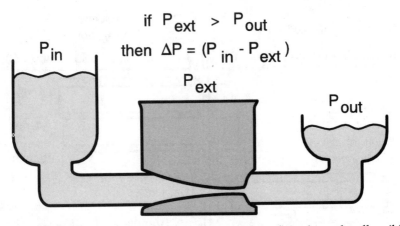

Figure 1.6. The influence of external compression on flow through collapsible tubes. P_{ext} = extravascular pressure, P_{out} = pressure at the tube outlet. P_{in} = inlet pressure, P_{out} = outlet pressure, P_{ext} = external pressure.

ticular concern in patients who require positive-pressure mechanical ventilation (14). In this situation, pressures in the alveoli can exceed pressures in the underlying pulmonary capillaries, and the resultant capillary compression changes the driving force for flow across the lungs, as illustrated in Figure 1.6. Thus, whereas the normal driving pressure for flow across the lungs is the difference between the mean pulmonary artery pressure and the left-atrial pressure (PAP − LAP), the driving pressure for flow when pulmonary capillaries are compressed is the difference between the pulmonary artery pressure and the alveolar pressure (PAP − Palv). The pulmonary vascular resistance (PVR) will then differ as follows:

$$\text{Normal: PVR = PAP − LAP/CO} \qquad (1.9)$$

$$\text{When Palv > LAP: PVR = PAP − Palv/CO} \qquad (1.10)$$

The problems created by vascular compression in the lungs are discussed in Chapters 11 and 26.

VISCOSITY

Solids resist being deformed (changing shape), whereas fluids deform continuously (i.e., flow) but resist changes in the rate of deformation (i.e., the flow rate). The inherent resistance of a fluid to changes in flow rate is expressed as the **viscosity** of the fluid (12,15). When a force is applied that changes flow rate (i.e., a shear force), the change in flow rate varies inversely with the viscosity of the fluid. Thus, as the viscosity of a fluid increases, the fluid flows less rapidly in response to a shear force. The influence of viscosity is easily demonstrated by comparing the flow of molasses (high viscosity) and the flow of water (low viscosity) when the force of gravity is applied (i.e., when both are spilled).

Blood Viscosity

The viscosity of whole blood is determined by the number and strength of interactions between plasma fibrinogen and the circulating erythrocytes (15,16). The concentration of circulating erythrocytes (i.e., the hematocrit) is the principal determinant of whole blood viscosity. The relationship between hematocrit and blood viscosity is shown in Table 1.2. Note that viscosity is expressed in absolute units (centipoise) and also as a relative value (the ratio of blood viscosity to the viscosity of water). Whole blood with a normal hematocrit (i.e., 40%) has a viscosity that is three to four times higher than that of water. Thus, to move whole blood with a normal hematocrit, the circulatory system must generate a pressure that is three to four times higher than the pressure needed to move water the same distance. The acellular blood (zero hematocrit) in Table 1.2 is equivalent to plasma, and has a viscosity that more closely approximates the viscosity of water. Thus, moving plasma does not require nearly the work involved in moving whole blood. This difference in work load can have significant implications in the patient with coronary disease or limited cardiac reserve.

Other factors that influence viscosity are body temperature and the flow rate (16). Viscosity rises in response to decreases in temperature and flow rate. The increase in blood viscosity in low flow states might represent an adaptive response aimed at promoting coagulation at sites of hemorrhage (15). However, the rise in viscosity can also serve to further reduce blood flow and thereby provoke ischemic injury. The tendency of viscosity to increase with decreases in blood flow is a potential problem in the ICU patient population, and deserves further study.

TABLE 1.2. BLOOD VISCOSITY AS A FUNCTION OF HEMATOCRIT

Hematocrit	Viscosity*	
	Relative	Absolute
0	1.4	
10	1.8	1.2
20	2.1	1.5
30	2.8	1.8
40	3.7	2.3
50	4.8	2.9
60	5.8	3.8
70	8.2	5.3

* Absolute viscosity expressed in centipoise (CP).
Data from Documenta Geigy Scientific Tables. 7th ed. Basel: Documenta Geigy, 1966:557–558.

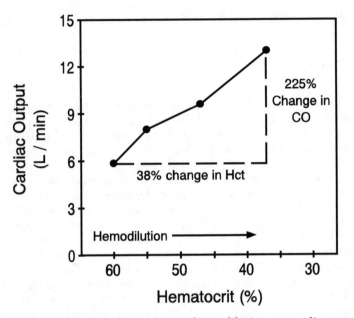

Figure 1.7. The influence of progressive hemodilution on cardiac output in a patient with polycythemia. *CO* = cardiac output. (From LeVeen HH et al. Lowering blood viscosity to overcome vascular resistance. Surg Gynecol Obstet 1980;150:139–149.)

Hemodynamic Effects

The Hagen–Poisseuille equation predicts that (all other variables constant) blood flow will change in the same proportion as the change in blood viscosity; that is, if viscosity is reduced by one-half, blood flow will double (15).

The graph in Figure 1.7 demonstrates the hemodynamic effects of a progressive decrease in blood viscosity. In this case, the subject was an elderly male with secondary polycythemia, and the reduction in viscosity was achieved by progressive (isovolemic) hemodilution. As shown in the graph, the progressive reduction in hematocrit was associated with a progressive rise in cardiac output. The disproportionate improvement in cardiac output may be caused by the fact that low flow rates can increase viscosity, and thus an increase in flow could itself produce a further increase in flow. The ability to modulate blood flow by manipulating the hematocrit is presented in more detail in Chapter 44.

Clinical Monitoring

Viscosity is measured by placing a fluid sample between two parallel plates that are sliding past each other, and recording the resistance or "stickiness" in the movement of the plates. The instrument that performs this task is called a viscometer. The units of measurement for viscosity are the poise (or dyne × second/cm^2) in the CGS system, and the pascal second (Pa s) in the SI system. To convert units, use the relationship 1 poise = 0.1 Pa s. Viscosity is also expressed in relative terms (relative to the viscosity of water), a method that may be preferred for its simplicity.

The major drawback in monitoring viscosity is the tendency of viscosity to vary with changes in temperature, hematocrit, and flow rate. As a result, local conditions in the microcirculation can produce changes in blood viscosity that will go undetected in the in vitro (viscometer) measurement of viscosity. In states of adequate blood flow, the measurement is considered to be reasonably accurate. However, for the critically ill patient with suspected low flow who might benefit from measurements of blood viscosity, the reliability of the measurement is likely to be uncertain. A more feasible application of the viscosity measurement would be to monitor the effects of packed cell transfusions on blood viscosity to determine the point at which hemoconcentration can be counterproductive in individual patients.

REFERENCES

GENERAL TEXTS

Guyton AC, Jones CE, Coleman TG. Circulatory physiology: cardiac output and its regulation. 2nd ed. Philadelphia: WB Saunders, 1973.
Nichols WW, O'Rourke M. McDonald's blood flow in arteries. 3rd ed. Baltimore: Williams & Wilkins, 1990.
Berne R, Levy M. Cardiovascular physiology. 6th ed. St. Louis: CV Mosby, 1992.
Warltier DC. Ventricular function. Baltimore: Williams & Wilkins, 1995.

CARDIAC OUTPUT

1. Vogel S. Vital circuits. New York: Oxford University Press, 1992:1–17.
2. Vogel S. Life in moving fluids. Princeton, NJ: Princeton University Press, 1981: 25–28.
3. Braunwald E, Sonnenblick EH, Ross J Jr. Mechanisms of cardiac contraction and relaxation. In: Braunwald E, ed. Heart disease: a textbook of cardiovascular medicine. 4th ed. Philadelphia: WB Saunders, 1992;351–392.
4. Parmley WM, Talbot L. The heart as a pump. In: Berne RM, ed. Handbook of physiology. The cardiovascular system. Bethesda, MD: American Physiological Society, 1979;429–460.
5. Gilbert JC, Glantz SA. Determinants of left ventricular filling and of the diastolic pressure-volume relation. Circ Res 1989;64:827–852.
6. Grossman W. Diastolic dysfunction in congestive heart failure. N Engl J Med 1991;325:1557–1564.
7. Pinsky MR. Cardiopulmonary interactions: the effects of negative and positive changes in pleural pressures on cardiac output. In: Dantzger DR, ed. Cardiopulmonary critical care. 2nd ed. Philadelphia: WB Saunders, 1991;87–120.
8. Weil MH, Gazmuri RJ, Rackow EC. The clinical rationale of cardiac resuscitation. Dis Mon 1990;36:423–468.
9. Finkelstein SM, Collins R. Vascular impedance measurement. Prog Cardiovasc Dis 1982;24:401–418.

10. Laskey WK, Parker G, Ferrari VA, et al. Estimation of arterial compliance in humans. J Appl Physiol 1990;69:112–119.
11. Lang RM, Borrow KM, Neumann A, et al. Systemic vascular resistance: an unreliable index of left ventricular afterload. Circulation 1986;74:1114–1123.

PERIPHERAL BLOOD FLOW

12. Chien S, Usami S, Skalak R. Blood flow in small tubes. In: Renkin EM, Michel CC, eds. Handbook of physiology. Section 2: the cardiovascular system. Vol. IV. The microcirculation. Bethesda: American Physiological Society, 1984; 217–249.
13. Little RC, Little WC. Physiology of the heart and circulation. 4th ed. Chicago: Year Book, 1989;219–236.
14. Gorback MS. Problems associated with the determination of pulmonary vascular resistance. J Clin Monit 1990;6:118–127.
15. Merrill EW. Rheology of blood. Physiol Rev 1969;49:863–888.
16. Lowe GOD. Blood rheology in vitro and in vivo. Bailleres Clin Hematol 1987; 1:597.

2

RESPIRATORY GAS TRANSPORT

Respiration is thus a process of combustion, in truth very slow, but otherwise exactly like that of charcoal.

Antoine Lavoisier

One of the basic elements of aerobic life is the combustion reaction, in which oxygen releases the energy stored in organic fuels and carbon dioxide is generated as a chemical byproduct. The business of aerobic metabolism is the combustion of nutrient fuels, and the circulatory system plays a dual role in supporting this process by delivering oxygen to drive the reaction and removing the carbon dioxide that is generated. Because both processes have a common purpose, the transport of oxygen and carbon dioxide in blood has been designated the *respiratory function of blood*. This chapter describes the basic features of each transport system, and demonstrates the central role of hemoglobin in the transport of both oxygen and carbon dioxide.

OXYGEN TRANSPORT

Oxygen is the most abundant element on the surface of the earth (1), yet because it does not dissolve readily in water, it is unavailable to cells in the interior of the body. Thus, we depend on a steady supply of this element to survive, yet we function as a natural barrier to its movement. A possible explanation for this is the role of oxygen in promoting oxidative damage, discussed in Chapter 3. For now, we will assume that oxygen is a wonderful element.

The transport system for oxygen is separated into four components: blood oxygen content, oxygen delivery in arterial blood, oxygen uptake from the microcirculation, and oxygen extraction ratio.

WHOLE BLOOD O_2 CONTENT

The concentration of oxygen in arterial blood (Ca_{O_2}), often called the oxygen content, is described by Equation 2.1.

$$Ca_{O_2} = (1.34 \times Hb \times Sa_{O_2}) + (0.003 \times Pa_{O_2}) \qquad (2.1)$$

The contribution of hemoglobin is described in the first term of the equation: $1.34 \times Hb \times Sa_{O_2}$. This relationship states that each gram of hemoglobin (Hb) will bind 1.34 mL O_2 when it is fully saturated with oxygen. The arterial O_2 saturation (Sa_{O_2}) is expressed as a fraction, not a percentage (i.e., 1.0 instead of 100%). One gram of hemoglobin can actually bind 1.39 mL O_2 at full saturation (2). However, a small fraction of the circulating hemoglobin is represented by forms that do not readily bind oxygen (i.e., methemoglobin and carboxyhemoglobin), so the lower binding capacity of 1.34 mL/g more accurately describes the behavior of the total pool of circulating hemoglobin. The oxygen bound by hemoglobin at a concentration of 15 g/dL and an O_2 saturation of 98% will then be

$$1.34 \ (mL/g) \times 15 \ (g/dL) \times 0.98 = 19.7 \ mL/100 \ mL \qquad (2.2)$$

Note that because hemoglobin concentration is expressed in g/dL (g/100 mL), the concentration of hemoglobin-bound oxygen is expressed in mL/100 mL (volume %). The contribution of the oxygen dissolved in plasma is defined by the solubility coefficients shown in Table 2.1. At a normal body temperature of 37 C, the solubility of oxygen in plasma is .028 mL/L/mm Hg. To express the concentration in mL/100 mL, the solubility coefficient is divided by 10, creating the second term shown in Equation 2.1: $0.003 \times Pa_{O_2}$. Thus, at a Pa_{O_2} of 100 mm Hg, the expected concentration of dissolved oxygen is

$$0.003 \ (mL/100 \ mL/mm \ Hg) \times 100 \ mm \ Hg = 0.3 \ mL/100 \ mL \qquad (2.3)$$

The total concentration of oxygen in arterial blood is then $19.7 + 0.3 = 20$ mL/100 mL, or 200 mL/L. Repeating this calculation using an O_2 saturation of 75% derives the O_2 content in mixed venous (pulmonary artery) blood, as shown in Table 2.2.

A comparison of the total and dissolved O_2 concentrations in Table 2.2 shows that hemoglobin carries 98.5% of the oxygen in arterial blood and 99.5% in mixed venous blood. If we were forced to rely solely on the 3 mL/L of dissolved oxygen in arterial blood, a cardiac output of

TABLE 2.1. SOLUBILITY OF O_2 AND CO_2 IN PLASMA		
Temp (°C)	mL O_2/L/mm Hg*	mL CO_2/L/mm Hg†
25	0.033	0.892
30	0.031	0.802
35	0.028	0.713
37	0.028	0.686
40	0.027	0.624

* From Christoforites C et al. J Appl Physiol 1969;26:56.
† From Severinghaus JW et al. J Appl Physiol 1956;9:189.

TABLE 2.2. CONCENTRATION OF O_2 AND CO_2 IN WHOLE BLOOD*			
	Arterial	**Venous**	**A − V Difference**
Po_2	90 mm Hg	40 mm Hg	50 mm Hg
Dissolved O_2	3 mL/L	1 mL/L	2 mL/L
Total O_2	200 mL/L	150 mL/L	50 mL/L
Pco_2	40 mm Hg	45 mm Hg	5 mm Hg
Dissolved CO_2	26 mL/L	29 mL/L	3 mL/L
Total CO_2	490 mL/L	530 mL/L	40 mL/L

* Temperature = 37° C, hemoglobin = 150 g/L.
Po_2 = oxygen pressure, Pco_2 = carbon dioxide pressure.

89 L/minute would be necessary to sustain a normal whole-body O_2 consumption of 250 mL/minute.

Hemoglobin versus Pao_2

To illustrate the relative strength of hemoglobin and Pao_2 in determining the O_2 content of blood, Table 2.3 shows the relative influence of anemia and hypoxemia on arterial oxygenation. A 50% reduction in hemoglobin (from 15 to 7.5 mg/dL) is fully expressed as a 50% reduction in Cao_2. However, a 50% reduction in Pao_2 (from 90 to 45 mm Hg) results in only a 20% decrease in Cao_2 (which is similar to the 18% decrease in Sao_2). These examples emphasize the following points:

Changes in hemoglobin concentration have a larger impact on arterial oxygenation than changes in Pao_2.
Hypoxemia (a decrease in Pao_2) has a relatively minor impact on arterial oxygenation if the accompanying change in Sao_2 is small.

Po_2 influences blood oxygenation only to the extent that it influences the saturation of hemoglobin with oxygen. Therefore, Sao_2 is a more reliable index of arterial oxygenation than Pao_2.

TABLE 2.3. RELATIVE INFLUENCE OF ANEMIA AND HYPOXEMIA ON ARTERIAL OXYGENATION			
Parameter	**Normal**	**Hypoxemia**	**Anemia**
Pao_2	90 mm Hg	45 mm Hg	90 mm Hg
Sao_2	98%	80%	98%
Hb	150 g/L	150 g/L	75 g/L
Cao_2	200 mL/L	163 mL/L	101 mL/L
% change in Cao_2		18.6%	49.5%

Pao_2 = arterial oxygen pressure, Sao_2 = arterial oxygen saturation, Hb = hemoglobin, Cao_2 = arterial oxygen concentration.

TABLE 2.4. PARAMETERS OF OXYGEN AND CARBON DIOXIDE TRANSPORT		
Parameter	Equations	Normal Range
Oxygen delivery (Do_2)	$Q \times 13.4 \times Hb \times Sao_2$	520–570 mL/minute/m^2
Oxygen uptake (Vo_2)	$Q \times 13.4 \times Hb \times (Sao_2 - Svo_2)$	110–160 mL/minute/m^2
Oxygen extraction ratio (O_2ER)	$(Sao_2 - Svo_2/Sao_2) \times 100$	20–30%
Carbon dioxide elimination (Vco_2)	$Q \times (Cvco_2 - Caco_2)$	90–130 mL/minute/m^2
Respiratory quotient (RQ)	Vco_2/Vo_2	0.75–0.85

Hb = hemoglobin, Sao_2 = arterial oxygen saturation, Svo_2 = venous oxygen saturation, $Cvco_2$ = venous carbon dioxide concentration, $Caco_2$ = arterial carbon dioxide concentration, Q = cardiac output.

The Hemoglobin Mass

The hemoglobin concentration is traditionally expressed in grams per deciliter rather than in grams per liter, and this tends to create an underappreciation for the size of the hemoglobin pool in blood. For example, a hemoglobin concentration of 15 g/dL means that there are 150 grams of hemoglobin per liter of whole blood. Thus, a normal blood volume of 5.5 liters contains 0.825 kg, or 1.85 lb, of hemoglobin! To place this in perspective, consider that the normal weight of the heart is 0.3 kg, or about one-third the mass of circulating hemoglobin. Therefore, the heart must push three times its weight to move hemoglobin through the circulatory system. This represents a substantial work load for the heart. The reason for the size of hemoglobin pool is not clear because there is much more than needed for oxygen transport. The answer may be that hemoglobin has other functions in addition to oxygen transport, as discussed later in the chapter.

OXYGEN DELIVERY (Do_2)

The oxygen transport parameters are shown in Table 2.4. Transport in arterial blood is described by oxygen delivery (Do_2), which is defined as the product of the cardiac output (Q) and the arterial oxygen content (Cao_2).

$$Do_2 = Q \times Cao_2 = Q \times (1.34 \times Hb \times Sao_2) \times 10 \quad (2.4)$$

Note that the dissolved oxygen component is eliminated. The factor 10 converts the final units to mL/minute. If the cardiac index (cardiac output divided by the body surface area) is used to derive the Do_2, the units are expressed as mL/minute/m^2. As shown in Table 2.4, the normal range for Do_2 is 520 to 570 mL/minute/m^2.

OXYGEN UPTAKE (Vo_2)

The oxygen uptake from the microcirculation is a function of the cardiac output and the difference in oxygen content between arterial

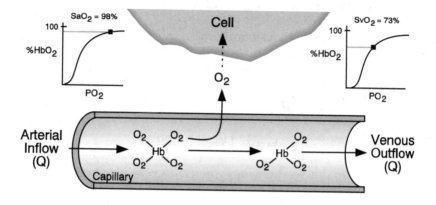

$$VO_2 = Q \times Hb \times 13.4 \times (SaO_2 - SvO_2)$$

Figure 2.1. Schematic view of oxygen uptake ($\dot{V}O_2$) from the microcirculation. SaO_2 = arterial oxygen saturation, SvO_2 = venous oxygen saturation, Hb = hemoglobin, PO_2 = oxygen pressure.

and venous blood; that is, $\dot{V}O_2 = Q \times (CaO_2 - CvO_2)$. Because CaO_2 and CvO_2 share the same term for hemoglobin binding ($1.34 \times Hb$), this term can be isolated to create Equation 2.5.

$$\dot{V}O_2 = Q \times 13.4 \times Hb \times (SaO_2 - SvO_2) \qquad (2.5)$$

The factor 1.34 has been multiplied by 10 to convert units. This relationship is depicted schematically in Figure 2.1. As indicated in Table 2.4, the normal range for the $\dot{V}O_2$ is $110 - 160$ mL/minute/m².

OXYGEN EXTRACTION RATIO (O_2ER)

The oxygen extraction ratio (O_2ER) is the ratio of O_2 uptake to O_2 delivery ($\dot{V}O_2/DO_2$), and is the fraction of the oxygen delivered to the microcirculation that is taken up into the tissues. The ratio can be multiplied by 100 to generate a percentage.

$$O_2ER = \dot{V}O_2/DO_2 \times 100 \qquad (2.6)$$

The normal O_2ER is 0.2 to 0.3 (20 to 30%), indicating that 20 to 30% of the oxygen delivered to the capillaries is taken up into the tissues. Thus, only a small fraction of the available oxygen in capillary blood is used to support aerobic metabolism. Oxygen extraction is adjustable, and in conditions where O_2 delivery is impaired, the O_2ER can increase to 0.5 to 0.6. In trained athletes, the O_2ER can be as high as 0.8 during maximal exercise (3). Adjustments in O_2 extraction play an important role in maintaining oxygen uptake when oxygen delivery is variable, as described in the next section.

CONTROL OF OXYGEN UPTAKE

The oxygen transport system normally operates to maintain a constant rate of oxygen uptake (V_{O_2}) in conditions where O_2 delivery (D_{O_2}) can vary widely (3). This is accomplished by compensatory adjustments in O_2ER in response to changes in D_{O_2}. The O_2ER describes the relationship between O_2 and D_{O_2}; that is, $O_2ER = V_{O_2}/D_{O_2}$, which can be rearranged as shown in Equation 2.7.

$$V_{O_2} = D_{O_2} \times O_2ER \qquad (2.7)$$

According to this relationship, when a decrease in D_{O_2} is accompanied by a proportional increase in O_2ER, the V_{O_2} remains constant. However, when the O_2ER is fixed, a decrease in D_{O_2} is accompanied by a proportional decrease in V_{O_2}. The adjustability of the O_2 extraction therefore defines the tendency for V_{O_2} to change in response to variations in O_2 delivery. The normal relationship between D_{O_2} and V_{O_2} is described in the next section.

THE D_{O_2}–V_{O_2} CURVE

The relationship between O_2 delivery and O_2 uptake is described by the curve in Figure 2.2, where O_2 delivery is the independent variable. As the O_2 delivery decreases below normal, the O_2ER increases

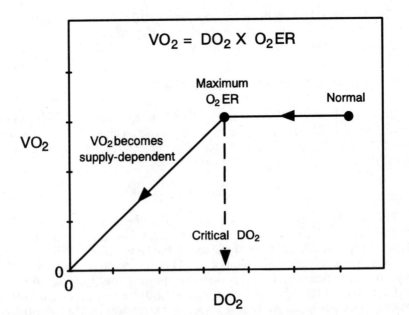

Figure 2.2. Graph describing the normal relationship between O_2 delivery (D_{O_2}) and O_2 uptake (V_{O_2}). O_2ER = oxygen extraction ratio.

proportionally and the V_{O_2} remains constant. When the O_2ER reaches its maximum level (0.5 to 0.6), further decreases in D_{O_2} are accompanied by proportional decreases in V_{O_2}. In the linear portion of the curve, the V_{O_2} is supply-dependent and the production of adenosine triphosphate (ATP) is limited by the supply of oxygen. This condition of oxygen-limited energy production is called *dysoxia* (4).

Critical O_2 Delivery

The D_{O_2} at which the V_{O_2} becomes supply-dependent is called the *critical oxygen delivery*, and is the point at which energy production in cells becomes oxygen-limited (dysoxia). The critical D_{O_2} in anesthetized subjects is in the vicinity of 300 mL/minute/m^2, but in critically ill patients, the critical D_{O_2} varies widely, from 150 to 1000 mL/minute/m^2 (3). Regardless of the source of this variability, it means that the critical D_{O_2} must be determined for each individual patient in the ICU.

Supply-Dependent V_{O_2}

In critically ill patients, the D_{O_2}–V_{O_2} relationship can be linear over a wide range, and the supply-dependent V_{O_2} in these patients can be the result of three possible conditions (3–6). One condition is pathologic supply dependency, where ATP production is limited by the supply of oxygen (dysoxia). This condition produces the supply dependency at very low levels of D_{O_2} in Figure 2.2. Another condition is physiologic supply dependency, where V_{O_2} is the independent variable and D_{O_2} changes in response to a primary change in the metabolic rate (6). This condition is responsible for the linear D_{O_2}–V_{O_2} relationship seen during exercise, and may be responsible for supply dependency in critically ill patients. Most importantly, it indicates that a linear D_{O_2}–V_{O_2} relationship may not be the result of a pathologic process. Finally, supply dependency may be an artifact produced when V_{O_2} is calculated and not directly measured. This latter possibility is discussed in more detail in Chapter 13.

The relationship between D_{O_2} and V_{O_2} is an important component of oxygen transport monitoring in the ICU, and can be used to identify tissue ischemia (e.g., pathologic supply dependency) or to create a therapeutic strategy (e.g., increasing D_{O_2} when the O_2 extraction is maximal). The applications of oxygen transport monitoring in the care of critically ill patients is described in Chapter 13.

CARBON DIOXIDE TRANSPORT

Carbon dioxide is the major end-product of oxidative metabolism (7) and, because it is capable of transforming into carbonic acid when hydrated, it can cause problems if allowed to accumulate. The value of CO_2 elimination is apparent in the operation of the ventilatory control system; that is, the ventilatory control system is designed to regulate carbon dioxide and to promote its elimination through the lungs. An increase in P_{CO_2} of 5 mm Hg can result in a twofold increase in minute ventilation. To produce an equivalent increment in ventilation, the arterial P_{O_2} must drop to 55 mm Hg (8). Thus, the ventilatory control system keeps a close eye on CO_2, but pays little attention to oxygen (whereas clinicians keep a close eye on oxygen and pay little attention to CO_2).

TOTAL BODY CO_2

Carbon dioxide is more soluble in water than oxygen, and thus moves more freely in the body fluids. However, the total body content of CO_2 is reported as 130 L (9), which seems to be quite a trick, considering that the average adult has no more than 40 to 50 L of water to spare. The explanation for this is that the CO_2 enters into a chemical reaction with water. This allows large volumes of CO_2 to enter a solution because the reaction with water dissociates CO_2 and maintains the gradient that drives the gas into solution. Opening a bottle of warm champagne or a warm beer demonstrates how much CO_2 can be present in a solution.

WHOLE BLOOD CO_2 CONTENT

Unlike oxygen, the CO_2 content of whole blood cannot be derived using simple equations. The reason for this will become apparent as the CO_2 transport process is revealed. However, the fraction of CO_2 dissolved in plasma can be defined using the solubility coefficients for CO_2 shown in Table 2.1. At a normal body temperature of 37° C, the concentration of dissolved CO_2 is 0.686 mL/L/mm Hg. At a P_{CO_2} of 40 mm Hg, the dissolved CO_2 in arterial blood is $(40 \times .68)$ 26 mL/L, as shown in Table 2.2. When compared with the total CO_2 content, it is apparent that only a small fraction of the CO_2 is present in the dissolved form.

TRANSPORT SCHEME

The centerpiece of CO_2 transport is the hydration reaction, and Figure 2.3 shows how the reaction participates in the transport process. The first step in the hydration reaction is the formation of carbonic acid (H_2CO_3). This is normally a slow reaction, and takes about 40 seconds to complete (10). The reaction speeds up considerably in the presence of the enzyme carbonic anhydrase, and takes less than 10 milliseconds to complete (10). Carbonic anhydrase is confined to the red cell, and is not present in plasma. Thus, CO_2 is rapidly hydrated only in the red cell, so CO_2 is drawn into the red cell.

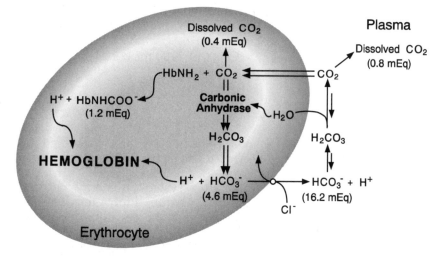

Figure 2.3. The chemical reactions involved in CO_2 transport. Values represent amounts in 1 L whole blood (venous). The double arrows indicate favored pathways. *Hb* = hemoglobin.

Carbonic acid dissociates to generate hydrogen and bicarbonate ions. A large fraction of the bicarbonate generated in the red cell is pumped back into the plasma in exchange for chloride. The hydrogen ion generated in the red cell is buffered by the hemoglobin. In this way, the CO_2 that enters the red cell is dismantled, and the parts stored (hemoglobin) or discarded (bicarbonate) to create room for more CO_2 to enter the red cell. These processes, along with the carbonic anhydrase–facilitated hydration reaction, create a sink for large volumes of CO_2 in the red cell.

A small fraction of CO_2 in the red cell reacts with free amino groups on hemoglobin. This produces carbamic acids, which dissociate into hydrogen ions and carbamino residues ($HbNHCOO^-$. This reaction is not a major component of CO_2 transport.

Unit Conversions

If the values in Figure 2.3 are added up, the total CO_2 content is 23 mEq/L in whole blood, with 17 mEq/L in plasma and 6 mEq/L in the red cell. Thus, most of the CO_2 appears to be in the plasma, but this is deceiving because much of the plasma component is in the form of bicarbonate that has been expelled from the red blood cell.

Because CO_2 is a ready source of ions (hydrogen and bicarbonate), the concentration of CO_2 is often expressed in mEq/L. This is the case in Figure 2.3. The conversion is based on the following: 1 mole of CO_2 has a volume of 22.3 L (STPD), so 1 mM CO_2 is approximately 22.3

mL and 1 mM/L CO_2 is approximately 22.3 mL/L or 2.23 mL/100 mL (vol%). Therefore,

$$CO_2 \text{ (mEq/L)} = CO_2 \text{ (mL/100 mL)}/2.23 \qquad (2.8)$$

HEMOGLOBIN AS A BUFFER

As mentioned earlier, the mass of hemoglobin in circulating blood is far greater than what is needed to transport oxygen, and moving this excess hemoglobin represents a considerable work load for the heart. This would make the circulatory system an energy-inefficient system unless the excess hemoglobin is required for some other vital function. As shown in Figure 2.3, hemoglobin has an important role in the transport of carbon dioxide. Considering the large volume of CO_2 in the blood, the large size of the hemoglobin pool becomes more understandable.

The function of hemoglobin in CO_2 transport is to act as a buffer for the hydrogen ions that are produced by the hydration of CO_2 in the red blood cell. The ability of hemoglobin to act as a buffer has been recognized since the 1930s, but this property of hemoglobin receives little attention. The buffer capacity of hemoglobin is shown in Table 2.5 (11). Note that **the total buffering capacity of hemoglobin is six times as great as the buffering capacity of all the plasma proteins combined.** A small part of this difference is due to the enhanced buffer capacity of the hemoglobin molecule, but most of the difference is due to the enormous size of the circulating hemoglobin pool.

The buffering actions of hemoglobin are caused by the histidine residues on the molecule. The imidazole group in histidine is responsible for the buffering actions, and is most effective at a pH of 7.0 (the dissociation constant of imidazole has a pK = 7.0, and buffers are most effective within 1 pH unit on either side of the pK). This means that hemoglobin is an effective buffer in the usual pH range of blood. In fact, hemoglobin should be more effective as a buffer than bicarbonate because the pK of carbonic acid is 6.1, which is outside the usual pH range of blood.

Thus, hemoglobin is the focal point of CO_2 transport because it can bind the acid equivalence of CO_2. The binding of hydrogen ions by hemoglobin creates a sink that maintains CO_2 flux into the red cell. Only because of its large mass can hemoglobin accomplish this.

TABLE 2.5. BUFFERING CAPACITY OF BLOOD PROTEINS		
	Hemoglobin	Plasma Proteins
Inherent buffering capacity	0.18 mEq H^+/g	0.11 mEq H^+/g
Concentration in whole blood	150 g/L	38.5 g/L
Total buffering capacity	27.5 mEq H^+/L	4.24 mEq H^+/L

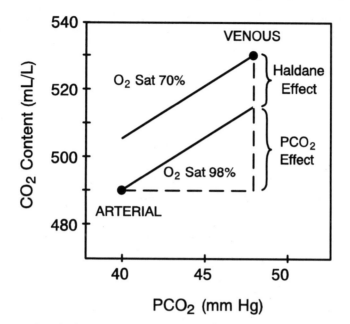

Figure 2.4. Graph showing the factors that contribute to the increase in CO_2 content from arterial to venous blood. *Sat* = saturation, PCO_2 = carbon dioxide pressure.

Haldane Effect

Hemoglobin has a greater buffer capacity when it is in the desaturated form, and blood that is fully desaturated can bind an additional 60 mL/L CO_2. The increase in CO_2 content that occurs when blood is desaturated is known as the *Haldane effect*. The graph in Figure 2.4 shows that the Haldane effect is responsible for a significant portion of the change in CO_2 content between arterial and venous blood. This reaffirms the important role played by hemoglobin in CO_2 transport.

CO_2 ELIMINATION (V_{CO_2})

Although CO_2 is dismantled for transport in the peripheral venous blood, it is reconstituted when the blood reaches the lungs. The next step is elimination through the lungs, and this process is described in Figure 2.5. The elimination of CO_2 (V_{CO_2}) is a Fick relationship, like V_{O_2}, but with the arterial and venous components reversed. Because there are no simple derivative equations for CO_2 content in blood, V_{CO_2} is usually measured directly. When V_{CO_2} is expressed as volume/time, the normal value is about 80% of the V_{O_2} (Table 2.4). The ratio $V_{CO_2}/$

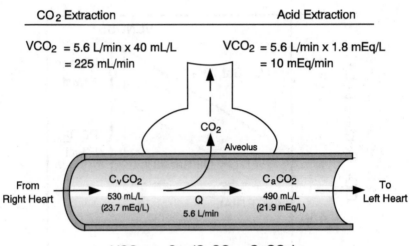

$$VCO_2 = Q \times (CvCO_2 - CaCO_2)$$

Figure 2.5. Schematic view of CO_2 elimination (VCO_2) via the lungs. The dotted line represents the alveolar–capillary interface. $CvCO_2$ = venous carbon dioxide concentration, $CaCO_2$ = arterial carbon dioxide concentration, Q = cardiac output.

VO_2 is thus 0.8 normally. This ratio is known as the respiratory quotient (RQ), and it varies according to the type of nutrient being metabolized. (See Chapter 46 for more information on the RQ.)

Acid Excretion

When VCO_2 is expressed in mEq/L, it describes the rate of volatile acid excretion. As shown in Figure 2.5, this rate is normally 10 mEq/minute, or 14,400 mEq/24 hours. During exercise, the excretion of volatile acids via the lungs can increase to 40,000 mEq/24 hours. Considering that the kidneys excrete only 40 to 80 mEq acid/24 hours, the major organ of acid excretion in the human body is the lungs, not the kidneys. This method of describing CO_2 elimination emphasizes the acid burden of metabolism. This emphasis on the production side of metabolism is an important addition to the current supply-dominant approach to metabolic support.

REFERENCES

GENERAL WORKS

Edwards JD, Shoemaker WC, Vincent J-L. Oxygen transport. Principles and practice. Philadelphia: WB Saunders, 1993.
Zander R, Mertzlufft F, eds. The oxygen status of arterial blood. Basel: S. Karger, 1991.

OXYGEN TRANSPORT

1. Pauling L. General chemistry. 3rd ed. Mineola NY: Dover Publications, 1988: 215.
2. Zander R. Calculation of oxygen concentration. In: Zander R, Mertzlufft F, eds. The oxygen status of arterial blood. Basel: S. Karger, 1991;203–209.
3. Leach RM, Treacher DF. The relationship between oxygen delivery and consumption. Dis Mon 1994;30:301–368.
4. Connett RJ, Honig CR, Gayeski TEJ, Brooks GA. Defining hypoxia: a systems view of V_{O_2}, glycolysis, energetics, and intracellular P_{O_2}. J Appl Physiol 1990; 68:833–842.
5. Russel JA, Phang PT. The oxygen delivery/consumption controversy. Approaches to management in the critically ill. Am Rev Respir Crit Care Med 1994;149:533–553.
6. Weissman C, Kemper M. Stressing the critically ill patient: the cardiopulmonary and metabolic responses to an acute increase in oxygen consumption. J Crit Care 1993;7:100–109.

CARBON DIOXIDE TRANSPORT

7. Nunn JF. Nunn's applied respiratory physiology. 4th ed. Stoneham, MA: Butterworth, 1993:219–246.
8. Lambertson CJ. Carbon dioxide and respiration in acid–base homeostasis. Anesthesiology 1960;21:642–651.
9. Henneberg S, Soderberg D, Groth T, et al. Carbon dioxide production during mechanical ventilation. Crit Care Med 1987;15:8–13.
10. Brahm J. The red cell anion-transport system: kinetics and physiologic implications. In: Gunn RB, Parker C, eds. Cell physiology of blood. New York: Rockefeller Press 1988;142–150.
11. Comroe JH Jr. Physiology of respiration. 2nd ed. Chicago: Year Book, 1974: 201–210.

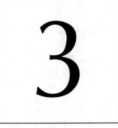

THE THREAT OF OXIDANT INJURY

All human things are subject to decay.
John Dryden

The treatment of critically ill patients is dominated by the notion that promoting the supply of oxygen to the vital organs is a necessary and life-sustaining measure. Oxygen is provided in a liberal and unregulated fashion, while the tendency for oxygen to degrade and decompose organic (carbon-based) matter is either overlooked or underestimated. In contrast to the notion that oxygen protects cells from injury in the critically ill patient, the accumulated evidence over the past 15 years suggests that oxygen is *responsible* for the cell injury that accompanies critical illness. Oxygen's ability to act as a lethal toxin has monumental implications for the way we treat critically ill patients.

THE OXIDATION REACTION

An oxidation reaction is a chemical reaction between oxygen and another chemical species. Because oxygen removes electrons from other atoms and molecules, **oxidation is** also described as **the loss of electrons by an atom or molecule.** The chemical species that removes the electrons is called an oxidizing agent or oxidant. The companion process (i.e., the gain of electrons by an atom or molecule) is called a reduction reaction, and the chemical species that donates the electrons is called a reducing agent. Because oxidation of one atom or molecule must be accompanied by reduction of another atom or molecule, the overall reaction is often called a *redox* reaction.

When an organic molecule (a molecule with a carbon skeleton) reacts with oxygen, electrons are removed from carbon atoms in the molecule. This disrupts one or more covalent bonds, and as each bond ruptures, energy is released in the form of heat and light (and sometimes sound). The organic molecule then breaks into smaller fragments. When oxidation is complete, the parent molecule is broken down into the smallest molecules capable of independent existence. Because organic matter is composed mainly of carbon and hydrogen, the end-products of oxidation are simple combinations of oxygen with carbon and hydrogen: carbon dioxide and water.

OXYGEN METABOLISM

Oxygen is a weak oxidizing agent, but some of its metabolites are potent oxidants capable of producing widespread and lethal cell injury (1). The mechanism whereby oxygen metabolism can produce more powerful oxidants than the parent molecule is related to the atomic structure of the oxygen molecule, which is described below.

THE OXYGEN MOLECULE

Oxygen in its natural state is a diatomic molecule, as shown by the familiar O_2 symbol at the top of Figure 3.1. The orbital diagram to the right of the O_2 symbol shows how the outer electrons of the oxygen molecule are arranged. The circles in the diagram represent orbitals. (An orbital is an energy field that can be occupied by electrons. It is distinct from an orbit, which is a path that represents a specific point in space and time.) The arrows in the diagram represent electrons that are spinning in the same or opposite directions (indicated by the direction of the arrows). Note that one of oxygen's orbitals contains two electrons with opposing spins, and the other two orbitals each contain a single electron spinning in the same direction. The orbital with the paired electrons is obeying one of the basic rules of the quantum atom: An electron orbital can be occupied by two electrons if they have opposing spins. Thus, the two outermost orbitals that contain single electrons are only half full, and their electrons are unpaired. **An atom or molecule that has one or more unpaired electrons in its outer orbitals is called a free radical** (2). (The term *free* indicates that the atom or molecule is capable of independent existence—it is free-living.)

Free radicals tend to be highly reactive chemical species by virtue of their unpaired electrons. However, not all free radicals are highly reactive. This is the case with oxygen, which is not a highly reactive molecule despite having two unpaired electrons.

The reason for oxygen's sluggish reactivity is the directional spin of its two unpaired electrons. No two electrons can occupy the same orbital if they have the same directional spin. Thus, an electron pair cannot be added to oxygen because one orbital would have two electrons with the same directional spin, which is a quantum impossibility. This spin restriction limits oxygen to single electron additions, and this not only increases the number of reactions needed to reduce molecular

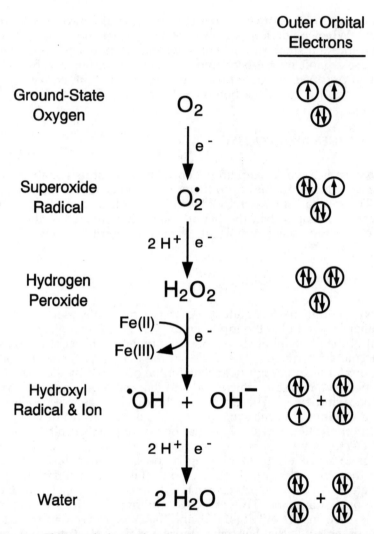

Figure 3.1. The metabolism of molecular oxygen to water. Orbital diagrams on the right side of the figure show the electron configuration (*arrows*) in the outer orbitals (*circles*) of each reactant. The highest orbitals in each diagram are furthest from the nucleus. Single electron reductions indicated by e^-.

oxygen to water, but it also produces more highly reactive intermediates.

THE METABOLIC PATHWAY

Oxygen is metabolized at the very end of the electron transport chain, where the electrons and protons that have completed the transport process are left to accumulate. The complete reduction of molecular oxygen to water requires the addition of four electrons and four protons, as shown in the reaction sequence in Figure 3.1. Each metabolite in this sequence is accompanied by an orbital diagram to demonstrate the changes occurring at each point in the pathway.

Superoxide Radical

The first reaction adds one electron to oxygen, and produces the superoxide radical.

$$O_2 + e^- \rightarrow O_2^{\bullet} \tag{3.1}$$

Note the superscript dot on the superoxide symbol. This signifies an unpaired electron, and is the conventional symbol for a free radical. The superoxide radical has one unpaired electron, and thus is less of a free radical than oxygen. Superoxide is neither a highly reactive radical nor a potent oxidant (3). Nevertheless, it has been implicated in conditions associated with widespread tissue damage, such as the reperfusion injury that follows a period of ischemia (2). The toxicity of superoxide may be caused by the large daily production, which is estimated at 1 billion molecules per cell, or 1.75 kg (4 lb) for a 70-kg adult (4).

Hydrogen Peroxide

The addition of one electron to superoxide creates hydrogen peroxide, a strong oxidizing agent (and the source of acid rain in the atmosphere) (5).

$$O_2^{\bullet} + e^- + 2H^+ \rightarrow H_2O_2 \tag{3.2}$$

Hydrogen peroxide is very mobile, and crosses cell membranes easily. It is a powerful cytotoxin and is well known for its ability to damage endothelial cells. It is not a free radical, but it may have to generate a free radical (a hydroxyl radical) to express its toxicity.

Hydrogen peroxide is loosely held together by a weak oxygen–oxygen bond (this bond is represented by the lower orbital in the orbital diagram for hydrogen peroxide). This bond ruptures easily, producing two hydroxyl radicals, each with one unpaired electron. An electron is donated to one of the hydroxyl radicals, creating one hydroxyl ion (OH^-) and one hydroxyl radical ($^{\bullet}OH$). The electron is donated by iron in its reduced form, Fe(II), which serves as a catalyst for the reaction. Iron is involved in many free radical reactions, and is considered a powerful pro-oxidant. The role of transition metals in free radical reactions is discussed again later in the chapter.

Hydroxyl Radical

The iron-catalyzed dissociation of hydrogen peroxide proceeds as follows:

$$H_2O_2 + Fe(II) \rightarrow OH^- + {}^{\bullet}OH + Fe(III) \tag{3.3}$$

(Note that Roman numerals are used instead of plus signs to designate the oxidation state of iron, as recommended by the International Union of Chemistry.) The hydroxyl radical is the ace of free radicals. It is one of the most reactive molecules in biochemistry and often reacts with another chemical species within five molecular diameters from its point of origin (2). This high degree of reactivity limits the mobility of the hydroxyl radical, and this may serve as a protective device to limit the toxicity of the hydroxyl radical. However, the hydroxyl radical is always dangerous because it can oxidize any molecule in the human body.

Hypochlorous Acid

The metabolism of oxygen in neutrophils has an additional pathway (not shown in Figure 3.1) that uses a myeloperoxidase enzyme to chlorinate hydrogen peroxide, creating hypochlorous acid (hypochlorite).

$$H_2O_2 + 2CL^- \rightarrow 2HOCL \tag{3.4}$$

When neutrophils are activated, the conversion of oxygen to superoxide increases twentyfold. This is called the respiratory burst, which is an unfortunate term because the increased O_2 consumption has nothing to do with energy metabolism. When the increased metabolic traffic reaches hydrogen peroxide, about 40% is diverted to hypochlorite production and the remainder forms hydroxyl radicals (6). Hypochlorite is the active ingredient in household bleach. It is a powerful germicidal agent and requires only milliseconds to produce lethal damage in bacteria (7).

Water

The final reaction in oxygen metabolism adds an electron to the hydroxyl radical and produces two molecules of water.

$$^\bullet OH + OH^- + e^- + 2H^+ \rightarrow 2H_2O \tag{3.5}$$

Therefore, the metabolism of one molecule of oxygen requires four chemical reactions, each involving the addition of a single electron. This process, then, requires four reducing equivalents (electrons and protons).

Under normal conditions, about 98% of the oxygen metabolism is completed, and less than 2% of the metabolites escape into the cytoplasm (3). This is a tribute to cytochrome oxidase, which carries on the reactions in a deep recess that effectively blocks any radical escape. This degree of suppression is necessary because of the ability of free radicals to start chain reactions (see next section).

Proposed Scheme

The superoxide radical is mobile but not toxic, whereas the hydroxyl radical is toxic but not mobile. Combining the advantages of each oxidant yields a scheme that has the mobile oxidant serving as a transport vehicle that can reach distant places. Once at the desired location, this metabolite could then generate hydroxyl radicals to produce local damage (3). This scheme is intuitively satisfying, regardless of its validity.

FREE RADICAL REACTIONS

The damaging effects of oxidation are largely the result of free radical reactions. This section describes the two basic types of free radical reactions: those involving free radicals and nonradicals and those involving two free radicals.

RADICAL AND NONRADICAL

When a free radical reacts with a nonradical, the nonradical loses an electron and is transformed into a free radical. Therefore, the union of a radical and a nonradical begets another radical (thus illustrating the survival value of the free radical). Because free radicals are often highly reactive in nature. This type of radical-regenerating reaction tends to become repetitive, creating a series of self-sustaining reactions known collectively as a **chain reaction** (3). The tendency to produce chain reactions is one of the most characteristic features of free radical reactions. A fire is one example of a chain reaction involving free radicals, and fires illustrate a very important feature of chain reactions: the tendency to produce widespread damage. A chain reaction that is capable of producing widespread organ damage is described below.

Lipid Peroxidation

The rancidity that develops in decaying food is the result of oxidative changes in polyunsaturated fatty acids (8). This same process, called lipid peroxidation, is also responsible for the oxidative damage of membrane lipids. The lipophilic interior of cell membranes is rich in polyunsaturated fatty acids (e.g., arachidonic acid) and the characteristic low melting point of these fatty acids may be responsible for the fluidity of cell membranes. Oxidation increases the melting point of membrane fatty acids and reduces membrane fluidity. The membranes eventually lose their selective permeability and become leaky, predisposing cells to osmotic disruption (8).

The peroxidation of membrane lipids proceeds as shown in Figure 3.2. The reaction sequence is initiated by a strong oxidant such as the hydroxyl radical, which removes an entire hydrogen atom (proton and electron) from one of the carbon atoms in a polyunsaturated fatty acid. This creates a carbon-centered radical ($C^\bullet$), which is then transformed into an oxygen-centered peroxy radical ($COO^\bullet$) that can remove a hydrogen atom from an adjacent fatty acid and initiate a new series of reactions. The final propagation reaction creates a self-sustaining chain

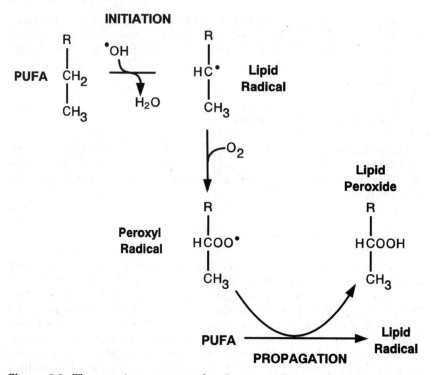

Figure 3.2. The reaction sequence for the peroxidation of polyunsaturated fatty acids (*PUFAs*) in cell membranes.

reaction that will continue until the substrate (i.e., fatty acid) is exhausted, or until something interferes with the propagation reaction. (The latter mechanism is the basis for the antioxidant action of vitamin E, which is described later.)

Implications

Free radical reactions have been implicated in the pathogenesis of more than 100 diseases (9), but it is not clear whether oxidant injury is a cause or a consequence of disease (9,10). However, **a chain reaction is an independent process** (i.e., independent of the initiating process), **and if it causes tissue injury it becomes an independent pathologic process (a primary illness).**

RADICAL AND RADICAL

Two radicals can react by sharing electrons to form a covalent bond. This eliminates the free radicals but does not necessarily eliminate the risk of toxicity. In the example below, the product of a radical–radical reaction is much more destructive than both radicals combined.

Nitric Oxide Transformation

Nitric oxide has been placed in a category of its own as a free radical because of its beneficial actions as a vasodilator, neurotransmitter, and bactericidal agent (11). The regard for nitric oxide has been so favorable that it was named "Molecule of the Year" by *Science Magazine* in 1992. However, despite its favorable profile, nitric oxide can become a toxin in the presence of superoxide. The reaction of superoxide with nitric oxide generates a powerful oxidant called peroxynitrite, which is 2000 times more potent than hydrogen peroxide as an oxidizing agent (12). Peroxynitrite can either cause direct tissue damage or can decompose and produce hydroxyl radicals and nitrogen dioxide.

$$NO^{\bullet} + O_2^{\bullet-} \rightarrow ONOOO^- \text{ (peroxynitrite)} \tag{3.6}$$

$$ONOOOH \rightarrow {}^{\bullet}OH + NO_2 \tag{3.7}$$

The transformation of nitric oxide into a source of oxidant injury demonstrates how free radicals can promote oxidant damage indirectly.

ANTIOXIDANT PROTECTION

Evidence for endogenous antioxidant protection is provided by the simple observation that accelerated decay begins at the moment of death. This section presents the substances that are believed to play a major role in this protection.

An antioxidant is defined as any chemical species that can reduce or delay the oxidation of an oxidizable substrate (2). The nonenzyme antioxidants are included in Table 3.1.

ENZYME ANTIOXIDANTS

There are three enzymes that function as antioxidants, shown in Figure 3.3. Note that the reaction sequence in this figure is the same as in Figure 3.1.

Superoxide Dismutase

The discovery of superoxide dismutase (SOD) enzyme in 1969 was the first indication of free radical activity in humans, and this began the frenzy of interest in free radicals. The role of SOD as an antioxidant is not clear. In fact, SOD promotes the formation of hydrogen peroxide, which is an oxidant. **How can an enzyme that promotes the formation of an oxidant be defined as an antioxidant?** In fact, if SOD increases

TABLE 3.1. ENDOGENOUS AND EXOGENOUS ANTIOXIDANTS

Antioxidant	Action(s)	Comments
Selenium	A cofactor for glutathione peroxidanse. Enzyme activity is depressed when selenium levels in blood are below normal.	Although an essential nutrient, it is not routinely provided. Can be given IV as selenite salt. RDA: 70 μg/d (M) 55 μg/d (F) Maximum safe dose: 200 μg/d
Glutathione	A reducing agent, by virtue of an SH group on a cysteine residue.	A major intracellular antioxidant. Synthesized de novo in cells. Does not easily cross cell membranes
N-Acetylcysteine	A commercially available mucolytic agent that acts as a glutathione analog.	Proven effective as an exogenous glutathione surrogate in acetaminophen overdose (see Chapter 53). Effective when given orally or IV. Only the oral route is approved in the United States.
Vitamin E	Blocks propagation of lipid peroxidation in cell membranes and circulating lipoproteins.	The major antioxidant protection against oxidant damage in membrane lipids. Serum levels (corrected for total lipids) frequently low in ICU patients, even in face of supplemental treatment.
Vitamin C	A reducing agent. Can return vitamin E to its active form (has a cooperative effect). Can act as a pro-oxidant by maintaining iron as Fe(II).	Antioxidant role not clear. May be important in eyes and lungs. Activity is mostly extracellular. Risk for pro-oxidant actions in the presence of transitional metals is a concern.
1. Caeruloplasmin 2. Transferrin 3. Albumin 4. Uric Acid	Major antioxidants in plasma. Most act by promoting the binding of iron (1, 2, 3, 4) and copper (1, 3, 4) Albumin is a potent scavenger of HOCL.	Major antioxidant action involves the removal of free iron and copper from the plasma. Caeruloplasmin accounts for most of the antioxidant activity in plasma.
Aminosteroids High-Dose Methylprednisolone (MP)	Inhibit lipid peroxidation by a nonglucocorticoid action. The dose of MP for this effect is 30 mg/kg IV (Ann Emerg Med 1993;22:1022–1027)	High-dose MP has been successful in acute spinal cord injury if given within 8 hours after injury (J Neurosurg 1992; 76:23–31). Aminosteroids (nonglucocortocoids) are being evaluated for brain and spinal cord injury.

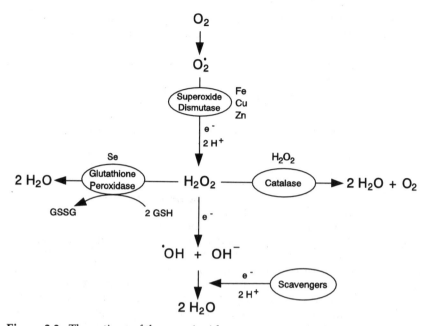

Figure 3.3. The actions of three antioxidant enzymes and a free radical scavenger. The reaction sequence depicts oxygen metabolism, as shown in Figure 3.1. Cofactors for superoxide dismutase are iron (Fe), zinc (Zn), and copper (Cu), but are never present as a triad on the same enzyme. Cofactor for glutathione peroxidase is selenium (Se). GSH = reduced glutathione, $GSSG$ = oxidized glutathione as a dipeptide.

the metabolic traffic flowing through hydrogen peroxide, and the catalase and peroxidase reactions are unable to increase their activity proportionally, the hydrogen peroxide levels may rise, and in this situation SOD functions as a pro-oxidant (13). Thus, SOD is not an antioxidant at least some of the time.

Catalase

Catalase is an iron-containing heme protein that reduces hydrogen peroxide to water. It is present in most cells, but is lowest in cardiac cells and neurones. Inhibition of the catalase enzyme does not enhance the toxicity of hydrogen peroxide for endothelial cells (14), so the role of this enzyme as an antioxidant is unclear.

Glutathione Peroxidase

The peroxidase enzyme reduces hydrogen peroxide to water by removing electrons from glutathione in its reduced form and then donating the electrons to hydrogen peroxide. Glutathione is returned to its reduced state by a reductase enzyme that transfers the reducing equivalents from NADPH. The total reaction can be written as follows:

$$\text{Peroxidase reaction: } H_2O_2 + 2GSH \rightarrow 2H_2O + GSSG \quad (3.8)$$

$$\text{Reductase reaction: } NADPH + H + GSSG \rightarrow 2GSH + NADP \quad (3.9)$$

where GSSG and GSH are oxidized and reduced glutathione, respectively.

Selenium

The activity of the glutathione peroxidase enzyme in humans depends on the trace element selenium. Selenium is an essential nutrient with a recommended dietary allowance of 70 µg daily for men and 55 µg daily for women (15). Despite this recommendation, selenium is not included in most total parenteral nutrition regimens. Because the absence of dietary selenium produces measurable differences in glutathione peroxidase activity after just 1 week (16), the routine administration of selenium seems justified. However, selenium, has no clear-cut deficiency syndrome in humans, so there is little impetus to provide selenium on a routine basis.

Selenium status can be monitored with whole blood selenium levels. The normal range is 0.5 to 2.5 mg/L. Selenium can be provided intravenously as sodium selenite (17). The highest daily dose that is considered safe is 200 µg, given in divided doses (50 µg intravenously every 6 hours).

NONENZYME ANTIOXIDANTS

Glutathione

One of the major antioxidants in the human body is a sulfur-containing tripeptide glutathione (glycine–cysteine–glutamine), which is present in molar concentrations (0.5 to 10 mM/L) in most cells (18,19). Glutathione is a reducing agent by virtue of a sulfhydryl group in the cysteine residue of the molecule. It is normally in the reduced state (GSH), and the ratio of reduced to oxidized forms is 10:1. The major antioxidant action of glutathione is to reduce hydrogen peroxide directly to water, which diverts hydrogen peroxide from producing hydroxyl radicals. Glutathione is found in all organs, but is particularly prevalent in the lung, liver, endothelium, and intestinal mucosa. It is primarily an intracellular antioxidant, and plasma levels of glutathione are three orders of magnitude lower than intracellular levels.

Glutathione does not cross cell membranes directly, but is broken down first into its constituent amino acids and then reconstituted on the other side of the membrane. It is synthesized in every cell of the body, and largely remains sequestered within cells. Exogenous glutathione has little effect on intracellular levels (20), which limits the therapeutic value of this agent.

N-Acetylcysteine

N-Acetylcysteine, a popular mucolytic agent (Mucomyst), is a sulfhydryl-containing glutathione analog capable of passing readily across cell membranes. N-Acetylcysteine is effective as a glutathione analog in acetaminophen toxicity, which is the result of an overwhelmed glutathione detoxification pathway (see Chapter 53). Therefore, N-acetylcysteine has a proven track record as an exogenous glutathione analog.

N-Acetylcysteine may prove to be a valuable antioxidant for therapeutic use. It protects the myocardium from ischemic injury, and has been successful in reducing the incidence of reperfusion injury during cardiac catheterization (21). It has also been used with some success in treating critically ill patients with acute respiratory distress syndrome and inflammatory shock syndromes (22,23).

Vitamin E

Vitamin E (α-tocopherol) is a lipid-soluble vitamin that functions primarily as an antioxidant that antagonizes the peroxidative injury of membrane lipids. It is the only antioxidant capable of halting the propagation of lipid peroxidation. The mechanism for this action is shown in Figure 3.4. Vitamin E inhabits the lipophilic interior of cell membranes, where the polyunsaturated fatty acids are also located. When a propagating wave of lipid peroxidation reaches vitamin E, it is oxidized to a free radical, thereby sparing any adjacent polyunsaturated fatty acids from oxidation. The vitamin E radical is poorly reactive, and this halts the propagation of the peroxidation reactions. This action has earned vitamin E the title of a *chain-breaking* antioxidant.

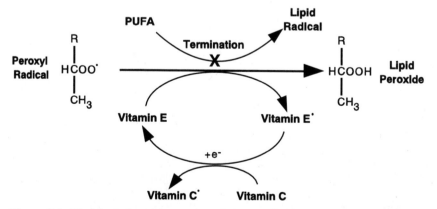

Figure 3.4. The chain-breaking action of vitamin E that terminates lipid peroxidation in cell membranes.

TABLE 3.2. CLINICAL CONDITIONS THAT ARE ACCOMPANIED BY OXIDANT STRESS*		
Target Organs	**Clinical Conditions**	**Comments**
Lung	Acute respiratory distress syndrome Asthma Reperfusion pulmonary edema Acid aspiration Pulmonary oxygen toxicity	The lung is vulnerable to oxidant injury from the airways (e.g., high inspired O_2) and from the microcirculation (e.g., WBC sequestration). Protection from O_2 is aided by high levels of glutathione and vitamin C in the epithelial lining of the lower airways.

Heart	Acute myocardial infarction
	Reperfusion injury due to:
	  Angioplasty
	  Cardioplegia
	  Coronary occlusion
	  Thrombolysis
		Oxidants most likely play a role in the "stunned" myocardium associated with reperfusion injury.

Nervous system	Stroke Traumatic brain injury Postresuscitation injury Spinal cord injury	Lipid peroxidation is a prominent form of oxidant injury in the brain and spinal cord. Steroids that inhibit lipid peroxidation are being evaluated for nervous system injury (see Table 3.1)
Gastrointestinal tract	Drug-induced mucosal injury Intestinal ischemia Peptic ulcer disease	The gut is susceptible to reperfusion injury, possibly due to the abundance of xanthine dehydrogenase (a source of O_2^- during ischemia) in the bowel wall.

Kidney	Acute renal failure due to:
	  Aminoglycosides
	  Ischemia
	  Myoglobinuria
		Hydrogen peroxide and iron may have important roles in oxidant injury involving the kidneys.

Multiple organs	Cardiopulmonary bypass Multiple organ dysfunction syndrome Multisystem trauma Postresuscitation injury Septic shock Thermal injury	Inflammation is a common source of oxidant production in these conditions. Nitric oxide may promote hypotension in septic shock. Agents that inhibit nitric oxide production are being evaluated in septic shock (Ann Pharmacother 1995;29:36–46).

* Includes only conditions that are prevalent in ICU patients.

The vitamin E radical is transformed back to vitamin E, and vitamin C can act as the electron donor in this reaction.

Vitamin E deficiency may be common in critically ill patients (24). The normal vitamin E level in plasma is 1 mg/dL, and a level below 0.5 mg/dL is evidence of deficiency (25). Considering the important role of vitamin E as an antioxidant, it seems wise to check the vitamin E status in patients who are at risk for oxidant injury (see Table 3.2).

Vitamin C

Vitamin C (ascorbic acid) is a reducing agent that can donate electrons to free radicals and fill their electron orbitals. It is a water-soluble antioxidant, and operates primarily in the extracellular space. Vitamin C is found in abundance in the lung, where it may play a protective role in inactivating pollutants that enter the airways.

The problem with vitamin C is its tendency to promote (rather than retard) the formation of oxidants in the presence of iron and copper (26–28). Vitamin C reduces iron to the Fe(II) state, and this normally aids in the absorption of iron from the intestinal tract. However, Fe(II) can promote the production of hydroxyl radicals, as described earlier. Thus, vitamin C can function as a pro-oxidant by maintaining iron in its reduced or Fe(II) state. The reactions involved are as follows:

$$\text{Ascorbate } + \text{ Fe(III)} \rightarrow \text{Fe(II)} + \text{ Dehydroascorbate} \qquad (3.10)$$

$$\text{Fe(II)} + H_2O_2 \rightarrow {}^{\bullet}OH + OH^- + \text{Fe(III)} \qquad (3.11)$$

Several conditions that are common in ICU patients can promote an increase in free iron. Among these are inflammation, blood transfusions, and reductions in binding proteins. The prevalence of these conditions raises serious concerns about the use of vitamin C as an exogenous antioxidant in the ICU patient population.

Plasma Antioxidants

The plasma components with antioxidant activity are listed at the very bottom of Table 3.2. Most of the antioxidant activity in plasma can be traced to two proteins that make up only 4% of total plasma protein pool (27): ceruloplasmin (the copper transport or storage protein) and transferrin. Transferrin binds iron in the Fe(III) state, and ceruloplasmin oxidizes iron from the Fe(II) to Fe(III) state. Therefore, ceruloplasmin helps transferrin to bind iron, and both proteins then act to limit free iron in the plasma. For this reason, iron sequestration has been proposed as the major antioxidant activity in plasma (24). This is consistent with the actions of Fe(II) to promote free radical production, as shown in Figure 3.1.

OXIDANT STRESS

The risk and severity of oxidation-induced tissue injury are determined by the balance between oxidant and antioxidant activities. When oxidant activity exceeds the neutralizing capacity of the antioxidants, the excess or unopposed oxidant activity can promote tissue injury. This condition of unopposed biological oxidation is known as *oxidant stress* (29).

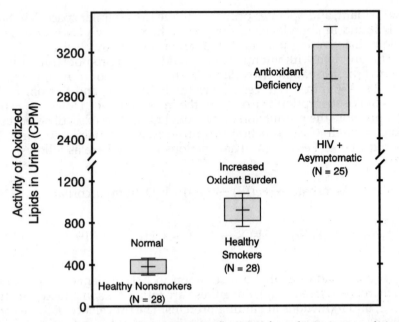

Figure 3.5. Box diagrams showing the influence of predisposing conditions on oxidant stress. The vertical axis shows the urinary activity of lipid hydroperoxides, measured as spontaneous chemiluminescence and recorded in counts per minute (*CPM*). The three groups represent age-matched adults, and N indicates the number of subjects in each group. The control group is represented on the left. *HIV* = human immunodeficiency virus. (From Millili J, Marino PL, Nusbaum M. The pattern of spontaneous chemiluminescence in humans and its use in measuring oxidant stress. Proceedings of the First International Conference on Clinical Chemiluminescence. Berlin: Humboldt University Press, 1994.)

PREDISPOSING CONDITIONS

Any imbalance in the activities of oxidants and antioxidants can result in unopposed oxidation. The box plots in Figure 3.5 show the effects of two conditions that promote oxidant–antioxidant imbalance on the level of oxidant stress in humans. The index of oxidant stress in this study is the activity of lipid hydroperoxides in urine, measured as spontaneous chemiluminescence and reported in counts per minute (CPM). Healthy, nonsmoking adults (the control group) show the lowest level of oxidant activity. The effects of an increase in oxidant burden is shown in a group of heavy smokers (one puff of a cigarette contains roughly one billion free radicals). The effects of a deficiency in antioxidant protection are shown for a group of patients with human immunodeficiency virus (HIV) infection (glutathione deficiency is common in HIV infections) (30). Each of the predisposing conditions is accompanied by a significant increase in oxidant activity in comparison to the activity in the healthy, control subjects. Note also that the HIV patients have ongoing oxidant stress when they are symptom-free.

This supports the notion that oxidant stress is a cause and not a consequence of pathologic organ injury.

CLINICAL DISEASE

As mentioned earlier, oxidants have been implicated in the pathogenesis of more than 100 clinical diseases (9); the ones most likely to be encountered in the ICU are listed in Table 3.2. Unopposed biological oxidation has been documented in each of these clinical conditions (9,10,30–35). This does not establish a causal role for oxidation (this will require evidence that antioxidant therapy can improve outcome), but the tendency for oxidation to cause independent and progressive tissue damage (e.g., in chain reactions) is reason enough to suspect that oxidant-induced injury plays a role in these illnesses.

Inflammation

Most of the clinical conditions in Table 3.2 are accompanied by inflammation, and the conditions with multiorgan involvement are often associated with a progressive, systemic inflammatory response. As a result, inflammation has been proposed as a principal offender in pathologic forms of oxidant injury. The release of free radicals from activated neutrophils and macrophages creates an oxidant-intense environment, and the ability of host cells to withstand this oxidative assault may be the important factor in determining the clinical course of inflammatory conditions. In the desirable world, leukocyte-derived oxidants would annihilate all invading microbes, but would not affect the host cells. In the undesirable world, the inflammatory oxidants would destroy both the invader and the host. This proposed scheme is intuitively appealing, and emphasizes the value of providing antioxidants routinely in inflammatory illnesses.

Antioxidant Therapy

The value of maintaining antioxidant protection is not a debatable issue because loss of antioxidant defenses is a known cause of tissue destruction; the best example of this is the accelerated decay that occurs after death. Therefore, antioxidant supplements should be considered as a routine measure in patients who spend more than a few days in the ICU. In patients with any of the clinical conditions in Table 3.2, it would be wise to monitor some of the endogenous antioxidants (vitamin E, vitamin C, and selenium). A reduced antioxidant level in blood (or any body fluid) may not indicate a deficiency state (it may indicate that the antioxidant is being used), but would certainly be an indication to provide supplements. The real value of antioxidant therapy will be determined by clinical studies, some of which are currently in progress.

METABOLIC SUPPORT

The tendency for aerobic metabolism to generate toxins has significant implications for the approach to metabolic support in critically ill patients. When metabolically-generated oxidants overwhelm the body's antioxidant defenses, the common practice of supporting metabolism by promoting the availability of oxygen and nutrients serves only to generate more toxic metabolites. The proper maneuver here is to support the antioxidant defenses. This approach adds another dimension to the concept of metabolic support by considering the output side of metabolism. Remember that metabolism is an engine (i.e., an energy converter) and like all engines, it has an exhaust that contains noxious byproducts of combustion. The exhaust from an automobile engine adds pollutants to the atmosphere; likewise, the exhaust from a metabolic engine adds pollutants to the "biosphere."

REFERENCES

GENERAL WORKS

Davies KJA, Ursini F, eds. The oxygen paradox. Padova, Italy: CLEUP University Press, 1995.

Grisham MB. Reactive metabolites of oxygen and nitrogen in biology and medicine. Austin, TX: RG Landes, 1992.

Halliwell B, Gutteridge JM. Free radicals in biology and medicine. 2nd ed. Oxford: Clarendon Press, 1989.

Moslen MT, Smith CV. Free radical mechanisms of tissue injury. Boca Raton, FL: CRC Press, 1992.

Sies H, ed. Oxidative stress II: oxidants and antioxidants. New York: Academic Press, 1991.

Yagi K, ed. Active oxygens, lipid peroxides, and antioxidants. Boca Raton, FL: CRC Press, 1993.

OXIDANTS

1. Chance B, Sies H, Boveris A. Hydroperoxide metabolism in mammalian organs. Physiol Rev 1979;59:527–605.
2. Halliwell B, Gutteridge JM. Free radicals in biology and medicine. 2nd ed. Clarendon: Oxford University Press, 1989:2–80.
3. Liochev SI, Fridovich I. The role of O_2 in the production of $HO^\bullet$ in vitro and in vivo. Free Radic Biol Med 1994;16:29–33.
4. Frei B. Reactive oxygen species and antioxidant vitamins: mechanisms of action. Am J Med 1994;97(Suppl 3A):5–23.
5. Thompson AM. The oxidizing capacity of the earth's atmosphere: probable past and future changes. Science 1992;256:1157–1165.
6. Anderson BO, Brown JM, Harken A. Mechanisms of neutrophil-mediated tissue injury. J Surg Res 1991;51:170–179.
7. Bernovsky C. Nucleotide chloramines and neutrophil-mediated cytotoxicity. FASEB J 1991;5:295–300.

8. Halliwell B, Gutteridge JM. Free radicals in biology and medicine. 2nd ed. Clarendon: Oxford University Press, 1989:188–204.
9. Gutteridge JMC. Free radicals in disease processes: a compilation of cause and consequence. Free Radic Res Commun 1993;19:141–158.
10. Halliwell B. Free radical, antioxidants, and human disease: curiosity, cause, or consequence. Lancet 1994;344:721–724.
11. Anggard E. Nitric oxide: mediator, murderer, and medicine. Lancet 1994;343: 1199–1206.
12. Freeman B. Free radical chemistry of nitric oxide. Looking at the dark side. Chest 1994;105(Suppl):79–84.

ANTIOXIDANTS

13. Michiels C, Raes M, Toussant O, Remacle J. Importance of Se-glutathione, peroxidase, catalase, and CU/ZN-SOD for cell survival against oxidative stress. Free Radic Biol Med 1994;17:235–248.
14. Suttorp N, Toepfer W, Roka L. Antioxidant defense mechanisms of endothelial cells: glutathione redox cycle versus catalase. Am J Physiol 1986;251:671–680.
15. National Research Council. Subcommittee on the tenth edition of the RDAs. Washington, DC: National Academic Press, 1989:220.
16. Sando K, Hoki M, Nezu R, et al. Platelet glutathione peroxidase activity in long-term total parenteral nutrition with and without selenium supplementation. J Parent Ent Nutr 1992;16:54–58.
17. World Health Organization. Selenium. Environmental Health Criteria 58. Geneva, Switzerland, 1987.
18. Meister A. On the antioxidant effects of ascorbic acid and glutathione. Biochem Pharmacol 1992;44:1905–1915.
19. Cantin AM, Begin R. Glutathione and inflammatory disorders of the lung. Lung 1991;169:123–138.
20. Robinson M, Ahn MS, Rounds JD, et al. Parenteral glutathione monoester enhances tissue antioxidant stores. J Parent Ent Nutr 1992;16:413–418.
21. Ferrari R, Ceconi C, Curello S, et al. Oxygen free radicals and myocardial damage: protective role of thiol containing agents. Am J Med 1991;91(Suppl 3C):95–112.
22. Henderson A, Hayes P. Acetylcysteine as a cytoprotective antioxidant in patients with severe sepsis: potential new use for an old drug. Ann Pharmacother 1994;28:1086–1088.
23. Suter PM, Domenighetti G, Schaller MD, et al. N-Acetylcysteine enhances recovery from acute lung injury in man: a randomized, double-blind placebo-controlled clinical study. Chest 1994;105:190–194.
24. Pincemail J, Bertrand Y, Hanique G, et al. Evaluation of vitamin E deficiency in patients with adult respiratory distress syndrome. Ann N Y Acad Sci 1989; 570:498–500.
25. Meydani M. Vitamin E. Lancet 1995;345:170–176.
26. Herbert V, Shaw S, Jayatilleke E. Vitamin C supplements are harmful to lethal for over 10% of Americans with high iron stores. FASEB J 1994;8:A678.
27. Halliwell B, Gutteridge JMC. Role of free radicals and catalytic metal ions in human disease. Methods Enzymol 1990;186:1–85.
28. Herbert V, Shaw S, Jayatilleke E, Stopler-Kasdan T. Most free-radical injury is iron-related: it is promoted by iron, hemin, haloferritin and vitamin C, and inhibited by desferrioxamine and apoferritin. Stem Cells 1994;12:289–303.

OXIDANT STRESS

29. Smith CV. Correlations and apparent contradictions in assessment of oxidant stress in vivo. Free Radic Biol Med 1991;10:217–224.
30. Staal FJ, Ela SW, Roederer M, et al. Glutathione deficiency and human immunodeficiency virus infection. Lancet 1992;339:909–912.
31. Weitz ZW, Birnbaum AI, Sobotka PA, et al. High breath pentane concentrations during acute myocardial infarction. Lancet 1991;337:933–936.
32. Cross CE, van der Vilet A, O'Neill CA, Eiserich JP. Reactive oxygen species and the lung. Lancet 1994;344:930–935.
33. Grace PA. Ischemia-reperfusion injury. Br J Surg 1994;81:637–647.
34. Deitch EA. Multiple organ failure. Ann Surg 1992;216:117–134.
35. Natanson C, Hoffman WD, Suffredini AF, et al. Selected treatment strategies for septic shock based on proposed mechanisms of pathogenesis. Ann Intern Med 1994;120:771–783.

section II
STANDARD PRACTICES IN PATIENT CARE

We are constantly misled by the ease with which our minds fall into the ruts of one or two experiences.

Sir William Osler

c h a p t e r

4

VASCULAR ACCESS

He who works with his hands is a laborer.
He who works with his head and his hands is a craftsman.
St. Francis of Assisi

The care of critically ill patients requires one or more pipelines to the vascular system, for both monitoring and interventions. This chapter presents some guidelines for the insertion of vascular catheters, including a brief description of the common percutaneous access routes (1–3). The emphasis here is on the craft of establishing vascular access. The labor of vascular cannulation is a skill learned at the bedside.

PREPARING FOR VASCULAR CANNULATION

HANDWASHING

Handwashing is mandatory (and often overlooked) before the insertion of vascular devices. Scrubbing with antimicrobial cleansing solutions does not reduce the incidence of catheter-related sepsis (4), so a simple soap-and-water scrub is sufficient.

UNIVERSAL PRECAUTIONS

In 1985, the Centers for Disease Control introduced a strategy for blood and body fluid precautions known as universal precautions (5). This strategy is based on the assumption that all patients are potential sources of human immunodeficiency virus (HIV) and other blood-borne pathogens (e.g., hepatitis viruses) until proven otherwise. The following recommendations apply to the insertion of vascular catheters.

53

Use protective gloves for all vascular cannulations.

Use sterile gloves for all cannulations except those involving the introduction of a short catheter into a peripheral vein.

Caps, gowns, masks, and protective eyewear are not necessary unless splashes of blood are anticipated (e.g., in a trauma victim). These measures do not reduce the incidence of catheter-related sepsis (6).

Avoid needlestick injuries. Do not recap needles or manually remove needles from syringes. Place all sharp instruments in puncture-resistant containers immediately after use.

If a needlestick injury is sustained during the procedure, follow the recommendations in Table 4.1.

Needlestick injuries are reported in up to 80% of medical students and interns (9). Therefore, in patients who are known risks for transmitting HIV or viral hepatitis, vascular cannulation should be performed only by an experienced senior-level resident or fellow.

LATEX ALLERGY

The increased use of rubber gloves (made of latex or vinyl) as protection against HIV infections has resulted in an increased recognition of **allergic reactions to latex** (10). These reactions can be manifest as a contact dermatitis (urticarial lesions of the hands and face), or as a conjunctivitis, rhinitis, or asthma. The latter three manifestations are reactions to airborne latex particles, and they **do not require direct physical contact with gloves.** They often appear when the affected individual enters an area where latex gloves are being used. Therefore, a latex allergy should be suspected in any ICU team member who develops atopic symptoms when in the ICU. When this occurs, a switch to vinyl gloves will eliminate the problem. Latex allergy can be manifest as anaphylaxis (10), so the transition to vinyl gloves for suspected latex allergy should not be delayed.

CLEANSING THE SKIN

Agents that reduce skin microflora are called antiseptics, whereas agents that reduce the microflora on inanimate objects are called disinfectants. Common antiseptic agents are listed in Table 4.2 (11,12). The most widely used antiseptic agents are alcohol and iodine, both of which have a broad spectrum of antimicrobial activity. Alcohol (commonly used as a 70% solution) may not work well on dirty skin (that is, it does not have a detergent action), so it is often used in combination with another antiseptic agent. The most popular antiseptic solution currently in use is a **povidone–iodine** preparation (e.g., Betadine), also known as an iodophor, a water-soluble complex of iodine and a carrier molecule. The iodine is released slowly from the carrier molecule, and this reduces the irritating effects of iodine on the skin. This preparation

TABLE 4.1. RECOMMENDATIONS FOR NEEDLESTICK INJURIES

Source	Exposed Person	Action
HBsAG-positive	Unvaccinated	Hepatitis B immune globulin 0.06 mL/kg IM within 24 hr Hepatitis B vaccine 1.0 mL within 7 days Repeat dose at 1 and 6 months.
	Vaccinated Anti-HBs titer unknown	Assay for anti-HBs: If anti-HBs levels are nonprotective • Give hepatitis B immune globulin 0.06 mL/kg IM within 24 hr. • Give a booster dose (1.0 mL) of hepatitis B vaccine.
	Vaccinated Anti-HBs titer protective within past 2 yr	Assay for anti-HBs: If anti-HBs levels are nonprotective, give a booster dose (1.0 mL) of hepatitis B vaccine.
Hepatitis B status unknown	Unvaccinated	Hepatitis B vaccine 1.0 mL within 7 days Repeat dose at 1 and 6 months.
	Vaccinated Anti-HBs titer unknown	Assay for anti-HBs: If anti-HBs levels are nonprotective, give a booster dose (1.0 mL) of hepatitis B vaccine.
HIV-positive	Risk of seroconversion less than 1 in 100 (7)	Consult your infection control service for recommendations on chemoprophylaxis. Exposed person should • Be tested for HIV status soon after exposure and again at 6, 12, and 24 weeks after exposure. • Report any febrile illness that occurs within 12 wk after exposure. • Refrain from blood donation and use appropriate protection for sexual intercourse for first 12 wk after exposure (5).
HIV status unknown	Risk of seroconversion estimated at 1 in 10,000 (8)	If source is high-risk for HIV infection, following recommendations above.

Hepatitis B recommendations taken from ACP Task Force on Adult Immunization and Infectious Disease Society of America. Guide for adult immunization. 3rd ed. Philadelphia: American College of Physicians, 1994 (with permission). *HBsAG* = hepatitis B surface antigen, *anti-HBs* = antibody to hepatitis B surface antigen, *HIV* = human immunodeficiency virus.

should be left in contact with the skin for at least 2 minutes to allow sufficient time for iodine to be released from the carrier molecule.

HAIR REMOVAL

Shaving is not recommended for hair removal because it abrades the skin and promotes bacterial colonization. If hair removal is necessary, the hair can be clipped or a depilatory can be applied (6).

TABLE 4.2. COMMON ANTISEPTIC AGENTS

Antiseptic Agent	Commercial Preparations	Antimicrobial Spectrum	Advantages	Disadvantages
Alcohol	50–90% ethyl alcohol or isopropyl alcohol	Bacteria (Gram-positive or Gram-negative) HIV Fungi Mycobacteria	Broad spectrum of activity Rapid acting	Little residual activity Requires a clean surface for optimal efficacy
Iodine	Tincture of iodine or povidone–iodine (Betadine)	Bacteria (Gram-positive or Gram-negative) HIV Fungi Mycobacteria	Broad spectrum of activity Good residual activity	Irritates skin and soft tissues Povidone–iodine not immediately effective
Chlorhexidine gluconate	Hibiclens (4% solution)	Bacteria (Gram-positive or Gram-negative)	Good residual activity Does not irritate the skin	Residual activity is diminished by soap An ocular irritant
Hexachlorophene	pHisoHex (3% solution)	Bacteria (Gram-positive)	Good residual activity	Limited spectrum of activity

HIV = human immunodeficiency virus.

CATHETER INSERTION DEVICES

Vascular cannulation can be performed by advancing the catheter over a needle or guidewire that is in contact with the lumen of a blood vessel.

CATHETER-OVER-NEEDLE

A catheter-over-needle device is shown in Figure 4.1. The catheter fits snugly over the insertion needle, and has a tapered end to minimize damage to the catheter tip and soft tissues during insertion. This device can be held like a pencil (i.e., between the thumb and forefinger) as it is inserted through the skin and directed to the target vessel. When the tip of the needle enters the lumen of a patent blood vessel, blood moves up the needle by capillary action and enters the flashback chamber. When this occurs, the catheter is threaded over the needle and into the lumen of the blood vessel as the needle is withdrawn.

The advantage of a catheter-over-needle device is the ability to can-

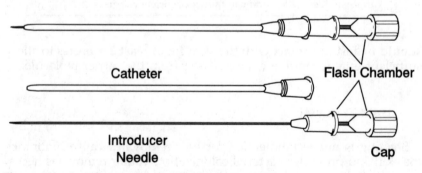

Figure 4.1. A catheter-over-needle device.

nulate vessels in a simple one-step procedure. The disadvantage is the tendency for the catheter tip to become frayed as it passes through the skin and soft tissues, and to subsequently damage the vascular endothelium and promote phlebitis and thrombosis. To minimize this risk, the catheter-over-needle device is usually reserved for cannulation of superficial vessels.

CATHETER-OVER-GUIDEWIRE

Guidewire-assisted vascular cannulation was introduced in the early 1950s and is often called the Seldinger technique, after its inventor. This technique is illustrated in Figure 4.2. A small-bore needle (usually 20 gauge) is used to probe for the target vessel. When the tip of the needle enters the vessel, a thin wire with a flexible tip (called a J-tip because of its shape) is passed through the needle and into the vessel lumen. The needle is then removed, leaving the wire in place to serve as a guide for cannulation of the vessel. When cannulating deep vessels, a rigid dilator catheter is first threaded over the guidewire and removed; this creates a tract that facilitates insertion of the vascular catheter.

The guidewire technique has the presumed advantage of minimizing damage to soft tissues and blood vessels by using a small-bore probe needle. However, the use of a rigid dilator catheter (as explained above) seems to nullify this advantage. Nevertheless, the guidewire technique is currently the preferred method for central venous and arterial cannulation (1,2).

THE CATHETERS

Vascular catheters are composed of plastic polymers impregnated with barium or tungsten salts to enhance radiopacity. Catheters intended for short-term cannulation (days) are usually made of polyurethane; catheters used for long-term venous access (weeks to months) are composed of a more flexible and less thrombogenic derivative of silicone. The silicone catheters (e.g., Hickman and Broviac catheters) are too flexible for routine percutaneous insertion, and are not appropriate for use in the ICU.

HEPARIN BONDING

Some vascular catheters are impregnated or coated with heparin to reduce thrombogenicity. However, this measure has not proven effective in reducing the incidence of catheter-associated thrombosis (13). Because heparin-coated catheters can be a source of heparin-induced thrombocytopenia (see Chapter 45), catheters used in the ICU should not be impregnated or coated with heparin.

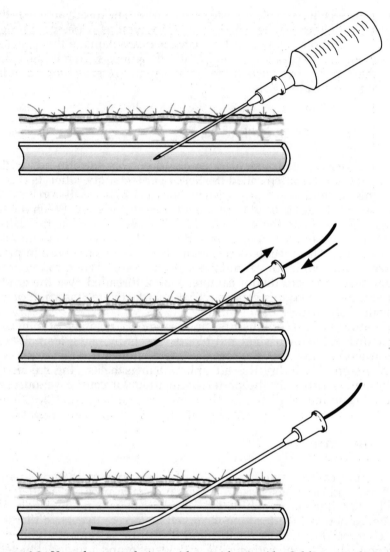

Figure 4.2. Vascular cannulation with a guidewire (the Seldinger technique).

CATHETER SIZE

The size of vascular catheters is commonly expressed in terms of the outside diameter, and the units of measurement are shown in Table 4.3. The French size is a metric derivative equivalent to the outside diameter in millimeters multiplied by 3; that is, French size = outside diameter (in mm) × 3. The gauge system was developed for wires and needles, and has been adopted for catheters. There is no simple mathematical relationship between gauge size and other units of measurement, and a table of reference values such as Table 4.3 is needed

TABLE 4.3. CATHETER SIZES AND COMPARATIVE FLOW RATES

Gauge	French Size	Outside Diameter Inches	Outside Diameter Millimeters	Flow Rate* (mL/min)
14	6.30	0.083	2.10	—
16	4.95	0.065	1.65	96.3
18	3.72	0.049	1.24	60.0
20	2.67	0.035	0.89	39.5
22	2.13	0.018	0.71	24.7
24	1.68	0.022	0.56	—

* Flow rates are for gravity flow of one unit of packed cells diluted with 250 mL normal saline passing through catheters of equal length. Data from de la Roche MRP, Gauthier L. Rapid transfusion of packed red blood cells: effects of dilution, pressure, and catheter size. Ann Emerg Med 1993;22:1551–1555.

to make the appropriate conversions (14). Gauge sizes usually range from 14 (largest diameter) to 27 (smallest diameter).

As described in Chapter 1, the steady or laminar flow through a rigid tube is influenced most by the radius of the tube (see the Hagen–Poisseuille equation in the section on peripheral blood flow in Chapter 1). The influence of tube diameter on flow rate is demonstrated in Table 4.3 for gravity flow of one unit of packed red blood cells diluted with 250 mL normal saline flowing through catheters of equal length (15). Note that a little more than a doubling of tube diameter (from 0.7 mm to 1.65 mm) is associated with almost a quadrupling of flow rate (from 24.7 to 96.3 mL/minute). Thus, catheter size (diameter) is an important consideration if rapid flow rates are desired.

MULTILUMEN CATHETERS

Multilumen catheters were introduced for clinical use in the early 1980s, and are now used routinely for central venous cannulation. The design of a triple-lumen catheter is shown in Figure 4.3. These catheters have an outside diameter of 2.3 mm (6.9 French) and may have three channels of equal diameter (usually 18 gauge) or may have one larger channel (16 gauge) and two smaller channels of equal diameter (18 gauge). The distal opening of each channel is separated from the other by at least 1 cm to help minimize mixing of infusate solutions.

Multilumen catheters have proven to be valuable aids because they minimize the number of venipunctures needed for monitoring and infusion therapy, yet they do not increase the risk of thrombosis or infection when compared with single-lumen catheters (13).

INTRODUCER CATHETERS

Another valuable addition to the family of vascular catheters is the introducer catheter, shown in Figure 4.3. These large-bore catheters (8

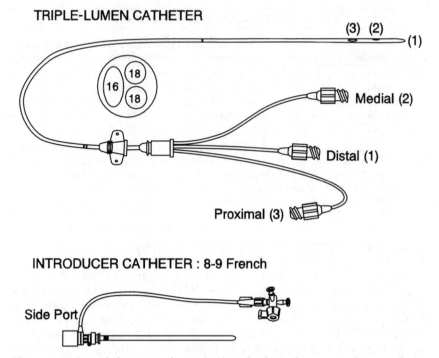

Figure 4.3. A multilumen catheter (*top*) and a large-bore introducer catheter (*bottom*).

to 9 French) can be used as conduits for insertion and removal of smaller vascular catheters (including multilumen catheters and pulmonary artery catheters) through a single venipuncture. The side-arm infusion port on the catheter provides an additional infusion line, and allows a continuous flush to prevent thrombus formation around smaller catheters that sit in the lumen of the introducer catheter. This side-arm infusion port also allows the introducer catheter to be used as a stand-alone infusion device (a rubber membrane on the hub of the catheter provides an effective seal when fluids are infusing through the side-arm port of the catheter). The large diameter of introducer catheters makes them particularly valuable as infusion devices when rapid infusion rates are necessary (e.g., in the resuscitation of massive hemorrhage).

ACCESS ROUTES

The following is a brief description of common vascular access routes in the arm (antecubital veins and radial artery), the thoracic inlet (subclavian and jugular veins), and the groin (femoral artery and vein).

ANTECUBITAL VEINS

The veins in the antecubital fossa provide rapid and safe vascular access for acute resuscitative therapy. Although long catheters can be inserted into the antecubital veins and advanced into the superior vena cava, such peripherally inserted central venous catheters (PICC devices) are more appropriate for home infusion therapy than for treating critically ill patients (16). Short catheters (5 to 7 cm) are preferred for acute resuscitation via the antecubital veins because they are more easily inserted and allow more rapid infusion rates than the longer PICC catheters.

Anatomy

The surface anatomy of the antecubital veins is shown in Figure 4.4. The basilic vein runs along the medial aspect of the antecubital fossa, and the cephalic vein is situated on the opposite side. The basilic vein is preferred for cannulation because it runs a straighter and less variable course up the arm than the cephalic vein.

Insertion Technique

The patient need not be supine, but the arm should be straight and abducted. The antecubital veins can be distended by tourniquet or by inflating a blood pressure cuff to just above the diastolic pressure (this allows arterial inflow while impeding venous outflow). Once the veins are visible or palpable, a catheter-over-needle device is used to insert a short 16- or 18-gauge catheter into the basilic or cephalic vein.

Blind Insertion

If the antecubital veins are neither visible nor palpable, palpate the brachial artery pulse at a point 1 inch above the antecubital crease. The basilic vein (or brachial vein) should lie just medial to the palpated pulse at this point, and can be entered by inserting the catheter-over-needle device through the skin at a 35° to 45° angle and advancing the needle until blood return is noted. This approach has a reported success rate of 80% (17). Injury to the median nerve (which is also medial to the artery, but deep to the veins) can occur with excessive movement of the probe needle.

Comment

Cannulation of the antecubital veins is recommended (18,19).

For rapid venous access (e.g., cardiopulmonary resuscitation)
For thrombolytic therapy in acute myocardial infarction
For trauma victims who require thoracotomy

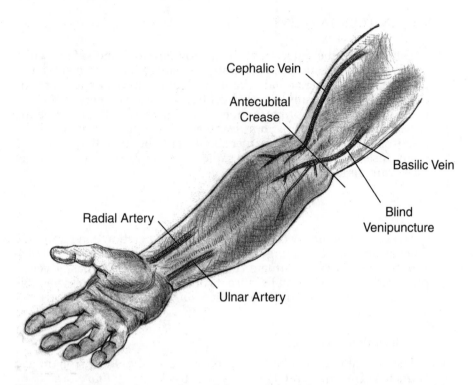

Figure 4.4. The vascular topology of the antecubital fossa and wrist.

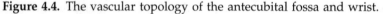

Remember that the shorter the catheter, the more rapid the flow rate through the catheter (see Chapter 1). Thus, insertion of short catheters into the antecubital veins permits more rapid volume resuscitation than insertion of the longer central venous catheters.

RADIAL ARTERY

The radial artery is a favored site for arterial cannulation because the vessel is superficial and accessible and the insertion site is easy to keep clean. The major disadvantage of the radial artery is its small size, which limits the success rate of cannulation and promotes vascular occlusion.

Anatomy

The surface anatomy of the radial and ulnar arteries is shown in Figure 4.4. The radial artery is usually palpable at a point just medial to the styloid process of the radius. The ulnar artery is on the opposite (medial) side of the wrist, just lateral to the pisiform bone. Although the radial artery is preferred, the ulnar artery is the larger of the two arteries and should be easier to cannulate (20).

The Allen Test

The Allen test evaluates the capacity of the ulnar artery to supply blood to the digits when the radial artery is occluded. The test is performed by first occluding the radial and ulnar arteries with the thumb and index finger. The patient is then instructed to raise the wrist above the head and to make a fist repeatedly until the fingers turn white. The ulnar artery is then released, and the time required for return of the normal color to the fingers is recorded. A normal response time is 7 seconds or less, and a delay of 14 seconds or greater is evidence of insufficient flow in the ulnar artery.

Although a positive Allen test (i.e., 14 seconds or longer for return of color to the digits) is often stated as a contraindication to radial artery cannulation, in numerous instances the Allen test has indicated inadequate flow in the ulnar artery, yet subsequent radial artery cannulation has been uneventful (2,21). Thus, a positive Allen test is not a contraindication to radial artery cannulation. Another limitation is the need for patient cooperation to perform the test. Therefore, this test is not worth the time it takes.

Insertion Technique

The wrist should be hyperextended to bring the artery closer to the surface. A short 20-gauge catheter is appropriate, and can be inserted by a catheter-over-needle device or by the guidewire technique. When using a catheter-over-needle device, the following through-and-through technique is recommended: When the needle tip first punctures the artery (and blood appears in the flashback chamber), the tip of the catheter is just outside the vessel. To position the catheter tip in the lumen of the vessel, the needle is passed completely through the artery and then withdrawn until blood returns again through the needle. At this point, the catheter tip should be in the lumen of the artery, and the catheter can be advanced while the needle is retracted. If two attempts at cannulation are unsuccessful, switch to an alternative site (to reduce trauma to the vessel).

Comment

Arterial occlusion occurs in as many as 25% of radial artery cannulations, but digital ischemia is rare (2,22). Despite being well tolerated in most patients, cannulation of the radial artery (or any artery) should be reserved for monitoring blood pressure, and is not to be used as a convenience measure for monitoring blood gases or other blood components (23).

THE SUBCLAVIAN VEIN

More than 3 million central venous cannulations are performed yearly in the United States (24), and a majority of these procedures are performed via the subclavian vein (25). The subclavian vein is well suited for cannulation because it is a large vessel (about 20 mm in diameter) and is prevented from collapsing by its surrounding structures. The immediate risks of subclavian vein cannulation include pneumothorax (1% to 2%) and hemothorax (less than 1%) (25). The incidence of bleeding is no different in the presence or absence of a coagulopathy (26); that is, **the presence of a coagulation disorder is not a contraindication to subclavian vein cannulation.**

Anatomy

The subclavian vein is a continuation of the axillary vein as it passes over the first rib, and the apical pleura lies about 5 mm deep to the vein at its point of origin. As shown in Figure 4.5, the subclavian vein runs most of its course along the underside of the clavicle. The vein runs along the outer surface of the anterior scalene muscle, which separates the vein from its companion artery on the underbelly of the muscle. At the thoracic inlet, the subclavian vein meets the internal jugular vein to form the brachiocephalic vein. The convergence of the right and left brachiocephalic veins forms the superior vena cava.

Anatomic Distances

The lengths of the vascular segments involved in subclavian (and internal jugular) vein cannulation are shown in Table 4.4. The average distance from venipuncture site to the right atrium is 14.5 cm and

TABLE 4.4. ANATOMIC DISTANCES IN CENTRAL VENOUS CANNULATION		
	Average Length (cm)	
Vascular Segment	**Right**	**Left**
Cannulated portion of subclavian or internal jugular veins	5	5
Brachiocephalic vein	2.5	6.5
Superior vena cava	7	7
Total distance to right atrium	14.5	18.5

From Warwick R, Williams PL, eds. Gray's anatomy. 35th ed. London: Longman, 1973:700–702; and Romanes GL. Cunningham's textbook of anatomy. 12th ed. New York: Oxford University Press, 1981:942–948.

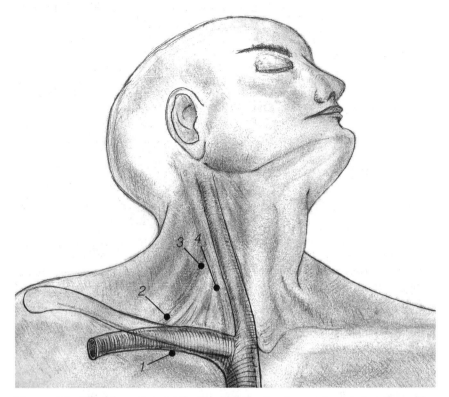

Figure 4.5. A surface view of the large central veins as they converge at the thoracic inlet. The circular markers indicate skin insertion sites for cannulation of the subclavian vein (1 and 2) and internal jugular vein (3 and 4).

18.5 cm for right-sided and left-sided cannulations, respectively. These distances are far shorter than catheter lengths recommended for right-sided (20 cm) and left-sided (30 cm) central venous cannulations, and are more consistent with a recent report showing that the average distance to the right atrium is 16.5 cm in central venous cannulation from either side in adults (27). Therefore, to avoid placing catheter tips in the right atrium (which can lead to cardiac perforation and fatal cardiac tamponade), **all central venous catheters should be no longer than 15 or 16 cm in length** (27).

INSERTION TECHNIQUE

The patient is placed supine, with arms at the sides and head faced away from the insertion site. A towel roll can be placed between the shoulder blades, but this is uncomfortable and unnecessary. Identify the clavicular insertion of the sternocleidomastoid muscle. The subclavian vein lies just underneath the clavicle where the muscle inserts onto the clavicle. The vein can be entered from either side of the clavicle.

Infraclavicular Approach (Insertion Site 1 in Figure 4.5). Identify the lateral margin of the sternocleidomastoid muscle as it inserts on the clavicle. The catheter is inserted in line with this margin, but below the clavicle. Insert the probing needle (18 or 20 gauge) with the bevel pointing upward (toward the ceiling) and advance the needle along the underside of the clavicle and toward the suprasternal notch. The path of the needle should be parallel to the patient's back. When the vein is entered, turn the bevel of the needle to 3 o'clock so the guidewire threads in the direction of the superior vena cava.

Supraclavicular Approach (Insertion Site 2 in Figure 4.5). Identify the angle formed by the lateral margin of the sternocleidomastoid muscle and the clavicle. The probe needle is inserted so that it bisects this angle. Keep the bevel of the needle facing upward and direct the needle under the clavicle in the direction of the opposite nipple. The vein should be entered at a distance of 1 to 2 cm from the skin surface (the subclavian vein is more superficial in the supraclavicular approach). When the vein is entered, turn the bevel of the needle to 9 o'clock so the guidewire threads in the direction of the superior vena cava.

Comment

Patient comfort and ease of insertion are the most compelling reasons to select the subclavian vein for central venous access. Selection of the infraclavicular versus supraclavicular approach is largely a matter of personal preference. Some recommend avoiding the subclavian vein in ventilator-dependent patients because of the risk of pneumothorax. However, the risk of pneumothorax is too small to justify abandoning the subclavian vein in patients with respiratory failure.

THE INTERNAL JUGULAR VEIN

Cannulation of the internal jugular vein reduces (but does not eliminate) the risk of pneumothorax, but introduces new risks (e.g., carotid artery puncture and thoracic duct injury).

Anatomy

The internal jugular vein is located under the sternocleidomastoid muscle in the neck and, as shown in Figure 4.5, the vein follows an oblique course as it runs down the neck. When the head is turned to the opposite side, the vein forms a straight line from the pinna of the ear to the sternoclavicular joint. Near the base of the neck, the internal jugular vein becomes the most lateral structure in the carotid sheath (which contains the carotid artery sandwiched between the vein laterally and the vagus nerve medially).

Insertion Technique

The right side is preferred because the vessels run a straighter course to the right atrium. The patient is placed in a supine or Trendelenburg position, with the head turned to the opposite side. The internal jugular vein can be entered from an anterior or posterior approach.

The Anterior Approach (Insertion Site 4 in Figure 4.5). The anterior approach is through a triangular region created by two heads of the sternocleidomastoid muscle. The carotid artery is palpated in the triangle and retracted medially. The probe needle is inserted at the apex of the triangle with the bevel facing up, and the needle is advanced toward the ipsilateral nipple, at a 45° angle with the skin surface. If the vein is not encountered by a depth of 5 cm, the needle is withdrawn 4 cm and advanced again in a more lateral direction. When a vessel is entered, look for pulsations. If the blood is red and pulsating, you have entered the carotid artery. In this situation, remove the needle and tamponade the area for 5 to 10 minutes. When the carotid artery has been punctured, no further attempts should be made on either side because puncture of both arteries can have serious consequences.

The Posterior Approach (Insertion Site 3 in Figure 4.5). The insertion site for this approach is 1 centimeter superior to the point where the external jugular vein crosses over the lateral edge of the sternocleidomastoid muscle. The probe needle is inserted with the bevel positioned at 3 o'clock. The needle is advanced along the underbelly of the muscle in a direction pointing to the suprasternal notch. The internal jugular vein should be encountered 5 to 6 cm from the skin surface with this approach (28).

Carotid Artery Puncture. If the carotid artery has been punctured with a probing needle, the needle should be removed and pressure should be applied to the site for at least 5 minutes (10 minutes is recommended for patients with a coagulopathy). No further attempts should be made to cannulate the internal jugular vein on either side, to avoid puncture of both carotid arteries. **If the carotid artery has been inadvertently cannulated, the catheter should not be removed,** as this could provoke serious hemorrhage. In this situation, a vascular surgeon should be consulted immediately.

Comment

As with the subclavian vein, cannulation of the internal jugular vein is safe and effective when performed by skilled operators. However, several disadvantages of internal jugular cannulation deserve mention. (*a*) Accidental puncture of the carotid artery is reported in 2 to 10% of attempted cannulations (28). (*b*) Awake patients often complain of the limited neck mobility when the internal jugular vein is cannulated. (*c*) In agitated patients, inappropriate neck flexion can result in thrombotic occlusion of the catheter and vein. (*d*) In patients with tracheostomies, the insertion site can be exposed to infected secretions that drain from the tracheal stoma.

THE EXTERNAL JUGULAR VEIN

Cannulation of the external jugular vein has two advantages: (*a*) There is no risk of pneumothorax, and (*b*) hemorrhage is easily controlled. The major drawback is difficulty advancing the catheter.

Anatomy

The external jugular vein runs along a line extending from the angle of the jaw to a point midway along the clavicle. The vein runs obliquely across the surface of the sternocleidomastoid muscle and joins the subclavian vein at an acute angle. This acute angle is the major impediment to advancing catheters that have been inserted into the external jugular vein.

Insertion Technique

The patient is placed in the supine or Trendelenburg position, with the head turned away from the insertion site. If necessary, the vein can be occluded just above the clavicle (with the forefinger of the non-dominant hand) to engorge the entry site. As many as 15% of patients so not have an identifiable external jugular vein, even under optimal conditions of vein engorgement (28).

The external jugular vein has little support from surrounding structures, so the vein should be anchored between the thumb and forefinger when the needle is inserted. The bevel of the needle should be pointing upward when it enters the vein. The recommended insertion point is midway between the angle of the jaw and the clavicle (see Fig. 4.5). Use a 16-gauge single-lumen catheter that is 10 to 15 cm in length. If the catheter does not advance easily, do not force it, as this may result in vascular perforation at the junction between the external jugular and subclavian veins.

Comment

This approach is best reserved for temporary access in patients with a severe coagulopathy, particularly when the operator is inexperienced and does not feel comfortable cannulating the subclavian or internal jugular veins. Contrary to popular belief, cannulation of the external jugular is not always easier to accomplish than central venous cannulation because of the difficulty in advancing catheters past the acute angle at the junction of the subclavian vein.

THE FEMORAL VEIN

The femoral vein is the easiest of the large veins to cannulate and also does not carry a risk of pneumothorax. The disadvantages associated with this route are venous thrombosis (10%), femoral artery puncture (5%), and limited ability to flex the hip (which can be bothersome for awake patients). Contrary to popular belief, the infection rate with femoral vein catheters is no different from that of subclavian or internal jugular vein catheters (28).

Anatomy

The anatomy of the femoral sheath is shown in Figure 4.6. The femoral vein is the most medial structure in the femoral sheath and is situated just medial to the femoral artery. At the inguinal ligament, the femoral vessels are just a few centimeters below the skin surface.

Insertion Technique

Palpate the femoral artery just below the inguinal crease and insert the needle (bevel up) 1 to 2 cm medial to the palpated pulse. Advance

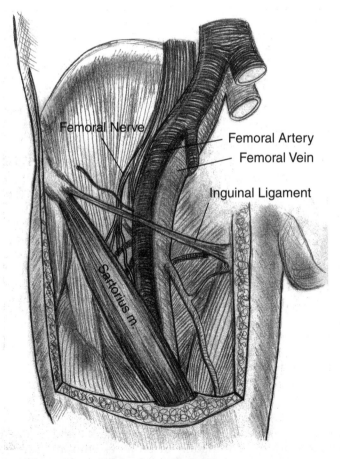

Figure 4.6. The anatomy of the femoral sheath.

the needle at a 45° angle to the skin surface, entering the vein at a depth of 2 to 4 cm. Once in the vessel, if the catheter or guidewire will not pass beyond the tip of the needle, tilt the needle so that it is more parallel to the skin surface (this may move the needle tip away from the far side of the vessel wall and into more direct contact with the lumen of the vessel). Femoral vein catheters should be at least 15 cm long.

Blind Insertion

If the femoral artery pulse is not palpable, draw an imaginary line from the anterior superior iliac crest to the pubic tubercle, and divide the line into three equal segments. The femoral artery lies at the junction between the middle and most medial segment, and the femoral vein is 1 to 2 cm medial to this point. This method of locating the femoral vein has a reported success rate of over 90% (29).

Comment

Femoral vein cannulation is usually reserved for patients who are paralyzed or comatose and immobile. This approach is **not recommended for cardiopulmonary resuscitation** (because of the delayed transit times for bolus drug injections) (18) **or in patients with bleeding disorders** (28).

THE FEMORAL ARTERY

Cannulation of the femoral artery is usually reserved for situations where radial artery cannulation is unsuccessful or contraindicated. Despite its reserve status, the femoral artery is larger than the radial artery, and is easier to cannulate. The complications of femoral artery cannulation are the same as for radial artery cannulation (thrombosis, bleeding, and infection). The incidence of infection is the same with radial and femoral artery catheters, and the incidence of thrombosis is lower with femoral artery cannulation (2). Thrombosis of the femoral artery, like that in the radial artery, only rarely results in troublesome ischemia in the distal extremity (2).

Localization and cannulation of the femoral artery proceeds as described in the section on femoral vein cannulation. The Seldinger technique is preferred for catheter insertion, and catheters should be 18 gauge in diameter and 15 to 20 cm long.

Comment

Femoral artery cannulation is a viable alternative and may be preferable to radial artery cannulation in patients who are paralyzed or otherwise immobile, unless they have a significant coagulopathy (in which case the radial artery is preferred). The incidence of thrombotic complications is lower in femoral artery cannulations, and the pressure in the femoral artery more closely approximates the pressure in the aorta than does the pressure in the radial artery (see Chapter 8).

IMMEDIATE CONCERNS

VENOUS AIR EMBOLISM

Inadvertent air entry is one of the most feared complications of central venous cannulation. The importance of maintaining a closed system during insertion is highlighted by the following statement:

> A pressure gradient of 4 mm Hg along a 14-gauge catheter can entrain air at a rate of 90 mL/second and can produce a fatal air embolus in 1 second (30).

Preventive Measures

Prevention is the hallmark of reducing the morbidity and mortality of venous air embolism. The most effective method of preventing air entry is to keep the venous pressure more positive than atmospheric pressure. This is facilitated by placing the patient in the Trendelenburg position with the head 15° below the horizontal plane. Remember that the **Trendelenburg position does not prevent venous air entry** because patients still generate negative intrathoracic pressures while in the Trendelenburg position. When changing connections in a central venous line, a temporary positive pressure can be created by having the patient hum audibly. This not only produces a positive intrathoracic pressure, but allows clinicians to hear when the intrathoracic pressure is positive. In ventilator-dependent patients, the nurse or respiratory therapist should initiate a mechanical lung inflation when changing connections.

Clinical Presentation

The usual presentation is acute onset of dyspnea that occurs during the procedure. Hypotension and cardiac arrest can develop rapidly. Air can pass across a patent foramen ovale and obstruct the cerebral circulation, producing an acute ischemic stroke. A characteristic "mill wheel" murmur can be heard over the right heart, but this murmur may be fleeting.

Therapeutic Maneuvers

If a venous air embolism is suspected, immediately place the patient with the left side down, and attempt to aspirate air directly from the venous line. In dire circumstances, a needle should be inserted through the chest wall and into the right ventricle to aspirate the air. Unfortunately, the mortality in severe cases of venous air embolism remains high despite these maneuvers.

PNEUMOTHORAX

Pneumothorax is a concern primarily with subclavian vein cannulation but can also complicate jugular vein cannulation (2,30). This is one reason that postinsertion chest films are recommended after all central venous cannulations (or attempts). If possible, postinsertion films should be obtained in the upright position and during expiration. **Expiratory films** facilitate the detection of small pneumothoraxes because expiration decreases the volume of air in the lungs, but not the volume of air in the pleural space. Thus, during expiration, the volume of air in the pleural space is a larger fraction of the total volume of the hemithorax, thereby magnifying the radiographic appearance of the pneumothorax (31).

Upright films are not always possible in ICU patients. When supine films are necessary, remember that **pleural air does not often collect at the apex of the lung when the patient is in the supine position** (32,33). In this situation, pleural air tends to collect in the subpulmonic recess and along the anteromedial border of the mediastinum (see Chapter 28).

Delayed Pneumothorax

Pneumothoraxes may not be radiographically evident until 24 to 48 hours after central venous cannulation (31,33). Therefore, the absence of a pneumothorax on an immediate postinsertion chest film does not absolutely exclude the possibility of a catheter-induced pneumothorax. This is an important consideration in patients who develop dyspnea or other signs of pneumothorax in the first few days after central venous cannulation. In the absence of signs and symptoms, there is little justification for serial chest films following central venous catheter placement.

CATHETER TIP POSITION

The properly placed central venous catheter should run parallel to the superior vena cava, and the tip of the catheter should be positioned above the junction of the superior vena cava and right atrium. The following conditions warrant corrective measures.

Tip Against the Wall of the Vena Cava

Catheters inserted from the left side must make an acute turn downward when they reach the superior vena cava. If they fail to make this turn, the catheters can end up in a position like the one shown in

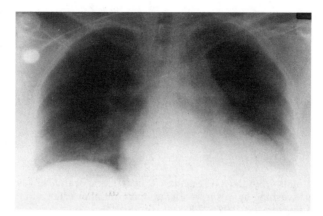

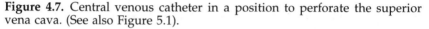

Figure 4.7. Central venous catheter in a position to perforate the superior vena cava. (See also Figure 5.1).

Figure 4.7. The tip of the catheter is up against the lateral wall of the vena cava, and in this position, the catheter tip can stab the vessel wall and perforate the vena cava. Therefore, catheters that abut the wall of the vena cava should be repositioned as soon as possible. (The problem of vascular perforation is discussed in more detail in Chapter 5.)

Tip in the Right Atrium

The Food and Drug Administration has issued a strong warning about the risk of cardiac perforation from catheter tips that are advanced into the heart (24). However, cardiac perforation is a rare complication of central venous cannulation (27), even though over half of central venous catheters may be misplaced in the right atrium (27). Nevertheless, tamponade is often fatal, so cardiac placement of catheters should be avoided. A few measures help to minimize the risk of cardiac perforation. The most effective measure is to use shorter catheters, as recommended earlier. The tip of indwelling catheters should be above the third right costal cartilage (this is the level where the vena cava meets the right atrium). If the anterior portion of the third rib cannot be visualized, keep the catheter tip at or above the tracheal carina.

REFERENCES

GENERAL TEXTS

Benumof JL, ed. Clinical procedures in anesthesia and intensive care. Philadelphia: JB Lippincott, 1992.
Rosen M, Latto P, Ng S. Handbook of percutaneous central venous catheterization. 2nd ed. Philadelphia: WB Saunders, 1992.

REVIEWS

1. Agee KR, Balk RA. Central venous catheterization in the critically ill patient. Crit Care Clin North Am 1992;8:677–686.
2. Clark VL, Kruse JA. Arterial catheterization. Crit Care Clin North Am 1992; 8:687–698.
3. Baranowski L. Central venous access devices. J Intraven Nurs 1993;16:167–194 (122 references).

PREPARATION

4. Doebbeling BN, Stanley GL, Sheetz CT, et al. Comparative efficacy of alternative hand-washing agents in reducing nosocomial infections in intensive care units. N Engl J Med 1992;327:88–93.
5. Centers for Disease Control. Guidelines for the prevention of transmission of human immunodeficiency virus and hepatitis B virus to health-care and public-safety workers. Morbid Mort Weekly Rev 1989;38:1–37.
6. Centers for Disease Control Working Group. Guidelines for prevention of intravascular infections. In: Guidelines for the prevention of nosocomial infections. Washington, DC: Department of Health & Human Services, Public Health Service, 1981.
7. Geberding JL. Risks to health care workers from exposure to hepatitis B virus, human immunodeficiency virus, and cytomegalovirus. Infect Dis Clin North Am 1989;3:735–745.
8. Malcolm JA, Dobson PM, Sutherland DC. Combination chemoprophylaxis after needlestick injury. Lancet 1993;341:112–113.
9. Needlesticks: preaching to the seroconverted. Lancet 1992;340:640–641 (editorial).
10. Buback ME, Reed CE, Fransway AF, et al. Allergic reactions to latex among health-care workers. Mayo Clin Proc 1992;67:1075–1079.
11. Larson EL. Guidelines for use of topical antimicrobial agents. APIC Guidelines for Infection Control Practice. Am J Infect Control 1988;16:253–266.
12. Wyatt WJ, Beckett TA, Bonet V, Davis SM. Comparative efficacy of surgical scrub solutions on control of skin microflora. Infect Surg 1990;9:17–21.

CATHETERS

13. Rosen M, Latto P, Ng S. Handbook of percutaneous central venous catheterization. 2nd ed. Philadelphia: WB Saunders, 1992;11–30.
14. Lawson M, Vertenstein MJ. Methods for determining the internal volume of central venous catheters. J Intraven Nurs 1993;16:148–155.
15. de la Roche MRP, Gauthier L. Rapid transfusion of packed red blood cells: effects of dilution, pressure, and catheter size. Ann Emerg Med 1993;22: 1551–1555.

ANTECUBITAL VEINS

16. Hadaway LC. An overview of vascular access devices inserted via the antecubital area. J Intraven Nurs 1989;13:297–306.
17. Vyskocil JJ, Kruse JA, Wilson RF. Alternative techniques for gaining venous access. J Crit Illness 1993;8:435–442.

18. American Heart Association. Textbook of advanced cardiac life support. Dallas: American Heart Association, 1994.
19. Rosa DH, Griffin CC, Flanagan JJ, Machiedo GW. A comparison of intravenous access sites for bolus injections during shock and resuscitation after emergency room thoracotomy with and without aortic cross-clamping. Am Surgeon 1990; 56:567–570.

ARTERIAL CANNULATION

20. Mathers LH. Anatomical considerations in obtaining arterial access. J Intensive Care Med 1990;5:110–119.
21. Thompson SR, Hirshberg A. Allen's test revisited. Crit Care Med 1988;16:915.
22. Slogoff, S, Keats AS, Arlund C. On the safety of radial artery cannulation. Anesthesiology 1983;59:42–47.
23. Tenholder MF. The pendulum and the arterial line. Chest 1993;104:1650–1651.

CENTRAL VENOUS CANNULATION

24. Food and Drug Administration. Precautions necessary with central venous catheters. FDA Drug Bull 1989;July:15–16.
25. Wegener ME. Complications of central venous line placement. Contemp Surg 1993;42:266–268.
26. Foster PF, Moore LR, Sankary HN, et al. Central venous catheterization in patients with coagulopathy. Arch Surg 1992;127:273–275.
27. McGee WT, Ackerman BL, Rouben LR, et al. Accurate placement of central venous catheters: a prospective, randomized, multicenter trial. Crit Care Med 1993;21:1118–1123.
28. Seneff MG. Central venous catheterization. A comprehensive review. Intensive Care Med 1987;2:163–175, 218–232.
29. Getzen LC, Pollack EW. Short-term femoral vein catheterization. Am J Surg 1979;138:875–877.

IMMEDIATE CONCERNS

30. Sladen A. Complications of invasive hemodynamic monitoring in the intensive care unit. Curr Probl Surg 1988;25:69–145.
31. Marino PL. Delayed pneumothorax: a complication of subclavian vein catheterization. J Parenter Enteral Nutr 1985;9:232.
32. Tocino IM, Miller MH, Fairfax WR. Distribution of pneumothorax in the supine and semirecumbent critically ill adult. Am J Radiol 1985;144:901–905.
33. Collin GR, Clarke LE. Delayed pneumothorax: a complication of central venous catheterization. Surg Rounds 1994;17:589–594.

5

THE INDWELLING VASCULAR CATHETER

This chapter is a continuation of Chapter 4, and describes the routine care and adverse complications of indwelling vascular catheters. The first section is devoted to the daily care of catheters and insertion sites, (1,2) and the final sections focus on catheter-related complications, with emphasis on catheter-related infections (3,4).

ROUTINE CATHETER CARE

The following practices are designed to prevent or limit the complications created by indwelling vascular catheters (1,2). Many of these preventive practices have little or no proven value.

PROTECTIVE DRESSINGS

Catheter insertion sites on the skin are covered at all times as a standard antiseptic measure (1,2). The different protective dressings and their comparative features are shown in Table 5.1. The standard dressing is a sterile gauze covering that is anchored to the skin by hypoallergenic tape and is replaced every 48 hours (1,2). Occlusive dressings made of transparent polyurethane or colloid gels have also become popular in recent years because they allow inspection of the catheter insertion site (for signs of infection) without breaking the protective seal on the skin. However, **occlusive dressings** have one disadvantage that deserves emphasis: They **promote microbial colonization on the underlying skin** (5–7). These dressings block the escape of water vapor from the underlying skin and create a moist environment that enhances the growth of skin microflora. Some occlusive dressings are more permeable to water vapor than others (see Table 5.1); however,

	Proprietary		Skin	Risk of
TABLE 5.1. COMPARATIVE FEATURES OF PROTECTIVE DRESSINGS				
Type of Dressing	**Names**	**Cost**	**Colonization**	**Septicemia**
Sterile gauze and tape		+	+	+
Occlusive dressings permeable to water vapor		+ + +	+ +	+
Occlusive dressings impermeable to water vapor	Op Site Tegaderm DuoDERM	+ + +	+ + +	+ +

Relative magnitudes are indicated by the number of plus signs (5–7).

all trap moisture on the skin to some extent, and all occlusive dressings promote skin colonization. However, only the dressings that are completely impervious to water vapor show a higher incidence of catheter-related septicemia (5,6).

Thus, occlusive skin dressings produce an effect that is opposite that desired from protective dressings. Based on this adverse effect and the added cost of occlusive dressings (which is about three times the cost of gauze dressings), **the routine use of occlusive dressings is not recommended.**

ANTIMICROBIAL OINTMENT

Another common antiseptic practice is the application of a polymicrobial ointment (such as polymyxin–neomycin–bacitracin) to the catheter insertion site on the skin. However, this practice has not been shown to reduce the incidence of catheter-related infections (4), and therefore is **not recommended.**

REPLACING CATHETERS

The incidence of catheter-associated infections is higher in catheters that remain in place for longer than 3 days (8). This observation led to the common practice of replacing vascular catheters (usually over a guidewire) every few days to reduce the risk of catheter-associated infections. However, replacement of vascular catheters at regular intervals, using either guidewire exchange or a new venipuncture site, does not reduce the incidence of catheter-related infections (9) and may actually increase the risk of catheter-associated complications (both mechanical and infectious) (10). Therefore, **routine replacement of indwelling vascular catheters is not recommended.**

INDICATIONS FOR REPLACING VASCULAR CATHETERS

When there is purulence or spreading erythema at the catheter insertion site, use a new venipuncture site.

When catheter-related infection is suspected, use guidewire exchange.

When the tip or intradermal portion of a previously removed catheter shows significant infection (more than 15 colony-forming units on semiquantitative culture), use a new venipuncture site.

When a catheter has been placed emergently (e.g. cardiopulmonary arrest), without strict aseptic technique, use guidewire exchange.

FLUSHING CATHETERS

All vascular catheters are flushed routinely to maintain patency, and the standard flush solution is heparinized saline (heparin concentration ranging from 10 to 1000 units/mL) (1,2,11). Indwelling catheters that are used only intermittently are capped and filled with heparinized saline when idle. (The cap that seals the proximal end of a catheter creates a partial vacuum that holds the flush solution in place; hence, the term *heparin lock* is used to describe this device.) Arterial catheters are flushed continuously (usual rate is 3 mL/hour using a pressurized bag to drive the flush solution through the catheter (12).

Alternatives to Heparin

There are two disadvantages to the use of heparinized saline as the standard flush solution. The first is the added cost of the heparin, which can exceed $65,000 per year for each hospital (11). The second disadvantage is the risk of heparin-induced thrombocytopenia (see Chapter 45).

The disadvantages of heparinized flushes can be eliminated by adopting alternative flush techniques such as the ones shown in Table 5.2. Saline (without heparin) has proved to be as effective as heparin-

TABLE 5.2. ALTERNATIVES TO HEPARINIZED FLUSHES		
Vascular Device	**Alternate Flush Technique**	**Indications**
Central and peripheral venous catheters	Flush with 0.9% sodium chloride, using the same volume (1–5 mL) and time interval (every 8–12 hours) used with heparin (11).	Standard protocol for all venous catheters
Peripheral venous catheters	Flush with 0.9% sodium chloride (1–5 mL) only after drug administration (13).	Standard protocol for peripheral catheters
Arterial catheters	Flush with 1.4% sodium citrate, using a continuous-flow technique (14).	Heparin-induced thrombocytopenia

ized saline for flushing venous catheters (11), and routine flushes may not be necessary for peripheral venous catheters (13). Saline is not always an effective alternative to heparinized saline for flushing arterial catheters (12). If there is a contraindication to the use of heparinized flushes (e.g., heparin-induced thrombocytopenia) a 1.4% sodium citrate solution can be used for flushing arterial catheters (14).

MECHANICAL COMPLICATIONS

The mechanical complications of indwelling catheters can be classified as occlusive (e.g., catheter or vascular occlusion) or erosive (e.g., vascular or cardiac perforation). The following are the more common or preventable mechanical complications.

CATHETER OCCLUSION

Sources of catheter occlusion include sharp angles or kinks and localized indentations along the catheter (these are usually created during catheter insertion), along with thrombi (from backwash of blood into the catheter) and insoluble precipitates in the infusion solutions (usually medications or inorganic salts). Signs of occlusion include limited flow (partial occlusion), total cessation of flow (complete occlusion), and unidirectional cessation of flow (withdrawal occlusion).

Insoluble Precipitates

The substances most likely to form insoluble precipitates in intravenous infusion solutions are as follows (15):

Medications: barbiturates, diazepam, digoxin, phenytoin, and trimethoprim-sulfa
Anion–cation complexes: calcium phosphate and heparin–aminoglycoside complexes

Precipitation is most often caused by inherent hydrophobic behavior in the native substance (e.g., diazepam or digoxin) and acid or alkaline pH in the infusion solutions (e.g., calcium and phosphate form insoluble complexes more readily as the pH becomes more alkaline).

Restoring Patency

Every effort should be made to relieve catheter occlusion and prevent catheter replacement. Guidewires should never be passed through catheters to relieve obstruction because of the risk of dislodging the obstructing mass and creating an embolus. When catheters are partially occluded (and there is some flow through the catheter), irrigation with a thrombolytic agent or dilute (0.1 N) hydrochloric acid can be successful in restoring catheter patency (16,17). Irrigation with acid is aimed primarily at improving the solubility of calcium phos-

TABLE 5.3. A PROTOCOL FOR RESTORING PATENCY IN PARTIALLY OCCLUDED CATHETERS

Solution A: Urokinase or streptokinase (5000 U/mL)
 Solution B: 0.1 N hydrochloric acid
 Volume: Internal volume of catheter, or 2.0 mL
 Follow the steps below in sequence.
   1. Inject solution A into the catheter and cap the proximal hub.
   2. Allow a dwell time of 10 minutes, then withdraw the solution.
   3. Flush catheter with 10 mL heparinized saline (100 U/mL)
   4. If occlusion persists, repeat steps 1–3 and increase dwell time to 1 hour.
   5. If occlusion persists, repeat steps 1–3 and increase dwell time to 2 hours.
   6. If occlusion persists, repeat steps 1–5 using solution B.
   7. If occlusion persists, replace the catheter.

phate precipitates, and cases of catheter occlusion refractory to thrombolytic agents have shown a beneficial response to dilute acid (17).

A protocol for chemical dissolution of catheter occlusions is shown in Table 5.3. The protocol uses a thrombolytic agent initially, but the dilute hydrochloric acid can be used initially if precipitates are evident in the infusion system or if one of the precipitation-prone medications is being used.

SUBCLAVIAN VEIN THROMBOSIS

Clinically apparent thrombosis of the subclavian vein occurs in 3% of patients with subclavian vein catheters (18). The hallmark of subclavian vein obstruction is unilateral arm swelling on the side of the catheter insertion. The evaluation for suspected subclavian vein thrombosis should begin with a noninvasive approach using Doppler ultrasound examination. This method has a high success rate for the diagnosis of occlusive thrombosis, and it can thus eliminate the need for more invasive contrast venography in many cases.

If a subclavian vein thrombosis is confirmed, the catheter should be removed. Because thrombi from the subclavian vein can extend into the superior vena cava, it seems wise to avoid all central venous cannulation for a few weeks, if possible. Heparin anticoagulation is often recommended in this setting (18). However, there is no evidence that anticoagulation reduces the incidence of pulmonary embolism or otherwise alters the clinical course in catheter-induced subclavian vein thrombosis (13). Symptomatic pulmonary emboli are uncommon (10%) in subclavian vein thrombosis, and thus anticoagulation should not be expected to provide much added benefit in this situation.

VASCULAR EROSIONS

Catheter-induced perforations of the superior vena cava and right atrium are uncommon, and many of the cases that do occur are consid-

ered avoidable (19,20). Attention to proper positioning of central venous catheters was mentioned at the end of Chapter 4, and an example
of a catheter position that has a high risk for perforation of the superior
vena cava was provided in Figure 4.7. Left-sided catheter insertions
are responsible for 70% of superior vena cava perforations (20), so
avoiding left-sided insertions is an important step for reducing the
risk of vena cava perforation.

Clinical Features

Perforation of the superior vena cava can occur at any time after
insertion of central venous catheters and can also occur after replacement of catheters over a guidewire (21). The most common time for
perforation is in the first 7 days after cannulation, but perforations can
be delayed for as long as 2 months after cannulation (19). The clinical
symptoms (substernal chest pain, cough, and dyspnea) are nonspecific, and suspicion of perforation is prompted by radiographic
changes such as the ones in Figure 5.1 (19). Note the mediastinal widening and pleural effusion, which are the radiographic hallmarks of

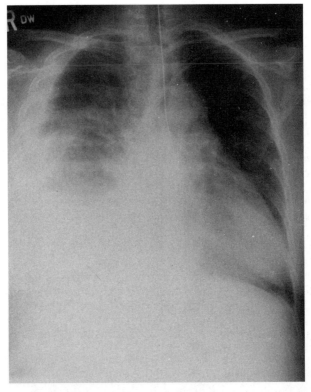

Figure 5.1. The radiographic features of superior vena cava perforation by a
central venous catheter. Note the mediastinal widening and the pleural effusion. Chest film courtesy of Dr. John E. Heffner (from reference 19).

vena cava perforation. In fact, **the sudden and unexpected appearance of a pleural effusion in a patient with a central venous catheter should raise suspicion of vascular perforation.** The pleural effusions can be unilateral (right- or left-sided) or bilateral.

Diagnosis

Thoracentesis is a valuable diagnostic procedure because the chemical composition of the pleural fluid should be similar to that of the intravenous fluid in cases of vascular perforation. (Pleural fluid glucose levels can be useful if the intravenous fluids contain dextrose.) The diagnosis can be confirmed by injecting radiocontrast dye through the distal port of the catheter. The presence of dye in the mediastinum (on a portable chest roentgenogram) confirms the perforation. Once the diagnosis is certain, the perforating catheter should be removed immediately. Contrary to what one might suspect, catheter removal does not promote bleeding in this setting (20).

INFECTIOUS COMPLICATIONS

Hospital-acquired (nosocomial) septicemia occurs 2 to 7 times more often in ICU patients than in other hospitalized patients, and indwelling vascular catheters are the second leading cause of nosocomial septicemia in the ICU (pneumonia is the first) (22). The appearance of a nosocomial septicemia can double the length of stay in the ICU, and can increase the likelihood of a fatal outcome by 25 to 35% (22). As these observations indicate, infections associated with vascular catheters have a significant impact on both morbidity and mortality in the ICU.

DEFINITIONS

The following definitions are applied to catheter-associated infections (3).

Catheter Colonization

This condition occurs when a microorganism is isolated from the intravascular segment of the catheter (the catheter tip), but either the organism is saprophytic or growth is considered too sparse to cause infection. There is no septicemia and no evidence of local or systemic inflammation.

Catheter-Related Infection

In this condition, a pathogen is isolated from the catheter tip, and growth is considered dense enough to cause infection. This condition is not accompanied by septicemia, but it can be a prelude to septicemia.

Signs of local inflammation (e.g., erythema or purulence at the insertion site) and systemic inflammation (e.g., fever or leukocytosis) may be present or absent. (This condition is not entirely satisfying because it is possible to have a catheter-related infection without clinical signs of infection or inflammation.)

Catheter-Related Septicemia

In this condition, the same pathogenic organism is found on the catheter tip and in the systemic circulation, and growth of the organism on the catheter is dense enough to indicate that the catheter is the primary source of the septicemia. Sparse growth of the organism on the catheter would indicate a distant site as the source of septicemia, with secondary seeding of the catheter tip.

PATHOGENESIS

The host response to a foreign body is aimed at degrading or encapsulating the foreign body (23). Because catheters are not biodegradable, the host response to these devices is to encapsulate them in a fibrin sheath. This sheath is a meshwork of fibrin strands that traps microorganisms and provides a protective environment that favors microbial proliferation.

Routes of Infection

The common routes of catheter-related septicemia are shown in Figure 5.2 (3,4). These routes are as follows, using the corresponding numbers in Figure 5.2:

1. Microbes can enter the internal lumen of vascular catheters through break points in the infusion system, such as stopcocks and catheter hubs. Infections via this route can be limited by maintaining a closed infusion system and avoiding unnecessary breaks in the system.

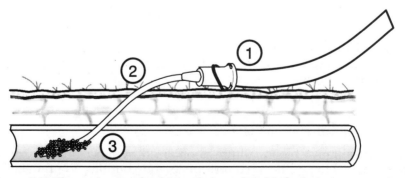

Figure 5.2. The routes involved in catheter-related infections.

2. Microbes on the skin can migrate along the subcutaneous tract created by indwelling catheters. This is considered the predominant route of catheter-related infections, but the evidence for this is not convincing (as discussed in the last section of this chapter).
3. Microorganisms in circulating blood can become trapped in the fibrin meshwork that surrounds the intravascular segment of indwelling catheters. The fibrin sheath thus acts like a filter for circulating blood, like the in-line filters used for blood transfusions. This route is often ignored, but may assume an important role in critically ill patients (see end of chapter).

Microbiology

The organisms involved in catheter-related septicemia are identified by the following list taken from 13 prospective studies of catheter-related septicemia (24): *Staphylococcus epidermidis* (27%), *S. aureus* (26%), *Candida* species (17%), *Klebsiella–Enterobacter* (11%), *Serratia* (5%), *Enterococcus* (5%), *Pseudomonas* species (3%), and others (8%). Thus, about half of the infections involve staphylococci and half involve fungi and various enteric pathogens. This microbial spectrum is important to consider when selecting empiric antimicrobial therapy.

CLINICAL FEATURES

Catheter-related septicemia usually becomes manifest as an unexplained fever in a patient who has had an indwelling vascular catheter for longer than 48 hours. There is often no evidence of local infection or inflammation at the catheter insertion site on the skin. The presence of erythema at the insertion site can heighten the suspicion of a catheter-related septicemia, but the presence of pus is required to confirm the diagnosis.

CULTURE METHODS

The diagnosis of catheter-related septicemia is a laboratory-based diagnosis, and the two culture methods that provide the most valuable diagnostic information are briefly described below (25–27).

Quantitative Blood Cultures

A quantitative blood culture is obtained by inoculating a known volume of blood onto a culture plate and counting the number of colonies that appear after incubation. The results are reported as num-

TABLE 5.4. THE QUANTITATIVE BLOOD CULTURE METHOD

Specimens: 10 mL blood withdrawn through the indwelling catheter and 10 mL blood from a site distal to the cannulation site. Place all specimens in evacuated culture tubes (e.g., Isolator System, Dupont Co.).
Diagnostic Criteria:
  I. Catheter-related septicemia (a or b):
    a. >100 CFU/mL in catheter blood
    b. CFU/mL in catheter blood >10 × CFU/mL in peripheral blood
  II. Septicemia from another site (a and b):
    a. <100 CFU/mL in catheter blood
    b. CFU/mL in catheter blood <10 × CFU/mL in peripheral blood
Performance: Sensitivity = 78%, specificity = 100%.
Comment: This method has a high diagnostic yield, and does not create the burden of removing and replacing indwelling catheters.

CFU = colony-forming unit.

ber of colony-forming units per milliliter (CFU/mL). The features of the quantitative blood culture technique are shown in Table 5.4. Two blood specimens are required: One specimen is withdrawn through the indwelling vascular catheter, and the other is obtained from a site distal to the catheter insertion site. The blood is not placed in the usual (broth) blood culture bottles, but it must be placed in specially designed evacuated bottles that contain an anticoagulant. These bottles are commercially available as Isolater bottles from Dupont Co. (Wilmington, DE), and come in adult (10 mL) and children's (1.5 mL) sizes.

The results of a quantitative culture are shown in Figure 5.3. In this case, the blood sample obtained through the indwelling catheter yielded the greatest number of colonies on incubation. This illustrates how the quantitative culture technique uses the differential growth in the two blood specimens to identify the source of the septicemia.

Catheter Tip Cultures

The standard diagnostic approach to catheter-related septicemia involves removing the index catheter and culturing the intravascular segment of the catheter. When catheter tips are placed in broth and cultured qualitatively (growth reported as present or absent, as in standard blood cultures), false-positive results are common (25). Therefore, qualitative broth cultures are never recommended. The culture method used is a semiquantitative technique that involves rolling the catheter tip across the surface of a culture plate and counting the number of colonies (CFUs) on the plate after the incubation period.

The principal features of the semiquantitative catheter culture technique are shown in Table 5.5 (27). A standard blood culture must be obtained from a distal site at the time of catheter removal. When the

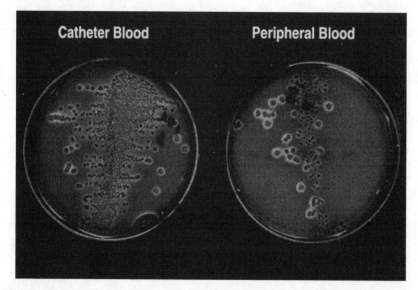

Figure 5.3. Quantitative cultures of blood aspirated through a central venous catheter (*Catheter Blood*) and blood obtained from a distant site (*Peripheral Blood*). The greater growth from the catheter blood specimen is evidence of catheter-related septicemia. (From Curtas S, Tramposch K. Culture methods to evaluate central venous catheter sepsis. Nutr Clin Pract 1991;6:43–51).

same organism is found in the blood and on the catheter tip, 15 colonies from the catheter tip is the threshold that identifies the source of the septicemia. Note that the sensitivity of this diagnostic method is quite low (36%), which means that a large number of cases of catheter-

---

TABLE 5.5. CATHETER TIP CULTURE: THE SEMIQUANTITATIVE METHOD

Specimens: Tip of the vascular catheter (distal 5 cm) in a sterile culturette tube, and one set of blood cultures from a site distal to the cannulation site.

Diagnostic Criteria:
    I. Catheter-related infection:
        >15 CFU from catheter tip and no organism in blood
    II. Catheter-related septicemia:
        >15 CFU from catheter tip and same organism in blood
    III. Septicemia from another site:
        <15 CFU from catheter tip and same organism in blood

Performance: Sensitivity = 36%, specificity = 100%.

Comment: This method requires frequent and often unnecessary removal of indwelling vascular catheters, and has a low sensitivity for the detection of catheter-related infections.

related septicemia will be missed. The sensitivity can be improved by plating the catheter tips at the bedside, immediately after removal (28).

WHICH METHOD IS PREFERRED?

The roll plate method for culturing catheter tips is the accepted method for evaluating catheter-related infections. However, it suffers from several disadvantages, including a low sensitivity and inability to detect infections on the inner luminal surface of catheters; most important, it requires removal of the catheters and insertion of replacement catheters. More than 50% of the catheters removed for suspected catheter-related infections show little growth on subsequent cultures. This means that catheter removal and replacement is unnecessary in the majority of cases of suspected catheter-related septicemia. This problem can be eliminated with the quantitative blood culture method, which does not require catheter removal. The quantitative blood culture method is also much more sensitive than the catheter culture method.

Thus, **the quantitative blood culture technique should be preferred** to the semiquantitative catheter tip culture. This latter culture technique is appropriate only when removal of indwelling catheters is indicated (i.e., when there is erythema or purulence at the catheter insertion site); when it is used, the catheter tip should be plated at the bedside to improve the diagnostic yield.

CATHETER GRAM STAIN

When catheters are removed for semiquantitative culture, a Gram stain of the catheter tip can help in the early decisions about diagnosis and management (29). The distal few centimeters of the catheter can be donated to the stain procedure, without compromising the 5-cm segment submitted for culture. The catheter segment to be stained is slit longitudinally, exposing the inner luminal surface of the catheter. Holding the catheter with sterile forceps while applying the stain allows both inner and outer surfaces of the catheter to be stained for inspection.

The benefits of this approach are obvious. The presence of organisms on the catheter is presumptive evidence of infection, and the morphology can help to identify the likely pathogens and select the appropriate antimicrobial therapy. Morphology may be particularly useful for identifying *Candida* infections (these organisms are large, Gram-positive round or oval forms). Finally, identifying organisms on the inside of the catheter is valuable for the interpretation of the catheter cultures

| TABLE 5.6. EMPIRIC ANTIMICROBIAL THERAPY: INDICATIONS AND REGIMENS ||
Condition	Antibiotics (Dose)*
Fever only	None
Pus at catheter insertion site	Vancomycin (1 g intravenously every 12 hours)
Prosthetic valve	Vancomycin and gentamicin (1 mg/kg intravenously every 8 hours)
Neutropenia ($<500/mm^3$)	Vancomycin, gentamicin, and ceftazidime (2 g intravenously every 8 hours)

Fever for 7 days despite empiric antibiotics, plus any one of the following:
    Candiduria
    Prolonged steroids
    Prosthetic valve
    Clinical deterioration
	Amphotericin B (0.5 mg/kg intravenously every day; total dose 5 mg/kg)

* Drug doses are for normal renal and hepatic function.	

because the roll plate method cultures only the outer surface of the catheter.

EMPIRIC ANTIMICROBIAL THERAPY

The decision to institute empiric antibiotic therapy is determined by the likelihood of catheter-related infection and the clinical condition of the patient. The clinical determinants of empiric antimicrobial therapy are shown in Table 5.6. In the patient with an unexplained fever and nothing else, antimicrobial therapy is not necessary if the catheter is removed (4). The remaining conditions in Table 5.6 warrant the empiric antibiotics indicated. Remember that S. epidermidis is often methicillin-resistant and thus is also resistant to the cephalosporins. Vancomycin is the drug of choice for this organism and should be included in all empiric antibiotic regimens (4). Adding an aminoglycoside is recommended for patients with prosthetic valves (aminoglycosides and vancomycin can be synergistic for S. epidermidis endocarditis), and ceftazidime is also added in neutropenic patients (for extra antipseudomonal activity).

PERSISTENT SEPSIS

Evidence of continuing infection or inflammation after antibiotic therapy is under way can signal the following conditions.

Disseminated Candidiasis

Persistent fever despite catheter replacement and broad-spectrum antimicrobial therapy may be a sign of disseminated candidiasis. Predisposing conditions include immunosuppression due to chemotherapy, steroids, human immunodeficiency virus infection, broad-spectrum antimicrobial therapy, prosthetic joints and heart valves, and vascular catheters (30). The diagnosis of disseminated candidiasis is often elusive because blood cultures are negative in over 50% of cases (30–32). Other laboratory methods for detecting systemic candidiasis include serum levels of enolase (a cytoplasmic antigen) and a latex agglutination test for a *Candida* cell wall antigen (titers 1:4 or higher suggest disseminated disease). However, these tests are not considered reliable enough to secure the diagnosis without other evidence of disseminated candidiasis (32).

Clinical markers of disseminated candidiasis include candiduria in the absence of indwelling urethral catheters, and endophthalmitis. Therefore, in cases of suspected candidiasis, examine or culture the urine and consult an ophthalmologist for a funduscopic examination of the eye. Heavy colonization of the urine in high-risk patients, even in the presence of an indwelling Foley catheter, can be used as an indication to initiate empiric antifungal therapy (31). Endophthalmitis can occur in up to 20% of cases of disseminated candidiasis (31), and evidence of ophthalmitis on the eye examination secures the diagnosis of candidemia and provides an indication to initiate antifungal therapy.

Empiric antifungal therapy is usually reserved for patients with persistent unexplained fever who are neutropenic or have a prosthetic heart valve, or high-risk patients who show evidence of progressive sepsis (i.e., organ dysfunction or hemodynamic instability). The antifungal agent of choice for empiric therapy is amphotericin B, 0.5 to 0.7 mg/kg daily (31). The addition of fluconazole (200 to 400 mg/day) has no proven benefit in this setting (31).

Suppurative Thrombophlebitis

Thrombosis surrounding the catheter tip is a common finding in patients with catheter-related septicemia (33), but in most cases the local thrombosis does not transform into a suppurative thrombophlebitis. The latter complication is suggested by persistently positive blood cultures despite catheter removal and appropriate antimicrobial therapy. (*Candida* suppurative thrombophlebitis may be associated with negative blood cultures.) Suppurative phlebitis in peripheral veins is often accompanied by local inflammation and purulent drainage from the catheter insertion site on the skin (34).

Therapy for this complication is surgical excision if a peripheral vessel is involved. In the large central veins, antimicrobial therapy combined with heparin anticoagulation can produce satisfactory results in 50% of cases (35).

ANOTHER PERSPECTIVE

The accepted practices for the prevention, recognition, and management of catheter-related infections are firmly rooted in the notion that microorganisms on the skin are the culprits in most cases of catheter-related infections. This notion is rarely disputed, yet there is no convincing evidence to support its claims. The remainder of the chapter attempts to show that there is a more likely source of septicemia than the skin in critically ill patients. Why is this important? Because we spend a lot of time scrubbing and cleaning the skin, and we may be cleaning the wrong surface.

A CASE AGAINST THE SKIN

The observations listed below do not support the notion that the skin is the principal source of catheter-related infections.

There is a poor correlation between organisms isolated from the skin around catheter insertion sites and organisms isolated from the bloodstream in cases of catheter-related septicemia (25,36). This is why surveillance cultures of the skin are not recommended as a predictive tool for identifying future inhabitants of the bloodstream.

Practices aimed at reducing the migration of skin microbes along the catheter tract (e.g., antimicrobial ointments, subcutaneous tunnels, and antimicrobial cuffs attached to the catheters) have had little or no impact on the incidence of catheter-related septicemias (4,37–39).

Half of the cases of catheter-related septicemia involve organisms that are not commonly found on the skin (i.e., enteric pathogens and *Candida* spp.) (24).

The prevalence of staphylococcal isolates cannot be used as evidence that the infections originate on the skin because staphylococci are also prominent bowel organisms, particularly in critically ill patients and patients receiving antibiotics (40). In fact, *S. epidermidis* is one of the most common isolates in the upper gastrointestinal tract of patients with multiorgan failure (41), so the species term for this organism (indicating an epidermal habitat) is misleading.

A Long Day's Journey

Another strike against the skin is the long distances that must be traveled in order for skin microbes to reach the intravascular segment of indwelling catheters. Staphylococci are nonmotile organisms and are only 0.001 mm in diameter. Thus, to reach the tip of a 20-cm central venous catheter, these organisms must travel a distance that is 2 million times their own length. This is equivalent to a 6-foot human being who must travel 2272 miles (roughly the distance between Atlanta and Los Angeles) without the aid of transportation or even legs (because the staphylococcus is nonmotile).

A CASE FOR THE BOWEL

The body surface with the highest density of pathogens is the bowel mucosa, not the skin (remember that the bowel mucosa is outside your

TABLE 5.7. CATHETER-RELATED SEPTICEMIA FROM THE BOWEL		
The cultures below are from a patient who developed a nosocomial fever on the seventh day after having an esophagogastrectomy. Note how the diagnostic impression changes when the bowel is included in the evaluation.		
Culture Specimen	**Growth**	**Diagnosis**
A. Peripheral blood (×4)	*Enterobacter cloacae*	A + B = Catheter-related
B. Subclavian catheter tip	*Enterobacter cloacae* (>100 CFUs)	septicemia
C. Gastric aspirate (×2)	*Enterobacter cloacae*	A–D = Bowel-related
D. Skin swab at catheter insertion site (×2)	No growth	septicemia
From Sing R, Marino PL. Bacterial translocation: an occult cause of catheter-related sepsis. Infect Med 1993;10:54–57.		

body), and enteric microbes must travel only a few millimeters to reach the bloodstream. The fact that enteric organisms are commonly involved in catheter-related septicemias suggests that the bowel route is active.

The case report in Table 5.7 shows how the bowel can act as an occult source of catheter-related septicemia (42). The cultures listed were obtained from a patient in the surgical ICU who developed a nosocomial fever on the seventh day following an esophagogastrectomy. The same organism (*Enterobacter cloacae*) was isolated from multiple blood cultures and from a semiquantitative central venous catheter culture. The colony count from the catheter (more than 100 CFUs) indicates a diagnosis of catheter-related septicemia. However, cultures were also obtained from the skin surrounding the catheter insertion site and from nasogastric aspirates, and these culture results suggest a diagnosis other than catheter-related septicemia. That is, the nasogastric aspirates grew the same type of organism that was isolated from the blood and the catheter tip, and this suggests that the septicemia originated from the bowel, with secondary seeding of the indwelling catheter. This illustrates how the diagnosis of catheter-related septicemia can be erroneous if the bowel is excluded in the diagnostic evaluation.

The role of the bowel as an occult source of catheter-related sepsis is unclear at present. However, critically ill patients are particularly prone to developing septicemia of bowel origin, and the conditions responsible for this predisposition are described in Chapter 6.

REFERENCES

REVIEWS

1. Intravenous Nurses Society. Intravenous Nursing Standards of Practice. Belmont, MA: Intravenous Nurses Society, 1990.
2. Perucca R. Intravenous monitoring and catheter care. In: Terry J, Baranowski L, Lonsway RA, Hedrick C, eds. Intravenous therapy. Philadelphia: WB Saunders, 1995;392–399.
3. Norwood S, Ruby A, Civetta J, Cortes V. Catheter-related infections and associated septicemia. Chest 1991;99:968–975.

4. Bjornson HS. Pathogenesis, prevention, and management of catheter-associated infections. New Horiz 1993;1:271–278.

PROTECTIVE DRESSINGS

5. Hoffman KK, Weber DJ, Samsa GP, et al. Transparent polyurethane film as intravenous catheter dressing. A meta-analysis of infection risks. JAMA 1992; 267:2072–2076.
6. Maki DG, Stolz SS, Wheeler S, Mermi LA. A prospective, randomized trial of gauze and two polyurethane dressings for site care of pulmonary artery catheters: implications for catheter management. Crit Care Med 1994;22: 1729–1737.
7. Marshall DA, Mertz PA, Eaglestein WH. Occlusive dressings. Arch Surg 1990; 125:1136–1139.

REPLACING CATHETERS

8. Ullman RF, Guerivich I, Schoch PE, Cunha BA. Colonization and bacteremia related to duration of triple-lumen intravascular catheter placement. Am J Infect Control 1990;18:201–207.
9. Eyer S, Brummitt C, Crossley K, et al. Catheter-related sepsis: prospective, randomized study of three methods of long-term catheter maintenance. Crit Care Med 1990;18:1073–1079.
10. Cobb DK, High KP, Sawyer RP, et al. A controlled trial of scheduled replacement of central venous and pulmonary artery catheters. N Engl J Med 1992; 327:1062–1068.

CATHETER FLUSHES

11. Peterson FY, Kirchhoff KT. Analysis of research about heparinized versus non-heparinized intravascular lines. Heart Lung 1991;20:631–642.
12. American Association of Critical Care Nurses. Evaluation of the effects of heparinized and nonheparinized flush solutions on the patency of arterial pressure monitoring lines: the AACN Thunder Project. Am J Crit Care 1993; 2:3–15.
13. Walsh DA, Mellor JA. Why flush peripheral intravenous cannulae used for intermittent intravenous injection? Br J Clin Pract 1991;45:31–32.
14. Branson PK, McCoy RA, Phillips BA, Clifton GD. Efficacy of 1.4% sodium citrate in maintaining arterial catheter patency in patients in a medical ICU. Chest 1993;103:882–885.

MECHANICAL COMPLICATIONS

15. Trissel LA. Drug stability and compatibility issues in drug delivery. Cancer Bull 1990;42:393–398.
16. Monturo CA, Dickerson RN, Mullen J. Efficacy of thrombolytic therapy for occlusion of long-term catheters. J Parent Ent Nutr 1990;14:312–314.
17. Shulman RJ, Reed T, Pitre D, Laine L. Use of hydrochloric acid to clear obstructed central venous catheters. J Parent Ent Nutr 1988;12:509–510.
18. Heffner JE. A 20-year-old woman with respiratory failure and a swollen right arm. J Crit Illness 1994;9:187–192.
19. Duntley P, Siever J, Korwes ML, et al. Vascular erosion by central venous catheters. Chest 1992;101:1633–1638.
20. Heffner JE. A 49-year-old man with tachypnea and a rapidly enlarging pleural effusion. J Crit Illness 1994;9:101–109.
21. Armstrong CW, Mayhall CG. Contralateral hydrothorax following subclavian catheter replacement using a guidewire. Chest 1983;84:231–233.

INFECTIOUS COMPLICATIONS

22. Pittet D, Tarara D, Wenzel RP. Nosocomial bloodstream infection in critically ill patients. JAMA 1994;271:1598–1601.
23. Vaudaux PE, Lew DP, Waldvogel FA. Host factors predisposing to foreign body infections. In: Bisno AL, Waldvogel FA, eds. Infections associated with indwelling medical devices. Washington, DC: American Society for Microbiology, 1989;3–26.
24. Hampton AA, Sheretz RJ. Vascular-access infections in hospitalized patients. Surg Clin North Am 1988;68:57–71.
25. Curtas S, Tramposch K. Culture methods to evaluate central venous catheter sepsis. Nutr Clin Pract 1991;6:43–48.
26. Benezra D, Kiehn TE, Gold JWM, et al. Prospective study of infections in indwelling central venous catheters using quantitative blood cultures. Am J Med 1988;85:495–498.
27. Maki DG, Weise CE, Sarafin HW. A semiquantitative culture method for identifying intravenous catheter-related infections. N Engl J Med 1977;296: 1305–1309.
28. Hnatiuk OW, Pike J, Stolzfus D, Lane W. Value of bedside plating of semiquantitative cultures for diagnosis of catheter-related infections in ICU patients. Chest 1993;103:896–899.
29. Cooper GL, Hopkins CC. Rapid diagnosis of intravascular catheter-associated infection by direct gram staining of catheter segments. N Engl J Med 1985; 312:1142–1145.
30. Magnussen CR. Disseminated *Candida* infection: diagnostic clues, therapeutic options. J Crit Illness 1992;7:513–525.
31. British Society for Antimicrobial Chemotherapy Working Party. Management of deep *Candida* infection in surgical and intensive care unit patients. Intensive Care Med 1994;20:522–528.
32. Rosemurgy AS, Sweeney JF, Albrink MH, et al. Implications of candida antigen tests in injured adults. Contemp Surg 1993;42:327–332.
33. Raad II, Luna M, Khali S-A, et al. The relationship between the thrombotic and infectious complications of central venous catheters. JAMA 1994;271: 1014–1016.
34. Garrison RN, Richardson JD, Frye DE. Catheter-associated septic thrombophlebitis. South Med J 1982;75:917–919.
35. Verghese A, Widrich WC, Arbeit RD. Central venous septic thrombophlebitis: the role of antimicrobial therapy. Medicine 1985;64:394–400.
36. Golledge C, McPherson M. Skin entry site swabbing a poor predictor of catheter-related sepsis. Infect Control Hosp Epidemiol 1988;9:54–62.
37. Sitges-Serra A, Linares J. Tunnels do not protect against venous catheter-related sepsis. Lancet 1984;1:459–460.
38. Norwood S, Hajjar G, Jenkins L. The influence of an attachable subcutaneous cuff for preventing triple lumen catheter infections in critically ill surgical and trauma patients. Surg Gynecol Obstet 1992;175:33–40.
39. Groeger JS, Lucas AB, Coit D, et al. A prospective, randomized evaluation of the effect of silver-impregnated subcutaneous cuffs for preventing tunneled chronic venous access catheter infections in cancer patients. Ann Surg 1993; 218:206–210.
40. Altemeier WA, Hummel RP, Hill EO. Staphylococcal enterocolitis following antibiotic therapy. Ann Surg 1963;157:847–858.
41. Marshall JC, Christou NV, Horn R, Meakins JL. The microbiology of multiple organ failure. Arch Surg 1988;123:309–315.
42. Sing R, Marino PL. Bacterial translocation: an occult cause of catheter-related sepsis. Infect Med 1993;10:54–57.

6

GASTROINTESTINAL PROPHYLAXIS

We are told the most fantastic biological tales. For example, that it is dangerous to have acid in your stomach.

JBS Haldane (1939)

We are preoccupied with the threat of microbial invasion through the skin and tend to neglect a similar threat of invasion through our "internal skin" in the gastrointestinal (GI) tract. The GI tract is outside the body (like the hole in a donut), and thus the mucosal surface of the GI tract must serve as a barrier to microbial invasion, much like the skin. Two observations suggest that the real threat of microbial invasion is from the GI tract, not the skin. First, the skin provides several layers of protection, whereas the GI mucosa is a single layer of cells only 0.01 mm thick. Second, the microbial population is far greater in the alimentary tract than on the skin. In fact, **the number of bacteria in 1 gram of stool** (10 to 100 billion) **is greater than the number of people on Earth** (5.7 billion in 1995). This chapter focuses on conditions that predispose critically ill patients to microbial invasion from the bowel, and describes some measures that can be used to counteract this threat.

THE THREAT OF TRANSLOCATION

There are 400 to 500 different species of bacteria and fungi in the human alimentary tract (1,2); the distribution of this indigenous microflora is shown in Table 6.1. The organisms in the mouth are constantly being swallowed in the saliva, but microbial density in the stomach is dramatically reduced by the bactericidal actions of gastric acid. The density of microbes then rises progressively through the small bowel and colon, and at the distal end of the GI tract, microbes make up as much as 40% of the total fecal mass (2).

TABLE 6.1. MICROBIAL DENSITY IN THE ALIMENTARY TRACT	
Segment	Population Density*
Oral cavity	10^5-10^6
Stomach	$<10^3$
Distal small bowel	10^7-10^9
Rectum	$10^{10}-10^{12}$

* Colony-forming units (CFUs) per gram or mL of luminal contents.
From Simon GL, Gorbach SL. Intestinal microflora. Med Clin North Am 1982;
66:557.

PROTECTIVE MECHANISMS

Several protective mechanisms prevent the microbes on our inner surface from invading us. First, many of the indigenous bacteria and fungi in the alimentary tract are saprophytes and show little tendency for invasive infection. Second, as already mentioned, the bactericidal action of gastric acid helps to curb the population of immigrant microbes from the oral cavity. A third factor is the intrinsic barrier function of the mucosal lining of the bowel. Finally, the reticuloendothelial system in the bowel (i.e., the lymphatic system and phagocytic cells) can trap and destroy organisms that breach the mucosal barrier. Roughly **two-thirds of the reticuloendothelial system in the body is located in the abdomen** (3), which suggests that microbial invasion across the bowel mucosa may be a common occurrence (3).

PREDISPOSING FACTORS

A defect in any of the protective mechanisms described above favors the movement, or *translocation*, of enteric pathogens into the systemic circulation (4). Figure 6.1 shows three conditions that favor bloodstream invasion by bowel microbes: microbial overgrowth in the bowel lumen, disruption of the surface mucosa, and defective clearance by submucosal lymphatics. The clinical conditions described in this chapter are characterized by one or more of these predisposing conditions, and the goal of gastrointestinal prophylaxis is to prevent these conditions from developing.

STRESS ULCERS

Stress ulcers are superficial erosions in the gastric mucosa that are commonplace in patients with acute, life-threatening diseases (5,6). These erosions are usually confined to the surface mucosa and are distinct from the lesions of peptic ulcer disease, which are deeper craters that can erode through the entire width of the bowel wall. Thus, the term *stress ulcer* is somewhat misleading.

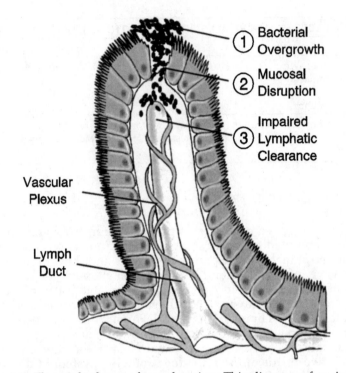

Figure 6.1. The triple threat of translocation. This diagram of an intestinal microvillus shows three conditions that predispose to bloodstream invasion by enteric pathogens.

PATHOGENESIS

The mucosal lining of the GI tract is normally shed and replaced every 2 to 3 days. When nutrient blood flow is inadequate to support the replacement process, the surface of the bowel becomes denuded, creating the superficial erosions known as stress ulcers. Although gastric acid can aggravate the condition, **the primary cause of stress ulceration is impaired blood flow, not gastric acidity** (5).

CLINICAL FEATURES

Gastric erosions are present in 10 to 25% of patients on admission to a medical and surgical intensive care unit, and in 90% of patients by the third day of the ICU stay (6,7). The risk of mucosal ulceration seems to be particularly high in patients with head injury and patients with thermal injury that involves at least 30% of the body surface area (5,6).

Although gastric erosions are commonplace in critically ill patients, they are often clinically silent. The two consequences of stress ulceration are disruption of the mucosal barrier (with subsequent risk of translocation and nosocomial septicemia) and hemorrhage from erosion through surface vessels. Perforation is rare with stress ulceration because of the superficial location of the lesions. The incidence of nosocomial septicemia from stress ulceration has not been studied. The **incidence of bleeding from stress ulcers** is almost 100% for clinically silent (occult) bleeding (8) **but is only about 5% for clinically apparent (overt) hemorrhage, and 1 to 2% for clinically important hemorrhage** (i.e., hemorrhage requiring blood transfusions) (8–10).

HIGH-RISK CONDITIONS

The low incidence of overt or clinically important bleeding from stress ulceration raises some question of whether preventive therapy for stress ulceration is justified in all patients. (The risk of translocation from stress erosions has not been considered in the debate over the value of stress ulcer prophylaxis). In general, the following conditions are considered high risk for stress ulcer-related bleeding, and thus are indications for prophylactic therapy (9).

INDICATIONS FOR PROPHYLAXIS

Head injury
Thermal injury involving at least 30% of the body surface area
Emergent or major surgery
Severe or multisystem trauma
Shock or multiorgan failure
Coagulopathy
Mechanical ventilation for more than 48 hours
Ongoing therapy with ulcerogenic drugs
History of ulcer-related bleeding

PREVENTIVE STRATEGIES

The following measures are considered effective for reducing the incidence of overt bleeding from stress ulcers (10). (Because stress ulcers are usually asymptomatic, prophylactic efficacy is usually evaluated by the incidence of hemorrhage from the lesions.) The preventive measures below are listed in order of preference.

Preserving Splanchnic Blood Flow

Because impaired nutrient blood flow is the inciting event in stress ulceration, preserving adequate mesenteric blood flow should be the optimal prophylaxis for stress ulcers. Unfortunately, few methods are available for monitoring mesenteric blood flow in the clinical setting. Gastric tonometry (this technique is described in Chapter 13) has been proposed as a method of monitoring the adequacy of gastric mucosal blood flow in critically ill patients, but this technique has limitations and has yet to gain widespread acceptance. The best strategy at present is to maintain adequate levels of systemic blood flow and oxygen transport, using conventional hemodynamic monitoring with pulmonary artery catheters, if possible.

Enteral Nutrition

Enteral tube feedings have a dual benefit: They reduce the risk of stress ulcer bleeding while providing daily nutrient requirements (11). The mechanism for the protective effect of tube feedings may be acid neutralization, or may result from the trophic effect of luminal nutrients on the functional integrity of the bowel mucosa. (The delivery of enteral tube feedings is described in Chapter 47.)

If full enteral nutrition is not possible, there are two pharmacologic approaches to stress ulcer prophylaxis. One approach uses a cytoprotective agent that maintains the functional integrity of the gastric mucosa; the other approach is based on suppression of gastric acid. The pharmacologic approach to stress ulcer prophylaxis is outlined in Table 6.2.

TABLE 6.2. PHARMACOLOGIC APPROACH TO STRESS ULCER PROPHYLAXIS		
Agent	**Actions**	**Dosage Recommendations**
Sucralfate	Cytoprotection	Dilute 1 g sucralfate in 5–10 mL sterile water and administer via nasogastric tube every 6 hr.
Cimetidine	Gastric acid suppression	1. Start with IV loading dose of 300 mg (over 5 min). 2. Follow with continuous infusion at 37.5 mg/hr. 3. Increase infusion rate in increments of 25 mg/hr until gastric pH is greater than 4. 4. Maximum infusion rate is 100 mg/hr. 5. If renal function is abnormal, use dose schedule in Chapter 54.
Ranitidine	Gastric acid suppression	1. Start with IV loading dose of 0.5 mg/kg (over 30 min). 2. Follow with continuous infusion at 0.125 mg/kg/hr. 3. Increase infusion rate in increments of 0.06 mg/kg/hr until gastric is greater than 4.
Antacids	Gastric acid neutralization	1. Give 30 mL antacid and check gastric pH in 1 hr. 2. If pH is less than 4.0, give 60 mL antacid and check pH in 1 hr. 3. Repeat step 2 until gastric pH is greater than 4. 4. Give maintenance antacid doses every 1–2 hr. Clamp NG tube for 30 min after each bolus dose.

Sucralfate

Sucralfate is an aluminum salt of sucrose sulfate that helps maintain the structural and functional integrity of the gastric mucosa (12). The drug is administered orally or via nasogastric tube at the dosage shown in Table 6.2. This agent has proven effective in reducing the incidence of stress ulcers (7) and reducing the incidence of hemorrhage from stress ulcers (8,10,12). The mechanism of sucralfate's protective effect is not known (12).

The bulk of evidence indicates that **sucralfate should be the preferred method of prophylaxis when full enteral nutrition is not feasible.** The drug is safe, inexpensive, and easy to administer (the only requirement is that the patient tolerate gastric installation of 5 to 10 mL of fluid every 4 to 6 hours). The advantages of sucralfate over other pharmacologic agents are discussed later.

Interactions. Sucralfate is capable of binding the medications listed in Table 6.3 (13). This can lead to reduced absorption and diminished bioavailability of the specified drugs. To minimize potential interactions, sucralfate should not be administered at the same time as these medications (this does not apply to parenteral drug administration). Because sucralfate contains aluminum, it can also bind and reduce phosphorous absorption from the bowel. Although sucralfate therapy has a reported association with hypophosphatemia (14), a cause-and-

TABLE 6.3. DRUG INTERACTIONS

Agent	Interactions	Recommendations
Sucralfate	Can bind the following drugs in the GI tract (reduces bioavailability) Cimetidine Norfloxacin Ciprofloxacin Phenytoin Coumadin Ranitidine Digoxin Theophylline	Avoid combination with oral fluoroquinolones and sucralfate. Give sucralfate 2 hr before enteral administration of the other drugs.
Cimetidine	Decreased hepatic metabolism of Coumadin Phenytoin Diazepam Propranolol Labetolol Theophylline Lidocaine Triazolam Metoprolol Verapamil Nifedipine	Monitor serum drug levels or clinical effects for evidence of drug toxicity.
Ranitidine	2.5 times less potent than cimetidine in reducing hepatic metabolism of the above agents.	No action usually necessary.
Antacids	Can reduce the absorption of Digoxin (Al, Mg) Ranitidine (Al) Iron (Al, Mg, Ca) Thyroxine (Al) Phenytoin (Ca) Vitamins A, D, E, K (Al) Prednisone (Al, Mg)	Avoid combination.

effect relationship has not been established. Nevertheless, it is wise to consider sucralfate as a possible culprit in any patient with unexplained hypophosphatemia. The aluminum content of sucralfate does not promote elevations in plasma aluminum levels (15).

Histamine H_2 Receptor Antagonists

One of the most popular methods of stress ulcer prophylaxis is to inhibit gastric acid production with histamine H_2-receptor antagonists. All histamine-blocking drugs are equally effective in reducing the incidence of stress ulcer bleeding (10). The drugs are usually given intravenously (although oral therapy is also effective), and continuous infusion therapy is more effective in maintaining the target pH (above 4) than bolus drug administration (16,17). Dosing regimens for continuous infusion of cimetidine and ranitidine are shown in Table 6.2. The dosage of cimetidine is altered in the presence of renal insufficiency (see Chapter 54 for dosage adjustments); continuous-infusion ranitidine has not been studied in renal insufficiency (13).

Interactions. Cimetidine interferes with the hepatic metabolism of several drugs used in the care of critically ill patients, and Table 6.3 contains a list of the pertinent agents (13). Ranitidine has a similar but less potent action (13), so ranitidine has gained favor over cimetidine. The potential for drug interactions must be considered when cimetidine is given concurrently with any of the drugs in Table 6.3.

Antacids

Neutralization of gastric acidity with antacids is the least desirable method of stress ulcer prophylaxis. Antacid titration using the regimen in Table 6.2 is time-consuming and offers no advantage over sucralfate or histamine H_2 blockers other than reduced cost. The potential for multiple drug interactions (see Table 6.3) should further discourage the use of antacids for stress ulcer prophylaxis.

SUCRALFATE VERSUS H_2 BLOCKERS

Sucralfate prophylaxis offers a number of advantages over the histamine H_2 blockers. The first is cost. The routine use of sucralfate instead of H_2 blockers carries an estimated cost savings of $30,000 per hospital bed per year (8), which translates to an estimated annual savings of $4 billion dollars yearly in the United States (8). (This amount is one-third of the total NIH budget for 1995!) The second most important advantage is the lower risk of gastric colonization with sucralfate. Suppression of gastric acidity with histamine H_2 blockers or antacids results in the overgrowth of bacteria and fungi in the stomach, and this colonization of the stomach can be a prelude to nosocomial pneumonia

(10,18) and translocation with nosocomial septicemia (19). Considering that stress ulceration is itself a risk factor for translocation (as shown in Figure 6.1), interventions that promote bacterial overgrowth in this setting add to the risk of translocation, and thus do not seem a wise choice.

THE ACID PHOBIA

As indicated in the introductory remark by JBS Haldane (a geneticist, not the physiologist who described the Haldane effect), our fear of gastric acid is based on legend more than scientific observation. Consider why we secrete gastric acid. It is not an important digestive aid, because patients with achlorhydria are not troubled with malabsorption (20). The function of gastric acid is revealed in the work of Sir Joseph Lister, who popularized the antiseptic approach to surgery by cleansing surgical wounds with carbolic acid (also known as phenol). The bactericidal actions of an acid pH are demonstrated in Figure 6.2. In this case, the common enteric organism *Escherichia coli* is completely eradicated in 1 hour when pH of the growth medium is reduced to 3; the same organism flourishes at a slightly higher pH of 5. Note that the threshold pH at which bacterial growth occurs (pH

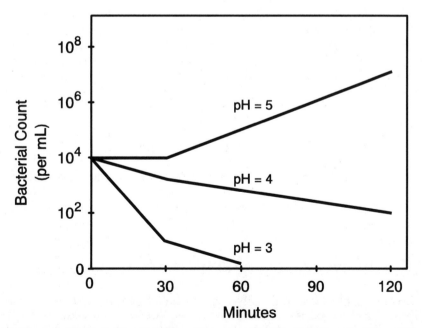

Figure 6.2. The influence of pH on the growth of *Escherichia coli*. (From Gianella J et al. Gut 1972;13:251.)

greater than 4) is the same as the target pH for stress ulcer prophylaxis with histamine H_2 blockers (see Table 6.2).

Thus, **gastric acid functions as an antibacterial defense mechanism that prevents immigrant microbes from gaining access to the alimentary tract.** This function applies not only to the bacteria that are swallowed in the saliva, but also to eradicating microbes that populate the food we ingest (this fact explains why food ingestion stimulates gastric acid secretion). Just as acid is used to eradicate *Salmonella* organisms in chickens, our own gastric acid serves a similar function of eradicating *Salmonella* organisms that we ingest. This explains why gastric acid suppression therapy is associated with recurrent *Salmonella* enteritis (21) and why achlorhydria is associated with an increased risk of enteric infections (20–22). In this sense, gastric acid is **an intrinsic mechanism for disinfecting the food we eat.**

The fear of gastric acid is based largely on the presumed association between gastric acid and peptic ulcer disease (and on the marketing skills of certain drug manufacturers). However, recent evidence indicates that many gastric and duodenal ulcers are the result of a local infection with *Helicobacter pylori* (23). As physicians become more aware that gastric acid is not the culprit in gastric mucosal injury, the unfounded and dangerous practice of gastric acid suppression in critically ill patients may finally be abandoned.

OCCULT BLOOD TESTING

Monitoring for occult blood in gastric secretions is a common practice in the prophylaxis for stress ulceration, but it has limited value. Nasogastric aspirates almost always contain occult blood in the presence of stress ulceration (8), and because few cases of stress ulceration are associated with gross (overt) hemorrhage, the presence of occult blood in a nasogastric aspirate has no predictive value for assessing the risk of significant bleeding. Because overt hemorrhage almost never appears when there is no occult blood in gastric secretions (24), a negative occult blood test has predictive value. However, this is unlikely to alter decisions regarding stress ulcer prophylaxis.

When evaluating gastric aspirates, the guaiac and Hemoccult tests are inappropriate because they give false-positive and false-negative results when the test solution has a pH less than 4 (25). The Gastroccult test (Smith, Kline Laboratories) is not influenced by pH (25), and thus is the appropriate test for occult blood in gastric aspirates.

SELECTIVE DIGESTIVE DECONTAMINATION

The microbes that normally inhabit the alimentary tract seem content with their existence and show little tendency to invade us. However, in the presence of disease, these microbes are replaced by more aggressive species, and this colonization serves as a prelude to nosocomial infections (such as pneumonias, urinary tract infections, and septicemia). The aim of selective digestive decontamination (SDD) is to prevent colonization of the alimentary tract by invasive pathogens, and thus prevent nosocomial infections. To accomplish this purpose, antibiotics designed to eradicate fungi and Gram-negative aerobic pathogens are placed in the oral cavity and GI tract on a regular basis. The antibiotics are nonabsorbable, and thus pose no threat of systemic toxicity. The normal, indigenous microflora (mostly anaerobes) are undisturbed, to limit colonization by resistant organisms.

THE METHOD

Several antibiotic regimens have been used for SDD, and one of the effective ones is as follows (26):

Oral cavity: A paste containing 2% polymyxin, 2% tobramycin, and 2% amphotericin is applied to the inside of the mouth with a gloved finger, and the application is repeated every 6 hours (the pharmacy will make the paste).

GI tract: A 10-mL solution containing 100 mg polymyxin E, 80 mg tobramycin, and 500 mg amphotericin is administered via a nasogastric tube every 6 hours.

This regimen eradicates most Gram-negative pathogens from the mouth and GI tract in just 1 week. It is then continued for as long as the patient resides in the ICU. After 10 years of clinical experience with SDD, there has been no problem with the emergence of antibiotic resistance during the course of therapy.

RESULTS

A recent review of 25 clinical trials showed that SDD was effective in reducing the incidence of nosocomial infections in patients in the ICU (27). The results of one study are shown in Figure 6.3. In this study, SDD was associated with significant reductions in the incidence of pneumonia, urinary tract infections, and catheter-related septicemia. (Note that SDD virtually eliminated catheter-related septicemia, which supports the notion that the bowel is an important source of catheter-related septicemias.) Despite impressive results such as those in Figure 6.3, SDD has not been embraced with enthusiasm in the United States. Much of the hesitancy is due to the fact that SDD has not been effective in reducing mortality in many (but not all) of the clinical studies (27). However, **the aim of SDD is to reduce nosocomial infections, and in this regard, SDD must be considered an effective method of infection control in the ICU.** The lack of association between nosocomial infections and mortality rate in the ICU is a separate issue (and one that adds to the long list of uncertainties in clinical medicine).

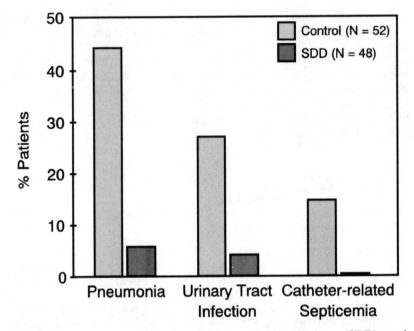

Figure 6.3. The effects of selective digestive decontamination (SDD) on the incidence of nosocomial infections in general medical-surgical ICU patients. (From Ulrich C et al. Intensive Care Med 1989;15:424.)

REFERENCES

GENERAL TEXTS

Hollander D, Tarnowski AS. Gastric cytoprotection: a clinician's guide. New York: Plenum, 1989.

Marston A, Bulkley GR, Fiddian-Green RG, Haglund UH, eds. Splanchnic ischemia and multiple organ failure. St. Louis: CV Mosby, 1989.

TRANSLOCATION

1. Simon GL, Gorbach SL. Intestinal microflora. Med Clin North Am 1982;66:557–574.
2. Borriello SP. Microbial flora of the gastrointestinal tract. In: Microbial metabolism in the digestive tract. Boca Raton, FL: CRC Press, 1989;2–19.
3. Langkamp-Henken B, Glezer JA, Kudsk KA. Immunologic structure and function of the gastrointestinal tract. Nutr Clin Pract 1992;7:100–108.
4. Alexander JW, Boyce ST, Babcock GF, et al. The process of microbial translocation. Ann Surg 1990;212:496–510.

STRESS ULCERS

5. Schiessel R, Feil W, Wenzel E. Mechanisms of stress ulceration and implications for treatment. Gastroenterol Clin North Am 1990;19:101–120.

6. Reusser P, Gyr K, Scheidegger D, et al. Prospective endoscopic study of stress erosions and ulcers in critically ill neurosurgical patients. Current incidence and effect of acid-reducing prophylaxis. Crit Care Med 1990;18:270–274.
7. Eddleston JM, Pearson RC, Holland J, et al. Prospective endoscopic study of stress erosions and ulcers in critically ill adult patients treated with either sucralfate or placebo. Crit Care Med 1994;22:1949–1954.
8. Maier RV, Mitchell D, Gentiello L. Optimal therapy for stress gastritis. Ann Surg 1994;220:353–363.
9. Cook DJ, Fuller MB, Guyatt GH. Risk factors for gastrointestinal bleeding in critically ill patients. N Engl J Med 1994;330:377–381.
10. Cook DJ, Reeve BK, Guyatt GH. Stress ulcer prophylaxis in critically ill patients. JAMA 1996;275:308–314.
11. Pingleton SR. Gastric bleeding and/or enteral feeding. Chest 1986;90:2–3.
12. McCarthy DM. Sucralfate. N Engl J Med 1990;325:1016–1025.
13. McEvoy GK, ed. AHFS Drug Information, 1995. Bethesda, MD: American Society of Health System Pharmacists, 1995:2021–2065.
14. Miller SJ, Simpson J. Medication–nutrient interactions: hypophosphatemia associated with sucralfate in the intensive care unit. Nutr Clin Pract 1991;6: 199–201.
15. Tryba M, Kurz-Muller K, Donner B. Plasma aluminum concentrations in long-term mechanically ventilated patients receiving stress ulcer prophylaxis with sucralfate. Crit Care Med 1994;22:1769–1773.
16. Ben-Menachem T, Fogel R, Patel RV, et al. Prophylaxis for stress-related gastric hemorrhage in the medical intensive care unit. Ann Intern Med 1994;121: 568–575.
17. Morris DL, Markham SJ, Beechey A, et al. Ranitidine-bolus or infusion prophylaxis for stress ulcer. Crit Care Med 1988;16:229–232.
18. Cook DJ, Laine LA, Guyatt GH, et al. Nosocomial pneumonia and the role of gastric pH. Chest 1991;100:7–13.
19. Garvey BM, McCambley JA, Tuxen DV. Effects of gastric alkalization on bacterial colonization in critically ill patients. Crit Care Med 1989;17:211–216.
20. Howden CW, Hunt RH. Relationship between gastric secretion and infection. Gut 1987;28:96–107.
21. Wingate DL. Acid reduction and recurrent enteritis. Lancet 1990;335:222.
22. Cook GC. Infective gastroenteritis and its relationship to reduced acidity. Scand J Gastroenterol 1985;20(Suppl 111):17–21.
23. Soli AH. Medical treatment of peptic ulcer disease. Practice guidelines. JAMA 1996;275:622–629.
24. Derrida S, Nury B, Slama R, et al. Occult gastrointestinal bleeding in high-risk intensive care unit patients receiving antacid prophylaxis: frequency and significance. Crit Care Med 1989;17:122–125.
25. Rosenthal P, Thompson J, Singh M. Detection of occult blood in gastric juice. J Clin Gastroenterol 1984;6:119.

SELECTIVE DIGESTIVE DECONTAMINATION

26. Stoutenbeek CP, van Saene HKF, Miranda DR, Zandstra DF. The effect of selective decontamination of the digestive tract on colonization and infection rate in multiple trauma patients. Intensive Care Med 1984;10:185–192.
27. Heyland DK, Cook DJ, Jaeschke R, et al. Selective decontamination of the digestive tract. An overview. Chest 1994;105:1221–1229.

c h a p t e r

7

VENOUS THROMBOEMBOLISM

Two words best characterize the mortality and morbidity due to venous thromboembolism in the United States: substantial and unacceptable.
Kenneth M. Moser, Am Rev Resp Dis, 1990

The threat of venous thrombosis and acute pulmonary embolism (i.e., venous thromboembolism) is an everyday concern in the care of critically ill patients. A variety of clinical conditions, many of them common in ICU patients, can be accompanied by venous thrombosis in the lower extremities. Thrombosis involving the deep venous system in the thighs is often a silent process, and becomes evident only when it sends thrombotic projectiles to the lungs. In more than two-thirds of cases of acute pulmonary embolism, the source of the problem (i.e., proximal leg vein thrombosis) goes unnoticed before the embolism (1–6). Because this thrombosis is such an insidious process, emphasis is placed on prevention to reduce the risks associated with venous thromboembolism.

The material in this chapter is presented in four parts. The first part identifies patients who are at risk for thromboembolism, and the second part describes the appropriate prophylaxis for each group of high-risk patients. The third part describes a diagnostic algorithm for patients with suspected acute pulmonary embolism, and the final part describes the early management of thromboembolism with anticoagulants and thrombolytic agents.

PATIENTS AT RISK

The clinical conditions that predispose to venous thromboembolism are listed by risk category in Table 7.1. Accompanying each category is the reported incidence of proximal deep vein thrombosis (proximal DVT) in the leg and fatal pulmonary embolism (fatal PE). The incidence of calf vein thrombosis is not included because thrombosis

TABLE 7.1. RISK CATEGORIES FOR VENOUS THROMBOEMBOLISM

Category	Conditions	Proximal DVT	Fatal PE
Low risk	Minor surgery (<30 min) Major surgery (>30 min) + age <40 yrs Medical illness (except MI, stroke)	<1%	<0.1%
Moderate risk	Major surgery + age >40 yrs Minor surgery + history DVT or PE Major trauma or burns Acute MI or stroke	1–10%	0.1–1%
High risk	Major surgery or major trauma + history of DVT or PE Cancer surgery (abdomen or pelvis) Hip or knee surgery Hip or pelvic fracture Lower limb paralysis	10–30%	1–10%

From the Thromboembolic Risk Factors Consensus Group. BMJ 1992;305:567.

below the knee is not considered an important source of pulmonary emboli (1).

SURGERY

Several factors promote thrombosis in the early period following major surgery. These include venous stasis, vascular injury, and a generalized hypercoagulable state (caused by thromboplastin release during surgery and depressed levels of antithrombin III that persist for 5 to 7 days after surgery). Orthopedic procedures involving the hip and knee represent a particularly high risk for thromboembolism, as does cancer-related surgery in the abdomen and pelvis.

TRAUMA

Trauma carries the same risk factors for thromboembolism as surgery (surgery is a form of controlled trauma). The high-risk conditions in trauma include multisystem involvement, acute spinal cord injury, and fractures involving the pelvis and lower extremities.

MEDICAL ILLNESS

Relatively few acute medical illnesses carry a high risk of venous thromboembolism. The most noted high-risk medical conditions are acute myocardial infarction, ischemic stroke, lower extremity paralysis (either pharmacologic or disease related), and cancer (particularly pelvic tumors).

METHODS OF PROPHYLAXIS

A variety of preventive measures have proven effective in reducing the incidence of thromboembolism in critically ill patients. As a result, **routine thromboprophylaxis is recommended for all patients in the moderate- and high-risk categories in Table 7.1 (2,7).** This point deserves emphasis because surveys reveal that physicians neglect thromboprophylaxis in 70 to 80% of patients who would benefit from the intervention (8). The preventive measures recommended in each type of clinical condition are shown in Table 7.2 (2). Each of these measures is described briefly in the paragraphs that follow.

GRADED COMPRESSION STOCKINGS

Graded compression stockings (also known as thromboembolism deterrent or TED stockings) promote venous flow in the legs by providing 18 mm Hg external compression at the ankles and 8 mm Hg external compression in the thigh (3). These stockings have proven effective in reducing the incidence of thromboembolism associated with major abdominal surgery and neurosurgery (9,10). Nevertheless, TED stockings are not recommended as the sole preventive measure in any moderate- or high-risk clinical condition (2).

TABLE 7.2. PREFERRED (P) AND ALTERNATIVE (A) METHODS OF THROMBOPROPHYLAXIS				
Condition	Pneumatic Boots	Low-Dose Heparin	LMW Heparin	Low-Dose Warfarin
Moderate-risk general surgery	A	P		
High-risk general surgery	A	P		
Neurosurgery	P	A		
Prostate surgery	P	A		
Total hip replacement			P	A
Hip fracture			A	P
Knee surgery	P		A	
Acute MI		P		
Ischemic stroke	A	P		
Spinal cord injury or paralysis			P	
From GP Clagget et al. Third ACCP Consensus Conference on Antithrombotic Therapy. Chest 1992;102(Suppl):391S–407S.				

INTERMITTENT PNEUMATIC COMPRESSION BOOTS

Intermittent pneumatic compression boots are inflatable devices that provide 35 mm Hg external compression at the ankle and 20 mm Hg external compression at the thigh. These devices are considered more effective than graded compression stockings, and can more than double the venous flow rate in the legs (2,3). Because there is no risk of bleeding with pneumatic boots, they are favored in neurosurgical patients and in patients undergoing prostatectomy (2,3). Pneumatic boots are also very effective in patients undergoing reconstructive surgery of the knee, and can be used as the sole prophylactic measure in these patients if there is no interference from immobilization casts.

LOW-DOSE HEPARIN

The major anticoagulant action of heparin is to activate antithrombin III, which then inhibits the conversion of prothrombin to thrombin. In the absence of active thrombosis, this action occurs at low doses of heparin, below the doses that interfere with other components of the coagulation process. As a result, low doses of heparin can inhibit thrombus formation without creating the risk of hemorrhage associated with full anticoagulation (11).

Dosing Regimen

The usual low-dose heparin regimen is 5000 IU subcutaneous every 12 hours. In surgical patients, the initial dose is given 2 hours before surgery, and therapy continues through the first postoperative week, or until the patient is ambulatory. Laboratory tests of coagulation status are not monitored.

Low-dose heparin is recommended as effective prophylaxis in major abdominal surgery and in acute medical illnesses with a risk of thromboembolism. It does not provide optimal prophylaxis in high-risk traumatic and orthopedic conditions.

LOW-MOLECULAR-WEIGHT HEPARIN

Conventional preparations of heparin contain a heterogeneous mix of polysaccharide molecules that vary widely in size, and only 30% of the molecules show anticoagulant activity (11,12). These molecules can be broken down (enzymatically) into smaller molecules of more uniform size. The low-molecular-weight (LMW) heparin has more anticoagulant activity and produces an anticoagulant effect at lower dosages than the conventional unfractionated heparin. The potential advantages of LMW heparin over unfractionated heparin include less frequent dosing, lower risk of bleeding, and a lower incidence of heparin-induced thrombocytopenia (11–13). At present, many of these advantages are more theoretical than actual. The disadvantage of LMW heparin is the cost. Prophylaxis with LMW heparin using the regimen shown below is 10 times more costly (per day) than low-dose heparin (13).

Dosing Regimen

For enoxaparin (Lovenox, Rhone-Poulenc Rorer Pharmaceuticals), the dosage for thromboprophylaxis is 30 mg subcutaneous every 12 hours. Laboratory tests of coagulation status are not monitored.

LMW heparin is more effective than low-dose heparin in hip fractures, reconstructive surgery of the hip and knee, and acute spinal cord injury with paralysis (Table 7.2) (2,12). It is not recommended in patients with active bleeding, or in documented cases of heparin-induced thrombocytopenia.

LOW-DOSE WARFARIN

Low-level anticoagulation with coumadin is an effective alternative to LMW heparin in patients with a high risk of thromboembolism. However, prophylaxis with coumadin is more cumbersome than LMW heparin because it requires dosage titration and monitoring of laboratory tests of coagulation status.

Dosing Regimen

The initial dose of coumadin is 10 mg orally, followed by a daily dose of 2 mg. The dosage is then adjusted to achieve a prothrombin time with an international normalized ratio (INR) of 2 to 3 (2). (See Reference 25 for a description of the INR).

Low-dose warfarin is recommended in the same high-risk clinical conditions as low-molecular-weight heparin. Because it has been shown to reduce the incidence of fatal pulmonary embolism in patients with hip fractures (2), low-dose warfarin may be the preferred method of prophylaxis for hip fractures.

VENA CAVA FILTERS

Meshlike filters can be placed in the inferior vena cava to prevent embolization of clots in the leg veins (14,15). The indications for placement of a vena caval filter are listed below.

Indications

    A. Documented iliofemoral vein thrombosis and
        1. Contraindication to anticoagulation (such as active hemorrhage)
        2. Documented pulmonary embolization during full anticoagulation
        3. Free-floating thrombus

4. High-risk condition for fatal pulmonary embolus (such as severe lung disease)
B. No iliofemoral vein thrombosis, but
1. Long-term prophylaxis is necessary (as in paraplegia)
2. High risk for both thromboembolism and hemorrhage

The Greenfield Filter

The most widely used vena caval filter in the United States is the Greenfield filter (Medi-Tech, Watertown, Mass.) shown in Figure 7.1. The conical shape of this filter is a structural advantage because as much as 75% of the basket can be filled with a thrombus without compromising the cross-sectional area of the vena cava. This design limits the risk for vena cava obstruction and troublesome leg edema.

Greenfield filters are inserted percutaneously, usually through the internal jugular vein or femoral vein, and are placed below the renal veins, if possible. Suprarenal placement is occasionally necessary when the thrombus extends to the level of the renal veins, and does not impair venous drainage from the kidneys.

The Greenfield filter has been the preferred vena cava filter in the United States for last 20 years, and has proven both safe and effective. The reported incidence of pulmonary embolism with a caval filter in place is 2 to 5% (14), and fatal embolism is rare. Complications are uncommon. Venous insufficiency occurs in only 5% of cases (14), and troublesome migration of the filters is rare. The cost of inserting these devices deserves mention. In 1992, the patient charge for percutaneous placement of a Greenfield filter was $5300 in one hospital (16).

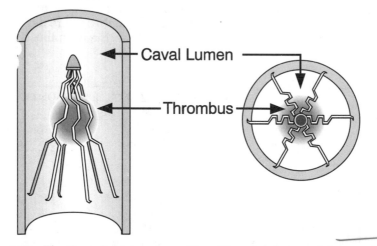

Figure 7.1. The Greenfield vena cava filter. Note the elongated shape, which allows the filter to trap thrombi without compromising the cross-sectional area of the vena cava.

DIAGNOSTIC APPROACH

As mentioned earlier, thrombosis in the deep veins of the thigh is often clinically silent, and the problem becomes evident only when a pulmonary embolus occurs. Therefore, the diagnostic evaluation of thromboembolism usually involves patients suspected of having an acute pulmonary embolism.

CLINICAL PRESENTATION

The clinical manifestations of acute pulmonary embolism are neither sensitive nor specific enough to be of diagnostic value. As shown in Table 7.3, no single clinical manifestation can reliably predict whether a pulmonary embolus is present. Of particular note is the observation that hypoxemia may be absent in 30% of patients with acute pulmonary embolism (i.e., negative predictive value = 0.70). Although not shown in Table 7.3, a normal alveolar–arterial Po_2 gradient also does not exclude the presence of an acute pulmonary embolism (17). Thus, **clinical presentation cannot be used to confirm or exclude the presence of pulmonary emboli.** When the clinical findings are suspicious for an acute pulmonary embolism, the diagnostic evaluation can proceed according to the algorithm in Figure 7.2.

VENOUS ULTRASOUND

The diagnostic evaluation in Figure 7.2 begins with a search for thrombosis in the proximal veins of the leg. This approach is based on the fact that **pulmonary embolism is not a primary illness, but is a secondary manifestation of an underlying venous thrombosis.** Because most pulmonary emboli originate from thrombi in the femoral veins (1), the evaluation begins with a search for thrombosis in the deep veins of the thigh.

TABLE 7.3. CLINICAL FINDINGS IN ACUTE PULMONARY EMBOLISM		
Manifestation	Positive Predictive Value	Negative Predictive Value
Dyspnea	0.37	0.75
Tachypnea	0.48	0.75
Pleuritic chest pain	0.39	0.71
Hemoptysis	0.32	0.67
Hypoxemia	0.34	0.70
Effusion on chest film	0.40	0.69
Infiltrate on chest film	0.33	0.71
From Hoellerich VL, Wigton RS. Diagnosing pulmonary embolism using clinical findings. Arch Intern Med 1986;146:1699–1704.		

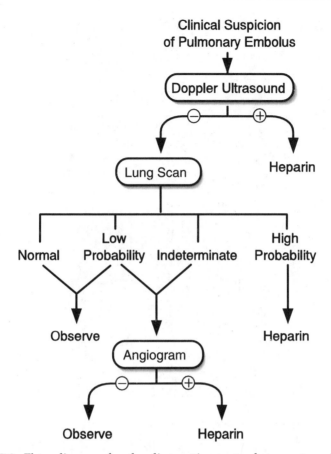

Figure 7.2. Flow diagram for the diagnostic approach to acute pulmonary embolism.

Although contrast venography is the most reliable method of documenting venous thrombosis in the legs, vascular ultrasound has proven to be a reliable noninvasive method for detecting proximal vein thrombosis in the legs. Vascular ultrasound offers two complementary techniques for the detection of venous thrombosis (18). The first technique is **venous compression ultrasound.** This method uses two-dimensional brightness modulation (B-mode) ultrasound to obtain a cross-sectional view of the femoral artery and vein, as shown in panel 1 of Figure 7.3. When a compressive force is created by pushing the ultrasound probe against the overlying skin, the vein becomes obliterated, as shown in panel 2 of Figure 7.3. When a vein is filled with a thrombus, external compression does not obliterate the vessel. Thus, failure to obliterate the femoral vein by external compression is indirect evidence of femoral vein thrombosis.

The second method is **Doppler ultrasound,** which relies on the well-known Doppler shift to detect the velocity of flow in an underlying vessel. This method is particularly valuable when it is difficult to dis-

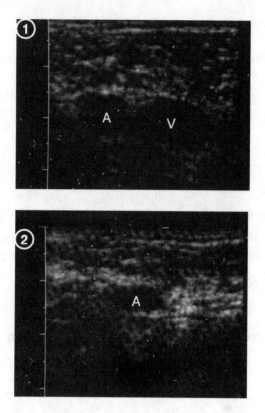

Figure 7.3. Ultrasound visualization of the femoral artery (*A*) and femoral vein (*V*). External compression of the overlying skin in panel 2 results in obliteration of the femoral vein. (Adapted from Cronan JJ, Murphy TP. A comprehensive review of vascular ultrasound for intensivists. J Intensive Care Med 1993;8:188.)

tinguish arteries and veins with two-dimensional B-mode ultrasound. **The combination of compression and Doppler methods is called duplex ultrasound.** This combined (duplex) method is more accurate than either of the individual ultrasound methods, and has a sensitivity of 90 to 100% and a specificity of 80 to 100% for the diagnosis of venous thrombosis in the thigh (18). Ultrasound is less reliable for the detection of calf-vein thrombosis because the veins below the knee are smaller and more difficult to visualize with ultrasound techniques.

Although most pulmonary emboli originate from thrombi in the proximal (iliofemoral) veins of the legs (1), as many as 30% of patients with acute pulmonary emboli show no evidence of venous thrombosis in the legs (19). As a result, **the absence of venous thrombosis in the legs does not exclude the possibility of an acute pulmonary embolus.** When the search for leg vein thrombosis is unrewarding, the next step is to obtain a radionuclide lung scan.

RADIONUCLIDE LUNG SCANS

The interpretation of ventilation–perfusion lung scans can be summarized as follows (20):

A normal lung scan excludes the presence of a (clinically important) pulmonary embolus. A high-probability lung scan means that the patient has an 85% chance of having a pulmonary embolism.

A low-probability lung scan may not reliably exclude the presence of a pulmonary embolism in patients with underlying cardiopulmonary disease. However, when a low-probability lung scan is combined with a negative evaluation for leg vein thrombosis, it is probably safe to observe the patient (and not proceed with pulmonary angiography).

An intermediate-probability or indeterminate lung scan has no value in predicting the presence or absence of a pulmonary embolus.

Using these interpretation guidelines, the lung scan should be the final diagnostic procedure in the majority of patients with suspected pulmonary embolism. Only patients with indeterminate or intermediate-probability lung scans should require further diagnostic evaluation.

PULMONARY ANGIOGRAPHY

Pulmonary angiography is the most accurate (but not infallible) method of confirming or excluding the presence of pulmonary emboli. However, when the diagnostic algorithm in Figure 7.2 is followed, only a minority of cases of suspected pulmonary embolism should require this invasive and expensive procedure.

ANTITHROMBOTIC THERAPY

ANTICOAGULATION

The mainstay of acute therapy for thromboembolism is anticoagulation with intravenous heparin. The goal is to achieve an activated partial thromboplastin time (PTT) that is 1.5 to 2.5 times control levels (21). **Therapeutic levels of anticoagulation should be achieved as soon as possible** because delays in reaching the therapeutic PTT range have been shown to increase the risk of progressive thrombosis and recurrent pulmonary embolism (21). Heparin dosing based on body weight has proven superior to conventional heparin dosing in achieving therapeutic levels of anticoagulation rapidly and safely (22). The recommended dosages of heparin based on (actual) body weight are

TABLE 7.4. WEIGHT-BASED HEPARIN DOSING REGIMEN

1 Prepare herparin infusion by adding 20,000 IU heparin to 500 mL diluent (40 IU/mL).

2 Give initial bolus dose of 80 IU/kg and follow with continuous infusion of 18 IU/kg/hr. (Use actual body weight.)

3 Check PTT 6 hr after start of infusion, and adjust heparin dose as indicated below:

PTT (sec)	PTT Ratio	Bolus Dose	Continuous Infusion
<35	<1.2	80 IU/kg	Increase by 4 IU/kg/hr.
35–45	1.2–1.5	40 IU/kg	Increase by 2 IU/kg/hr.
46–70	1.5–2.3	—	—
71–90	2.3–3.0	—	Decrease by 2 IU/kg/hr.
>90	>3	—	Stop infusion for 1 hour, then decrease by 3 IU/kg.hr.

4 Check PTT 6 hr after each dose adjustment. When in the desired range (46–70 sec), monitor daily.

From Raschke RA et al. The weight-based heparin dosing nomogram compared with the "standard care" nomogram. Ann Intern Med 1993;119:874.

shown in Table 7.4. One point worth noting is that weight-based heparin-dosing nomograms have been derived from patients weighing less than 130 kg (22). In morbidly obese patients (body weight > 130 kg), weight-based heparin dosage can result in excessive anticoagulation (23), so it is important to monitor anticoagulation carefully when using weight-based heparin dosing in the morbidly obese.

Oral anticoagulation with **coumadin can be started on the first day of heparin therapy.** When the prothrombin time reaches an international normalized ratio (INR) of 2 to 3, the heparin can be discontinued. (The INR is a more standardized measurement of the prothrombin time, and has been adopted to reduce the variability in prothrombin time determinations in different clinical laboratories. See Reference 25 for a more detailed description of the INR method.) Although the standard duration of heparin therapy for thromboembolism is 10 to 14 days, recent evidence indicates that **5 days of heparin therapy is as effective as the traditional 10- to 14-day regimen** (24).

Laboratory Abnormalities

Two nonhemorrhagic side effects of heparin treatment deserve mention. The first is **elevation of serum aminotransferase levels,** which has been reported in as many as 80% of patients receiving heparin (26). The increase in serum transaminase levels usually occurs 5 to 10 days after onset of heparin therapy, and peak transaminase levels can be 15 times higher than the normal range. This laboratory abnormality is not associated with liver dysfunction, and it disappears after the drug is discontinued. Therefore, an elevation in serum transaminase levels during heparin treatment should prompt further diagnostic studies unless there is other evidence of liver dysfunction.

The other complication is **hyperkalemia,** which occurs in 5 to 10% of patients receiving heparin (27), and is the result of heparin-induced aldosterone suppression. The hyperkalemia can appear within a few days after the onset of heparin therapy, and has been reported with heparin dosages as low as 5000 IU twice a day (the same dosage used

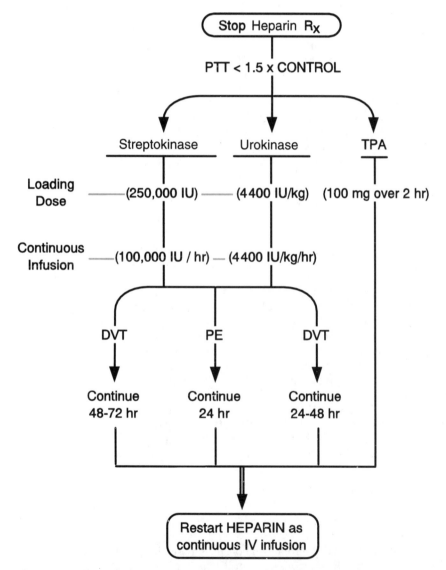

Figure 7.4. Thrombolytic therapy for venous thromboembolism. (From Hyers TM et al. Antithrombotic therapy for venous thromboembolic disease. Chest 1992;102(Suppl):408S.)

in low-dose heparin thromboprophylaxis). The potential for hyperka-lemia has prompted the recommendation that serum potassium levels be monitored periodically in patients receiving heparin for more than 3 days (27).

THROMBOLYTIC THERAPY

Early therapy with thrombolytic agents is associated with more rapid and more complete resolution of venous thromboemboli than anticoagulation therapy with heparin (28,29). Despite this advantage, thrombolytic therapy has not gained widespread favor in the acute management of venous thromboembolism. Several factors contribute to this lack of enthusiasm. Foremost is the risk of hemorrhage, which contraindicates thrombolytic therapy in a large number of hospitalized patients. In one study, 93% of patients with leg vein thrombosis had at least one contraindication to thrombolytic therapy (30). (See Chapter 19 for the contraindications to thrombolytic therapy.) In addition, thrombolytic therapy has not had a significant impact on mortality and (early) morbidity associated with venous thromboembolism (28). A final drawback is the brief therapeutic window for thrombolytic therapy: Thrombolytic agents are effective only if given within the first 7 days after the onset of thromboembolism (28). Because proximal leg vein thrombosis is often clinically silent (and thus the time of onset is not known), it is often not known whether thrombolytic therapy will fall in the appropriate therapeutic window.

The recommended dosages of three thrombolytic agents in venous thrombosis and pulmonary embolism are shown in Figure 7.4. All three agents should be considered equivalent in efficacy and risk of hemorrhage (28). If streptokinase is administered, a thrombin time should be obtained a few hours after the onset of drug therapy. Prolon-gation of the thrombin time to twice control values provides evidence for a proteolytic state in the plasma (29). If the thrombin time is not sufficiently prolonged, give a second loading dose that is double the initial dose (to overcome binding by streptokinase antibodies), and recheck the thrombin time 2 to 3 hours later. Failure to achieve an adequate lytic state after the second loading dose is reason to switch to another lytic agent. Thrombolytic therapy should always be fol-lowed by anticoagulation therapy with heparin and warfarin. (For more information on thrombolytic therapy, see Chapter 19.)

REFERENCES

REVIEWS

1. Moser KM. Venous thromboembolism. Am Rev Respir Dis 1990;141:235–249 (199 references).
2. Claggett GP, Anderson FA, Levine MN, et al. Prevention of venous thrombo-embolism. In: Dalen JE, Hirsh J, eds. Third ACCP Consensus Conference on Antithrombotic Therapy. Chest 1992;102(Suppl):391S–407S (210 references).

3. Goldhaber SZ, Marpurgo M, for the WHO/ISFC Task Force on Pulmonary Embolism. Diagnosis, treatment and prevention of pulmonary embolism. JAMA 1992;268:1727–1733 (57 references).
4. Weinmann EE, Salzman EW. Deep-vein thrombosis. N Engl J Med 1994;331:1630–1641 (215 references).

CONCISE REVIEWS

5. Cowen J, Kelley MA. Pulmonary embolism in the critically ill: strategies for prevention and management. J Crit Illness 1994;9:988–991.
6. Rosenow EC III. Venous and pulmonary thromboembolism: an algorithmic approach to diagnosis and management. Mayo Clin Proc 1995;70:45–49.

THROMBOPROPHYLAXIS

7. Thromboembolic Risk Factors (THRIFT) Consensus Group. Risk of and prophylaxis for venous thromboembolism in hospitalized patients. BMJ 1992;305:567–574.
8. Anderson FA Jr, Wheeler B, Goldberg RJ, et al. Physician practices in the prevention of venous thromboembolism. Ann Intern Med 1991;115:591–596.
9. Wells PS, Lensing AW, Hirsh J. Graduated compression stockings in the prevention of postoperative venous thromboembolism. A meta-analysis. Arch Intern Med 1994;154:67–72.
10. Turpie AG, Hirsh J, Gent M, et al. Prevention of deep vein thrombosis in potential neurosurgical patients. Arch Intern Med 1989;149:679–681.
11. Hirsh J, Dalen JE, Deykin D, Poller L. Heparin: mechanism of action, pharmacokinetics, dosing considerations, monitoring, efficacy and safety. Chest 1992;102(Suppl):337S–351S.
12. Hirsh J, Levine MN. Low-molecular-weight heparin. Blood 1992;79:1–17.
13. Warkentin TE, Levine MN, Hirsh J, et al. Heparin-induced thrombocytopenia in patients treated with low-molecular-weight heparin or unfractionated heparin. N Engl J Med 1995;332:1330–1335.
14. Becker DM, Philbrick JT, Selby B. Inferior vena cava filters. Indications, safety, effectiveness. Arch Intern Med 1992;152:1985–1994.
15. Smith BA. Vena cava filters. Emerg Med Clin North Am 1994;12:645–656.
16. Magnant JG, Walsh DB, Juravsky LI, Cronenwett JL. Current use of inferior vena cava filters. J Vasc Surg 1992;16:701–706.

DIAGNOSTIC APPROACH

17. Stein PD, Goldhaber SZ, Henry JW. Alveolar–arterial oxygen gradient in the assessment of acute pulmonary embolism. Chest 1995;107:139–143.
18. Stewart JH, Grubb M. Understanding vascular ultrasonography. Mayo Clin Proc 1992;67:1186–1196.
19. Hull RD, Hirsh J, Carter CJ, et al. Pulmonary angiography, ventilation lung scanning, and venography for clinically suspected pulmonary embolism with abnormal perfusion scans. Ann Intern Med 1983;98:891–899.
20. Kelley MA, Carson JL, Palevsky HI, Schwartz S. Diagnosing pulmonary embolism: new facts and strategies. Ann Intern Med 1991;114:300–306.

ANTITHROMBOTIC THERAPY

21. Hull RD, Raskob GE, Rosenbloom D, et al. Optimal therapeutic level of heparin therapy in patients with venous thrombosis. Arch Intern Med 1992;152: 1589–1595.
22. Raschke RA, Reilly BM, Guidry JR, et al. The weight-based heparin dosing nomogram compared with a "standard care" nomogram. Ann Intern Med 1993;119:874–881.
23. Holliday DM, Watling SM, Yanos J. Heparin dosing in the morbidly obese patient. Ann Pharmacother 1994;28:1110–1111.
24. Hull RD, Raskob GE, Rosenbloom D, et al. Heparin for 5 days compared with 10 days in the initial treatment of proximal venous thrombosis. N Engl J Med 1990;322:1260–1264.
25. Le DT, Weibert RT, Sevilla BK, et al. The international normalized ratio (INR) for monitoring warfarin therapy: reliability and relation to other monitoring methods. Ann Intern Med 1994;120:552–558.
26. Salomon F, Schmid M. Heparin. N Engl J Med 1991;325:1585.
27. Oster JR, Singer I, Fishman LM. Heparin-induced aldosterone suppression and hyperkalemia. Am J Med 1995;98:575–586.
28. Hyers TM, Hull RD, Weg JG. Antithrombotic therapy for venous thromboembolic disease. Chest 1992;102(Suppl):408S–425S.
29. Rogers LQ, Lutcher CL. Streptokinase therapy for deep vein thrombosis: a comprehensive review of the English literature. Am J Med 1990;88:389–395.
30. Markel A, Manzo RA, Strandess E Jr. The potential role of thrombolytic therapy in venous thrombosis. Arch Intern Med 1992;152:1265–1267.

8

ANALGESIA AND SEDATION

Men do not fear death, they fear the pain of dying.
Apsley Cherry-Garrard

Contrary to popular perception, our principal function in patient care is not to save lives (because this is impossible on a consistent basis), but to relieve suffering. And there is no location in the hospital that can match the suffering experienced by both patients and families than the intensive care unit. To get an idea of how well prepared we are to relieve pain and suffering in the ICU, look at Figure 8.1.

This chapter focuses on the available methods for establishing patient comfort in the ICU with parenterally administered analgesic and sedative medications. For more information on this important topic, a number of general reviews are included at the end of the chapter (1–7).

PAIN IN THE ICU

PREVALENCE

Although a majority of patients in the ICU receive parenteral analgesics routinely (8,9), pain is a prominent part of the patient experience in the ICU. Anywhere from 30 to 70% of patients are bothered by pain during their ICU stay (10–12), and the pain is described as moderate, severe, or excruciating in over half of the cases (10,12). In a survey of patients discharged from an ICU, half of the respondents identified pain as their worst memory of the ICU experience (13). (For a vivid, first-hand account of the pain involved in being an ICU patient, as experienced by a critical care physician, see Reference 14.) It appears

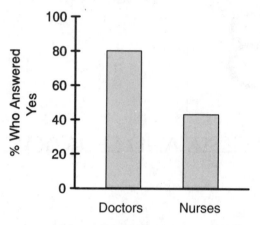

Figure 8.1. Percentage of house staff physicians and ICU nurses who answered incorrectly when asked whether diazepam (Valium) is an analgesic. (From Loper KA et al. Paralysed with pain: the need for education. Pain 1989; 37:315.)

that the incidence of inadequate analgesia in the ICU is the same today as it was 30 years ago (11).

OPIOPHOBIA

The problem of inadequate pain control is caused largely by misconceptions about the addictive potential of narcotic analgesics and about the appropriate dosage needed to achieve effective analgesia (15). The following statements are directed at these misconceptions.

Opiate use in hospitalized patients does not create drug addicts (16).

The effective dosage of a narcotic analgesic is determined by the patient response, not by some perception of what an effective dosage should be (2–4).

Avoiding irrational fears about narcotic analgesics is an important step in learning to provide adequate pain relief for ICU patients.

MONITORING PAIN

Pain severity can be recorded using a variety of pain intensity scales such as the ones shown in Figure 8.2 (1). The uppermost scale (Adjective Rating Scale) uses descriptive terms, the middle scale (Numerical

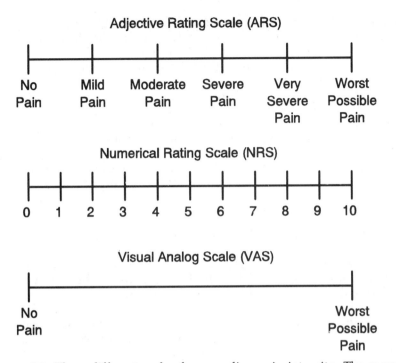

Figure 8.2. Three different scales for recording pain intensity. The recommended length for the numeric scales (NRS and VAS) is 10 cm. For more information on recording pain intensity, see Reference 1.

Ranking Scale) uses whole numbers, and the lower scale (Visual Analog Scale) records pain intensity as a discrete point placed along a line between two ends of the pain intensity spectrum. The Visual Analog Scale is the one most commonly used in clinical studies of analgesic regimens (1), but there is no evidence that any one scale is superior to the others.

Pain intensity scales are used to evaluate the effect of analgesic regimens in individual patients. A numerical score of 3 or less on the Numerical Rating Scale or Visual Analog Scale can be used as evidence of effective analgesia (3). However, it seems easier to just ask the patient whether he or she has pain, and whether he or she would like something to relieve it. Direct communication with patients is not only the best method of determining comfort needs, it is itself a source of comfort to patients.

OPIOID ANALGESIA

Chemical derivatives of opium are called opiates. These substances are also called narcotics (sleep-inducers), but this term has become stigmatized by law enforcement agencies (who use the term to refer to illicit drugs) and is no longer useful. Opiates produce their effects by stimulating discrete receptors in the central nervous system called opioid receptors. There are at least three types of opioid receptors: μ, κ, and σ. Stimulation of μ receptors produces analgesia, euphoria, bradycardia, constipation, and respiratory depression. κ-Receptor stimulation produces sedation and pupillary constriction. σ receptors produce dysphoria, delirium, and hallucinations. Opiates and other chemical substances that stimulate opioid receptors are called opioids.

Opioids are the most commonly administered agents for pain relief *and* sedation in the ICU (8,9). The opioids used most often are morphine and fentanyl, delivered via intravenous, intrathecal, or epidural routes.

INTRAVENOUS OPIOIDS

The intravenous administration of morphine and fentanyl is described in Table 8.1 (1–4,17–19). The response to opioids varies in individual patients (3), and a wide range of dosages may be necessary to achieve effective analgesia in individual patients. As mentioned earlier, **the effective opioid dosage should be determined by patient response, not by the numerical values of the dosage.** The dosages shown in Table 8.1 are the usual effective dosages but may not apply to all patients.

Fentanyl versus Morphine

In surveys including both medical and surgical ICUs, morphine was the most common agent given for *both* analgesia and sedation (8,9). Although fentanyl seems less popular, it may be the preferred opioid agent for analgesia in the ICU. One of the most noted differences between fentanyl and morphine is their lipid solubility. Fentanyl is roughly 40 times more lipid soluble than morphine, so fentanyl is

TABLE 8.1. INTRAVENOUS OPIOID ANALGESIA (3, 17, 18)		
	Morphine	**Fentanyl**
Loading dose	5–15 mg	50–150 μg
Maintenance infusion	1–6 mg/hr	30–100 μg/hr
Lipid solubility	$\times$	40 $\times$
Onset of action	10–20 min	1–2 min
Duration of action	4 hr	1 hr
Therapeutic index*	70	2727
Wholesale cost	$0.57 per 10 mg	$2.81 per 100 μg
Patient-Controlled Analgesia		
Dose	0.2–3 mg	20–100 μg
Lockout interval	8–10 min	5–8 min

* Therapeutic index is the ratio of the lethal dose to the effective dose.
From references 3,17,18.

taken up into the (lipid-laden) central nervous system much more readily than morphine. This makes fentanyl a more potent analgesic than morphine. In general, fentanyl produces equivalent analgesia at 1/100 the dose of morphine. Fentanyl is also more rapidly acting than morphine, and thus can be titrated more rapidly. Both opioids should be given by continuous infusion, preceded by a loading dose. Intermittent as needed (PRN) dosing is never recommended for pain control in the ICU (2–4) because of the high incidence of inadequate analgesia with PRN dosing schedules.

Opioids are metabolized primarily in the liver, and the metabolites are excreted in the urine. Morphine has an active metabolite that can accumulate in renal failure, and for this reason, the dosage of morphine should be reduced by 50% in patients with renal failure (i.e., creatinine clearance less than 10 mL/min) (19). The recommendations for fentanyl dosing in renal failure are inconsistent. One source recommends a 50% reduction in the fentanyl dosage in renal failure (19), and another source recommends no change in dosage (20).

For patients **with unstable or compromised hemodynamic function, fentanyl is preferred to morphine** for two reasons. The first reason is more rapid titration with fentanyl, as mentioned earlier. The second reason is tendency for morphine to promote histamine release, which promotes vasodilation and hypotension. Fentanyl shows much less tendency to stimulate histamine release, so fentanyl use eliminates the risk of adverse hemodynamic effects produced by histamine.

Patient-Controlled Analgesia

For patients who are awake and aware, a method known as patient-controlled analgesia (PCA) can be used for pain control. This method involves intermittent intravenous doses of an opioid delivered on-demand by the patient, using a self-activating infusion pump. A mandatory time interval is set between successive doses. This time interval is called the "lockout interval" because the patient is unable to deliver a dose of the drug during this time.

The recommended dosage regimens for PCA are included in Table 8.1. The lockout interval for each drug is close to the time required for the onset of drug action. Common lockout intervals are 5 minutes for fentanyl and 10 minutes for morphine. The intermittent dose and the lockout interval must be specified when the orders for PCA are written.

Patient satisfaction is often greater with PCA than with conventional intravenous dosing (21,22), and the technique is particularly popular in postoperative patients.

EPIDURAL OPIOIDS

Epidural installation of opioids is a popular method of pain control in the early postoperative period following thoracic and abdominal surgery. Catheters are placed in the epidural space at the cervical,

TABLE 8.2. EPIDURAL ANALGESIA AND ANESTHESIA			
		Infusion Rate (mL/hr)	
Agent	Concentration*	Thoracic	Lumbar
Morphine	20–60 μg/mL	6–10	8–15
Fentanyl	1–10 μg/mL	6–10	8–15
Bupivacaine	0.0625–0.25%	4–8	6–15

* Use concentrations in the lower end of each range when opioids are used with bupivacaine, and use concentrations in the higher end of the range when opioids are used alone.
From Hamill RJ, Rowlingson JC. Handbook of critical care pain management. New York: McGraw-Hill, 1994;218.

thoracic, or lower lumbar level while the patient is in the operating room, and the analgesics are administered through these catheters for the first few postoperative days. The dosing regimens for epidural analgesia are shown in Table 8.2 (23). The opioids can be given as intermittent bolus doses but are more commonly given as a continuous infusion along with a local anesthetic such as bupivacaine. The addition of the local anesthetic provides more effective analgesia. To minimize the risk of impaired motor function and local sympathectomy (with hypotension) that accompany epidural anesthesia, only dilute solutions of local anesthetics are instilled.

Benefits

There is little evidence that the epidural route provides any advantage over the intravenous route for opioid analgesia. When a local anesthetic is added to the epidural regimen, the analgesia seems to be more effective than with intravenous opioids (24). However, epidural opioids alone do not provide better analgesia than intravenous opioids (24). More important, epidural analgesia does not reduce postoperative morbidity (cardiovascular, pulmonary, or gastrointestinal) when compared with intravenous analgesia (24).

Adverse Effects

Adverse effects of epidural analgesia are more common with morphine than with fentanyl. Epidural opioids can produce respiratory depression, but the reaction is delayed. The incidence of respiratory depression is 1% for epidural morphine and 0.9% for intravenous morphine (24). More prevalent side effects of epidural analgesia include pruritus (28 to 100%), nausea (30 to 100%), and urinary retention (15 to 90%) (24). The pruritus from epidural opioids is discussed in the section of this chapter on adverse effects of opioids.

Intrathecal Opioids

Opioids can also be placed in the subarachnoid space around the lower lumbar spine (in lower doses) to produce analgesia. However, there is a risk of arachnoiditis if catheters are left in place, so the epidural route is favored.

ADVERSE EFFECTS OF OPIOIDS

There is a long list of adverse reactions to opioids; the most important are discussed here. (For a more comprehensive review of opioid side effects, see References 25 and 26.) The opioid antagonist naloxone is mentioned here, but the use of naloxone is described in Chapter 53.

Respiratory Depression

The same receptor that mediates the analgesic actions of opiates also produces respiratory depression. Therefore, some degree of respiratory depression is expected with opioid analgesia. Decreases in respiratory rate and tidal volume are common, but these changes can represent a general sedative effect, not specific inhibition of brainstem respiratory neurones (26). In fact, the use of opioids does not seem to increase the frequency of hypoxemic episodes in postoperative patients (27). Patients with sleep-apnea syndrome, however, can develop more frequent apneic episodes with severe oxygen desaturation (i.e., SaO_2 below 80%) during sleep (26).

Cardiovascular Effects

Decreases in blood pressure and heart rate are common side effects of opioid analgesia. However, like respiratory depression, these changes often result from a generalized decrease in sympathetic nervous system activity and are not pathologic changes. Opioid-induced hypotension is well tolerated, at least in the supine position, and usually requires no intervention (26). The same is true of the bradycardia produced by opioids, which is usually asymptomatic at rest.

Intestinal Motility

The depression of gastrointestinal motility associated with opioid use can be a problem in patients in the ICU, who have other conditions that depress bowel motility (the postoperative state). Parenteral naloxone can antagonize this opioid effect, but there is also loss of the analgesic effects. The oral administration of naloxone has been successful in treating constipation from chronic opioid use without producing systemic opioid antagonism (28). The starting dose is 1 mg every 6 hours, titrated upward to a maximum dose of 4 mg every 6 hours.

Pruritus

As mentioned, pruritus is common with epidural opioids, particularly morphine. This effect is resistant to treatment with antihistamines but can be eliminated with naloxone (29). Naloxone at a dosage of 1 to 2 μg/kg/hr can block the pruritus without antagonizing the analgesic actions of the opioids (Dr. Kenneth Sutin, MD, personal communication). Low doses of propofol (10 mg) have also resulted in prompt resolution of the pruritus associated with epidural opioids (30), by an unknown mechanism.

Meperidine

Meperidine (Demerol, Pethidine) was not among the opioid analgesics presented here. The reason for excluding this agent is the risk of neurotoxicity. Meperidine is metabolized to normeperidine in the liver, and this metabolite is excreted very slowly in the urine (elimination half-life of 17 hours). Normeperidine is a neurotoxin, and when it accumulates, it can produce a syndrome characterized by delirium, hallucinations, psychosis, and generalized seizures (31). Normeperidine can accumulate with repeated doses of meperidine, and the accumulation is more pronounced when renal function is impaired. Because there are several conditions in critically ill patients that can impair renal function the risk of neurotoxicity should be particularly high in these patients. Therefore, it does not seem wise to use meperidine as an analgesic in the ICU.

NONOPIOID ANALGESIA

There are few alternatives to the opioids for providing analgesia via the parenteral route. In fact, there is only one alternative, ketorolac.

KETOROLAC

Ketorolac is a nonsteroidal antiinflammatory drug (NSAID) introduced in 1990 as a parenteral analgesic agent for postoperative pain. Because ketorolac had none of the troublesome side effects of the opioids, it became an overnight hit. By the end of 1992, over 26 million patients had received the drug. The popularity of this agent has waned since then, due to a combination of limited efficacy and troublesome side effects.

Actions

Ketorolac is like other NSAIDs (aspirin-like drugs) and has analgesic and antiinflammatory actions. It is more of an analgesic agent, and is 350 times more potent than aspirin (32). Like other NSAIDs, ketorolac inhibits platelet adhesion and can damage the gastric mucosa.

Ketorolac can be given orally, or by intramuscular (IM) or intravenous (IV) injection. After IM injection, analgesia becomes evident at 1 hour, peaks at 2 hours, and lasts 5 to 6 hours. The drug is partly metabolized in the liver and excreted in the urine. Elimination is prolonged in renal impairment and old age.

Efficacy

For postoperative analgesia, 30 mg ketorolac IM is equivalent to 100 mg meperidine IM or 12 mg morphine IM. Ketorolac is usually not given alone, but it is added to opioid analgesia. Often this allows the opioid dosage to be reduced (33). This is the opiate-sparing effect of ketorolac.

Dosing Regimen

IM or IV (34):

10 mg initial dose, then
10 to 30 mg every 4 to 6 hours
Maximum duration: 2 days
Maximum daily dosage: 60 mg for the elderly, 90 mg for the others

This dosing regimen is a restricted version of the original regimen and was amended because of the risk of gastric mucosal injury (34). Although the drug is usually given by IM injection, this can result in hematoma formation (35). The IV route is safer (33). Ketorolac has been given by continuous IV infusion (5 mg/hour), resulting in more effective analgesia than intermittent IV doses (33).

Adverse Effects

Common side effects include somnolence (7%), nausea (7%), dizziness (6%), headaches (4%), and dyspepsia (2%) (32). The bleeding time is prolonged, but there is little evidence of abnormal bleeding. Although gastric ulceration is a concern, the risk is poorly documented. One case of anuric renal failure (onset 1 hour after IM ketorolac) has been reported (36).

ANXIETY IN THE ICU

ANXIETY DISORDERS

Anxiety and related disorders (agitation and delirium) are almost universal in the ICU patient population, with as many as 90% of patients in the ICU showing evidence of an anxiety disorder (7). Anxiety is characterized by a sense of foreboding or doom that is magnified beyond that expected from external circumstances (7,37). The process is thus driven more by internal mechanisms than by external events. If the internal process becomes autonomous and cannot be controlled, the anxiety becomes pathological (i.e., thought processes become counterproductive). Agitation is a combination of anxiety and increased motor activity, and delirium is a specific syndrome complex that may or may not have anxiety as a component (delirium is described in detail in Chapter 50).

SEDATION

Sedation is the process of establishing a state of relaxation or well-being (38). It does not, as often assumed, necessarily involve a depressed level of consciousness. Surveys of sedative drug use in medical ICUs indicate that no fewer than 18 different pharmacologic agents are used for sedation in the ICU (9). The drugs most commonly used are benzodiazepines and opioid analgesics (8,9). The opioids have a prominent sedative effect, and they can be used alone or in combination with benzodiazepines. The benzodiazepines have no analgesic effects, and thus cannot be used alone in patients who have pain as part of their anxiety state. When benzodiazepines are given to patients with pain, they can produce a dysphoric state that adds to the underlying anxiety.

Monitoring

Unfortunately, there is no objective measure of anxiety or sedation, so it is impossible to monitor therapy with sedatives in a quantitative or standardized manner. A few clinical scoring methods are available for anxiety and sedation, but they are not considered reliable enough to be of any value (39).

SEDATION WITH BENZODIAZEPINES

Benzodiazepines seem well-suited for the ICU because they have amnesic effects (anterograde amnesia) and because they are safe to use. Of the 13 benzodiazepines available for clinical use, 3 can be given intravenously: diazepam, lorazepam, and midazolam. Table 8.3 presents some pertinent information on the intravenous benzodiazepines.

DRUG COMPARISONS

The following are some characteristics shared by all of the intravenous benzodiazepines.

All are lipid soluble to some degree.
All are metabolized in the liver and excreted in the urine.

TABLE 8.3. SEDATION WITH INTRAVENOUS BENZODIAZEPINES			
	Diazepam	Lorazepam	Midazolam
Relative lipid solubility	×	0.48×	1.54×
Intravenous dose	0.1–0.2 mg/kg	0.04 mg/kg	0.025–0.35 mg/kg
Dosing interval	3–4 hr	6–12 hr	1–4 hr
Onset of action	1–3 min	5–15 min	1–3 min
Unit Cost*	$0.35/mg	$4.17/mg	$1.40/mg
Cost of equipotent dose in 70-kg adult*	$1.75	$8.34	$8.40

* Armstrong DK, Crisp CB. Pharmacoeconomic issues in sedation, analgesia, and neuromuscular blockade in critical care. New Horiz 1994;2:85.

The pharmacokinetic description does not always correlate with the clinical performance of the drug. For example, the elimination half-life of diazepam is 20 to 50 hours, and is only 2 hours for midazolam, yet the time of recovery from sedation is the same with both agents (40).

The sedative effects of benzodiazepines are more pronounced in old age, general debility, heart failure, and hepatic insufficiency.

Although they do not cause respiratory depression in healthy subjects, benzodiazepines can cause respiratory depression in elderly patients and patients with chronic CO_2 retention.

Diazepam (Valium) is the least favored of the intravenous benzodiazepines because of a tendency for oversedation with repeated drug administration. After a single intravenous dose of diazepam, onset of sedation occurs in 1 to 2 minutes, and the sedative effect lasts 6 to 12 hours (41). Repeated dosing results in accumulation of the drug and its active metabolite, and this accumulation leads to more pronounced sedation with repeated use of the drug.

Certain precautions are required when administering diazepam intravenously. The drug is not water soluble, and nonpolar solvents such as propylene glycol must be added to the commercial preparation to keep the drug in solution. Adding the drug to intravenous fluids can result in precipitation, so the drug should be injected as close to the hub of the catheter as possible (38). The drug is also very irritating, so fluid should be flowing through the catheter during and after the injection. Also, injection into a large central vein is preferred. The rate of injection should not exceed 5 mg/minute.

Lorazepam (Ativan) has the slowest onset and longest duration of action of the intravenous benzodiazepines. After a single intravenous dose of lorazepam, onset of sedation occurs at 5 to 15 minutes, and the sedative effect lasts 10 to 20 hours (41). Because of its long duration of action, lorazepam is best suited for prolonged sedation of stable patients (e.g., chronic ventilator-dependent patients). The same precautions for drug delivery described for diazepam also apply to lorazepam.

Midazolam (Versed) is the benzodiazepine of choice for short-term sedation in the ICU. This agent has the highest lipid solubility,

TABLE 8.4. SEDATION BY CONTINUOUS INFUSION THERAPY		
	Midazolam	Propofol
Loading dose	0.025–0.1 mg/kg	0.25–1 mg/kg
Maintenance infusion		
Light sedation	0.03–0.04 mg/kg/hr	1–3 mg/kg/hr
Deep sedation	0.06–0.15 mg/kg/hr	3–6 mg/kg/hr
Onset of action	1–2 min	<1 min
Time to arousal	Varies with infusion time	<10 min
Daily cost*	$168/24 hr	$180/24 hr
	@ 5 mg/hr	@150 mg/hr

*Based on an average wholesale cost of $1.40/mg for midazolam and $.05/mg for propofol (18).

the fastest onset, and the shortest duration of action of all the intravenous benzodiazepines. Because of its short elimination half-life (1 to 2 hours), midazolam is commonly given by continuous infusion, using the dosages shown in Table 8.4. However, **midazolam often accumulates and produces excessive sedation after prolonged periods of infusion** (i.e., longer than 48 hours) (3,42). This tendency to accumulate is caused partly by the high lipid solubility of the drug and partly by prolonged clearance in critically ill and elderly patients (43). Midazolam accumulation is particularly prominent in obese patients because of the lipophilic nature of the drug. Therefore, **in obese patients, the ideal body weight,** not the actual body weight, should be used to determine the appropriate dosage of midazolam (2).

The tendency for midazolam to accumulate more readily than suspected is caused partly by a misconception about the short elimination half-life of the drug. The rapid elimination of midazolam from the blood partly represents reuptake of the drug into tissues, and thus does not mean rapid elimination from the body. Therefore, the elimination half-life of the drug should not be taken as a reflection of excretion.

TOXIC EFFECTS

The principal toxicity of the benzodiazepines is excessive sedation with depressed consciousness (44). Although ventilation is not suppressed in normal subjects, oversedation with benzodiazepines has been associated with delayed weaning from mechanical ventilation (43,45). The manifestations and treatment of benzodiazepine toxicity are described in Chapter 53.

Withdrawal Syndrome

Abrupt termination of chronic benzodiazepine intake can produce a withdrawal syndrome consisting of extreme agitation, disorientation, paranoid delusion, and hallucinations. Benzodiazepine withdrawal can be a source of unexplained delirium in the first few days after admission to the ICU (46). The risk of withdrawal from long-term benzodiazepine sedation in the ICU is not clear. Gradual withdrawal has been recommended after 1 month of midazolam sedation to prevent this complication (38).

Drug Interactions

Several drugs can interfere with the oxidative metabolism of diazepam and midazolam in the liver, and these are listed in Table 8.5. (These interactions do not apply to lorazepam, which is metabolized by a different mechanism.) **The interaction between erythromycin and midazolam is significant,** and erythromycin should be avoided when possible during midazolam sedation, or the dosage of midazolam should be reduced by 55 to 75% during erythromycin therapy (47).

The interaction between theophylline and the benzodiazepines also deserves mention. **Theophylline antagonizes benzodiazepine sedation** (possibly by adenosine blockade) (48,49), and intravenous aminophylline (110 mg over 5 minutes) has been reported to cause more rapid awakening from benzodiazepine sedation in postoperative patients (48). This is likely to be a significant interaction, so it is wise to avoid theophylline in patients receiving benzodiazepine sedation. This should not be a difficult decision because theophylline is not the most effective bronchodilator available (see Chapter 25).

TABLE 8.5. DRUG INTERACTIONS WITH BENZODIAZEPINES			
Drugs	Mechanism	Significance	Recommendations
Drug Interactions that ENHANCE Benzodiazepine Efficacy			
Cimetidine Erythromycin Isoniazid Ketoconazole Metoprolol Propranolol Valproate	Interfere with hepatic metabolism of diazepam and midazolam.	Interaction between midazolam and erythromycin may be most significant.	Avoid erythomycin and midazolam, or decrease midazolam dosage by 50 to 75%. Otherwise, adjust dosage only when clinically indicated.
Drug Interactions That REDUCE Benzodiazepine Efficacy			
Rifampin	Enhances hepatic metabolism of diazepam and midazolam.	Clinical significance unclear.	Dosage adjustment only when clinically indicated.
Theophylline	Antagonizes benzodiazepine actions, possibly by adenosine blockage.	Clinically proven interaction.	Avoid theophylline (should be possible).

OTHER SEDATIVES

PROPOFOL

Propofol (Deprivan) is a rapid acting sedative that was introduced as an anesthetic induction agent and has since been proposed for short-term sedation in the ICU (50). The major advantage of propofol is rapid awakening, and the major disadvantage is expense. The daily cost of propofol is shown in Table 8.4 (18).

Actions

Propofol is a lipid-soluble agent with a rapid onset and short duration of action. A single intravenous dose of propofol produces sedation within 1 minute of injection. The sedative effect peaks at 2 minutes, and lasts 4 to 8 minutes (50). Recovery from sedation usually occurs within 10 minutes and is not prolonged by prolonged drug administration (51). Propofol is rapidly converted to inactive metabolites in the liver.

Propofol has no analgesic effects. The sedative effects can be accompanied by significant respiratory depression and vasodilation. The vasodilator actions can lead to a decrease in blood pressure, which occurs more often after bolus administration of the drug, or in patients who are hypovolemic or have a labile blood pressure (50,51).

Uses

Propofol has been recommended for short-term sedation in the early postoperative period. Some reports show more rapid weaning from mechanical ventilation associated with propofol sedation compared with midazolam sedation (52). However, this is not a consistent observation (53). At present, the proposed advantage of propofol in promoting more rapid weaning from mechanical ventilation is not documented well enough to justify the extreme expense of the drug.

Preparation and Dosage

Propofol is not water soluble, and the drug is available as a 1% solution (10 mg/mL) in 10% Intralipid (soybean oil, glycerol, and egg lecithin). The recommended dosages of propofol are shown in Table 8.4. Due to its short duration of action, the drug is given by continuous infusion. Because it is very lipophilic, propofol tends to accumulate in obese patients. Therefore, as with midazolam, the dosage of propofol **in obese patients** should be based on **ideal body weight,** not actual body weight (50).

Adverse Effects

The major adverse effects of propofol are respiratory depression and hypotension. Because of the risk of respiratory depression, propofol should be used only in patients who are receiving mechanical ventilation (38,50). The risk of hypotension is greatest after bolus drug administration, and for this reason the loading dose of the drug is sometimes eliminated. Propofol should not be used in patients who are hemodynamically unstable.

HALOPERIDOL

Haloperidol (Haldol) has gained popularity as a sedative in the ICU because of the low risk of cardiorespiratory depression. Although the drug is effective for generalized sedation, it **may be particularly valuable in the patient with delirium** (i.e., confusional anxiety). The disadvantages of the drug include a slow onset of action and the inability for rapid titration of drug dosage. The intravenous route has yet to receive approval by the FDA, but intravenous haloperidol has been proven safe and effective in repeated clinical trials (54,55).

Actions

Intravenous haloperidol has a prolonged distribution time (11 minutes or even longer in critically ill patients) (55), so the onset of action is slow, but the drug can be given by rapid intravenous push. A sedative effect should be evident within 20 minutes after drug injection. The sedation is not accompanied by respiratory depression, and hypotension is unusual unless the patient is hypovolemic or receiving a β-receptor antagonist (55). Extrapyramidal reactions are not common with the intravenous route of drug administration (55,56).

Uses

Because of its delayed onset of action, haloperidol is **not indicated for rapid control of the anxiety state.** A benzodiazepine (e.g., lorazepam, 1 mg) can be added to achieve more rapid sedation (56). Haloperidol is often targeted for the patient with delirium. However, because of the lack of respiratory depression, we use the drug for sedation of ventilator-dependent patients. Because the dosage cannot be titrated rapidly, we reserve the drug for chronic ventilator-dependent patients who are otherwise stable.

Dosage

The dosing recommendations for intravenous haloperidol are shown in Table 8.6. The dosages are higher than the traditional intramuscular dosages of haloperidol. Individual patients show a wide variation in serum drug levels after a given dose of haloperidol (57).

TABLE 8.6. INTRAVENOUS HALOPERIDOL	
Severity of Anxiety	**Dose**
Mild	0.5–2 mg
Moderate	5–10 mg
Severe	10–20 mg
1. Administer by IV push.	
2. Allow 20 minutes for response:	
a. If no response, double the dose.	
b. If partial response, add 1 mg lorazepam.	
3. If no response to 2 doses, switch to another agent.	

If there is no evidence of a sedative response after 20 minutes, the dosage should be doubled. If there is a partial response at 20 to 30 minutes, a second dose can be given along with 1 mg lorazepam (56). Lack of response to a second dose of haloperidol should prompt a switch to another agent.

Adverse Effects

There are two serious but uncommon reactions to haloperidol. One is the **neuroleptic malignant syndrome** (NMS) (58), a potentially fatal condition characterized by hyperthermia, muscle rigidity, autonomic dysfunction, and mental confusion. The muscle rigidity is widespread, and is often associated with rhabdomyolysis and myoglobinuric renal failure. This condition is a variant of the malignant hyperthermia syndrome, and responds to early treatment with the muscle relaxant dantrolene (see Chapter 30). NMS is an idiosyncratic response to haloperidol and is independent of drug dosage or duration of therapy (58). Early recognition is mandatory for successful treatment with dantrolene.

Haloperidol prolongs the QT interval, and this predisposes to the second serious reaction, **torsade de pointes** (polymorphic ventricular tachycardia). This is an uncommon complication, with a reported incidence of 0.4% in patients receiving intravenous haldol in the ICU (59). Nevertheless, because of the risk of this complication, it is wise to avoid haloperidol in patients with a prolonged QT interval and in those with a history of torsade de pointes.

REFERENCES

GENERAL TEXTS

Hamill RJ, Rowlingson JC, eds. Handbook of critical care pain management. New York: McGraw-Hill, 1994.

Park GR, Sladen RN, eds. Sedation and analgesia in the critically ill. Oxford: Blackwell Scientific Publications, 1995.

SYMPOSIA

Hansen-Flaschen J, ed. Improving patient tolerance of mechanical ventilation. Critical Care Clinics, Vol. 10. Philadelphia: WB Saunders, 1994 (October).

Hoyt JW, ed. Pain management in the ICU. Critical Care Clinics, Vol. 6. Philadelphia: WB Saunders, 1990 (April).

CLINICAL PRACTICE GUIDELINES

1. Acute Pain Management Guideline Panel. Acute pain management: operative or medical procedures and trauma. Clinical practice guideline. AHCPR Pub. No. 92-0032. Rockville, MD: Agency for Health Care Policy and Research, Public Health Service, U.S. Department of Health and Human Services, Feb. 1992.

REVIEWS

2. Levine RL. Pharmacology of intravenous sedatives and opioids in critically ill patients. Crit Care Clin 1994;10:709–731 (98 References).
3. Murray MJ, Plevak DJ. Analgesia in the critically ill patient. New Horiz 1994; 2:56–63 (34 References).
4. Wheeler A. Sedation, analgesia, and paralysis in the intensive care unit. Chest 1993;104:566–577 (184 References).
5. Durbin CG. Sedation in the critically ill patient. New Horiz 1994;2:64–74 (66 References).
6. Crippen DW. Pharmacologic treatment of brain failure and delirium. Crit Care Clin 1994;10:733–766 (110 References).
7. Bone RC, Hayden WR, Levine RL, et al. Recognition, assessment, and treatment of anxiety in the critical care patient. Dis Mon 1995;31:296–359 (169 References).

THE PAIN EXPERIENCE

8. Dasta JF, Fuhrman TM, McCandles C. Patterns of prescribing and administering drugs for agitation and pain in patients in a surgical intensive care unit. Crit Care Med 1994;22:974–980.
9. Hansen-Flaschen JH, Brazinsky S, Lanken PN. Use of sedating drugs and neuromuscular blocking agents in patients requiring mechanical ventilation for respiratory failure. JAMA 1991;266:2870–2875.
10. Donovan M, Dillon P, McGuire L. Incidence and characteristics of pain in a sample of medical-surgical inpatients. Pain 1987;30:69–78.
11. Stevens DS, Edwards WT. Management of pain in the critically ill. J Intensive Care Med 1990;5:258–291.
12. Puntillo KA. Pain experiences in ICU patients. Heart Lung 1990;19:526–533.
13. Paiement B, Boulanger M, Jones CW, Roy M. Intubation and other experiences in cardiac surgery: the consumer's views. Can Anesth Soc J 1979;26:173–180.
14. Hayden WR. Life and near-death in the intensive care unit. Crit Care Clin 1994;10:651–658.
15. Zenz M, Willweber-Strumpf A. Opiophobia and cancer pain in Europe. Lancet 1993;341:1075–1076.
16. Porter J, Jick H. Addiction rare in patients treated with narcotics. N Engl J Med 1980;302:123–128.

OPIOID ANALGESIA

17. Willens JS, Myslinski NR. Pharmacodynamics, pharmacokinetics, and clinical uses of fentanyl, sufentanil, and alfentanil. Heart Lung 1993;22:239–251.
18. Armstrong DK, Crisp CB. Pharmacoeconomic issues of sedation, analgesia, and neuromuscular blockade in critical care. New Horiz 1994;2:85–93.
19. Bennett WM, Aronoff GR, Golper TA, et al., eds. Drug prescribing in renal failure. 2nd ed. Philadelphia: American College of Physicians, 1991;63.
20. St. Peter WL, Halstenson CE. The pharmacologic approach in patients with renal failure. In: Chernow B, ed. The pharmacologic approach to the critically ill patient. 3rd ed. Baltimore: Williams & Wilkins, 1994;41–79.

21. Smythe M. Patient-controlled analgesia: a review. Pharmacotherapy 1992;12: 133–141.
22. Egbert AM, Lampros LL, Parks LL. Effects of patient-controlled analgesia on postoperative anxiety in elderly men. Am J Crit Care 1993;2:118–124.
23. Rowlingson JC, Hamill RJ. Techniques of narcotic and local anesthetic administration. In: Hamill RJ, Rowlingson JC, eds. Handbook of critical care pain management. New York: McGraw-Hill, 1994;207–228.
24. Liu S, Carpenter RL, Neal JM. Epidural anesthesia and analgesia. Anesthesiology 1995;82:1474–1506.
25. Buck ML, Blumer JL. Opioids and other analgesics. Adverse effects in the intensive care unit. Crit Care Clin 1991;7:615–637.
26. Schug SA, Zech D, Grond S. Adverse effects of systemic opioid analgesics. Drug Safety 1992;7:200–213.
27. Bailey PL. The use of opioids in anesthesia is not especially associated with nor predictive of postoperative hypoxemia. Anesthesiology 1992;77:1235.
28. Culpepper-Morgan JA, Inturrisi CE, Portenoy RK, et al. Treatment of opioid-induced constipation with oral naloxone: a pilot study. Clin Pharmacol Ther 1992;52:90–95.
29. Gowan JD, Hurtig JB, Fraser RA, et al. Naloxone infusion after prophylactic epidural morphine: effects on incidence of postoperative side-effects and quality of analgesia. Can J Anesth 1988;35:143–148.
30. Borgeat A, Wilder-Smith OHG, Salah M, Rifat K. Subhypnotic doses of propofol relieve pruritus induced by epidural and intrathecal morphine. Anesthesiology 1992;76:510–512.
31. Shochet RB, Murray GB. Neuropsychiatric toxicity of meperidine. J Intensive Care Med 1988;3:246–252.
32. Buckley M, Brogden RN. Ketorolac. A review of its pharmacodynamic and pharmacokinetic properties and therapeutic potential. Drugs 1990;39:86–109.
33. Ready LB, Brown CR, Stahlgren LH, et al. Evaluation of intravenous ketorolac administered by bolus or infusion for treatment of postoperative pain. Anesthesiology 1994;80:1277–1286.
34. Drug Update. Ketorolac doses reduced. Lancet 1993;342:105.
35. Garcha IS, Bostwick J. Postoperative hematomas associated with toradol. Plast Reconstr Surg 1991;88:919–920.
36. Boras-Uber LA, Brackett NC. Ketorolac-induced acute renal failure. Am J Med 1992;92:450–452.

ANXIETY IN THE ICU

37. Hansen-Flaschen J. Improving patient tolerance of mechanical ventilation. Crit Care Clin 1994;10:659–671.
38. Sladen RN. Sedation in the intensive care unit: clinical considerations. In: Reves JG, Greenblatt DJ, Sladen RV, eds. Drug infusion for sedation in the intensive care unit. Boston: Tufts University School of Medicine, 1994;24–36.
39. Hansen-Flaschen J, Cowan J, Polomano RC. Beyond the Ramsay scale: need for a validated measure of sedating drug efficacy in the intensive care unit. Crit Care Med 1994;22:732–733.

INTRAVENEOUS BENZODIAZEPINES

40. Ariano R, Kassum D, Aronson K. Comparison of sedative recovery time after midazolam versus diazepam administration. Crit Care Med 1994;22: 1492–1496.

41. Greenblatt DJ, Ehrenberg DJ, Gunderman J, et al. Kinetic and dynamic study of intravenous lorazepam: comparison with intravenous diazepam. J Pharmacol Exp Ther 1989;250:134–140.
42. Byatt CM, Lewis LD, Dawling S, et al. Accumulation of midazolam after repeated dosage in patients receiving mechanical ventilation in an intensive care unit. BMJ 1984;289:799–800.
43. Malacrida R, Fritz M, Suter P, et al. Pharmacokinetics of midazolam administered by continuous infusion to intensive care unit patients. Crit Care Med 1992;20:1123–1126.
44. Gaudreault P, Guay J, Thivierge RL, Verdy I. Benzodiazepine poisoning. Drug Safety 1991;6:247–265.
45. Shalansky SJ, Naumann TL, Englander FA. Therapy update: effect of flumazenil on benzodiazepine-induced respiratory depression. Clin Pharmacol 1993;12:483–487.
46. Moss JH. Sedative and hypnotic withdrawal states in hospitalized patients. Lancet 1991;338:575 (letter).
47. Olkkola KT, Aranko K, Luurila H, et al. A potentially hazardous interaction between erythromycin and midazolam. Clin Pharmacol Ther 1993;53:298–305.
48. Hoegholm A, Steptoe P, Fogh B, et al. Benzodiazepine antagonism by aminophylline. Acta Anesthesiol Scand 1989;33:164–166.
49. Gallen JS. Aminophylline reversal of midazolam sedation. Anesth Analg 1985; 69:268 (letter).

PROPOFOL

50. Barr J. Propofol: a new drug for sedation in the intensive care unit. Int Anesthesiol Clin 1993;31:131–154.
51. Carrasco G, Molina R, Costa J, et al. Propofol vs. midazolam in short-, medium-, and long-term sedation of critically ill patients. A cost–benefit analysis. Chest 1993;103:557–564.
52. Roekaerts PMHJ, Huygen FJPM, DeLange S. Infusion of propofol versus midazolam for sedation in the intensive care unit following coronary artery surgery. J Cardiothorac Vasc Anesth 1993;7:142–147.
53. Higgins TL, Yared J-P, Estafanous FG, et al. Propofol versus midazolam for intensive care unit sedation after coronary artery bypass grafting. Crit Care Med 1994;22:1415–1423.

HALOPERIDOL

54. Tesar GE, Stern TA. Rapid tranquilization of the agitated intensive care unit patient. J Intensive Care Med 1988;3:195–201.
55. Cassem EH, Lake CR, Boyer WF. Psychopharmacology in the ICU. In: Chernow B, ed. The pharmacologic approach to the critically ill patient. 3rd ed. Baltimore: Williams & Wilkins, 1994;651–665.
56. Sanders KM, Minnema AM, Murray GB. Low incidence of extrapyramidal symptoms in the treatment of delirium with intravenous haloperidol and lorazepam in the intensive care unit. J Intensive Care Med 1989;4:201–204.
57. Lawson GM. Monitoring of serum haloperidol. Mayo Clin Proc 1994;69: 189–190.
58. Sing RF, Branas CC, Marino PL. Neuroleptic malignant syndrome in the intensive care unit. J Am Osteopath Assoc 1993;93:615–618.
59. Wilt JL, Minnema AM, Johnson RF, Rosenblum AM. Torsade de pointes associated with the use of intravenous haloperidol. Ann Intern Med 1993;119: 391–394.

section III
HEMODYNAMIC MONITORING

Errors are not in the art but in the artificers.
Sir Isaac Newton

9

ARTERIAL BLOOD PRESSURE

It should be clearly recognized that arterial pressure cannot be measured with
precision by means of sphygmomanometers.
American Heart Association, Committee for Arterial Pressure Recording, 1951

The arterial blood pressure is one of the most common and most unreliable measurements in modern medicine. The folly of the blood pressure measurement is demonstrated in the following scenario. The most common medical disorder in the United States is hypertension, which affects 20% of Americans over the age of 6 years (1,2). About 80% of patients with hypertension have no evidence of end-organ involvement (1), which means that in the majority of cases of hypertension, the presence of the disorder is based solely on the blood pressure measurement. The standard method for measuring the blood pressure (i.e., sphygmomanometry) is well recognized for its inaccuracy (3), as pointed out by the warning issued by the American Heart Association in the introductory statement. Thus, **the most common medical disorder in the United States (high blood pressure) owes its existence to a technique that was disputed by expert opinion almost 50 years ago.**

This chapter describes the methods used to monitor the arterial blood pressure in critically ill patients. The first section describes some of the shortcomings of indirect pressure recordings, and the final section describes the direct method of recording pressures with intravascular catheters.

INDIRECT MEASUREMENTS

Indirect measurements of arterial pressure are obtained with a device that consists of a cloth cuff with an inflatable rubber bladder on the inner surface. The cloth cuff is wrapped around the arm or leg, and the bladder is inflated to generate a pressure that compresses the underlying artery and veins. The bladder is then slowly deflated, allowing the compressed artery to open, and the arterial pressure is determined either by detecting sounds that are generated (auscultation method) or by recording vascular pulsations (oscillometric method). The accuracy of these indirect pressure determinations is influenced by the size of the inflatable bladder relative to the girth of the compressed limb.

DIMENSIONS OF THE CUFF BLADDER

The inflatable cuff should produce uniform compression of the underlying artery to ensure optimal recordings when the artery is allowed to open. The ability of cuff inflation to produce uniform arterial compression is a function of the size of the inflatable bladder relative to the size of the limb. Figure 9.1 shows the optimal dimensions of the cuff bladder for indirect measurements of brachial artery pressure. The length of the bladder should be at least 80% of the circumference of the upper arm, and the width of the bladder should be at least 40% of the upper arm circumference (3,4). If the bladder size is too small for the arm circumference, the indirect pressure measurements will be falsely elevated (1–5).

The use of inappropriate-sized cuffs is one of the most common sources of error in indirect blood pressure measurements (1–5), so attention to this matter is important. A simple bedside method for evaluating cuff size is described below.

Bedside Method

The following maneuver is recommended for each patient before recording indirect pressures in the arm or leg. First, align the cuff so that its long axis is parallel to the long axis of the arm. Then turn the cuff around so that the inner surface (bladder side) is facing outward. Now wrap the cuff around the upper arm. The bladder (width) should

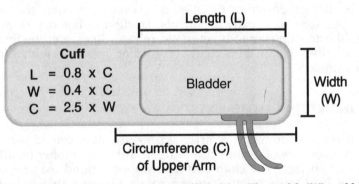

Figure 9.1. Optimal dimensions of the cuff bladder. The width (*W*) and length (*L*) of the bladder are expressed in relation to the circumference (*C*) of the upper arm.

encircle half of the upper arm (circumference). If the bladder encompasses less than half of the upper arm with this maneuver, select a larger cuff for the pressure measurements. No change in cuff size is necessary if the bladder encircles more than half of the upper arm with this maneuver because large cuffs (on thin limbs) do not produce considerable errors in blood pressure recording.

The following is a brief description of two indirect methods of blood pressure recording.

AUSCULTATORY METHOD

The standard method of measuring blood pressure involves manual inflation of an arm cuff placed over the brachial artery. The cuff is then gradually deflated, and the pressure is determined by sounds (called Korotkoff sounds) that are generated when the artery begins to open. The details of this method are not be presented in detail here; see References 3–5 for a review.

The Korotkoff Sounds

One of the fundamental problems of the auscultatory method is the ability to hear the Korotkoff sounds. The threshold frequency for sound detection by the human ear is 16 Hz, and the frequency range of the Korotkoff sounds is just above this threshold at 25 to 50 Hz (6). (Human speech occurs at frequencies of 120 to 250 Hz, whereas optimum sound detection by the human ear occurs at frequencies of 2000 to 3000 Hz.) Thus, **the human ear is almost deaf to the sounds it must hear to measure blood pressure.**

Stethoscope Head

Bell-shaped transducer stethoscope heads are designed to detect lower-frequency sounds than flat, diaphragm-shaped transducer heads. Therefore, to optimize detection of the low-frequency Korotkoff sounds, the American Heart Association recommends that a **bell-shaped stethoscope head be used to measure blood pressure** (2,4). This preference often is not appreciated, as illustrated by the fact that some stethoscopes are manufactured without a bell-shaped head.

Low Flow States

When systemic blood flow is reduced, the auscultatory method can significantly underestimate the actual blood pressure. This is illus-

TABLE 9.1. BLOOD PRESSURE MEASUREMENT IN SHOCK	
Systolic BP Difference (Direct BP − Cuff BP)	% Patients
0–10 mm Hg	0
10–20 mm Hg	28
20–30 mm Hg	22
>30 mm Hg	50

For patients with hypotension and low cardiac output. From Cohn JN. JAMA 1967;119:118–122.

trated in Table 9.1, which shows the difference between systolic pressures measured by auscultation of Korotkoff sounds and systolic pressures recorded with intraarterial catheters in hypotensive patients with low cardiac outputs. In half of the patients, the auscultatory method underestimated the actual systolic blood pressure by at least 30 mm Hg. According to the American Association for Medical Instrumentation, indirect pressure measurements should be within 5 mm Hg of directly recorded pressures to be considered accurate (7). Thus, there was not a single accurate pressure recording with the auscultatory method in the study results shown in Table 9.1.

The poor performance of the auscultatory method in low flow states is not surprising because Korotkoff sounds are generated by the flow of blood through partially constricted arteries. Thus, as flow diminishes, the Korotkoff sounds become less audible, and the earliest sounds that signal the systolic pressure might not be detected. **The potential for large measurement errors** such as those shown in Table 9.1 **is the reason the auscultatory method should never be used to monitor arterial pressures in hemodynamically unstable patients.**

OSCILLOMETRIC METHOD

The oscillometric method is based on the principle of plethysmography to detect pulsatile pressure changes in a nearby artery. When an arm cuff is inflated, pulsatile pressure changes in an underlying artery produce periodic pressure changes in the inflated cuff. The oscillometric method thus measures periodic pressure changes (i.e., oscillations) in an inflated cuff as an indirect measure of pulsatile pressure in an underlying artery (8). The most recognized oscillometric device is the Dinamap (device for indirect assessment of mean arterial pressure), first introduced for clinical use in 1976. The original device could detect only mean arterial pressures, but more modern devices are capable of measuring both systolic and diastolic pressures.

Reliability

Although considered more reliable than the auscultatory method, the oscillometric method also suffers from a limited and variable accu-

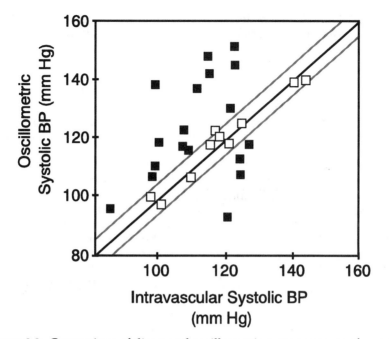

Figure 9.2. Comparison of direct and oscillometric measurements of systolic pressure in the brachial artery. (From Gravlee GP, Brockschmidt JK. Accuracy of four indirect methods of blood pressure measurement, with hemodynamic correlations. J Clin Monitor 1990;6:284–298.)

racy. This is demonstrated in Figure 9.2, which shows a comparison of systolic pressures measured with an automated oscillometric device and systolic pressures recorded with brachial artery catheters in patients undergoing cardiopulmonary bypass surgery. The dark line is the line of unity, where pressures obtained with both recording techniques are identical. The lighter lines are placed 5 mm Hg above and below the line of unity, and (because indirect pressures should be within 5 mm Hg of directly recorded pressures) the area bounded by the lighter lines represents the zone of acceptable accuracy for oscillometric pressure measurements. Note that most of the points fall outside the zone bounded by the lighter lines, (filled squares) indicating that a majority of the oscillometric measurements are inaccurate.

Automated oscillometric devices have gained widespread popularity in recent years, both in hospitals and in outpatient clinics, so it is important to be aware of their limitations.

INTRAVASCULAR PRESSURES

Direct recording of intravascular pressures is recommended for all patients in the ICU who require careful monitoring of arterial pressure. Unfortunately, direct arterial pressure monitoring has its own shortcomings. The following description is intended to help reduce errors in interpretation of directly recorded arterial pressures.

PRESSURE VERSUS FLOW WAVES

Although there is a tendency to consider arterial pressure an index of blood flow, pressure and flow are distinct physical entities. Ejection of the stroke volume generates both a pressure wave and a flow wave. Under normal conditions, the pressure wave travels 20 times faster than the flow wave (10 m/second versus 0.5 m/second), and thus the pulse pressure recorded in a peripheral artery precedes the corresponding stroke volume by a matter of seconds (9). When vascular impedance (i.e., compliance and resistance) is increased, the velocity of transmission of the pressure wave is increased while the velocity of transmission of the flow wave is decreased. (When vascular impedance is reduced, pressure can be diminished while flow is enhanced.) Thus, **when vascular impedance is abnormal, the arterial pressure is not a reliable index of arterial flow.** This discrepancy between pressure and flow is one of the major limitations of arterial pressure monitoring.

THE ARTERIAL PRESSURE WAVEFORM

The contour of the arterial pressure waveform changes as the pressure wave moves away from the proximal aorta. This is shown in Figure 9.3. Note that **as the pressure wave moves toward the periph-**

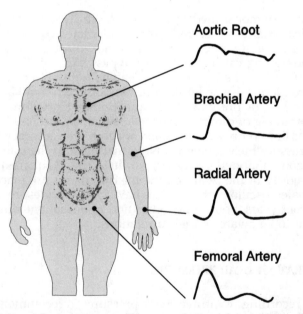

Figure 9.3. Arterial pressure waveforms at designated points in the arterial circulation.

ery, the systolic pressure gradually increases and the systolic portion of the waveform narrows. The systolic pressure can increase as much as 20 mm Hg from the proximal aorta to the radial or femoral arteries. This increase in peak systolic pressure is offset by the narrowing of the systolic pressure wave, so that **the mean arterial pressure remains unchanged.** Therefore, the mean arterial pressure is a more accurate measure of central aortic pressure.

Systolic Amplification

The increase in systolic pressure in peripheral arteries is the result of pressure waves that are reflected back from the periphery (10). These reflected waves originate from vascular bifurcations and from narrowed blood vessels. As the pressure wave moves peripherally, wave reflections become more prominent, and the reflected waves add to the systolic pressure wave and amplify the systolic pressure. **Amplification of the systolic pressure is particularly prominent when the arteries are noncompliant,** causing reflected waves to bounce back faster. This is the mechanism for systolic hypertension in the elderly (10). Because a large proportion of patients in the ICU are elderly, systolic pressure amplification is probably commonplace in the ICU.

RECORDING ARTIFACTS

Fluid-filled recording systems can produce artifacts that further distort the arterial pressure waveform. Failure to recognize recording system artifacts can lead to errors in interpretation.

RESONANT SYSTEMS

Vascular pressures are recorded by fluid-filled plastic tubes that connect the arterial catheters to the pressure transducers. This fluid-filled system can oscillate spontaneously, and the oscillations can distort the arterial pressure waveform (11,12).

The performance of a resonant system is defined by the resonant frequency and the damping factor of the system. The resonant frequency is the inherent frequency of oscillations produced in the system when it is disturbed. When the frequency of an incoming signal approaches the resonant frequency of the system, the resident oscillations add to the incoming signal and amplify it. This type of system is called an underdamped system. The damping factor is a measure of the tendency for the system to attenuate the incoming signal. A resonant system with a high damping factor is called an overdamped system.

WAVEFORM DISTORTION

Three waveforms obtained from different recording systems are shown in Figure 9.4. The waveform in panel *A*, with the rounded

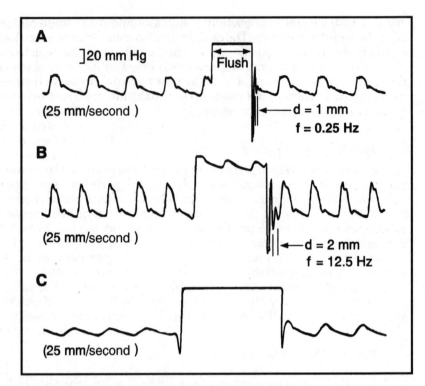

Figure 9.4. The rapid flush test. **A,** Normal test. **B,** Underdamped system. **C,** Overdamped system.

peak and the dicrotic notch, is the normal waveform expected from a recording system with no distortion. The waveform in panel *B*, with the sharp systolic peak, is from an underdamped recording system. The recording systems used in clinical practice are naturally underdamped, and these systems can amplify the systolic pressure by as much as 25 mm Hg (13). The systolic amplification can be minimized by limiting the length of the connector tubing between the catheter and the pressure transducer.

The waveform in panel *C* of Figure 9.4 shows an attenuated systolic peak with a gradual upslope and downslope and a narrow pulse pressure. This waveform is from an overdamped system. Overdamping reduces the gain of the system and is sometimes the result of air bubbles trapped in the connector tubing or in the dome of the pressure transducer. Flushing the hydraulic system to evacuate air bubbles should improve an overdamped signal.

Unfortunately, it is not always possible to identify underdamped and overdamped systems using the arterial pressure waveform. The test described in the next section can help in this regard.

THE FLUSH TEST

A brief flush to the catheter-tubing system can be applied to determine whether the recording system is distorting the pressure waveform (12,14). Most commercially available transducer systems are equipped with a one-way valve that can be used to deliver a flush from a pressurized source. Figure 9.4 shows the results of a flush test in three different situations. In each case, the pressure increases abruptly when the flush is applied. However, the response at the end of the flush differs in each panel. In panel *A*, the flush is followed by a few oscillating waveforms. The frequency of these oscillations is the resonant frequency (*f*) of the recording system, which is calculated as the reciprocal of the time period between the oscillations. When using standard strip-chart recording paper divided into 1-mm segments, *f* can be determined by measuring the distance between oscillations and dividing this into the paper speed (11); that is, *f* (in Hz) = paper speed (in mm/second) divided by the distance between oscillations (in mm). In the example shown in panel *A*, the distance (*d*) between oscillations is 1.0 mm and the paper speed is 25 mm/second, so *f* = 25 Hz (25 mm/second divided by 1.0 mm).

Signal distortion is minimal when the resonant frequency of the recording system is five times greater than the major frequency in the arterial pressure waveform. Because the major frequency in the arterial pulse is approximately 5 Hz (15), the resonant frequency of the recording system in panel *A* (25 Hz) is five times greater than the frequency in the incoming waveform, and the system will not distort the incoming waveform.

The flush test in panel *B* of Figure 9.4 reveals a resonant frequency of 12.5 Hz (*f* = 25/2). This is too close to the frequency of arterial pressure waveforms, so this system will distort the incoming signal and produce systolic amplification.

The flush test shown in panel *C* of Figure 9.4 does not produce any oscillations. This indicates that the system is overdamped, and this system will produce a spuriously low pressure recording. When an overdamped system is discovered, the system should be flushed thoroughly (including all stopcocks in the system) to release any trapped air bubbles. If this does not correct the problem, the arterial catheter should be repositioned or changed.

MEAN ARTERIAL PRESSURE

The **mean arterial pressure** has two features that make it **superior to the systolic pressure for arterial pressure monitoring.** First, the mean pressure is the true driving pressure for peripheral blood flow. Second, the mean pressure does not change as the pressure waveform moves distally, nor is it altered by distortions generated by recording systems (11).

The mean arterial pressure can be measured or estimated. Most electronic pressure monitoring devices can measure mean arterial pressure by integrating the area under the pressure waveform and dividing this by the duration of the cardiac cycle. The electronic measurement is preferred to the estimated mean pressure, which is derived as the diastolic pressure plus one-third of the pulse pressure. This formula is based on the assumption that diastole represents two-thirds of the cardiac cycle, which corresponds to a heart rate of 60 beats/minute. Therefore, heart rates faster than 60 beats/minute, which are common in critically ill patients, lead to errors in the estimated mean arterial pressure.

Cardiopulmonary Bypass

In most circumstances, the mean pressures in the aorta, radial artery, and femoral artery are within 3 mm Hg of each other. However in patients undergoing cardiopulmonary bypass surgery, the mean radial artery pressure can be significantly (more than 5 mm Hg) lower than the mean pressures in the aorta and femoral artery (16). This condition may be caused by a selective decrease in vascular resistance in the hand, because compression of the wrist often abolishes the pressure difference. An increase in radial artery pressure of at least 5 mm Hg when the wrist is compressed (distal to the radial artery catheter) suggests a discrepancy between radial artery pressure and pressures in other regions of the circulation (17).

REFERENCES

INDIRECT MEASUREMENTS

1. Fifth annual report of the Joint National Committee on the Detection, Evaluation, and Treatment of High Blood Pressure. Arch Intern Med 1993;153: 154–183.
2. Reeves RA. Does this patient have hypertension? How to measure blood pressure. JAMA 1995;273:1211–1218.
3. Pickering TG. Blood pressure measurement and detection of hypertension. Lancet 1994;344:31–35.
4. Frolich ED, Grim C, Labarthe DR, et al. Recommendations for human blood pressure determination by sphygmomanometers: report of a special task force appointed by the steering committee, American Heart Association. Hypertension 1988;11:210a–221a.
5. American Society for Hypertension. Recommendations for routine blood pressure measurement by indirect cuff sphygmomanometry. Am J Hypertens 1992; 5:207–209.
6. Ellestad MH. Reliability of blood pressure recordings. Am J Cardiol 1989;63: 983–985.
7. Davis RF. Clinical comparison of automated auscultatory and oscillometric and catheter-transducer measurements of arterial pressure. J Clin Monitor 1985;1:114–119.
8. Ramsey M. Blood pressure monitoring: automated oscillometric devices. J Clin Monitor 1991;7:56–67.

INTRAVASCULAR PRESSURES

9. Darovic GO, Vanriper S. Arterial pressure recording. In: Darovic GO, ed. Hemodynamic monitoring. 2nd ed. Philadelphia: WB Saunders, 1995;177–210.

10. Nichols WW, O'Rourke MF. McDonald's blood flow in arteries. 3rd ed. Philadelphia: Lea & Febiger, 1990;251–269.
11. Gardner RM. Direct blood pressure measurement dynamic response requirements. Anesthesiology 1981;54:227–236.
12. Darovic GO, Vanriper S, Vanriper J. Fluid-filled monitoring systems. In Darovic GO, ed. Hemodynamic monitoring. 2nd ed. Philadelphia: WB Saunders, 1995;149–175.
13. Rothe CF, Kim KC. Measuring systolic arterial blood pressure. Crit Care Med 1980;8:683–689.
14. Kleinman B, Powell S, Kumar P, Gardner RM. The fast flush test measures the dynamic response of the entire blood pressure monitoring system. Anesthesiology 1992;77:1215–1220.
15. Bruner JMR, Krewis LJ, Kunsman JM, Sherman AP. Comparison of direct and indirect methods of measuring arterial blood pressure. Med Instr 1981;15:11–21.
16. Rich GF, Lubanski RE Jr, McLoughlin TM. Differences between aortic and radial artery pressure associated with cardiopulmonary bypass. Anesthesiology 1992;77:63–66.
17. Pauca AL, Wallenhaupt SL, Kon ND. Reliability of the radial arterial pressure during anesthesia. Chest 1994;105:69–75.

chapter

10

THE PULMONARY ARTERY CATHETER

A searchlight cannot be used effectively without a fairly thorough knowledge of the territory to be searched.

Fergus Macartney, FRCP

The pulmonary artery catheter is not just important for the specialty of critical care, it is *responsible* for the specialty of critical care. This catheter is so much a part of patient care that it is impossible to function properly in the ICU without a clear understanding of this catheter and the information it provides. The pulmonary artery catheter is very much like a politician: it seems to function in the best interest of the population it serves, but you are never certain that what it tells you is completely trustworthy.

This chapter introduces the information generated by pulmonary artery catheters (1–4). Most of the hemodynamic variables in this chapter are described in detail in Chapters 1 and 2, so it may help to review these chapters before proceeding further. Remember that the power of the pulmonary artery catheter is based not on its ability to generate information, but on the clinician's ability to understand that information. This may seem to be a trivial point, but surveys indicate that physicians have an inadequate understanding of the measurements provided by pulmonary artery catheters (5).

CATHETER DESIGN

The birth of the pulmonary artery (PA) catheter is described here by HJC Swan, the cardiologist responsible for the original concept of the catheter.

In the fall of 1967, I had occasion to take my (then young) children to the beach in Santa Monica. . . . It was a hot Saturday, and the sailboats on the water were becalmed. However, about half-a-mile offshore, I noted a boat with a large spinnaker well set and moving through the water at a reasonable velocity. The idea then came to put a sail or parachute on the end of a highly flexible catheter and thereby increase the frequency of passage of the device into the pulmonary artery (1).

Three years later (in 1970), a PA catheter was introduced with a small balloon at its tip. When inflated, the balloon serves as a sail that allows the flow of venous blood to carry the catheter through the right side of the heart and out into the pulmonary artery. This balloon flotation principle allows a right heart catheterization to be performed at the bedside, without fluoroscopic guidance.

BASIC FEATURES

A basic PA catheter is illustrated in Figure 10.1. The catheter is 110 cm long and has an outside diameter of 2.3 mm (7 French). There are two internal channels: One channel runs the entire length of the catheter and opens at the very tip of the catheter (the distal port), and the

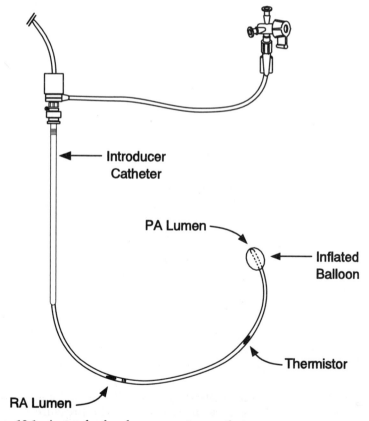

Figure 10.1. A standard pulmonary artery catheter.

other channel is shorter, with an opening 30 cm from the catheter tip (the proximal port). The tip of the catheter is equipped with a balloon with a 1.5-mL capacity. As shown, the fully inflated balloon creates a recess for the tip of the catheter, and this prevents the catheter tip from perforating the vascular structures as the catheter is advanced. Finally, there is a thermistor (i.e., a transducer device that senses changes in temperature) located on the outer surface of the catheter 4 cm from the catheter tip. The thermistor can measure the flow of a cold fluid that is injected through the proximal port of the catheter, and this flow rate is equivalent to the cardiac output (see Chapter 12).

ADDITIONAL ACCESSORIES

Other accessories are available on specially designed PA catheters:

An extra channel that opens 14 cm from the catheter tip and that can be used as an infusion channel or for passing temporary pacemaker leads into the right ventricle (6)

A fiberoptic system that allows continuous monitoring of mixed venous oxygen saturation (7)

A rapid-response thermistor that can measure the ejection fraction of the right ventricle (8)

A thermal filament that generates low-energy heat pulses and allows continuous thermodilution measurement of the cardiac output (9)

The large variety of gadgets available on the PA catheter makes this instrument akin to a Swiss Army knife for the critical care specialist.

INSERTING THE CATHETER

The PA catheter is inserted into the subclavian or internal jugular veins. (A large-bore introducer catheter like the one shown in Figure 10.1 is often used to facilitate insertion and removal of PA catheters.) Just before insertion, the distal port of the catheter is connected to a pressure transducer and oscilloscope monitor. Pressure tracings are monitored continuously while the catheter is inserted to help identify the location of the catheter tip. When the catheter tip first enters the vessel lumen, oscillations appear on the pressure tracing from the distal port of the catheter. When this occurs, the balloon should be fully inflated with 1.5 mL of air. The catheter is then advanced while the balloon is inflated. The pressure waveforms encountered as the catheter is advanced through the right side of the heart are shown in Figure 10.2 (10).

1. The superior vena cava pressure is identified by the appearance of oscillations in the pressure recording. The pressure recorded from the vena cava remains unchanged when the catheter tip

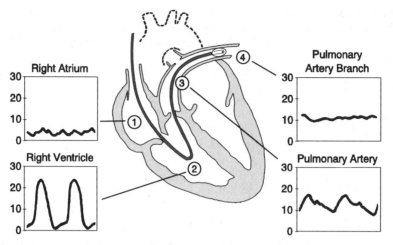

Figure 10.2. The pressure waveforms encountered during insertion of a pulmonary artery catheter.

is advanced into the right atrium. (Normal superior vena cava pressure is 1 to 6 mm Hg.)

2. When the catheter tip is advanced across the tricuspid valve and into the right ventricle, a pulsatile systolic pressure appears. The diastolic pressure on the pulsatile waveform is equal to the right-atrial pressure. (Normal right-ventricular systolic pressure is 15 to 30 mm Hg.)

3. When the catheter is carried across the pulmonic valve and into the pulmonary artery, the diastolic pressure suddenly rises, whereas the systolic pressure remains unchanged. (Normal pulmonary artery diastolic pressure is 6 to 12 mm Hg.)

4. As the catheter is advanced along the pulmonary artery, the systolic component of the waveform suddenly disappears. The pressure that remains is known as the pulmonary capillary wedge pressure (PCWP), and it is usually in the same range as the pulmonary artery diastolic pressure. (Normal wedge pressure is 6 to 12 mm Hg.)

5. When the wedge pressure tracing appears, stop advancing the catheter and deflate the balloon. The pulsatile pulmonary artery pressure should reappear.

BALLOON INFLATION

The balloon at the tip of the PA catheter should be deflated at all times while the catheter is left in place in the pulmonary artery. Balloon inflation is reserved for measurements of the pulmonary artery wedge pressure. When the balloon is inflated for a wedge pressure measurement, do not fully inflate the balloon (with 1.5 mL air) all at once. The balloon should be slowly inflated until a wedge pressure tracing appears on the oscilloscope monitor. Once a satisfactory wedge pressure is recorded, the balloon should be fully deflated. (Detaching the syringe from the balloon injection port will help prevent undetected balloon inflation while the catheter is in place.)

COMMON PROBLEMS

The following are some problems that may appear during the placement of a PA catheter.

Catheter Will Not Advance into the Right Ventricle

In this instance, no pulsatile pressure (from the right ventricle) is obtained even if the catheter is advanced more than 20 cm (see Table 4.4 for the cannulation distances to the right atrium). One maneuver that might resolve this problem is to fill the balloon with 1.5 mL fluid (sterile) instead of air (11). Then position the patient with the left side down and advance the catheter slowly. The fluid adds mass (weight) to the balloon, and this can help the balloon to drop into the right ventricle. The added mass also makes it more difficult for the balloon to be repelled by elevated pressures in the right ventricle. When the right ventricle is entered, the fluid should be removed and the balloon should be reinflated with air.

Catheter Will Not Advance into the Pulmonary Artery

This problem is usually caused by coiling of the catheter in the right ventricle. This problem can be resolved by simply withdrawing the catheter into the superior vena cava and readvancing the catheter. When advancing the catheter through the right ventricle, avoid rapid thrusts. Use slower, more continuous motions to advance the catheter. This allows the catheter to float along with the flow of blood into the pulmonary artery. If repeated attempts to advance the catheter are unsuccessful, consider giving a bolus of calcium sulfate through the distal port of the catheter to stimulate ventricular contraction. The only reported experience with this maneuver is limited and anecdotal; that is, it has been successful in each of three occasions when used by this author.

Arrhythmias

Atrial and ventricular arrhythmias are common during placement of PA catheters (arrhythmias appeared in over 50% of catheter placements in one report) (2). However, the arrhythmias are almost never harmful, and treatment is rarely necessary. If an arrhythmia is noted, withdraw the catheter into the vena cava, and the arrhythmia should disappear. The only rhythm disturbances that warrant immediate intervention are complete heart block (which should be treated with a temporary transvenous pacemaker) and sustained ventricular tachycardia (which should be treated with lidocaine or other suitable antiar-rhythmic agent). Fortunately, these malignant arrhythmias are rarely encountered during PA catheter insertion.

Unable to Obtain a Wedge Pressure

In about one-fourth of PA catheter insertions, the pulsatile PA pressure does not disappear even when the catheter is advanced the maximum distance along the pulmonary artery. This finding may be caused by nonuniform balloon inflation, but the true cause is unknown. When this occurs, the pulmonary artery diastolic pressure can be used as a substitute for the pulmonary capillary wedge pressure (the two pressures should be the same in all patients except those with pulmonary hypertension). Reinsertion of a new PA catheter is not necessary unless the patient has high PA pressures and the physician wants to determine whether the problem is left heart failure.

HEMODYNAMIC PARAMETERS

The most appealing feature of the PA catheter is its ability to generate a large number of (measured and derived) hemodynamic variables. There are 10 different parameters of cardiovascular performance and 4 parameters of systemic oxygen transport. Each of the physiologic variables generated by the PA catheter is described in detail in Chapters 1 and 2 (see Tables 1.1 and 2.4).

BODY SURFACE AREA

Hemodynamic variables are often expressed in relation to body size. Instead of mass (weight), the index of body size that is used is the body surface area (BSA), which incorporates both height (Ht) and weight (Wt). The BSA is obtained by using standard nomograms, or is calculated using a cumbersome equation known as the DuBois formula (see Appendix).

Either method can be replaced by using this simple equation (12):

$$\text{BSA (m}^2) = [\text{Ht (cm)} + \text{Wt (kg)} - 60]/100 \qquad (10.1)$$

The BSA derived by this formula has a 99% correlation with the BSA derived by the standard DuBois formula (13). The average-sized adult has a BSA of 1.6 to 1.9 m^2.

CARDIOVASCULAR PERFORMANCE

The parameters of cardiovascular performance are shown in Table 10.1 (see also Table 1.1). Those expressed in relation to body surface

TABLE 10.1. PARAMETERS OF CARDIOVASCULAR PERFORMANCE		
Parameter	**Abbreviation**	**Normal Range**
Central venous pressure	CVP	1–6 mm Hg
Pulmonary capillary wedge pressure	PCWP	6–12 mm Hg
Cardiac index	CI	2.4–4.0 L/min/m²
Stroke volume index	SVI	40–70 mL/beat/m²
Left-ventricular stroke work index	LVSWI	40–60 g·m/m²
Right-ventricular		
Stroke work index	RVSWI	4–8 g·m/m²
Ejection fraction	RVEF	46–50%
End-diastolic volume	RVEDV	80–150 mL/m²
Systemic vascular resistance index	SVRI	1600–2400 dynes·sec·m²/cm⁵
Pulmonary vascular resistance index	PVRI	200–400 dynes·sec·m²/cm⁵

area (BSA) are denoted by the term *index* (e.g., when cardiac output is expressed relative to BSA, it is called the cardiac index).

Central Venous Pressure

This pressure is recorded from the proximal port of the PA catheter situated in the superior vena cava or right atrium. Central venous pressure (CVP) is equal to the pressure in the right atrium. The right-atrial pressure (RAP) should be equivalent to right-ventricular end-diastolic pressure (RVEDP) when there is no obstruction between the right atrium and ventricle.

$$CVP = RAP = RVEDP \qquad (10.2)$$

Pulmonary Capillary Wedge Pressure

This pressure is measured as described in the last section. Because the PCWP is measured when there is no flow between the catheter tip and the left atrium (because the balloon on the PA catheter tip is inflated), the PCWP should be the same as the left-atrial pressure (LAP). The LAP should also be equivalent to the left-ventricular end-diastolic pressure (LVEDP) when there is no obstruction between left atrium and ventricle.

$$PCWP = LAP = LVEDP \qquad (10.3)$$

Cardiac Index

The thermistor at the distal end of the PA catheter provides a measure of cardiac output (CO) by recording the change in temperature of blood flowing in the pulmonary artery when the blood temperature is reduced by injecting a volume of cold fluid through the proximal port of the PA catheter in the right atrium. This is known as the thermodilution technique, and it measures cardiac output as a mean volumetric blood flow. The cardiac output is expressed as the cardiac index (CI) when it is divided by the BSA.

$$CI = CO/BSA \qquad (10.4)$$

Stroke Volume

The stroke volume index (SVI) is the volume ejected by the ventricles during systole. It is easily derived as the CI divided by the heart rate (HR).

$$SVI = CI/HR \qquad (10.5)$$

Right-Ventricular Ejection Fraction

The ejection fraction is the fraction of ventricular volume that is ejected during systole. The ejection fraction of the right ventricle (RVEF) can be measured with a specialized PA catheter that is equipped with a rapid-response thermistor. The resulting measurement is an index of the ratio between the stroke volume (SV) and the right-ventricular end-diastolic volume (RVEDV).

$$RVEF = SV/RVEDV \qquad (10.6)$$

Right-Ventricular End-Diastolic Volume

When the RVEF is measured, the RVEDV can be determined by rearranging the formula for RVEF shown above.

$$RVEDV = SV/RVEF \qquad (10.7)$$

Left-Ventricular Stroke Work Index

The left-ventricular stroke work index (LVSWI) is the work performed by the ventricle to eject the stroke volume into the aorta. Work is determined by force or pressure (Mean arterial pressure − PCWP) and the corresponding mass or volume (SV) that is moved. The factor 0.0136 converts pressure and volume to units of work.

$$LVSWI = (MAP - PCWP) \times SVI \ (\times \ 0.0136) \qquad (10.8)$$

Right-Ventricular Stroke Work Index

The right-ventricular stroke work index (RVSWI) is the work needed to move the stroke volume across the pulmonary circulation. It is derived as the pressure developed by the right ventricle during systole (Pulmonary artery pressure − CVP) to eject the stroke volume.

$$RVSWI = (PAP - CVP) \times SVI \, (\times \, 0.0136) \qquad (10.9)$$

Systemic Vascular Resistance Index

The systemic vascular resistance index (SVRI) is the vascular resistance across the whole of the systemic circulation. It is proportional to the pressure gradient from the aorta to the right atrium (MAP − CVP), and is inversely related to blood flow (CI). (The factor of 80 is necessary to convert units.)

$$SVRI = (MAP - RAP) \times 80/CI \qquad (10.10)$$

Pulmonary Vascular Resistance Index

The pulmonary vascular resistance index (PVRI) is proportional to the pressure gradient across the entire lungs, from the pulmonary artery (PAP) to the left atrium (LAP). Because the wedge pressure (PCWP) is equivalent to the LAP, the pressure gradient across the lungs can be expressed as (PAP − PCWP). The PVRI can then be derived using the following equation.

$$PVRI = (PAP - PCWP) \times 80/CI \qquad (10.11)$$

SYSTEMIC OXYGEN TRANSPORT

The parameters of systemic oxygen transport are shown in Table 10.2 (see also Table 2.4).

Oxygen Delivery

This is the rate of oxygen transport in arterial blood, and is the product of the cardiac output and the oxygen concentration in arterial

TABLE 10.2. OXYGEN TRANSPORT PARAMETERS		
Parameter	Symbol	Normal Range
Mixed venous oxygen saturation	Sv_{O_2}	70–75%
Oxygen delivery	D_{O_2}	520–570 mL/min·m^2
Oxygen uptake	V_{O_2}	110–160 mL/min·m^2
Oxygen extraction ratio	O_2ER	20–30%

blood. The arterial O_2 delivery (Do_2) is defined by Equation 10.12, where Hb is hemoglobin and Sao_2 is the arterial O_2 saturation (see Chapter 2 for the derivation of this equation).

$$Do_2 = CI \times 13.4 \times Hb \times Sao_2 \qquad (10.12)$$

Mixed Venous Oxygen Saturation

The oxygen saturation in pulmonary artery (mixed venous) blood can be monitored continuously with a specialized PA catheter, or it can be measured in vitro with a blood sample obtained from the distal port of the catheter. (See Chapter 22 for a description of the O_2 saturation measurement.) The Svo_2 varies inversely with the amount of oxygen extracted from the peripheral microcirculation; that is, $Svo_2 = 1/O_2$ extraction.

Oxygen Uptake

Oxygen uptake (Vo_2) is the rate of oxygen taken up from the systemic microcirculation and is the product of the cardiac output and the difference in oxygen concentration between arterial and mixed venous blood. The formula for O_2 uptake shown below is derived in Chapter 2.

$$Vo_2 = CI \times 13.4 \times Hb \times (Sao_2 - Svo_2) \qquad (10.13)$$

Oxygen Extraction Ratio

The oxygen extraction ratio (O_2ER) is the fractional uptake of oxygen from the systemic microcirculation, and is equivalent to the ratio between O_2 delivery and O_2 uptake. This ratio can be multiplied by 100 to express it as a percentage.

$$O_2ER = Vo_2/Do_2 \ (\times 100) \qquad (10.14)$$

HEMODYNAMIC PROFILES

The parameters just described can be organized to provide profiles of specific aspects of cardiovascular performance. Some examples of hemodynamic profiles are presented below.

HEART FAILURE

The performance of the right and left sides of the heart can be evaluated by the relationship between the ventricular filling pressure, the cardiac output (or stroke volume), and the outflow vascular resistance. The following are examples of profiles expected in severe heart failure.

Right Heart Failure	**Left Heart Failure**
High RAP	High PCWP
Low CI	Low CI
High PVRI	High SVRI

HYPOTENSION

The mean arterial pressure is a function of the cardiac output and the systemic vascular resistance: MAP = CI × SVRI. The cardiac output, in turn, depends on the venous return. If the CVP is used as an index of venous return, then there are three variables that can be used to evaluate the source of hypotension: CVP, CI, and SVRI. The following are profiles of these variables in the three classic types of hypotension.

Hypovolemic	**Cardiogenic**	**Vasogenic**
Low CVP	High CVP	Low CVP
Low CI	Low CI	High CI
High SVRI	High SVRI	Low SVRI

CLINICAL SHOCK

Clinical shock syndromes are all characterized by inadequate tissue oxygenation. The parameters of systemic oxygen transport provide an indirect evaluation of peripheral (tissue) oxygenation, and thus can help to identify a shock state. An example of how oxygen transport parameters can identify a shock state is shown below.

Heart Failure	**Cardiogenic Shock**
High CVP	High CVP
Low CI	Low CI
High SVRI	High SVRI
Normal V_{O_2}	Low V_{O_2}

Without the V_{O_2} measurement in the above profiles, it is impossible to differentiate a low cardiac output state from cardiogenic shock. This illustrates how oxygen transport monitoring can be used to determine the consequences of hemodynamic abnormalities on peripheral oxygenation. The uses and limitations of oxygen transport monitoring are described in more detail in Chapter 13.

COMPUTERIZED PROFILES

The numerous calculations involved in creating hemodynamic profiles make computer implementation well-suited to this task (14,15). A computer program written in BASIC that generates 10 hemodynamic parameters, including body surface area, is available from this author on request:

REFERENCES

GENERAL TEXTS

Daily EK, Schroeder JS. Techniques in bedside hemodynamic monitoring. 5th ed. St. Louis: CV Mosby, 1994.
Darovic GO, ed. Hemodynamic monitoring: invasive and noninvasive clinical application. 2nd ed. Philadelphia: WB Saunders, 1995.

REVIEWS

1. Swan HJ. The pulmonary artery catheter. Dis Mon 1991;37:473–543.
2. Ermakov S, Hoyt JW. Pulmonary artery catheterization. Crit Care Clin 1992; 8:773–806 (115 References).
3. American Society of Anesthesiologists Task Force on Pulmonary Artery Catheterization. Practice guidelines for pulmonary artery catheterization. Anesthesiology 1993;78:380–394 (89 References).
4. Darovic GO. Pulmonary artery pressure monitoring. In: Darovic GO, ed. Hemodynamic monitoring: invasive and noninvasive clinical application. 2nd ed. Philadelphia: WB Saunders, 1995;253–322 (84 References).

SELECTED REFERENCES

5. Iberti TJ, Fischer EP, Leibowitz AB, et al. A multicenter study of physicians' knowledge of the pulmonary artery catheter. JAMA 1990;264:2928–2932.
6. Halpern N, Feld H, Oropello JM, Stern E. The technique of inserting an RV port PA catheter and pacing probe. J Crit Illness 1991;6:1153–1159.
7. Armaganidis A, Dhainaut JF, Billard JL, et al. Accuracy assessment for three fiberoptic pulmonary artery catheters for SvO_2 monitoring. Intensive Care Med 1994;20:484–488.
8. Vincent JL, Thirion M, Brimioulle S, et al. Thermodilution measurement of right ventricular ejection fraction with a modified pulmonary artery catheter. Intensive Care Med 1986;12:33–38.
9. Yelderman M, Ramsay MA, Quinn MD, et al. Continuous thermodilution cardiac output measurement in intensive care unit patients. J Cardiothorac Vasc Anesth 1992;6:270–274.
10. Amin DK, Shah PK, Swan HJC. The technique of inserting the Swan–Ganz catheter. J Crit Illness 1993;8:1147–1156.
11. Venus B, Mathru M. A maneuver for bedside pulmonary artery catheterization in patients with right heart failure. Chest 1982;82:803–804.
12. Jacobson B. Medicine and clinical engineering. Englewood Cliffs, NJ: Prentice Hall, 1977;388.
13. Mattar JA. A simple calculation to estimate body surface area in adults and its correlation with the Dubois formula. Crit Care Med 1989;846–847.
14. Marino PL, Krasner J. Computerized interpretation of hemodynamic profiles in the ICU. Crit Care Med 1984;12:601–602.
15. Vyskocil JJ, Kruse JA. Hemodynamics and oxygen transport: using your computer to manage data. J Crit Illness 1994;9:447–459.

c h a p t e r

11

CENTRAL VENOUS PRESSURE AND WEDGE PRESSURE

It is what we think we know already that often prevents us from learning.
Claude Bernard

Monitoring central venous pressure (CVP) and pulmonary artery occlusion (wedge) pressure are routine practices in critical care (1–3). Like all familiar practices, these measurements are not often scrutinized. As a result, they are often misinterpreted (4,5). Attention to the material in this chapter will help reduce errors in interpretation of these two measurements.

SOURCES OF VARIABILITY

BODY POSITION

The zero reference point for venous pressures in the thorax is a point on the external thorax where the fourth intercostal space intersects the midaxillary line (i.e., the line midway between the anterior and posterior axillary folds). This point (called the phlebostatic axis) corresponds to the position of the right and left atrium when the patient is in the supine position. It is not a valid reference point in the lateral position, so **CVP and wedge pressure should not be recorded when patients are placed in lateral positions** (6).

CHANGES IN THORACIC PRESSURE

The vascular pressure recorded at the bedside is an *intravascular pressure;* i.e., the pressure in the vessel lumen relative to atmospheric (zero) pressure. However, the vascular pressure that determines ventricular preload (stretch on the ventricular muscle) and the rate of

166

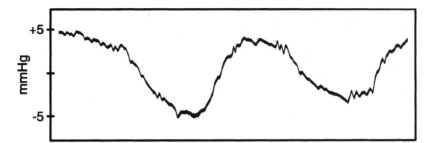

Figure 11.1. Respiratory variations in central venous pressure. Intravascular pressure is changing, but transmural pressure may be constant throughout the respiratory cycle.

edema formation is *transmural pressure;* i.e., the difference between the intravascular and extravascular pressures. Changes in thoracic pressures can cause a discrepancy between intravascular and transmural pressures. This discrepancy is illustrated by the respiratory variations in the CVP tracing shown in Figure 11.1. The intravascular pressure changes in this tracing are caused by respiratory variations in intrathoracic pressure that are transmitted into the lumen of the superior vena cava. If the changes in intrathoracic pressure are completely transmitted across the wall of the vessel, the transmural pressure remains constant throughout the respiratory cycle. (Because it is not possible to determine how much of the change in thoracic pressure is transmitted into the blood vessel in any individual patient, it is not possible to determine whether transmural pressure is absolutely constant.) Thus, **changes in intravascular pressures in the thorax may not reflect physiologically important (transmural) pressure changes** (7).

End-Expiration

Intravascular pressures should be equivalent to transmural pressures when the extravascular pressure is zero. In the thorax, the extravascular pressure should be close to zero (i.e., atmospheric pressure) at the end of expiration. Therefore, **intravascular pressures in the thorax should be measured at the end of expiration** (1–3,7). The intrathoracic pressure at the end of expiration is positive relative to atmospheric pressure in patients who are actively exhaling (e.g., by grunting) and in the presence of positive end-expiratory pressure (PEEP) (8). In the latter situation, the vascular pressures should be measured while the patient is briefly removed from PEEP, or the level of PEEP should be subtracted from the pressures measured at end-expiration. The influence of active exhalation on end-expiratory pressures cannot be determined in individual patients without inducing muscle paralysis.

Pressure Monitors

If the oscilloscope display screens in the ICU are equipped with horizontal grids, the CVP and wedge pressures should be measured directly from the pressure tracings on the screen. The measurements obtained with this method are more accurate than digitally displayed pressures (9). If only digital pressure readings are available, the systolic pressure should be used in patients who are breathing spontaneously and the diastolic pressure should be used in patients receiving positive-pressure mechanical ventilators. The reason is that the digital display on most pressure monitors represents the pressure measured over specific time intervals (usually 4 seconds, or the time for one sweep across the oscilloscope screen). The systolic pressure is the highest pressure, the diastolic pressure is the lowest pressure, and the mean pressure is the integrated area under the pressure wave in each time period (Fig. 11.1). During spontaneous breathing, the pressure at the end of expiration is the highest pressure (i.e., systolic pressure), and during positive-pressure mechanical ventilation, the end-expiratory pressure is the lowest pressure (i.e., diastolic pressure). Therefore, systolic pressure should be used as the end-expiratory vascular pressure in patients who are breathing spontaneously, whereas diastolic pressure should be used in patients receiving mechanical ventilation. **The mean pressure should never be used as a reflection of transmural pressure when there are respiratory variations in intravascular pressure** (1–3,7).

SPONTANEOUS VARIATIONS

Like any physiologic variable, vascular pressures in the thorax can vary spontaneously, without a change in the clinical condition of the patient. The spontaneous variation in wedge pressure is 4 mm Hg or less in 60% of patients, but it can be as high as 7 mm Hg in any individual patient (10). In general, **a change in CVP or wedge pressure of less than 4 mm Hg should not be considered a clinically significant change.**

MANOMETER PRESSURES

Most vascular pressures are measured with electronic pressure transducers that record the pressure in millimeters of mercury (mm Hg). An alternative method of measuring pressure (usually reserved for CVP) is water manometry, where pressure is recorded in cm H_2O (11). Because mercury is 13.6 times more dense than water (see Appendix 1), pressures measured in cm H_2O are divided by 1.36 to convert the units to mm Hg:

$$CVP \text{ (in cm } H_2O)/1.36 = CVP \text{ (in mm Hg)} \qquad (11.1)$$

The pressure correlations in cm H_2O and mm Hg are shown in Table 11.1.

TABLE 11.1. CONVERSION OF cm H_2O to mm Hg*			
cm H_2O	mm Hg	cm H_2O	mm Hg
1–2	1	12	9
3	2	13–14	10
4	3	15	11
5–6	4	16	12
7	5	17–18	13
8	6	19	14
9–10	7	20–21	15
11	8	22	16
* Pressures in mm Hg are the nearest whole number.			

WEDGE PRESSURE

Few pressures in the ICU are misinterpreted as frequently, and as consistently, as pulmonary capillary wedge pressure (4,5,12). Probably the most important feature of the wedge pressure is what it is *not:*

Wedge pressure is *not* left-ventricular preload.
Wedge pressure is *not* pulmonary capillary hydrostatic pressure.
Wedge pressure is *not* a reliable measure for differentiating cardiogenic from noncardiogenic pulmonary edema.

These limitations are explained in the description of wedge pressure that follows.

WEDGE PRESSURE TRACING

When the pulmonary artery catheter is properly positioned, inflation of the balloon at the tip of the catheter causes the pulsatile pressure to disappear. This is demonstrated in Figure 11.2. As mentioned, the

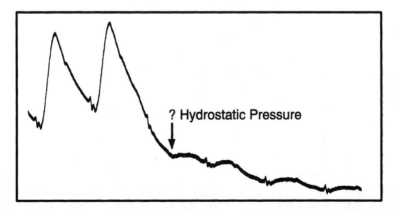

Figure 11.2. Pressure tracing showing the transition from a pulsatile pulmonary artery pressure to a balloon occlusion (wedge) pressure. The inflection point may represent capillary hydrostatic pressure.

nonpulsatile pressure created by balloon inflation is considered to be the pressure in the pulmonary microcirculation; hence it is called pulmonary capillary wedge pressure (PCWP). The wedge pressure shown in Figure 11.2 is lower than the pulmonary artery diastolic pressure because the pressure tracing is from a patient with pulmonary hypertension. In the absence of pulmonary artery hypertension, the wedge pressure is usually within a few mm Hg of the pulmonary artery diastolic pressure (13). (The inflection point in Figure 11.2, indicated as the possible hydrostatic pressure, is explained later.)

PRINCIPLE

The rationale for the wedge pressure measurement is illustrated in Figure 11.3 (13). Inflation of the balloon at the tip of pulmonary artery catheter obstructs blood flow and creates a static column of blood between the catheter tip and the left atrium. In this situation, the pressure at the tip of the pulmonary artery catheter should be the same as the pressure in the left atrium.

This condition is expressed by the hydraulic equation below (where P_c is capillary pressure, P_{LA} is left-atrial pressure, Q is pulmonary blood flow, and R_v is pulmonary venous resistance).

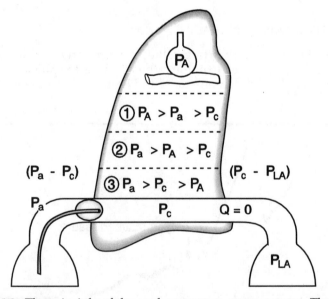

Figure 11.3. The principle of the wedge pressure measurement. The lung is divided into three zones based on the relationship between alveolar pressure (P_A), (mean) pulmonary artery pressure (P_a), and pulmonary capillary pressure (P_c). Wedge pressure is an accurate reflection of left-atrial pressure (P_{LA}) only in zone 3, where P_c is greater than P_A. Q = pulmonary blood flow.

$$P_c - P_{LA} = Q \times R_v$$

if $Q = 0$, $P_c - P_{LA} = 0$, and   (11.2)

$$P_c = P_{LA}$$

Thus, balloon inflation allows the pulmonary artery catheter to measure the pressure in the left atrium. Because left-atrial pressure is normally the equivalent of left-ventricular end-diastolic pressure (LVEDP), the pulmonary capillary wedge pressure can be used as a measure of left-ventricular filling pressure. What the wedge pressure actually measures is the focus of the remainder of this chapter.

PULMONARY CAPILLARY WEDGE PRESSURE AS PRELOAD

The wedge pressure is often used as a reflection of left-ventricular filling during diastole (i.e., ventricular preload). In Chapter 1, preload was defined as the force that stretched a muscle at rest, and the preload for the intact ventricle was identified as end-diastolic volume (EDV). However, wedge pressure is a measure of end-diastolic pressure, and end-diastolic pressure may not be an accurate reflection of preload (EDV) when the compliance (distensibility) of the ventricle is abnormal (see Fig. 1.1). Therefore, **wedge pressure is a reflection of left-ventricular preload only when compliance of the ventricle is normal or constant** (13,14).

Several conditions can alter ventricular compliance in patients in the ICU, such as ventricular hypertrophy, positive pressure ventilation, myocardial ischemia, and myocardial edema (e.g., after cardiopulmonary bypass surgery). Therefore, wedge pressure may not be a reliable index of left-ventricular preload in a large number of patients in the ICU.

PULMONARY CAPILLARY WEDGE PRESSURE
AS LEFT-ATRIAL PRESSURE

The following conditions can influence the accuracy of the wedge pressure as a measure of left-atrial pressure.

Lung Zones

If the pressure in the surrounding alveoli exceeds capillary (venous) pressure, the pressure at the tip of the pulmonary artery (PA) catheter may reflect the alveolar pressure more than the pressure in the left atrium. This is illustrated in Figure 11.3. The lung in this figure is divided into three zones based on the relationship between alveolar pressure and the pressures in the pulmonary circulation (1–3,13). The most dependent lung zone (zone 3) is the only region where capillary (venous) pressure exceeds alveolar pressure. Therefore, **wedge pres-**

sure is a reflection of left-atrial pressure only when the tip of the pulmonary artery catheter is located in zone 3 of the lung.

Catheter Tip Position

Although the lung zones shown in Figure 11.3 are based on physiologic rather than anatomic criteria, the lung regions below the left atrium are considered to be in lung zone 3 (1–3). Therefore, **the tip of the pulmonary artery catheter should be positioned below the level of the left atrium** to ensure that the wedge pressure is measuring left-atrial pressure. Most PA catheters are advanced into lung regions below the level of the left atrium (because of the higher blood flow in dependent lung regions). However, as many as 30% of PA catheters are positioned with their tips above the level of the left atrium (13). When patients are supine, routine portable (anteroposterior) chest x rays cannot be used to identify the catheter tip position relative to the left atrium. Rather, a lateral view of the chest is needed. However, lateral films have not gained favor for this use in most ICUs, probably because they are too time-consuming for the small percentage of improperly located catheter tips that will be revealed. Instead, catheter tips can be assumed to be positioned in zone 3 of the lung in all but the following conditions: when there are marked respiratory variations in the wedge pressure, and when PEEP is applied and wedge pressure increases by 50% or more of the applied PEEP (13).

Positive End-Expiratory Pressure

The presence of PEEP can reduce the area of zone 3 in the lung. In fact, when PEEP is combined with a low wedge pressure, there may be no zone 3 conditions in the lung, even in the most dependent lung regions. When this occurs, the wedge pressure is not an accurate reflection of left-atrial pressure, even when the catheter tip is below the level of the left atrium (13). Therefore, when PEEP is being applied, the wedge pressure should be measured while PEEP is temporarily discontinued (if this can be done without causing dangerous decreases in arterial oxygenation). PEEP can also be generated internally by patients who have inadequate emptying of the lungs during expiration (see Chapter 28). This type of intrinsic or *auto-PEEP* is common in patients with obstructive lung disease, particularly when they are breathing rapidly or receiving large inflation volumes during mechanical ventilation. A bedside maneuver that can help detect auto-PEEP is presented in Chapter 28.

Wedged Blood Gases

As many as 50% of the nonpulsatile pressures produced by balloon inflation represent damped PA pressures rather than pulmonary capillary pressures (15). Aspiration of blood from the catheter tip during balloon inflation can be used to identify a true wedge (capillary) pres-

TABLE 11.2. CRITERIA FOR WEDGE PRESSURE VALIDATION
• (Wedge P_{O_2} − Arterial P_{O_2}) ≥ 19 mm Hg • (Arterial P_{CO_2} − Wedge P_{CO_2}) ≥ 11 mm Hg • (Wedge pH − Arterial pH) ≥0.008
From Morris AH, Chapman RH (12).

sure using the three criteria shown in Table 11.2. Although this is a cumbersome practice that is not used routinely, it seems justified when making important diagnostic and therapeutic decisions based on the wedge pressure measurement.

PULMONARY CAPILLARY WEDGE PRESSURE AS LEFT-VENTRICULAR END-DIASTOLIC PRESSURE

Even when wedge pressure is an accurate reflection of left-atrial pressure, there may be a discrepancy between wedge (left-atrial) pressure and LVEDP. This can occur under the following conditions (13).

Aortic insufficiency: LVEDP can be higher than PCWP because the mitral valve closes prematurely while retrograde flow continues to fill the ventricle.

Noncompliant ventricle: Atrial contraction against a stiff ventricle produces a rapid rise in end-diastolic pressure that closes the mitral valve prematurely. The result is a PCWP that is lower than LVEDP.

Respiratory failure: PCWP can exceed LVEDP in patients with pulmonary disease. The presumed mechanism is constriction of small veins in lung regions that are hypoxic (17).

PULMONARY CAPILLARY WEDGE PRESSURE AS A HYDROSTATIC PRESSURE

Wedge pressure is often assumed to be a measure of hydrostatic pressure in the pulmonary capillaries. The problem with this assumption is that the wedge pressure is measured in the absence of blood flow. When the balloon is deflated and blood flow resumes, **the pressure in the pulmonary capillaries is equivalent to the left-atrial (wedge) pressure only when hydraulic resistance in the pulmonary veins is negligible.** This is expressed below, where P_c is capillary hydrostatic pressure, R_v is the hydraulic resistance in the pulmonary veins, Q is blood flow, and wedge pressure (PCWP) is substituted for left-atrial pressure.

$$P_c - \text{PCWP} = Q \times R_v$$

If $R_v = 0$, $\quad\quad P_c - \text{PCWP} = 0 \quad\quad\quad\quad\quad (11.3)$

$$P_c = \text{PCWP}$$

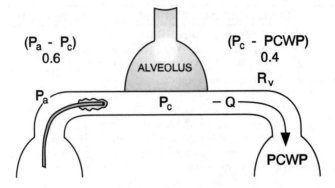

Figure 11.4. The distinction between capillary hydrostatic pressure (P_c) and wedge pressure (PCWP). When the balloon is deflated and flow (Q) resumes, P_c and PCWP are equivalent only when the hydraulic resistance in the pulmonary veins (R_v) is negligible. P_a = pulmonary artery pressure. If the pulmonary venous resistance (R_v) is greater than zero, the capillary hydrostatic pressure (P_c) will be higher than the wedge pressure.

Pulmonary Venous Resistance

Unlike the systemic veins, the pulmonary veins contribute a significant fraction to the total vascular resistance across the lungs. (This is a reflection more of a low resistance in the pulmonary arteries than of a high resistance in the pulmonary veins.) As shown in Figure 11.4, 40% of the pressure drop across the pulmonary circulation occurs on the venous side of the circulation, which means that the pulmonary veins contribute 40% of the total resistance in the pulmonary circulation (16). Although this is derived from animal studies, the contribution in humans is probably similar in magnitude.

The contribution of the hydraulic resistance in the pulmonary veins may be even greater in critically ill patients because several conditions that are common in patients in the ICU can promote pulmonary venoconstriction. These conditions include hypoxemia, endotoxemia, and the acute respiratory distress syndrome (17,18). These conditions further magnify differences between wedge pressure and capillary hydrostatic pressure, as demonstrated below.

Wedge–Hydrostatic Pressure Conversion

Equation 11.4 can be used to convert wedge pressure (PCWP) to pulmonary capillary hydrostatic pressure (P_c). This conversion is based on the assumption that the pressure drop from the pulmonary capillaries to the left atrium $(P_c - P_{LA})$ represents 40% of the pressure drop from the pulmonary arteries to the left atrium $(P_a - P_{LA})$. Substituting wedge pressure for left-atrial pressure (i.e., P_{LA} = PCWP) yields the following relationship:

$$P_c - \text{PCWP} = 0.4\,(P_a - \text{PCWP})$$

$$P_c = \text{PCWP} + 0.4\,(P_a - \text{PCWP})$$

(11.4)

For a normal (mean) pulmonary artery pressure of 15 mm Hg and a wedge pressure of 10 mm Hg, this relationship predicts the following:

$$\text{Normal lung: } P_c = 10 + 0.4 \times (15 - 10)$$

$$P_c = 12 \text{ mm Hg}$$

(11.5)

$$P_c - \text{PCWP} = 2 \text{ mm Hg}$$

Thus, in the normal lung, wedge pressure is equivalent to capillary hydrostatic pressure. However, in the presence of pulmonary venoconstriction and pulmonary hypertension (e.g., in acute respiratory distress syndrome, ARDS), there can be a considerable difference between wedge pressure and capillary hydrostatic pressure. The example below is based on a mean PA pressure of 30 mm Hg and a venous resistance that is 60% of the total pulmonary vascular resistance.

$$\text{ARDS: } P_c = 10 + 0.6 \times (30 - 10)$$

$$P_c = 22 \text{ mm Hg}$$

(11.6)

$$P_c - \text{PCWP} = 12 \text{ mm Hg}$$

Unfortunately, pulmonary venous resistance cannot be measured in critically ill patients, and this limits the accuracy of the wedge pressure as a measure of capillary hydrostatic pressure.

OCCLUSION PRESSURE PROFILE

The transition from pulsatile pulmonary artery pressure to nonpulsatile wedge pressure in Figure 11.2 shows an initial rapid phase followed by a slower, more gradual pressure change. The initial rapid phase may represent the pressure drop across the pulmonary arteries, whereas the slower phase represents the pressure drop across the pulmonary veins. If this is the case, the inflection point marking the transition from the rapid to the slow phase represents the capillary hydrostatic pressure. Although this method can provide a more definitive determination of the capillary hydrostatic pressure than the equations used above, an inflection point is not often recognizable (19,20).

SUMMARY

There are numerous sources of error in the interpretation of CVP and wedge pressure. Fortunately, with the ability to monitor cardiac output (Chapter 12) and systemic oxygen transport (Chapter 13), these pressures have become less important in the evaluation of hemodynamic status.

REFERENCES

GENERAL TEXTS

Ahrens TS, Taylor LA. Hemodynamic waveform analysis. Philadelphia: WB Saunders, 1992.

Daily EK, Schroeder JS. Hemodynamic waveforms. 2nd ed. St. Louis: CV Mosby, 1990.

Darovic GO, ed. Hemodynamic monitoring. Invasive and noninvasive clinical applications. 2nd ed. Philadelphia: WB Saunders, 1995.

REVIEWS

1. Schwenzer KJ. Venous and pulmonary pressures. In: Lake C, ed. Clinical monitoring. Philadelphia: WB Saunders, 1990;147–198 (166 References).
2. Bridges EJ, Woods SL. Pulmonary artery pressure measurement: state of the art. Heart Lung 1993;22:99–111 (62 References).
3. Darovic GO. Pulmonary artery pressure monitoring. In: Darovic GO, ed. Hemodynamic monitoring. Invasive and noninvasive clinical applications. 2nd ed. Philadelphia: WB Saunders, 1995:253–322 (71 References).

SELECTED REFERENCES

4. Nadeau S, Noble WH. Misinterpretation of pressure measurements from the pulmonary artery catheter. Can Anesth Soc J 1986;33:352–363.
5. Komandina KH, Schenk DA, LaVeau P, et al. Interobserver variability in the interpretation of pulmonary artery catheter pressure tracings. Chest 1991;100: 1647–1654.
6. Kee LL, Simonson JS, Stotts NA, et al. Echocardiographic determination of valid zero reference levels in supine and lateral positions. Am J Crit Care 1993; 2:72–80.
7. Schmitt EA, Brantigen CO. Common artifacts of pulmonary artery and pulmonary artery wedge pressures. Recognition and management. J Clin Monit 1986; 2:44–52.
8. Pinsky M, Vincent J-L, De Smet J-M. Estimating left ventricular filling pressure during positive end-expiratory pressure in humans. Am Rev Respir Dis 1991; 143:25–31.
9. Dobbin K, Wallace S, Ahlberg J, Chulay M. Pulmonary artery pressure measurement in patients with elevated pressures: effect of backrest elevation and method of measurement. Am J Crit Care 1992;2:61–69.
10. Nemens EJ, Woods SL. Normal fluctuations in pulmonary artery and pulmonary capillary wedge pressures in acutely ill patients. Heart Lung 1982;11: 393–398.
11. Halck S, Walther-Larsen S, Sanchez R. Reliability of central venous pressure measured by water column. Crit Care Med 1990;18:461–462.
12. Morris AH, Chapman RH, Gardner RM. Frequency of wedge pressure errors in the ICU. Crit Care Med 1985;13:705–708.

13. O'Quin R, Marini JJ. Pulmonary artery occlusion pressure: clinical physiology, measurement, and interpretation. Am Rev Respir Dis 1983;128:319–326.
14. Diebel LN, Wilson RF, Tagett MG, Kline RA. End-diastolic volume. A better indicator of preload in the critically ill. Arch Surg 1992;127:817–822.
15. Morris AH, Chapman RH. Wedge pressure confirmation by aspiration of pulmonary capillary blood. Crit Care Med 1985;13:756–759.
16. Michel RP, Hakim TS, Chang HK. Pulmonary arterial and venous pressures measured with small catheters. J Appl Physiol 1984;57:309–314.
17. Tracey WR, Hamilton JT, Craig ID, Paterson NAM. Effect of endothelial injury on the responses of isolated guinea pig pulmonary venules to reduced oxygen tension. J Appl Physiol 1989;67:2147–2153.
18. Kloess T, Birkenhauer U, Kottler B. Pulmonary pressure–flow relationship and peripheral oxygen supply in ARDS due to bacterial sepsis. Second Vienna Shock Forum, 1989:175–180.
19. Cope DK, Grimbert F, Downey JM, et al. Pulmonary capillary pressure: a review. Crit Care Med 1992;20:1043–1056.
20. Gilbert E, Hakim TS. Derivation of pulmonary capillary pressure from arterial occlusion in intact conditions. Crit Care Med 1994;22:986–993.

12

THERMODILUTION: METHODS AND APPLICATIONS

An exact science is dominated by the idea of approximation.
Bertrand Russell

A few years after its introduction, the pulmonary artery (PA) catheter was upgraded by incorporating a thermistor at the catheter tip to measure blood flow using the thermodilution principle. This single addition to the PA catheter increased its monitoring capacity from 2 parameters (i.e., central venous pressure and wedge pressure) to 10 parameters (see Tables 10.1 and 10.2). More recent refinements in thermodilution methodology have further increased the monitoring capacity of the PA catheter, adding the ability to measure the ejection fraction of the right ventricle and to monitor cardiac output continuously. This chapter describes each of the thermodilution methods for monitoring cardiac performance.

BASIC THERMODILUTION METHOD

Thermodilution is an indicator-dilution method of measuring blood flow. This method is based on the premise that when an indicator substance is added to circulating blood, the rate of blood flow is inversely proportional to the change in concentration of the indicator over time. The indicator substance can be a dye (dye-dilution method) or a fluid with a different temperature than blood (thermodilution method). The thermodilution method of measuring cardiac output

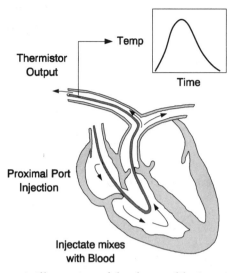

Figure 12.1. Schematic illustration of the thermodilution method for measuring cardiac output.

with a PA catheter is shown in Figure 12.1 (1–3). A dextrose or saline solution that is colder than blood is injected through the proximal port of the catheter in the right atrium. The cold fluid mixes with blood in the right heart chambers, and the cooled blood is ejected into the pulmonary artery and flows past the thermistor on the distal end of the catheter. The thermistor records the change in blood temperature with time and sends this information to an electronic instrument that records and displays a temperature–time curve like the one shown in Figure 12.1. The area under this curve is inversely proportional to the rate of blood flow in the pulmonary artery. In the absence of intracardiac shunts, this flow rate is equivalent to the (average) cardiac output.

THERMODILUTION CURVES

Examples of thermodilution curves are shown in Figure 12.2. The low cardiac output curve (upper panel) has a gradual rise and fall, whereas the high output curve (middle panel) has a rapid rise, an abbreviated peak, and a steep downslope. Note that the area under the low cardiac output curve is greater than the area under the high output curve; that is, the area under the curves is inversely related to the flow rate. Electronic cardiac monitors integrate the area under the temperature–time curves and provide a digital display of the calculated cardiac output. There is a tendency to rely on this digital display of the calculated cardiac output without examining the temperature–time curve, and this can lead to errors in interpretation.

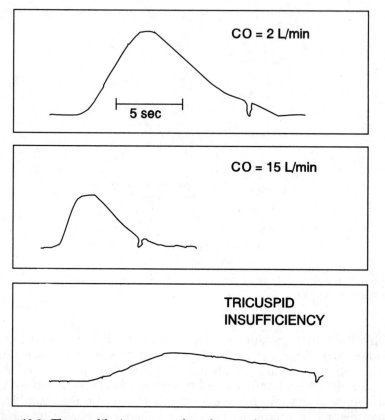

Figure 12.2. Thermodilution curves for a low cardiac output (*upper panel*), a high cardiac output (*middle panel*), and tricuspid insufficiency (*lower panel*). The sharp inflection in each curve marks the end of the measurement period. *CO* = cardiac output.

TECHNICAL CONSIDERATIONS

PATIENT POSITION

Cardiac output can be 30% higher in the supine position than in the semierect position (4). Therefore, consecutive cardiac output determinations should be performed with each patient in a uniform position, or the position of the patient should be recorded with each cardiac output determination.

INJECTING THE INDICATOR

Indicator Solution

Bolus injection of normal saline (0.9% sodium chloride) or 5% dextrose-in-water produces the most satisfactory measurements (3). Other injectate solutions can produce variable results (because of their varying specific heats) and are not recommended.

Injectate Volume and Temperature

The indicator solution can be cooled in ice or injected at room temperature, and can be administered in a volume of 5 mL or 10 mL. In general, higher-volume, lower-temperature injectates produce the highest signal-to-noise ratios, and thus the most accurate measurements (1–3,5). However, **room temperature injectates** (which are less tedious to administer than iced injectates) **produce reliable measurements in most critically ill patients** (6–9). When the indicator fluid is injected at room temperature, the large (10 mL) injection volume produces the most reliable results. When using smaller injectate volumes, using iced injectates increases the reliability of the measurements. Using small volumes of room temperature injectates can yield inaccurate results in low cardiac output states (5), and is thus not recommended.

Injection Time

Optimal results are produced when the bolus injection is completed within 2 seconds (10), but satisfactory results are obtained with injection times up to 4 seconds. Longer injection times can produce falsely low measurements.

Injection Timing

Cardiac output can vary significantly during the respiratory cycle, particularly during mechanical ventilation. Random thermodilution measurements obtained in different phases of the respiratory cycle can vary by more than 10%, whereas injections that are timed to the end of expiration can reduce the variability to 5% (11). This has led to the recommendation that thermodilution cardiac outputs always be recorded at end-expiration. However, it is very difficult to time injections so that the thermodilution curve is recorded at precisely the same time in the respiratory cycle. In fact, the injection time can be longer than the duration of the respiratory cycle in patients with rapid breathing; for example, at a respiratory rate above 15 breaths/minute, an injection time of 4 seconds is longer than the duration of each respiratory cycle (less than 4 seconds). It is best in such cases to **begin injecting the indicator solution at the same part of the respiratory cycle for each cardiac output measurement.**

Alternative Injection Ports

If the proximal (right-atrial) port of the PA catheter is obstructed, the injectate can be introduced through an alternative infusion port on the catheter (if one is available) (8) or through the side arm of the introducer catheter (see Fig. 10.1) (9).

ACCURACY AND RELIABILITY

NUMBER OF MEASUREMENTS

Serial measurements are recommended for each cardiac output determination. Three measurements are sufficient if they differ by 10% or less. Cardiac output is determined by averaging the serial measurements. The initial measurement is often falsely elevated (7), so for optimal accuracy, the initial measurement should be discarded. **Serial measurements that differ by more than 10% should be considered unreliable** (12).

TRICUSPID REGURGITATION

Tricuspid regurgitation causes the cold indicator fluid to be recycled back and forth across the tricuspid valve. This produces a prolonged, low-amplitude thermodilution curve like the one shown in the lower panel of Figure 12.2. This type of curve is an exaggerated version of a low-output curve (with a large area under the curve), so **tricuspid regurgitation produces a falsely low thermodilution cardiac output** (13). Tricuspid regurgitation may be common in mechanically ventilated patients because of the high right-sided cardiac pressures created by positive-pressure lung inflations. Therefore, this condition may be a common source of error in thermodilution cardiac outputs in the ICU.

LOW-OUTPUT STATES

Low cardiac outputs produce low-amplitude temperature–time curves, and this can affect the accuracy of thermodilution cardiac outputs by decreasing the signal-to-noise ratio. Accuracy is most affected when room temperature indicator solutions are injected in low (5 mL) volumes. In this situation, thermodilution can underestimate cardiac output by as much as 30% (5). In low-output states (cardiac index below 2.5 L/minute/m^2), an iced injectate gives the most accurate measurements if low injectate volumes are used.

INTRACARDIAC SHUNTS

Intracardiac shunts produce falsely high thermodilution cardiac output measurements. In right-to-left shunts, a portion of the cold indicator fluid passes through the shunt, thereby creating an abbreviated thermodilution curve (similar to the abbreviated high-output curve). In left-to-right shunts, the thermodilution curve is abbreviated because the shunted blood increases the blood volume in the right heart chambers, and this dilutes the indicator solution that is injected.

VARIABILITY

Thermodilution cardiac output can vary by as much as 10% without a change in the clinical condition of the patient (14). This means that a baseline cardiac output of 5 L/min can vary spontaneously from 4.5 to 5.5 L/min (or a baseline cardiac index of 3 L/min/m^2 can vary from 2.7 to 3.3 L/min/m^2) without representing a change in the clinical condition of the patient. Therefore, **the thermodilution cardiac output (or cardiac index) must change by more than 10% for the change to be considered clinically significant.**

THERMODILUTION EJECTION FRACTION

In the mid-1980s, a PA catheter was introduced with a fast-response thermistor capable of measuring the ejection fraction of the right ventricle (15). This added the ability to evaluate right-ventricular function at the bedside.

METHOD

Rapid-response thermistors can record the temperature changes associated with each cardiac cycle. This produces a ramplike thermodilution curve like the one shown in Figure 12.3. The change in temperature between each plateau on the curve is caused by dilution of the cold indicator fluid by venous blood that fills the ventricle during

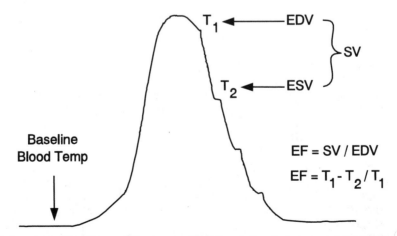

Figure 12.3. The thermodilution method for determining ventricular ejection fraction (*EF*) using thermal equivalents for end-diastolic volume (*EDV*), end-systolic volume (*ESV*), and stroke volume (*SV*).

diastole. Because the volume that fills the ventricles during diastole is equivalent to the stroke volume, the temperature difference $T_1 - T_2$ is the thermal equivalent of the stroke volume. Thus, the points at each end of the temperature change can be taken as the thermal equivalents of the end-diastolic volume (T_1) and end-systolic volume (T_2), respectively. Because the ejection fraction is the ratio of stroke volume (SV) to end-diastolic volume (EDV), the right-ventricular ejection fraction (RVEF) can be derived using the appropriate thermal equivalents:

$$RVEF = SV/EDV \qquad (12.1)$$

$$RVEF = (T_1 - T_2)/T_1$$

Normal thermodilution RVEF is 0.45 to 0.50. This is slightly lower than radionuclide RVEF (the gold standard), but the difference is less than 10% (16). Thermodilution RVEF can be measured reliably using a room temperature injectate (given as a 10-mL bolus) (17).

End-Diastolic Volume

Because the thermodilution PA catheter can measure stroke volume, RVEF can be used to derive the right-ventricular end-diastolic volume (RVEDV):

$$RVEDV = SV/RVEF \qquad (12.2)$$

This allows for a determination of ventricular preload (end-diastolic volume) at the bedside, and bypasses the shortcomings of end-diastolic pressure (e.g., the central venous pressure) as a reflection of preload (18).

CONTINUOUS CARDIAC OUTPUT

The most recent development in the thermodilution method has led to the introduction of a PA catheter that can monitor cardiac output continuously, without the need for intermittent bolus injections of indicator fluid (19). This catheter (Baxter Edwards Critical Care, Irvine, California) is equipped with a 10-cm thermal filament located 15 to 25 cm from the catheter tip. The filament generates low-energy heat pulses that are transmitted to the surrounding blood. The resulting change in blood temperature is then used to generate a thermodilution curve for determining cardiac output. Although the output is called continuous cardiac output, the measurement is an average cardiac output recorded over 3-minute time intervals and updated every 30 to 60 seconds.

Continuous thermodilution cardiac output monitoring has proven to be both safe and reliable (19,20). However, it has yet to gain widespread popularity, probably because of the added cost of the newer technology. Nevertheless, the advantages of a continuous measure of cardiac output (e.g., more on-line information regarding trends in cardiac output) seem to justify the additional cost of the technology in patients with unstable or severely compromised hemodynamic function.

REFERENCES

GENERAL TEXTS

Robertson JIS, Birkenhager WH, eds. Cardiac output measurement. Philadelphia: WB Saunders, 1991.

REVIEWS

1. Gardner PE. Cardiac output. Theory, technique, and troubleshooting. Crit Care Nurs Clin North Am 1989;1:577–587 (71 References).
2. Daily EK, Schroeder JS. Cardiac output measurements. In: Techniques in bedside hemodynamic monitoring. 5th ed. St. Louis: CV Mosby, 1994;173–194 (57 References).
3. Darovic GO, Yacone-Morton LA. Monitoring cardiac output. In: Darovic GO, ed. Hemodynamic monitoring. Invasive and noninvasive clinical applications. 2nd ed. Philadelphia: WB Saunders, 1995;323–346 (27 References).

BASIC THERMODILUTION METHOD

4. Driscoll A, Shanahan A, Crommy L, Gleeson A. The effect of patient position on the reproducibility of cardiac output measurements. Heart Lung 1995;24: 38–44.
5. Renner LE, Morton MJ, Sakuma GY. Indicator amount, temperature, and intrinsic cardiac output affect thermodilution cardiac output accuracy and reproducibility. Crit Care Med 1993;21:586–597.
6. Nelson LD, Anderson HB. Patient selection for iced versus room temperature injectate for thermodilution cardiac output determinations. Crit Care Med 1985;13:182–184.
7. Pearl RG, Rosenthal MH, Nielson L, et al. Effect of injectate volume and temperature on thermodilution cardiac output determinations. Anesthesiology 1986;64:798–801.
8. Pesola GR, Ayala B, Plante L. Room-temperature thermodilution cardiac output: proximal injectate lumen versus proximal infusion lumen. Am J Crit Care 1993;2:132–133.
9. Pesola HR, Pesola GR. Room-temperature thermodilution cardiac output. Central venous versus side port. Chest 1992;103:339–341.
10. Conway J, Lund-Johansen P. Thermodilution method for measuring cardiac output. In: Robertson JIS, Birkenhager WH, eds. Cardiac output measurement. Philadelphia: WB Saunders, 1991;17–20.
11. Stevens JH, Raffin TA, Mihm FG, et al. Thermodilution cardiac output measurement. Effects of respiratory cycle on its reproducibility. JAMA 1985;253: 2240–2242.

12. Nadeau S, Noble WH. Limitations of cardiac output measurement by thermodilution. Can J Anesth 1986;33:780–784.
13. Konishi T, Nakamura Y, Morii I, et al. Comparison of thermodilution and Fick methods for measurement of cardiac output in tricuspid regurgitation. Am J Cardiol 1992;70:538–540.
14. Sasse SA, Chen PA, Berry RB, et al. Variability of cardiac output over time in medical intensive care unit patients. Chest 1994;22:225-232.

THERMODILUTION EJECTION FRACTION

15. Vincent JL, Thirion M, Brimioulle S, et al. Thermodilution measurement of right ventricular ejection fraction with a modified pulmonary artery catheter. Intensive Care Med 1986;12:33–38.
16. Vincent JL. The measurement of right ventricular ejection fraction. Intensive Care World 1990;7:133–136.
17. Safcsak K, Nelson LD. Thermodilution right ventricular ejection fraction measurements: room temperature versus cold temperature injectate. Crit Care Med 1994;22:1136–1141.
18. Diebel LN, Wilson RF, Tagett MG, Kline RA. End-diastolic volume. A better indicator of preload in the critically ill. Arch Surg 1992;127:817–822.

CONTINUOUS CARDIAC OUTPUT

19. Yelderman M, Ramsay MA, Quinn MD, et al. Continuous thermodilution cardiac output measurement in intensive care unit patients. J Cardiothorac Vasc Anesth 1992;6:270–274.
20. Boldt J, Menges T, Wollbruck M, et al. Is continuous cardiac output measurement using thermodilution reliable in the critically ill patient? Crit Care Med 1994;22:1913–1918.

TISSUE OXYGENATION

No animal can live in an atmosphere where a flame does not burn.
Leonardo da Vinci, 1500

Despite good intentions, much of what we do to patients in the name of aerobic support is without documented need or documented benefit. This is a reflection of the inability to obtain a direct measurement of tissue oxygen tensions. As a result, decisions about oxygen are often based on surrogate measures of tissue oxygenation that are inappropriate (such as arterial blood gases).

The invasive nature of patient care in the ICU creates approaches to evaluating tissue oxygenation that are not available in other areas of the hospital. This chapter reviews some of these approaches, along with a more standard marker of tissue oxygen balance (i.e., blood lactate). The oxygen transport variables in this chapter are described in more detail in Chapter 2.

TISSUE OXYGEN BALANCE

The determinants of tissue oxygenation are illustrated in Figure 13.1. The oxygen supply to tissues is shown as the rate of O_2 uptake from the microcirculation (i.e., V_{O_2}). The metabolic requirement for oxygen (MR_{O_2}) is the rate at which oxygen is metabolized to water in the mitochondria. Because oxygen is not stored in tissues, V_{O_2} must match MR_{O_2} for aerobic metabolism to continue undisturbed. When this occurs, glucose is completely oxidized, as shown in Figure 13.1, and the energy yield is 36 moles of ATP (673 kcal) per mole glucose. When V_{O_2} cannot match MR_{O_2}, a portion of the glucose metabolism is diverted to the production of lactate, with an energy yield of 2 moles ATP (47 kcal) per mole glucose. Thus, when the O_2 supply is inadequate, the energy yield from substrate metabolism drops precipitously. This **con-**

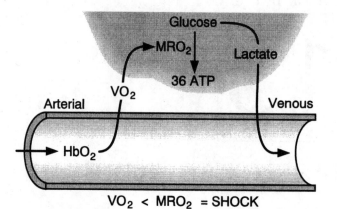

Figure 13.1. Schematic diagram of the relationship between oxygen uptake ($\dot{V}O_2$) and the metabolic requirement for oxygen (MRO_2). When $\dot{V}O_2$ matches MRO_2, glucose is completely oxidized to CO_2 and water. When $\dot{V}O_2$ is less than MRO_2, glucose forms lactate. Shock is defined as a condition where $\dot{V}O_2$ is lower than MRO_2.

dition, **in which the production of ATP is limited by the supply of oxygen,** is called dysoxia (1), and when cell dysoxia produces a measurable change in organ function, the condition **is commonly known as shock.**

OXYGEN TRANSPORT MONITORING

As described in Chapter 2, two variables are used to describe oxygen transport: the rate of oxygen delivery (DO_2) and the rate of oxygen uptake ($\dot{V}O_2$), also known as oxygen consumption. These are global measures of the oxygen supply (DO_2) and oxygen utilization ($\dot{V}O_2$) in the systemic circulation. Oxygen uptake ($\dot{V}O_2$) is equivalent to the oxygen supply identified in Figure 13.1. Oxygen transport monitoring therefore provides information about the oxygen supply to tissues (2), but it provides no information about the adequacy of tissue oxygenation (because that requires a measurement of metabolic rate).

INTERPRETATIONS

The important transport parameter is $\dot{V}O_2$, which can be interpreted as follows (see Table 13.1):

Low $\dot{V}O_2$: indicates tissue oxygen deficits (oxygen debt)

Normal V_{O_2}: A blood lactate level is required to determine whether tissue oxygenation is adequate.

V_{O_2} DEFICIT

If a decrease in oxygen uptake is not accompanied by a proportional decrease in metabolic rate, the oxygen supply will be inadequate to support aerobic metabolism. Because hypometabolism is uncommon in critically ill patients, **a V_{O_2} that falls below the normal range (below 100 mL/minute/m^2) can be used as evidence of impaired tissue oxygenation.**
An example of a low V_{O_2} that serves as a marker of inadequate tissue oxygenation is shown in Figure 13.2. The data in this figure are taken from a patient who underwent abdominal aortic aneurysm

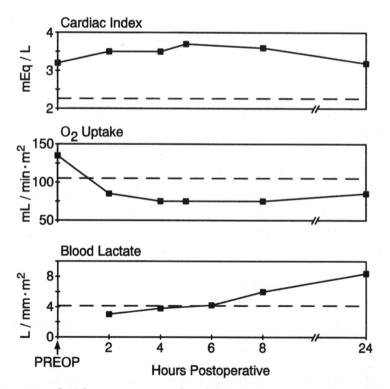

Figure 13.2. Serial measurements of cardiac index, oxygen uptake, and blood lactate levels before and after abdominal aortic aneurysm surgery. The first postoperative measurement reveals a deficit in oxygen uptake that persists and is accompanied by a progressive rise in blood lactate levels. Dotted lines indicate threshold values separating normal from abnormal measurements.

surgery. At the first postoperative recording (2 hours), V_{O_2} is below normal, and thereafter, V_{O_2} never returns to the normal range. At 6 hours, the serum lactate rises above the normal range. The lactate levels continue to rise steadily thereafter, reaching 9 mEq/L at 24 hours after surgery. The progressive rise in blood lactate is evidence that the low V_{O_2} indicates a widespread tissue oxygen deficit. Note that the cardiac index remains normal despite the ongoing ischemia. This high-lights the fact that cardiac output monitoring does not evaluate tissue oxygenation.

OXYGEN DEBT

The area under the dotted line in the V_{O_2} curve reflects the total V_{O_2} deficit over time. The cumulative V_{O_2} deficit (derived by integrating the V_{O_2} deficit over time) is known as the oxygen debt. Studies of the oxygen debt after resuscitation from hemorrhagic shock (3) and in postoperative patients (4) show a direct relationship between the magnitude of the oxygen debt and the risk of multiorgan failure and death. These correlations are evidence that the V_{O_2} deficit is a marker of tissue ischemia and that early correction of V_{O_2} deficits is warranted to limit the magnitude of the ischemic insult.

CORRECTING V_{O_2} DEFICITS

The flow diagram in Figure 13.3 shows a management strategy that can be used to correct a V_{O_2} deficit. This approach begins with a focus on blood volume.

Step 1: Central Venous Pressure or Wedge Pressure

1. If low, infuse volume to normalize the filling pressures.
2. For normal or high pressures, go to Step 2.

Correcting volume deficits is essential to maintain cardiac filling volume.

Step 2: Cardiac Output

1. If low, and filling pressures not high, infuse volume until central venous pressure (CVP) is 10 to 12 mm Hg or wedge pressure is 18 to 20 mm Hg.
2. If low, and filling pressures high, start dobutamine infusion at 3 $\mu g/kg/minute$ and titrate to cardiac index above 3.0 $L/min/m^2$. If blood pressure (BP) is low, use dopamine at starting dose of 5 $\mu g/kg/minute$.
3. For cardiac index over 3.0 $L/min/m^2$, go to Step 3.

Volume is preferred to adrenergic drugs, so volume is infused to high filling pressures, if needed. Dobutamine is the preferred inotrope

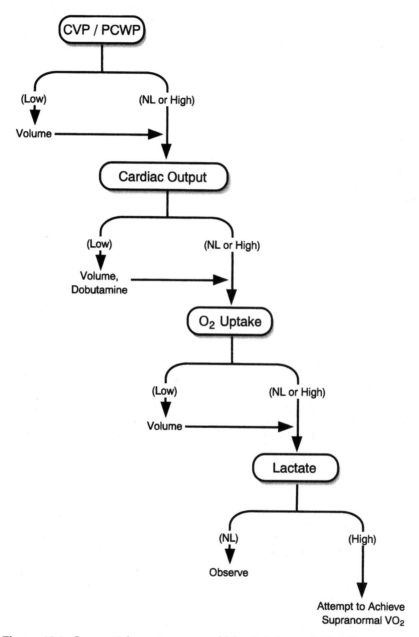

Figure 13.3. Sequential management of blood volume, blood flow, oxygen transport, and tissue oxygenation.

and is also less thermogenic than the other adrenergic drugs (and thus has less tendency to stimulate metabolism).

Step 3: Oxygen Uptake

1. If Vo_2 is less than 100 mL/min/m^2, use volume (to CVP = 8 to 10 or wedge pressure = 18 to 20) and inotropic therapy to achieve a cardiac index above 4.5 L/min/m^2. Correct anemia if Hb is less than 8 g/dL.
2. For Vo_2 greater than 100 mL/min/m^2, go to Step 4.

If Vo_2 does not readily increase when volume is adequate and cardiac index is high, the prognosis is poor. Correcting anemia usually does not increase Vo_2, but it can be used as a last resort. When Vo_2 is normal, the lactate is used to determine whether Vo_2 is matched to the metabolic rate.

Step 4: Blood Lactate Level

1. If lactate is greater than 4 mmol/L and other signs of shock (organ failure, low BP) are present, options include decreasing metabolic rate (through sedation or stopping feedings) and increasing Vo_2 above 160 mL/min/m^2 (if possible).
2. For lactate below 4 mmol/L, observe.

An elevated lactate indicates that Vo_2 is less than the metabolic rate, so the approach is to either decrease the metabolic rate or increase Vo_2. Achieving a supranormal Vo_2 is difficult to accomplish and can lead to unwanted cardiac and metabolic stimulation. Therefore, decreasing metabolic rate is preferred if possible. At this point in the management, if the prognosis is poor, there may be nothing more to do.

IMPENDING Vo_2 DEFICIT

As described in Chapter 2 and shown in Figure 13.4, Vo_2 is kept constant when Do_2 is reduced because of reciprocal adjustments in O_2ER (5,6). When O_2ER increases to a level of 0.5 to 0.6, Vo_2 becomes

TABLE 13.1. INDIRECT MEASURES OF TISSUE OXYGEN BALANCE		
Parameter	Usual Range	? O$_2$ Deficit
Oxygen uptake (mL/min/m^2)	110–160	< 100
Oxygen extraction ratio	0.2–0.3	> 0.5*
Blood lactate	< 2 mmol/L	> 4 mmol/L
Gastric intramucosal pH	7.35–7.41	< 7.32
* Applies only to conditions where O$_2$ delivery is impaired.		

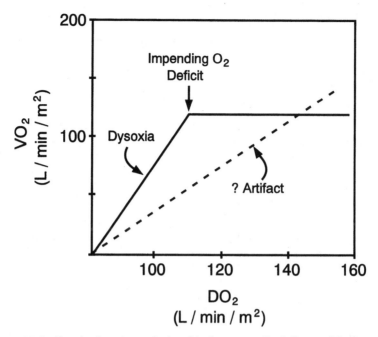

Figure 13.4. Graph showing relationship between O_2 delivery (Do_2) and O_2 uptake (Vo_2) in normal subjects (*solid line*) and in critically ill patients (*dashed line*).

supply dependent as Do_2 is further reduced. When this occurs, cellular energy production is oxygen-limited (dysoxia). Thus, in the setting of impaired O_2 delivery (e.g., low cardiac output or anemia) an O_2ER above 0.5 indicates a high risk of developing impaired tissue oxygenation. In this situation, measures aimed at increasing the Do_2 are protective. This principle has been applied to patients with normovolemic anemia, where an O_2ER above 50% is recommended as an indication for blood transfusion (7).

SUPPLY-DEPENDENT Vo_2

The Do_2–Vo_2 relationship in critically ill patients can differ from the normal pattern, as shown in Figure 13.4. The normal Do_2–Vo_2 relationship (described in Chapter 2) shows a constant Vo_2 over a wide range of variations in Do_2. In critically ill patients, the Do_2–Vo_2 curve is predominantly linear, and the slope is reduced (indicating a low O_2ER). This covariance was originally attributed to dysoxia and was called **pathologic supply dependency.** However, it now seems that in most cases, this phenomenon **is not the result of a pathologic derangement in oxygen metabolism,** but it is a manifestation of the processes described below (5,6,8,9).

Physiologic Coupling

A linear Do_2–Vo_2 relationship can occur when there is a primary change in metabolic rate and Do_2 changes proportionally to match the newly created oxygen requirements. In this situation, the covariance of Do_2 and Vo_2 is a normal adaptive response and is not a sign of impaired tissue oxygenation. Changes in metabolic rate occur commonly in patients in the ICU. The metabolic response to activity is often exaggerated in critically ill patients, and even routine ICU interventions (e.g., portable chest x-ray) can cause significant (20% or greater) increases in metabolic rate (9).

Mathematical Coupling

The **abnormal supply dependency in patients in the ICU** occurs almost exclusively when Do_2 and Vo_2 are calculated, and it **disappears when Vo_2 is directly measured** by gas exchange (8,10–13). This indicates that the abnormal link between Do_2 and Vo_2 is an artifact related to the calculations used to derive these parameters. One possible source of the problem is mathematical coupling because the equations for Do_2 and Vo_2 share three variables (i.e., hemoglobin, cardiac output, and arterial O_2 saturation). Thus, a change in any of these shared variables could affect both calculations and produce an artifactual link.

The source of the artifactual link between Do_2 and Vo_2 is still not clear, but the problem demonstrates that the calculations used to derive O_2 delivery and O_2 uptake can affect the reliability of oxygen transport monitoring. This warrants a brief look at calculated versus measured transport variables.

CALCULATED VERSUS MEASURED Vo_2

The Vo_2 is usually derived (and not measured) using Equation 13.1.

$$Vo_2 = Q \times 13.4 \times Hb \times (Sao_2 - Svo_2) \qquad (13.1)$$

The derivation is based on four measured variables: cardiac output (Q), hemoglobin concentration (Hb), arterial O_2 saturation (Sao_2), and mixed venous O_2 saturation (Svo_2). Each of these measurements varies, and their summed contribution can lead to considerable variability in the calculated Vo_2. This is shown in Table 13.2 (14).

The variability of each component is expressed by the coefficient of variation (CV), which is the standard deviation expressed as a percentage of the mean. Because the standard deviation is expressed on either side of the mean, the CV also expresses a range that is $2 \times CV$, and this range is indicated for each measurement. Laboratory measurements are considered reproducible if they have a CV below 5%, and each of the individual measurements has a CV that is within this range or not far removed. However, the sum of the individual variations creates a large variability in the calculated Vo_2. Considering the range

TABLE 13.2. VARIABILITY IN THE CALCULATED AND MEASURED VO$_2$

Variable	Coefficient of Variation (CV)	Range (2 × CV)
Thermodilution cardiac output	7.35%	14.7%
Whole blood hemoglobin	5.25	10.5
Arterial O$_2$ saturation	0.99	1.9
Mixed venous O$_2$ saturation	2.85	5.7
Calculated VO$_2$	16.44%	32.8%
Measured VO$_2$	3.95%	7.9%
From Schneeweiss B et al. (14).		

of variation, the calculated VO$_2$ could change by 30% without a change in the metabolic condition of the patient.

The calculated VO$_2$ is considered to have a range of error that is 15% on either side of the mean for individual determinations (15). This is consistent with the variability in Table 13.2 and forms the basis for the recommendation that **the calculated VO$_2$ should change at least 15% to be considered a physiologically significant change.**

Gas Exchange

VO$_2$ can also be measured as the oxygen concentration difference in inhaled and exhaled gas multiplied by the respiratory rate. A number of instruments are available that can measure VO$_2$ at the bedside. Many of these instruments can also measure carbon dioxide production (VCO$_2$) and are used by nutrition support services to measure daily energy requirements. As shown in Table 13.2, the measured VO$_2$ is much less variable than the calculated VO$_2$, and thus has less of a tendency for error. Because gas exchange measurements have a CV below 5%, **a change in the measured VO$_2$ that exceeds 5% can be considered physiologically significant.**

Whole Body versus Systemic VO$_2$

Although the calculated and measured VO$_2$ are often compared, they should not be considered equivalent because the gas exchange method measures the whole body VO$_2$, whereas the calculated VO$_2$ measures only systemic VO$_2$. Thus, the measured VO$_2$ is higher than the calculated VO$_2$ by the VO$_2$ in the lungs. Normally, the VO$_2$ in the lungs accounts for less than 5% of the whole body VO$_2$ (16). However, in patients with inflammatory lung injury (i.e., acute respiratory distress syndrome), 20% of the whole body VO$_2$ can take place in the lungs (17). This corresponds to a difference of 25 mL/minute/m^2 between whole body VO$_2$ and calculated VO$_2$. This difference deserves consideration when comparing measured and calculated parameters.

TABLE 13.3 CORRELATIONS WITH OUTCOME IN PATIENTS WITH SEPTIC SHOCK			
	Survivors	Nonsurvivors	Difference
Cardiac index (L/min/m^2)	3.8	3.9	2.6%
Oxygen uptake (mL/min/m^2)	173	164	5.2%
Arterial lactate (mmol/L)	2.6	7.7	296%

Measurements in nonsurvivors are the last ones recorded before death. From Bakker J et al. (20).

BLOOD LACTATE CONCENTRATION

As mentioned, blood lactate levels help determine whether Vo_2 is adequate for the needs of aerobic metabolism. Thus, adding lactate determinations to oxygen transport monitoring provides a more complete assessment of tissue oxygen balance. Because lactate levels in whole blood and plasma are equivalent (18), both measurements are called blood lactate.

BLOOD LACTATE AND SURVIVAL

One of the reasons the blood lactate is such popular test is its ability to predict outcome. A comparison of lactate with cardiac output and oxygen uptake is shown in Table 13.3 for patients with septic shock (19). Neither cardiac output nor oxygen uptake differs significantly in survivors and nonsurvivors, whereas the lactate levels are three times as high in the nonsurvivors. The predictive value of blood lactate levels is consistently better than any measure of hemodynamics or oxygen transport (20), but the ability of lactate to predict mortality is limited mostly to patients with shock.

Optimal Threshold

As shown in Table 13.1, the normal blood lactate concentration is less than 2 mmol/L, but the threshold for an elevated blood lactate is higher, at 4 mmol/L. The reason for this difference is shown in Table 13.4 (18). This table shows the relationship between the cutoff level

TABLE 13.4. INFLUENCE OF LACTATE THRESHOLD ON MORTALITY PREDICTIONS		
Ability to Identify a Fatal Outcome	Whole Blood or Plasma Lactate	
	> 2 mmol/L	> 4 mmol/L
Sensitivity	89%	62%
Specificity	42	88
Positive predictive value	58	80

Observations pertain to hypotensive patients only. From Aduen J et al. (18).

for an elevated blood lactate and the reliability of an elevated lactate level for predicting mortality. The lower threshold of 2 mmol/L is very sensitive but not specific, which means that a considerable fraction of lactate levels in this range will be false positives. On moving to the higher threshold of 4 mmol/L, sensitivity declines by 27% but specificity is much (46%) higher, as is the ability to predict outcome (i.e., the positive predictive value). Thus, the higher threshold is preferred for the clinical definition of hyperlactatemia.

OTHER SOURCES OF LACTATE

Anaerobic metabolism is not the only source of lactate. Other causes of hyperlactatemia include hepatic insufficiency (caused by impaired clearance of lactate by the liver), thiamine deficiency (blocks pyruvate entry into mitochondria), alkalosis (stimulates glycolysis), and production by enteric microbes (D-lactic acid).

Sepsis

Evidence suggests that the lactate accumulation in sepsis is not the result of oxygen deprivation. The culprit may be endotoxin, which blocks the actions of the pyruvate dehydrogenase enzyme that moves pyruvate into mitochondria. Pyruvate then accumulates in the cell cytoplasm and is converted to lactate. The ability of endotoxin to promote lactate formation is shown in the graph in Figure 13.5 (21). This graph is taken from a study in which animals were subjected to a 1-

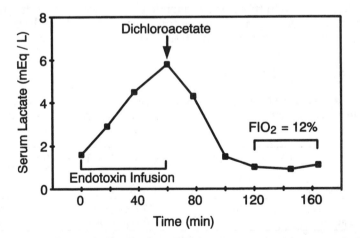

Figure 13.5. Influence of endotoxin, dichloroacetate, and hypoxic challenge on arterial lactate levels. Response to dichloroacetate indicates that endotoxin-associated lactic acidosis is not caused by anaerobic conditions. (From Curtis SE, Cain SM. Regional and systemic oxygen delivery/uptake relations and lactate flux in hyperdynamic, endotoxin-treated dogs. Am Rev Respir Dis 1992;145:348–354.)

hour infusion of endotoxin. As indicated on the graph, the endotoxin infusion was associated with a progressive rise in blood lactate. After the endotoxin infusion, the animals were given dichloroacetate, a substance that activates pyruvate dehydrogenase, but only in the presence of oxygen. The dichloroacetate was able to reduce the lactate levels to normal, indicating that oxygen was present in cells to permit the activation of pyruvate dehydrogenase. Furthermore, when hypoxia was induced by having the animals breathe a low-oxygen gas mixture (on the right side of the graph), the lactate levels failed to rise. This study shows that oxygen deprivation can be unrelated to lactate production in a setting that mimics sepsis.

LACTATE AS A FUEL

A final word about lactate that deserves mention is the possibility that lactate might serve as an oxidative fuel. The energy yield from the oxidation of lactate is shown in Table 13.5. Also shown is the energy yield from the oxidation of glucose. The energy yield from glucose oxidation is twice that of lactate, but glucose is twice the size of lactate (i.e., 6 carbons versus 3 carbons, respectively). Because each mole of glucose produces 2 moles of lactate, the energy yield from glucose metabolism is about the same when glucose is directly oxidized and when glucose is converted to lactate and the lactate is oxidized. A number of organs can oxidize lactate to derive energy, including the heart, brain, liver, and skeletal muscle (22,23).

If the lactate generated during periods of oxygen deprivation can undergo oxidation at a later time, when tissue oxygenation is restored, then the energy yield of glucose oxidation (i.e., oxidative metabolism) will be preserved. In this context, lactate production would be a mechanism for preserving nutrient energy during periods of hypoxia or ischemia, when prevailing conditions do not favor oxidation.

GASTRIC TONOMETRY

The oxygen transport variables and blood lactate levels are global (whole body) measures that cannot identify oxygen deficits in individ-

TABLE 13.5. LACTATE AS AN OXIDATIVE FUEL			
Substrate	Molecular Weight	Heat of Combustion	Caloric Value
Glucose	180	673 kcal/mole	3.74 kcal/g
Lactate	90	326 kcal/mole	3.62 kcal/g

$$\text{Glucose} \xrightarrow{\text{Oxidation}} 673 \text{ kcal}$$
$$\downarrow$$
$$(2) \text{ Lactate} \xrightarrow{\text{Oxidation}} 652 \text{ kcal}$$

From Lehninger AL. Bioenergetics. New York: WA Benjamin, 1965;16.

TABLE 13.6. THE GASTRIC TONOMETRY METHOD
1. A saline-filled balloon, permeable to CO_2, is placed in contact with the gastric mucosa. The CO_2 in the adjacent mucosa equilibrates with the saline in the balloon, and the Pco_2 in the saline is used as a measure of the Pco_2 in the gastric mucosa.
2. The bicarbonate concentration in arterial blood is used as a measure of the bicarbonate in the gastric mucosa.
3. The intramucosal pH is then derived with the Henderson–Hasselbach equation. $$pHi = 6.1 + \log_{10} \frac{\text{Arterial } HCO_3^-}{\text{Saline } Pco_2 \times 0.03}$$

ual organs. This limitation became a concern upon the discovery that splanchnic hypoperfusion is common in critically ill patients and may be the prelude to multiorgan failure (24). This led to the development of the method described here for evaluating oxygenation in the gastrointestinal tract (25,26).

METHOD

The basic elements of this method are outlined in Table 13.6. This method uses an indirect measurement of the pH in the gastric mucosa to evaluate the adequacy of tissue oxygenation (i.e., oxygen deficits produce a local acidosis). This measurement is derived using the Henderson–Hasselbach equation and an indirect measure of the gastric mucosal carbon dioxide pressure (Pco_2), obtained with a tonometer.

The tonometer is a CO_2-permeable silicone balloon affixed to the distal end of a standard 16-French nasogastric tube. The apparatus is placed in the stomach in the usual fashion, and the balloon is partially filled with saline (2.5 mL) and left that way for at least 30 minutes. During this time, the balloon is in contact with the gastric mucosa, and the CO_2 in the adjacent mucosa moves into the balloon. The CO_2 eventually equilibrates between the tissues and the saline in the balloon. When this occurs, the Pco_2 in the saline approximates the Pco_2 in the gastric mucosa, and thus the saline Pco_2 is measured and used as the intramucosal Pco_2. The pH calculation also requires a measure of the tissue bicarbonate, and the bicarbonate concentration in an arterial blood sample is used for this purpose. The normal gastric intramucosal pH has a mean of 7.38 and a standard deviation (SD) of 0.3, so the range is 7.35 to 7.41 (1 SD on either side of the mean). The threshold for an abnormal pH is 7.32, which is 2 SDs from the mean (Table 13.1).

PERFORMANCE

The advantage of monitoring pH in the gastric mucosa is illustrated by the case depicted in Figure 13.6. The line plots represent the tem-

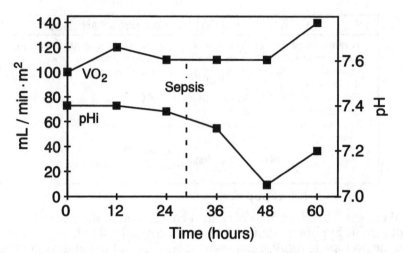

Figure 13.6. Postoperative changes in oxygen uptake (Vo_2) and gastric intra-mucosal pH (*pHi*) in a patient with postoperative sepsis. Onset of sepsis syndrome is indicated by the dashed line. Patient returned to operating room at 48 hours. (From Gutierrez G. Cellular energy metabolism during hypoxia. Crit Care Med 1991;19:619–626.)

poral changes in the systemic oxygen uptake (Vo_2) and the gastric intramucosal pH (pHi) in the early postoperative period following renal transplantation. Both measures are in the normal range during the first postoperative day. However, at approximately 30 hours after surgery, the patient developed a sepsis syndrome (indicated by the dashed line). Thereafter, the intramucosal pH dropped precipitously, while the Vo_2 remained unchanged. The patient was returned to the operating room 12 hours after the onset of sepsis, and an infected renal implant was removed. The sepsis subsequently resolved and the patient survived. At no time during this rocky postoperative course did the Vo_2 provide any hint of danger, whereas the gastric mucosal pH showed evidence of progressive ischemia as the sepsis progressed.

In keeping with the observations in Figure 13.6, the gastric mucosal pH has proven superior to the global measures of tissue oxygenation (O_2 transport variables and lactate) for predicting outcome in critically ill patients (25–28).

PROBLEMS

A number of shortcomings associated with gastric tonometry deserve mention. Descriptions of the major ones follow.

Gastric Acid Secretion

Acid secretion in the stomach is a confounding variable that must be eliminated when using gastric mucosal pH as a marker of tissue oxygenation. Routine doses of histamine H_2 blockers may not achieve adequate acid suppression. Administration of ranitidine 100 mg intravenously 1 hour before measurements effectively blocks acid secretion for 2 to 4 hours (29). Raising gastric pH carries the risk of gastric colonization, which is not a desirable condition in critically ill patients (as discussed in Chapter 6).

Acid–Base Disorders

Systemic acid–base disorders can also influence the pH of the gastric mucosa (30). This is a particular concern because metabolic acidosis can be common in patients with circulatory shock, and these patients represent a large target population for gastric mucosal pH monitoring. Also of concern is respiratory alkalosis, which is common in mechanically ventilated patients.

Arterial versus Mucosal Bicarbonate

The use of arterial bicarbonate as a measure of mucosal bicarbonate is problematic because the two are not equivalent in low flow states (because of local accumulation of acid) (24). Thus, in low flow states, where accuracy is most important, arterial bicarbonate measurements are likely to produce the least accurate results.

MANAGEMENT

The treatment of abnormal mucosal pH is not well defined. The few studies available on treatment use volume infusions followed by dobutamine. The volume is given in aliquots, with no clear endpoint. Dobutamine has consistently increased mucosal blood flow, but its effects on mucosal pH are variable. Individual studies of dobutamine show increased pH (31,32), no change in pH (33), and even decreased pH (34). The response to dobutamine therefore must be determined on an individual basis.

REFERENCES

GENERAL TEXTS

Edwards JD, Shoemaker WC, Vincent JL, eds. Oxygen transport. Principles and practice. Philadelphia: WB Saunders, 1993.
Marston A, Bulkley GB, Fiddian-Green RG, Haglund UH, eds. Splanchnic ischemia and multiple organ failure. St. Louis: CV Mosby, 1989.

TISSUE OXYGEN BALANCE

1. Connett RJ, Honig CR, Gayeski TEJ, Brooks GA. Defining hypoxia: a systems view of V_{O_2}, glycolysis, energetics, and intracellular P_{O_2}. J Appl Physiol 1990; 68:833–842.

OXYGEN TRANSPORT

2. Shoemaker WC, Kram HB, Appel PL. Therapy of shock based on pathophysiology, monitoring, and outcome prediction. Crit Care Med 1990;18(Suppl): S19–S25.
3. Dunham CM, Seigel JH, Weireter L, et al. Oxygen debt and metabolic acidemia as quantitative predictors of mortality and the severity of the ischemic insult in hemorrhagic shock. Crit Care Med 1991;19:231–243.
4. Shoemaker WC, Appel PL, Krom HB. Role of oxygen debt in the development of organ failure, sepsis, and death in high-risk surgical patients. Chest 1992; 102:208–215.
5. Leach RM, Treacher DF. The relationship between oxygen delivery and consumption. Dis Mon 1994;30:301–368.
6. Dantzker DR, Foresman B, Gutierrez G. Oxygen supply and utilization relationships. Am Rev Respir Dis 1991;143:675–679.
7. Levy P, Chavez RP, Crystal GJ, et al. Oxygen extraction ratio: a valid indicator of transfusion need in limited coronary vascular reserve? J Trauma 1992;32: 769–774.
8. Russell JA, Phang PT. The oxygen delivery/consumption controversy. Am Rev Respir Crit Care Med 1994;149:533–537.
9. Weissman C, Kemper M. The oxygen uptake–oxygen delivery relationship during ICU interventions. Chest 1991;99:430–435.
10. Hanique G, Dugernier T, Laterre PF, et al. Significance of pathologic oxygen supply dependence in critically ill patients: comparison between measured and calculated methods. Intensive Care Med 1994;20:12–18.
11. Ronco JJ, Phang PT, Walley KR, et al. Oxygen consumption is independent of changes in oxygen delivery in severe adult respiratory distress syndrome. Am Rev Respir Dis 1991;143:1267–1273.
12. Romco JJ, Fenwick JC, Wiggs BR, et al. Oxygen consumption is independent of increases in oxygen delivery by dobutamine in septic patients who have normal or increased lactate. Am Rev Respir Dis 1993;147:25–31.
13. Marik PE, Sibbald W. Effect of stored-blood transfusion on oxygen delivery in patients with sepsis. JAMA 1993;269:3024–3029.
14. Schneeweiss B, Druml W, Graninger W, et al. Assessment of oxygen-consumption by use of reverse Fick principle and indirect calorimetry in critically ill patients. Clin Nutr 1989;8:89–93.
15. Bartlett RH, Dechert RE. Oxygen kinetics: pitfalls in clinical research. J Crit Care 1990;5:77–80.
16. Nunn JF. Non-respiratory functions of the lung. In: Nunn JF, ed. Applied respiratory physiology. 4th ed. Kent, England: Butterworth, 1993;306–317.
17. Jolliet P, Thorens JB, Nicod L, et al. Relationship between pulmonary oxygen consumption, lung inflammation, and calculated venous admixture in patients with acute lung injury. Intensive Care Med 1996;22:277–285.

BLOOD LACTATE

18. Aduen J, Bernstein WK, Khastgir T, et al. The use and clinical importance of a substrate-specific electrode for rapid determination of blood lactate concentrations. JAMA 1994;272:1678–1685.
19. Mizock BA, Falk JL. Lactic acidosis in critical illness. Crit Care Med 1992;20: 80–93.
20. Bakker J, Coffernils M, Leon M, et al. Blood lactate levels are superior to oxygen-derived variables in predicting outcome in septic shock. Chest 1991; 99:956–962.

21. Curtis SE, Cain SM. Regional and systemic oxygen delivery/uptake relations and lactate flux in hyperdynamic, endotoxin-treated dogs. Am Rev Respir Dis 1992;145:348–354.
22. Brooks GA. Lactate production under fully aerobic conditions: the lactate shuttle during rest and exercise. Fed Proc 1986;45:2924–2929.
23. Maran A, Cranston I, Lomas J, et al. Protection by lactate of cerebral function during hypoglycemia. Lancet 1994;343:16–20.

GASTRIC TONOMETRY

24. Fiddian-Green RG. Studies in splanchnic ischemia and multiple organ failure. In: Marston A, Bulkley GB, Fiddian-Green RG, Haglund UH, eds. Splanchnic ischemia and multiple organ failure. St. Louis: CV Mosby, 1989;349–364.
25. Fiddian-Green RG. Tonometry: theory and applications. Intensive Care World 1992;9:60–65.
26. Gutierrez G, Brown SD. Gastric tonometry: a new monitoring modality in the intensive care unit. J Intensive Care Med 1995;10:34–44.
27. Marik PE. Gastric intramucosal pH. A better predictor of multiorgan dysfunction syndrome and death than oxygen-derived variables in patients with sepsis. Chest 1993;104:225–229.
28. Maynard N, Bihari D, Beale R, et al. Assessment of splanchnic oxygenation by gastric tonometry in patients with acute circulatory failure. JAMA 1993; 270:1203–1210.
29. Kolkman JJ, Groeneveld ABJ, Meuwissen SGM. Effect of ranitidine on basal and bicarbonate enhanced intragastric P_{CO_2}: a tonometric study. Gut 1994;35: 737–741.
30. Benjamin E, Polokoff E, Oropello JM, et al. Sodium bicarbonate administration affects the diagnostic accuracy of gastrointestinal tonometry in acute mesenteric ischemia. Crit Care Med 1992;20:1181–1183.
31. Silverman HJ, Tuma P. Gastric tonometry in patients with sepsis: effects of dobutamine infusions and packed red blood cell transfusions. Chest 1992;102: 184–188.
32. Gutierrez G, Clark C, Brown SD, et al. Effect of dobutamine on oxygen consumption and gastric mucosal pH in septic patients. Am Rev Respir Crit Care Med 1994;150:324–329.
33. Uusaro A, Ruokonen E, Takala J. Splanchnic oxygen transport after cardiac surgery: evidence for inadequate tissue perfusion after stabilization of hemodynamics. Intensive Care Med 1996;22:26–33.
34. Parviainen I, Ruokonen E, Takala J. Dobutamine-induced dissociation between changes in splanchnic blood flow and gastric intramucosal pH. Br J Anesth 1995;74:277–284.

section IV
DISORDERS OF CIRCULATORY FLOW

Movement is the cause of all life.
Leonardo da Vinci

chapter

14

HEMORRHAGE AND HYPOVOLEMIA

The dominant concern in the bleeding patient is the human body's intolerance to acute blood loss. The human cardiovascular system operates with a small volume and a steep Starling curve, which seems to be an energy-efficient design, but does not bode well in acute blood loss. Although we are more than half fluid by weight, only 12 to 13% of this fluid is located in the bloodstream. Because the acute loss of 40% of the blood volume can be fatal, the loss of only 5% (0.4 × 12%) of our total fluid volume can prove fatal. When confronted with acute hemorrhage, the task is to intervene before this small aliquot of fluid is lost.

This chapter introduces some of the fundamental concerns in the initial management of acute hemorrhage (1–9). The next chapter describes the different types of intravenous fluids. The material in these two chapters provides a fundamental knowledge of the principles of volume resuscitation.

BODY FLUIDS AND BLOOD LOSS

The relationship between total fluid volume and blood volume in adults is shown in Table 14.1 (10). The total volume of body fluids represents 60% of lean body weight (or 600 mL/kg) in men and 50% of lean body weight (or 500 mL/kg) in women. The volume of whole blood is 6.0 to 6.6% of lean body weight (or 60 to 66 mL/kg), which means that only 11 (i.e., 66/600) to 12% (60/500) of the total body fluid volume is in the intravascular compartment. Approximately 60% of the blood volume is in the plasma fraction, and the remaining 40% represents the erythrocyte volume. The corresponding volumes for an average-size adult man (weighing 80 kg or 176 lbs) and adult woman (weighing 60 kg or 132 lbs) is shown below.

TABLE 14.1. BODY FLUID AND BLOOD VOLUMES		
Fluid	Men	Women
Total body fluid	600 mL/kg	500 mL/kg
Whole blood	66 mL/kg	60 mL/kg
Plasma	40 mL/kg	36 mL/kg
Erythrocytes	26 mL/kg	24 mL/kg

Values expressed for lean body weights.
American Association of Blood Banks Technical Manual. 10th ed. Arlington, VA: American Association of Blood Banks, 1990:650.

	80-kg Man	60-kg Woman
Total body fluids	48 L	30 L
Whole blood	5.3 L	3.6 L
Plasma	3.2 L	2.2 L
Erythrocytes	2.1 L	1.4 L

Adjustments

The American Association of Blood Banks recommends the following adjustments for estimating blood, plasma, and erythrocyte volumes based on body weight (10).

1. For obese and elderly patients, estimate the volumes based on lean body weight and reduce the values by 10%.
2. For patients with a marked weight loss within 6 months, use the premorbid weight loss to estimate volumes.

RESPONSE TO MILD BLOOD LOSS

The principles of volume resuscitation are based on the normal body response to hemorrhage. This response has been examined in mild hemorrhage (< 15% loss in blood volume), when volume resuscitation is not necessary. The response is described in three stages (4).

Stage 1. The first hours after the onset of blood loss is characterized by movement of interstitial fluid into the capillaries. This *transcapillary refill* helps maintain blood volume but leaves an interstitial fluid deficit.

Stage 2. The loss of body fluids leads to activation of the renin–angiotensin–aldosterone system. This results in sodium conservation by the kidneys. Because sodium distributes primarily in the interstitial space, the retained sodium replenishes the interstitial fluid deficit.

Stage 3. Within a few hours after the onset of hemorrhage, the marrow begins to increase the production of erythrocytes. This response occurs more gradually, and complete replacement of erythrocytes can take up to 2 months (4).

According to the response to mild hemorrhage described above, the goal of acute volume resuscitation for blood loss should be to replenish interstitial fluid deficits (3,4). This is why crystalloid (electrolyte) fluids are used in the resuscitation of acute blood loss (3), as is discussed later.

CLINICAL CONSEQUENCES

The clinical consequences of hypovolemia are determined by the rapidity and magnitude of volume loss and by the responsiveness of individual patients to volume loss. Most cases of mild blood loss are relatively free of clinical manifestations. In fact, **hypovolemia may be clinically silent until the volume loss exceeds 30% of the blood volume.**

The American College of Surgeons identifies four categories of acute blood loss based on the percent loss of blood volume (11). These are shown in Table 14.2.

Class I. Loss of 15% or less of the total blood volume. This degree of blood loss is usually fully compensated by transcapillary refill. Because blood volume is maintained, clinical manifestations of hypovolemia are minimal or absent.

Class II. Loss of 15 to 30% of the blood volume. The clinical findings at this stage may include resting tachycardia and orthostatic changes in heart rate and blood pressure. However, **resting tachycardia can be an inconsistent finding, and orthostatic changes in pulse and blood pressure are too insensitive to be considered reliable manifestations** (5a,6,12). A positive tilt test, defined as an increase in pulse rate greater than 30 beats/minute or a drop in systolic pressure greater than 30 mm Hg on assuming the upright position (12), can be used as corroborative evidence for blood loss, but a negative result has no meaning. When the tilt test is performed, the lower legs must be in a dependent position (sitting without legs dangling is inappropriate). Also, because changes in pulse and pressure are variable within the first minute after changing positions

TABLE 14.2. CLASSIFICATION OF HEMORRHAGE BASED ON EXTENT OF BLOOD LOSS				
Parameter	Class I	Class II	Class III	Class IV
% Loss of blood volume	< 15%	15–30%	30–40%	> 40%
Pulse rate	< 100	> 100	> 120	> 140
Supine blood pressure	Normal	Normal	Decreased	Decreased
Urine output (mL/hr)	> 30	20–30	5–15	< 5
Mental status	Anxious	Agitated	Confused	Lethargic
Committee on Trauma. Advanced trauma life support student manual. Chicago: American College of Surgeons, 1989:57.				

(13), a waiting period of at least 1 minute after changing positions is recommended before the vital signs are recorded.

Class III. Loss of 30 to 40% of the blood volume usually marks the onset of hypovolemic shock, with a decrease in blood pressure and urine output. There is evidence that the tachycardia–vasoconstrictor response to hemorrhage can be lost at this stage of blood loss (5a). When this occurs, the decrease in blood pressure can be sudden and profound.

Class IV. Loss of more than 40% of blood volume is a harbinger of circulatory collapse. Therefore, when hypovolemia is accompanied by marked hypotension, oliguria, or other evidence of organ failure, prompt volume resuscitation is mandatory.

CLINICAL MONITORING

The clinical evaluation of blood loss is far from precise, even when employing invasive hemodynamic monitoring. The following are some important points regarding the clinical parameters used to evaluate patients with suspected or documented blood loss.

BLOOD PRESSURE

The systemic blood pressure is not a sensitive marker of blood loss, as shown in Table 14.2. However, when blood loss is severe enough to produce hypotension, the blood pressure can be a valuable guide in the resuscitative effort. As mentioned in Chapter 9, the **noninvasive methods of measuring blood pressure often yield spuriously low measurements in patients with hypovolemia** (presumably because of the vasoconstrictor response to volume loss) (6). Therefore, when hypovolemia begins to produce a change in noninvasive blood pressure measurements, the pressure should be monitored by direct intra-arterial recordings.

CARDIAC FILLING PRESSURES

Although **cardiac filling pressures** (i.e., the central venous pressure [CVP] and wedge pressure) are monitored routinely in patients with acute blood loss, these pressures **show a poor correlation with the presence and extent of volume loss** (14,15). In particular, these pressures often show little change until the blood loss is severe (i.e., greater than 30% of the blood volume). This insensitivity can be explained in two ways. First, the CVP and wedge pressures are normally low pressures (particularly the CVP, which is normally less than 5 mm Hg), and thus there is little margin for a detectable change in hypovolemia. Second, hypovolemia can be accompanied by a decrease in ventricular distensibility (presumably as a result of sympathetic activation) (16), and when this occurs, the CVP and wedge pressures will be higher than expected at any given ventricular volume. In one animal study of hypovolemia, decreases in ventricular compliance resulted in a two-fold increase in the wedge (left-ventricular end-diastolic) pressure despite a 50% reduction in the end-diastolic volume (16).

Positional changes in cardiac filling pressures may be a more sensitive marker of hypovolemia. In one report, hypovolemia failed to produce a change in the CVP when it was measured in the supine position; however, when the patients were placed in an upright position, the CVP decreased 4 to 5 mm Hg (17). Therefore, performing orthostatic maneuvers may help improve the sensitivity of cardiac filling pressures in hypovolemia.

OXYGEN EXTRACTION

As explained in Chapter 2, the normal response to a decrease in cardiac output (O_2 delivery) is an increase in oxygen extraction in the systemic microcirculation. This is a compensatory response aimed at keeping oxygen uptake normal when oxygen delivery is compromised. However, there is a limit to the increase in oxygen extraction, and when this limit is reached, decreases in cardiac output are accompanied by proportional decreases in oxygen uptake into the tissues (see Fig. 2.2). Therefore, an increase in O_2 extraction can be a marker of systemic hypoperfusion, and a maximum increases in O_2 extraction can be a marker of hypovolemic shock.

Oxygen extraction can be monitored without a pulmonary artery catheter by combining pulse oximetry (for arterial O_2 saturation) with measurements of oxygen saturation in blood samples obtained from a CVP catheter (the O_2 saturation in the superior vena cava is normally close to the mixed venous O_2 saturation). The expected changes in O_2 extraction and mixed venous O_2 saturation in progressive hypovolemia are shown below.

	Sao_2	Svo_2	$Sao_2 - Svo_2$
Normal	>95%	>65%	20–30%
Hypovolemia	>95%	50–65%	30–50%
Hypovolemic shock	>95%	<50%	>50%

The transition from compensated hypovolemia to hypovolemic shock takes place when the oxygen extraction reaches 50 to 60% and the mixed venous O_2 saturation falls to 50%. Therefore, **an O_2 extraction greater than 30% is a marker of hemodynamically significant hypovolemia, and an O_2 extraction greater than 50% indicates possible hypovolemia shock.** When the O_2 extraction exceeds 50%, a blood lactate level will help identify hypovolemic shock (a lactate level greater than 4 mmol/L indicates a shock state). Oxygen extraction can also be increased by hypermetabolism or in response to anemia, and these conditions must also be considered in the interpretation of an increased O_2 extraction.

END-EXPIRATORY CO_2

A decrease in cardiac output will decrease the P_{CO_2} in exhaled gas(18), and because the P_{CO_2} in exhaled gas can be measured noninvasively (see Chapter 22), this provides a potentially useful method for monitoring the severity of hypovolemia. Intubation is not necessary, because exhaled CO_2 can be monitored using standard nasal cannulas used to deliver supplemental oxygen (described in Chapter 22).

The changes in end-expiratory (end-tidal) P_{CO_2} in hypovolemia and volume resuscitation are shown in Figure 14.1 (6). The data in this figure are from a patient who presented with hypovolemic shock. The end-tidal P_{CO_2} before volume infusion is very low at 10 mm Hg (the end-tidal P_{CO_2} is normally within 3 mm Hg of the arterial P_{CO_2}). After volume resuscitation with 4.5 L of intravenous fluids, the end-tidal P_{CO_2} has risen to 30 mm Hg, indicating that the cardiac output has increased in response to the volume infusion. Because the end-tidal P_{CO_2} is measured on a breath-by-breath basis, it provides an on-line measure of the success or failure of volume resuscitation.

End-tidal CO_2 monitoring has been recommended for evaluating the response to cardiopulmonary resuscitation, and it should have a similar role in the evaluation of hypovolemia.

The Hematocrit

Both physicians and nurses share a common propensity to use the hematocrit as an estimate of acute blood loss. The error of this practice is indicated in the following statement taken from the Advanced

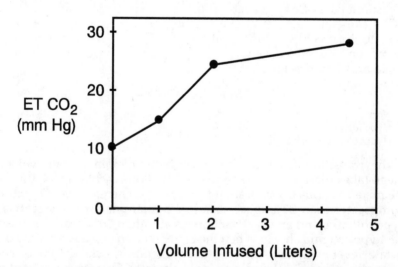

Figure 14.1. Serial changes in the end-tidal P_{CO_2} (ET CO_2) during volume resuscitation of a patient with hypovolemic shock. Horizontal axis represents cumulative volume infused. (From Falk JL et al. Fluid resuscitation in traumatic hemorrhagic shock. Crit Care Clin 1992;8:323–340.)

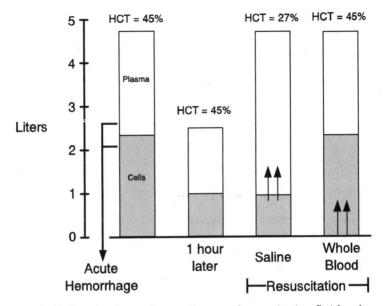

Figure 14.2. Influence of acute hemorrhage and resuscitation fluid on hematocrit. Each vertical bar is partitioned to indicated contribution of plasma and blood cells to total blood volume. Hematocrit indicated at the top of each vertical bar. (See text for further explanation.)

Trauma Life Support Course student manual, published by the American College of Surgeons: **"Use of the hematocrit to estimate acute blood loss is unreliable and inappropriate"** (11). Changes in hematocrit show a poor correlation with blood volume deficits and red cell volume deficits in acute hemorrhage (15). In fact, loss of whole blood is not expected to change the hematocrit because the relative proportions of plasma and red cell volume are unchanged. The decrease in hematocrit occurs when the kidney begins to conserve sodium (as described previously), which takes 8 to 12 hours to become evident. Another factor that drops the hematocrit in acute hemorrhage is the administration of intravenous (asanguinous) fluids.

The influence of volume resuscitation on the hematocrit is illustrated in Figure 14.2. Each column in this figure is partitioned to indicate the relative proportions of plasma and erythrocytes in the blood. The columns on the left show that acute blood loss decreases blood volume but does not change the hematocrit. The columns on the right show the influence of blood and asanguinous fluids on the hematocrit. Saline infusion increases the plasma volume selectively and thereby decreases the hematocrit. Infusion of whole blood expands the plasma and erythrocyte fractions proportionately, and thus does not alter the hematocrit. Therefore, in the first hours after the onset of blood loss, the hematocrit is a reflection of the resuscitation effort, not the extent of blood loss. The administration of intravenous (asanguinous) fluids is expected to produce a dilutional decrease in the hematocrit, even in the absence of blood loss (19), and thus a decrease in the hematocrit during volume resuscitation is a dilutional effect, and it is not an indication of ongoing blood loss.

RATE OF VOLUME RESUSCITATION

The mortality in hypovolemic shock is directly related to the magnitude and duration of the ischemic insult (6), and thus prompt replacement of volume deficits is the hallmark of successful management. The ability to infuse volume rapidly is thus an important consideration in the management of hypovolemia. The following is a brief description of the factors that influence the rate of volume infusion.

VASCULAR ACCESS SITE

Although there is a tendency to cannulate the large central veins for volume resuscitation, cannulation of peripheral veins is preferred. The larger size of the central veins is not an important consideration in volume resuscitation because **the rate of volume infusion is determined by the dimensions of the vascular catheter, not by the size of the vein.** Cannulation of the large central veins requires catheters that are at least 5 inches in length, whereas cannulation of peripheral veins can be accomplished with catheters that are 2 inches in length. Shorter catheters permit more rapid rates of volume infusion, and thus cannulation of peripheral veins is more favorable for rapid volume resuscitation. Central venous cannulation is reserved for monitoring cardiac filling pressures and venous O_2 saturation unless very-large-bore *introducer catheters* are used for volume resuscitation.

Catheter Dimensions

The determinants of flow through rigid tubes is described in Chapter 1. According to the Hagen-Poiseuille equation (presented in the latter part of Chapter 1 and depicted schematically in Figure 1.4), the rate of laminar or streamlined flow will vary directly with the fourth power of the inner radius of the catheter. Thus, if the radius of a catheter is doubled, the flow rate through the catheter will increase sixteenfold; that is, $(2r)^4 = 16r$. Changes in catheter length will have a proportional influence on flow rate; that is, if the length is doubled, the infusion rate will decrease by one-half. Because central venous catheters are 3 to 4 times longer than peripheral venous catheters, **the infusion rate through central catheters will be as much as 75% less than the infusion rate through peripheral catheters (of equal diameter).**

The influence of catheter size on infusion rate is shown in Figure

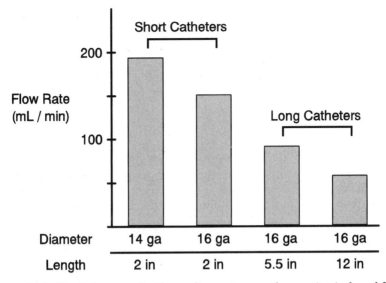

Figure 14.3. The influence of catheter dimensions on the gravity-induced flow rate of tap water. Catheter dimensions are indicated below the horizontal axis of the graph. (From Mateer JR et al. Rapid fluid resuscitation with central venous catheters. Ann Emerg Med 1983;12:149–152.)

14.3 (21). The fluid in this case is water, and the gradient for flow is the force of gravity. Note that for catheters of equivalent diameter (16 gauge), flow is 1.5 to 3 times faster in the shorter (2 inch) catheter. This demonstrates why shorter peripheral catheters are preferred for the resuscitation of hemorrhage.

Rapid Infusion

Because the radius of a tube has a much stronger influence on flow rate than the length of the tube, rapid infusion rates are more easily achieved by increasing the diameter of a catheter rather than decreasing its length. Rapid volume infusion, defined as the infusion of at least 5 L of fluid hourly (20), is thus best accomplished by using large-bore introducer catheters normally used in conjunction with multilumen central venous catheters. Introducer catheters are described in Chapter 4 (see Figure 4.3). These devices are 5 to 6 inches in length and are available in 8.5 French (2.7 mm outer diameter) and 9 French (3 mm outer diameter) sizes. They are normally used as intravascular conduits or sheaths for multilumen central venous and pulmonary artery catheters, and they allow these catheters to be inserted and removed without sacrificing the central venous access site. However, introducer catheters can be used as stand-alone infusion devices when rapid infusion is desirable. As shown in Table 14.3, flow through introducer catheters is almost as rapid as flow through standard intrave-

TABLE 14.3. RAPID VOLUME INFUSION	
Conduit	Flow Rate[1]
3-mm Intravenous tubing	1030 mL/min
9-French introducer catheter	838 mL/min
Side port of introducer catheter	238 mL/min

[1] Gravity flow of tap water.
From Hyman SA et al. Anesth Analg 1991;75:573.

nous tubing. However, as also shown in Table 14.3, the side infusion ports on introducer catheters create an impediment to flow (22). Thus, **when introducer catheters are used for rapid volume infusion, the side infusion port on the catheter must be bypassed.**

VISCOSITY

Viscosity is described in Chapter 1 as the property of a fluid that resists changes in flow rate. As shown in Table 1.2, the viscosity of blood is primarily a function of the erythrocyte density (i.e., hematocrit). The graph in Figure 14.4 shows the influence of cell density (viscosity) on the infusion rate of different resuscitation fluids (23). The force responsible for flow in this case is gravity, and the infusion device is a 16-gauge, 2-inch catheter similar to the ones used to cannulate peripheral veins. The acellular fluids (i.e., water and 5% albumin) have

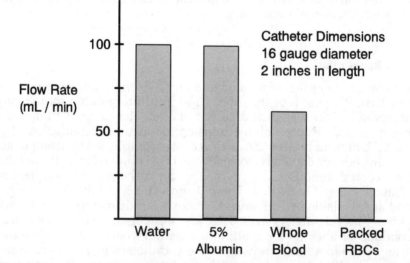

Figure 14.4. Gravity-driven infusion rates of blood products and intravenous fluids flowing through the same sized catheter. (From Dula DJ et al. Flow rate variance of commonly used IV infusion techniques. J Trauma 1981;21: 480–482.)

the highest flow rates, whereas the erythrocyte concentrate (packed RBCs) has the slowest flow rate. This demonstrates the inverse relationship between viscosity and flow rate in the Hagen–Poiseuille equation (see Chapter 1).

There is a popular misconception that colloid fluids such as plasma or albumin solutions flow more sluggishly than water or electrolyte solutions. However, because viscosity is primarily a function of cellular density, all acellular fluids should have equivalent flow properties. This is demonstrated by the equivalent flow rates for water and 5% albumin shown in Figure 14.4. Therefore, colloid solutions (containing large molecular weight substances) will infuse just as rapidly as crystalloid (electrolyte) solutions.

AUTOTRANSFUSION

Autotransfusion maneuvers are meant to promote venous return by shifting blood volume from the legs toward the heart. There are two autotransfusion methods: body tilt and pneumatic compression. Unfortunately, neither method is successful in achieving the desired effect, as described below.

THE TRENDELENBURG POSITION

Elevation of the pelvis above the horizontal plane in the supine position was introduced in the latter part of the 19th century as a method of facilitating surgical exposure of the pelvic organs. The originator was a surgeon named Friedrich Trendelenburg, who specialized in the surgical correction of vesicovaginal fistulas (5). The body position that now bears his name was later adopted as an *antishock position* during World War I and gained widespread popularity despite a lack of evidence for its efficacy. This popularity continues, as does the lack of evidence for efficacy (24–27).

Hemodynamic Effects

The hemodynamic effects of the Trendelenburg position (legs elevated and head below the horizontal plane) are shown in Table 14.4.

Parameter	Supine	Legs Up, Head Down	Change %	Change p	Effect
TABLE 14.4. HEMODYNAMIC EFFECTS OF THE TRENDELENBURG POSITION IN HYPOVOLEMIC ICU PATIENTS					
Mean arterial blood pressure (mm Hg)	64	71	11	< .001	↑
Wedge pressure (mm Hg)	4.6	7.2	57	< .001	↑
Cardiac index (L/min · m²)	2.1	1.9	9	NS	↔
Systemic vascular resistance (dyne · sec/cm⁵m²)	2347	2905	24	< .001	↑
Sing R et al. Ann Emerg Med 1994;23:564.					

The data in this table are from a study we performed on postoperative patients with indwelling pulmonary artery catheters who had evidence of severe hypovolemia (i.e., low cardiac filling pressures and hypotension) (24). The hemodynamic measurements were obtained in the supine position, and then repeated after the patients were placed in a position with the legs elevated 45 degrees above the horizontal plane and the head placed 15 degrees below the horizontal plane. As shown in the table, the change in position was associated with significant increases in the mean arterial pressure, wedge (left-ventricular filling) pressure, and systemic vascular resistance, while the cardiac output remained the same. This lack of an effect on the cardiac output indicates that the **Trendelenburg position does *not* promote venous return to the heart.** The increase in the wedge pressure can be due to an increase in intrathoracic pressure (transmitted into the pulmonary capillaries) caused by cephalad displacement of the diaphragm during the body tilt. The increase in blood pressure during body tilt is likely due to systemic vasoconstriction (indicated by the rise in systemic vascular resistance). These observations are consistent with other studies in animals and humans (25–27).

Why the Trendelenburg Position Cannot Work

The inability of the Trendelenburg position to augment cardiac output is not surprising, and it is explained by the high capacitance (distensibility) of the venous circulation. To augment cardiac output, the Trendelenburg position must increase the pressure gradient from peripheral to central veins, which would then increase venous return. However, the venous system is a high-capacitance system designed to absorb pressure and act as a volume reservoir. Thus, when pressure is applied to a vein, the vein distends and increases its volume capacity. This distensibility then limits any change in venous pressure, and this, in turn, counteracts any increase in the pressure gradient between peripheral and central veins. The venous system is more likely to transmit pressure when the veins are volume overloaded and less distensible. In other words, the Trendelenburg position is more likely to be effective (i.e., to augment venous return) during volume *overload*, not volume depletion.

Thus, the Trendelenburg position has not been, and never will be, effective in promoting venous return (cardiac output) in hypovolemia. As such, **this maneuver should be abandoned for the management of hypovolemia.** It remains axiomatic that the effective treatment for hypovolemia is volume replacement.

PNEUMATIC COMPRESSION

Pneumatic compression of leg veins has also been used to promote venous return in acute hemorrhage. However, as described for the Trendelenburg position, pneumatic compression of peripheral veins seems to augment the blood pressure by increasing peripheral vascular resistance (particularly in the abdomen), and not by increasing venous return (28). In fact, this maneuver can actually promote blood loss in penetrating thoracic injuries (28). At the present time, pneumatic "antishock" trousers are used predominantly for prehospital stabilization of trauma victims (i.e., when inflated, pneumatic trousers can produce a tourniquet effect that helps control pelvic and intraabdominal hemorrhage).

RESUSCITATION STRATEGIES

The universal goal of resuscitation is to maintain oxygen uptake (Vo_2) into the vital organs and thereby sustain aerobic metabolism (29). The determinants of oxygen uptake are identified in the equation shown below (as described in Chapter 2).

$$Vo_2 = Q \times Hb \times 13 \times (Sao_2 - Svo_2) \qquad (14.1)$$

The factors that pose a risk to the Vo_2 in acute blood loss are the cardiac output (Q) and the hemoglobin concentration (Hb). The consequences of a low cardiac output are far more threatening than the consequences of anemia. Therefore, the first priority in acute blood loss is to preserve blood flow (cardiac output), while correcting erythrocyte deficits is a secondary goal.

FLOW-DIRECTED RESUSCITATION

The ability of different resuscitation fluids to promote the cardiac output is shown in Figure 14.5 (29). Each of the fluids was infused in

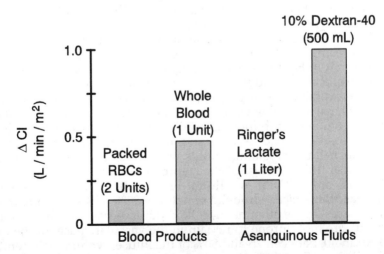

Figure 14.5. The ability of different resuscitation fluids to promote cardiac output. (From Shoemaker WC. Intensive Care Med 1987;13:230–243.)

the volume indicated over 60 minutes, and the height of the columns indicates the change in cardiac index recorded at the end of the infusion period. The volumes of whole blood, packed cells, and dextran-40 are equivalent (500 mL), whereas the infusion volume of lactated Ringer's (1 L) is double that of the other fluids. The most potent fluid for promoting the cardiac output is the dextran-40, and the least potent resuscitation fluid is the erythrocyte concentrate (packed RBCs).

Blood Products

If promoting cardiac output is the first priority in the management of acute hemorrhage, then blood is not the ideal resuscitation fluid for acute blood loss because blood products do not promote blood flow as well as some acellular fluids (such as dextran-40 in Figure 14.5). **The density of erythrocytes impedes the ability of blood products to promote blood flow** (a viscosity effect). In fact, **the administration of erythrocyte concentrates (packed cells) can reduce blood flow and aggravate tissue oxygen deficits** (30,31).

Asanguinous Fluids

There are two types of fluids other than blood products shown in Figure 14.5. The dextran-40 represents one type of fluid, which is characterized by the presence of large molecular weight substances that do not pass easily from one fluid compartment to another. These large molecules with limited mobility prevent the egress of water, and this maintains the volume of the fluid compartment. Fluids of this type that restrict water movement are called colloids (from the Greek word for glue). The other type of fluid is the lactated Ringer's solution, which is an electrolyte solution devoid of large molecules that impede water movement. Fluids of this type that allow water to move freely from one fluid compartment to another are called crystalloids.

The graph in Figure 14.5 reveals a marked difference in the ability of colloid and crystalloid fluids to augment blood flow. This difference cannot be explained by viscosity, because both types of fluids are acellular and have negligible viscosities. The difference is due to the differences in volume distribution. Crystalloid fluids are primarily sodium chloride solutions, and because sodium is distributed evenly in the extracellular fluid, crystalloid fluids will also distribute evenly in the extracellular fluid. Because plasma represents only 20% of the extracellular fluid, **only 20% of an aliquot of crystalloid fluid will remain in the vascular space, while the remaining 80% will add to the interstitial space.** On the other hand, colloid fluids, because of their limited mobility, are more prone to remain in the vascular space. In the case of dextran-40, between 75 and 80% of the infused volume will remain in the plasma. Therefore, **the enhanced effect of colloids on the cardiac output is due to the greater tendency of colloid fluids to increase**

the plasma volume. The increase in plasma volume augments cardiac output not only by increasing ventricular preload (volume effect) but also by decreasing ventricular afterload (dilutional effect on blood viscosity).

The following statements summarize some **salient features of resuscitation fluids** (6,8,9,29).

1. Colloid fluids are superior to blood products and crystalloid fluids for promoting blood flow (cardiac output).
2. Erythrocyte concentrates (packed cells) do not increase (and can decrease) blood flow, and thus they should never be used for volume resuscitation.
3. Crystalloid fluids primarily fill the interstitial space.
4. To have equivalent effects on cardiac output, the volume of crystalloid fluid infused must be at least three times greater than the volume of colloid infusion.

Despite the superior performance of colloid fluids, crystalloid fluids are more popular for volume resuscitation. This preference is partly due to the lower cost of crystalloid fluids, and partly due to habit. Chapter 15 expands further on the various likes and dislikes of colloid and crystalloid fluids.

Fluid Administration

The standard approach to volume resuscitation in hypovolemic shock is to **rapidly administer 2 L of crystalloid fluid as a bolus** (11), **or infuse crystalloid at a rate of 6 mL/min/kg** (31a). If a favorable response is seen, then crystalloid fluids are continued using the endpoints discussed below. If there is not a favorable response, then colloid fluids and blood products are added to the regimen. The rate of infusion is dictated by the clinical condition of the patient and will vary widely. Infusion rates as high as 2.5 mL/second can be delivered through introducer catheters (22). **A rough estimate of the resuscitation volume can be derived as follows** (see Table 14.5).

TABLE 14.5. A SIMPLE METHOD FOR DETERMINING RESUSCITATION VOLUME	
Sequence	Description
1. Estimate normal blood volume (BV)	See Table 14.1
2. Estimate % loss of blood volume	See Table 14.2
3. Calculate volume deficit (VD)	$VD = BV \times \%$ Loss
4. Determine resuscitation volume (RV)	Whole Blood $RV = VD$
	Colloid $RV = 1.5 \times VD$
	Crystalloid $RV = 4 \times VD$

1. **Estimate the normal blood volume** using Table 14.1. Remember to use lean body weight and to adjust for obesity and advanced age.
2. **Estimate the percent volume loss** using the classification system in Table 14.2. Clinical manifestations may not be prominent in mild volume loss, but aggressive volume infusion is not indicated in that setting. Once blood pressure drops in the supine position, there is at least a 30% decrease in blood volume.
3. **Calculate the volume deficit** by multiplying the estimated normal blood volume and the percent loss. This is a quantitative estimate of the volume needs in each patient.
4. **Determine the resuscitation volume** of specific fluids using the rules listed below.
    a. Blood replacement is usually not necessary for Class I and Class II hemorrhage (Table 14.2).
    b. Although colloid fluids can differ in their ability to remain in the vascular compartment, a general rule of thumb is to assume that no less than 50% and no more than 75% of infused colloid will remain in the vascular space. This translates to a replacement volume for colloid fluids that is 1.5 to 2 times the volume deficit.
    c. The resuscitation volume for crystalloid fluids is 4 times the volume deficit, or 3 times the resuscitation volume for colloids (8).

ENDPOINTS

The following are common endpoints of volume resuscitation:

1. CVP = 15 mm Hg (32)
2. Wedge pressure = 10 to 12 mmHg (33)
3. Cardiac index > 3 L/min/m^2
4. Oxygen uptake (V_{O_2}) > 100 mL/min/m^2
5. Blood lactate < 4 mmol/L
6. Base deficit -3 to $+3$ mmol/L

These endpoints represent normal hemodynamic parameters for adults.

Base Deficit

The base deficit (millimoles of base needed to correct the pH of 1 L of whole blood to 7.40) has been shown to correlate with volume deficits and with mortality in trauma victims (34). As a result, this parameter has been recommended as a valuable guide to volume therapy. The base deficit is routinely calculated by many automated blood gas analyzers, and the calculated base deficit is included in many blood gas reports. The normal range for the base deficit is 3 mmol/L on either side of zero. Elevations in base deficit can be classified as mild (2 to 5 mmol/L), moderate (6 to 14 mmol/L), or severe (> 15 mmol/L).

The base deficit that remains elevated during volume infusion is an indication of ongoing tissue ischemia. This measurement is probably a poor man's lactate determination, and it shows promise as a readily available and easy-to-use index of ischemic acid production in tissues.

ERYTHROCYTE RESUSCITATION

In the second stage of management, attention is directed to deficits in oxygen carrying capacity. The use of blood transfusions to correct normovolemic anemia is discussed in detail in Chapter 44. **The current practice of transfusing red blood cells based on hemoglobin determinations has absolutely no scientific basis** (35,36). A serum hemoglobin concentration provides no information about tissue oxygenation, nor is it synonymous with oxygen carrying capacity. To illustrate the latter point, when dehydration increases the serum hemoglobin concentration, does it also increase the oxygen carrying capacity of blood?

The move away from hemoglobin and hematocrit is apparent in the *Clinical Guideline on Elective Red Cell Transfusions* published by the American College of Physicians (35). The guideline states that for asymptomatic patients with anemia, "In the absence of patient risks (e.g., active coronary disease), transfusion is not indicated, *independent of hemoglobin level*"(italics mine).

Oxygen Transport Variables

A more rational approach to red cell transfusions is to employ the oxygen transport variables and the blood lactate level to assess tissue oxygenation (as described in Chapter 13) (37). The following conditions would be **indications for transfusion in normovolemic anemia:**

1. Oxygen uptake (Vo_2) below the normal range (indicating an oxygen debt)
2. Blood lactate greater than 4 mmol/L (regardless of the Vo_2)
3. Oxygen extraction ratio (O_2ER) greater than 0.5

The Vo_2 can also be used to evaluate the response to transfusion therapy. An increase in Vo_2 after transfusion of one unit of blood or packed cells indicates a beneficial response. Transfusion of single units of blood can then be continued until the Vo_2 is no longer augmented. (For more information on the correction of anemia see Chapter 44.)

OTHER CONCERNS

RESUSCITATION-INDUCED HEMORRHAGE

Although the prevailing opinion favors aggressive volume resuscitation for hemorrhage, evidence from both animal studies (38) and clinical trials (39) indicates that volume resuscitation to normotension can actually promote continued blood loss. This is an important observation for two reasons. First, it indicates that the blood pressure is not an appropriate endpoint for the resuscitation of hypovolemic shock (not, at least, until holes in blood vessels are sealed). Second, and more important, it implies that therapy aimed at achieving normal clinical parameters (which is the general approach in modern medicine) is not appropriate when the human body is subjected to abnormal conditions. Normal clinical parameters are a desirable goal only when abnormal (pathologic) conditions are corrected.

POST-RESUSCITATION INJURY

Injury to the major organs can continue unabated following apparently successful resuscitation of hypovolemic shock. This postresuscitation injury can be progressive and can involve several organs (the brain and intestinal tract appear to be most susceptible). Two processes have been implicated in the pathogenesis of this disorder: the no-reflow phenomenon and reperfusion injury.

No-Reflow Phenomenon

Defects in microvascular perfusion can persist despite the resuscitation of hypovolemic shock to premorbid levels of blood pressure and cardiac output (40–44). Several mechanisms have been proposed for this phenomenon, including calcium-induced vasoconstriction (42), leukocyte plugging (43), and vascular compression from the accumulation of edema fluid (43,44). Persistent hypoperfusion in the splanchnic circulation can lead to translocation of intestinal pathogens and postresuscitation septicemia (45). At present, there is no therapy that prevents the no-reflow phenomenon. Because its occurrence and severity seem to be related to the duration of ischemia, prompt resuscitation should help to prevent this complication.

Reperfusion Injury

Postresuscitation injury is also attributed to toxic metabolites that accumulate during the period of ischemia and are washed away during reperfusion, causing damage to remote tissues. Toxic oxygen metabolites have been implicated in this process (46). Two potential sources of enhanced oxidant production are neutrophil activation and generation of superoxide radicals from the oxidation of hypoxanthine (44,46). Despite the proposed role of oxidant injury in the reperfusion period, preliminary studies using antioxidants to prevent this phenomenon have been disappointing (46).

REFERENCES

GENERAL TEXTS

Committee on Trauma. American College of Surgeons. Early care of the injured patient. Philadelphia, B.C. Decker, 1990.

Geller ER (ed). Shock and resuscitation. New York, McGraw-Hill, 1993

CLASSIC STUDIES

1. Crowell JW, Smith EE. Oxygen deficit and irreversible hermorrhagic shock. Am J Physiol. 1964;206:313–316.
2. Weil MH, Afifi AA. Experimental and clinical studies on lactate and pyruvate as indicators of the severity of acute circulatory failure (shock). Circulation 1970;41:989–1001.
3. Moore FD. Effects of hemorrhage on body composition. New Engl J Med 1965; 273:567–577.
4. Shires GT, Coln D, Carrico J, Lightfoot S. Fluid therapy in hemorrhagic shock. Arch Surg 1964;88:688–693.
5. Trendelenburg F. The elevated pelvic position for operations within the abdominal cavity. Med Classics 1940;4:964–968. (Translation of original manuscript.)

REVIEWS

5a. Schadt JC, Ludbrook J. Hemodynamic and neurohumoral responses to acute hypovolemia in conscious animals. Am J Physiol 1991;260:H305–318.
6. Falk JL, O'Brien JF, Kerr R. Fluid resuscitation in traumatic hemorrhagic shock. Crit Care Clin 1992;8:323–340. (123 References).
7. Nacht A. The use of blood products in shock. Crit Care Clin 1992;8:255–293. (141 References).
8. Imm A, Carlson RW. Fluid resuscitation in circulatory shock. Crit Care Clin 1993;9:313–333. (73 References).
9. Domsky MF, Wilson RF. Hemodynamic resuscitation. Crit Care Clin 1993;9: 715–726 . (47 References).

CLINICAL PRESENTATION

10. Walker RH (ed). Technical manual of the American Association of Blood Banks. 10th ed., Arlington, VA, American Association of Blood Banks, 1990: 650.

11. Committee on Trauma. Advanced trauma life support student manual. Chicago, American College of Surgeons, 1989:47–59.
12. Williams TM, Knoop R. The clinical use of orthostatic vital signs. In Roberts JR, Hedges JR (eds). Clinical procedures in emergency medicine. Philadelphia, W.B. Saunders, 1991:445–449.
13. Moore KI, Newton K. Orthostatic heart rates and blood pressures in healthy young women and men. Heart & Lung 1986;611–617.
14. Shippy CR, Appel PL, Shoemaker WC. Reliability of clinical monitoring to assess blood volume in critically ill patients. Crit Care Med 1984;12:107–112.
15. Cordts PR, LaMorte WW, Fisher JB, et al. Poor predictive value of hematocrit and hemodynamic parameters for erythrocyte deficits after extensive vascular operations. Surg Gynecol Obstet 1992;175:243–248.
16. Walley KR, Cooper DJ. Diastolic stiffness impairs left ventricular function during hypovolemic shock in pigs. Am J Physiol 1991;260:H702–712.
17. Amoroso P, Greenwood RN. Posture and central venous pressure measurements in circulatory volume depletion. Lancet 1989;i:258–260.
18. Weil MH, Bisera J, Trevino RP, Rackow EC. Cardiac output and end-tidal carbon dioxide. Crit Care Med 1985;13:907–909.
19. Stamler KD. Effect of crystalloid infusion on hematocrit in nonbleeding patients, with applications to clinical traumatology. Ann Emerg Med 1989;18: 747–749.

RATE OF VOLUME REPLACEMENT

20. Buchman TG, Menker JB, Lipsett PA. Strategies for trauma resuscitation. Surg Gynecol Obstet 1991;172:8–12.
21. Mateer JR, Thompson BM, Aprahamian C, Darin JC. Rapid fluid resuscitation with central venous catheters. Ann Emerg Med 1983;12:149–152.
22. Hyman SA, Smith DW, England R, et al. Pulmonary artery catheter introducers: Do the component parts affect flow rate? Anesth Analg 1991;73:573–575.
23. Dula DJ, Muller A, Donovan JW. Flow rate of commonly used IV techniques. J Trauma 1981;21:480–482.

AUTOTRANSFUSION

24. Sing R, O'Hara D, Sawyer MAJ, Parino PL. Trendelenburg position and oxygen transport in hypovolemic adults. Ann Emerg Med 1994;23:564–568.
25. Taylor J, Weil MH. Failure of Trendelenburg position to improve circulation during clinical shock. Surg Gynecol Obstet 1967;122:1005–1010.
26. Bivins HG, Knopp R, dos Santos PAL. Blood volume distribution in the Trendelenburg position. Ann Emerg Med 1985;14:641–643.
27. Gaffney FA, Bastian BC, Thal ER, Atkins JM. Passive leg raising does not produce a significant autotransfusion effect. J. Trauma 1982;22:190–193.
28. Ali J, Vanderby B, Purcell C. The effect of pneumatic antishock garment (PASG) on hemodynamics, hemorrhage, and survival in penetrating thoracic aortic injury. J Trauma 1991;31:846–851.

RESUSCITATION STRATEGIES

29. Shoemaker WC. Relationship of oxygen transport patterns to the pathophysiology and therapy of shock states. Intensive Care Med 1987;213:230–243.

30. Marik PE, Sibbald WJ. Effect of stored-blood transfusion on oxygen delivery in patients with sepsis. JAMA 1993;269:3024–3029.
31. Silverman HJ, Tuma P. Gastric tonometry in patients with sepsis. Effects of dobutamine infusions and packed red blood cell transfusions. Chest 1992;102:184–188.
31a.Dula DJ, Lutz P, Vogel MF, et al. Rapid flow rates for the resuscitation of hypovolemic shock. Ann Emerg Med 1985;14:303–306.
32. Shoemaker WC, Fleming AW. Resuscitation of the trauma patient. Restoration of hemodynamic functions using clinical algorithms. Ann Emerg Med 1986;12:1437–1444.
33. Packman MI, Rackow EC. Optimum left heart filling pressures during fluid resuscitation of patients with hypovolemic and septic shock. Crit Care Med 1983;11:165–169.
34. Davis JW, Shackford SR, Holbrook TL. Base deficit as a sensitive indicator of compensated shock and tissue oxygen utilization. Surg Gynecol Obstet 1991;173:473–478.
35. American College of Physicians. Practice strategies for elective red blood cell transfusion. Annals Intern Med 1992;116:403–406.
36. Consensus Conference. Perioperative red blood cell transfusion. JAMA 1988;260:2700–2703.
37. Levy PS, Chavez RP, Crystal GJ, et al. Oxygen extraction ratio: A valid indicator of transfusion need in limited coronary vascular reserve. J Trauma 1992;32:769–774.

OTHER CONCERNS

38. Stern SA, Dronen SC, Birrer P, Wang X. Effect of blood pressure on hemorrhage volume and survival in a near-fatal hemorrhage model incorporating a vascular injury. Ann Emerg Med 1993;22:155–163.
39. Bickell WH, Wall MJ, Pepe PE, et al. Immediate versus delayed fluid resuscitation for hypotensive patients with penetrating torso injuries. New Engl J Med 1994;331:1105–1109.
40. Ames A, III, Wright RL, Kowada M, et al. Cerebral ischemia; the no-reflow phenomenon. Am J Pathol 1968;52:437–442.
41. Wang P, Hauptman JG, Chaudry IH. Hemorrhage produces depression of microvascular blood flow which persists despite fluid resuscitation. Circ Shock 1990;32:307–318.
42. Wang P, Zheng FB, Dean RE, Chaudry IH. Diltiazem administration after crystalloid resuscitation restores active hepatocellular function and hepatic blood flow after severe hemorrhagic shock. Surgery 1991;110:390–397.
43. Carden DL, Smith K, Kortyhuis RJ. Neutrophil-mediated microvascular dysfunction in postischemic canine skeletal muscle. Circ Res 1990;66:1436–1444.
44. Mellow CG, Knight KR, Angel MF. The biochemical basis of secondary edema. J Surg Res 1992;52:226–232.
45. Koziol JM, Rush BF, Smith SM, Machiedo GW. Occurrence of bacteremia during and after hemorrhagic shock. J Trauma 1988;28:10–16.
46. Grace PA. Ischemia-reperfusion injury. Br J Surg 1994;81:637–647.

chapter

15

COLLOID AND CRYSTALLOID RESUSCITATION

In 1861, Thomas Graham's investigations on diffusion led him to classify substances as crystalloids or colloids based on their ability to diffuse through a parchment membrane. Crystalloids passed readily through the membrane, whereas colloids (from the Greek word for glue) did not. Intravenous fluids are similarly classified based on their ability to pass through barriers separating body fluid compartments, particularly the one between intravascular and extravascular (interstitial) fluid compartments. This chapter describes the salient features of crystalloid and colloid fluids, both individually and as a group. This is a must-know topic in the care of hospitalized patients, and several reviews are included at the end of the chapter to supplement the text (1–4).

CRYSTALLOID FLUIDS

The principal component of crystalloid fluids is the inorganic salt sodium chloride (NaCl). Sodium is the most abundant solute in the extracellular fluids, and it is distributed uniformly throughout the extracellular space. Because 75 to 80% of the extracellular fluids are located in the extravascular (interstitial) space, a similar proportion of the total body sodium is in the interstitial fluids. Exogenously administered sodium follows the same distribution, so 75 to 80% of the volume of sodium-based intravenous fluids are distributed in the interstitial space. This means that **the predominant effect of volume resuscitation with crystalloid fluids is to expand the interstitial volume rather than the plasma volume.**

VOLEMIC EFFECTS

The change in interstitial volume and plasma volume associated with crystalloid fluid resuscitation is shown in Figure 15.1. As indi-

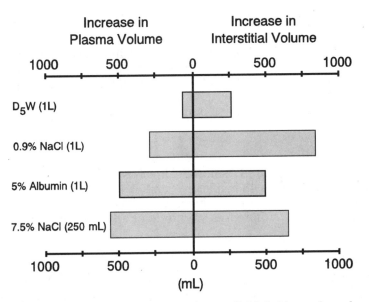

Figure 15.1. The influence of colloid and crystalloid fluids on the volume of the extracellular fluid compartments. (Data from Imm A, Carlson RW. Fluid resuscitation in circulatory shock. Crit Care Clin 1993;9:313.)

cated by the horizontal bar that is second from the top, infusion of 1 L of 0.9% sodium chloride (isotonic saline) adds 275 mL to the plasma volume and 825 mL to the interstitial volume (4). Note that the total volume expansion (1100 mL) is slightly greater than the infused volume. This is the result of a fluid shift from the intracellular to extracellular space, which occurs because isotonic saline is actually hypertonic to the extracellular fluids. The salient features of isotonic saline and other crystalloid fluids are summarized in Table 15.1 (along with some comparative features of plasma).

	\multicolumn{6}{c}{**TABLE 15.1. COMPOSITION OF INTRAVENOUS CRYSTALLOID FLUIDS**}		
	\multicolumn{6}{c}{mEq/L}		Osmolality
Fluid	Na	CL	K	Ca	Mg	Buffers	pH	(mOsm/L)
Plasma*	141	103	4–5	5	2	Bicarb (26)	7.4	289
0.9% NaCL	154	154					5.7	308
7.5% NaCL[†]	1283	1283					5.7	2567
Lactated Ringer's	130	109	4	3		Lactate (28)	6.4	273
Normosol or Plasma-Lyte	140	98	5		3	Acetate (27) Gluconate (23)	7.4	295

* From Brenner BM, Rector FC Jr, eds. The kidney. Philadelphia: WB Saunders, 1981;95.
† From Stapczynski JS et al. Emerg Med Reports 1994;15:245.

ISOTONIC SALINE

The prototype crystalloid fluid is 0.9% sodium chloride (NaCl), also called isotonic saline or normal saline. The latter term is inappropriate because a one normal (1 N) NaCl solution contains 58 g NaCl per liter (the combined molecular weights of sodium and chloride), whereas isotonic (0.9%) NaCl contains only 9 g NaCl per liter.

Features

As shown in Table 15.1, isotonic saline has higher concentrations of sodium and chloride than plasma, and it is slightly hypertonic to plasma. The pH of isotonic saline is also considerably lower than the plasma pH. These differences are rarely of any clinical significance.

Disadvantages

The chloride content of isotonic saline is particularly high relative to plasma (154 mEq/L versus 103 mEq/L, respectively), so hyperchloremic metabolic acidosis is a potential risk with large-volume isotonic saline resuscitation. Hyperchloremia has been reported, but acidosis is rare (1,5).

LACTATED RINGER'S

Ringer's solution was introduced in 1880 by Sydney Ringer, a British physician and research investigator who studied mechanisms of cardiac contraction (6). The solution was designed to promote the contraction of isolated frog hearts, and contained calcium and potassium in a sodium chloride diluent. In the 1930s, an American pediatrician named Alexis Hartmann proposed the addition of sodium lactate buffer to Ringer's solution for the treatment of metabolic acidoses. The lactated Ringer's solution, also known as Hartmann's solution, gradually gained in popularity and eventually replaced the standard Ringer's solution for routine intravenous therapy. The composition of lactated Ringer's solution is shown in Table 15.1.

Features

Lactated Ringer's solution contains potassium and calcium in concentrations that approximate the free (ionic) concentrations in plasma. The addition of these cations requires a reduction in sodium concentration for electrical neutrality, so lactated Ringer's solution has less sodium than isotonic saline. The addition of lactate (28 mEq/L) similarly requires a reduction in chloride concentration, and the chloride in lactated Ringer's more closely approximates plasma chloride levels than does isotonic saline.

Despite the differences in composition, there is no evidence that

TABLE 15.2. INCOMPATIBILITIES WITH RINGER'S SOLUTIONS*			
Definite	**Probable**	**Possible**	
Amicar	Ampicillin	Amikacin	Penicillin
Amphotericin	Doxycycline	Azlocillin	Procainamide
Blood products[†]		Bretylium	Propranolol
Cefamandole		Clindamycin	SoluMedrol
Metaraminol		Cyclosporin	Trimethoprim–
Thiopental		Mannitol	sulfamethoxazole
		Nitroglycerin	Vancomycin
		Nitroprusside	Vasopressin
		Norepinephrine	Urokinase

* Griffith CA (6).
† American Association of Blood Banks Technical Manual (7).

lactated Ringer's provides any benefit over isotonic saline. Furthermore, there is no evidence that the lactate in Ringer's solution provides any buffer effect.

Disadvantages

The calcium in lactated Ringer's can bind to certain drugs and reduce their bioavailability and efficacy. A list of intravenous products that may be incompatible with lactated Ringer's solution is shown in Table 15.2 (6). Of particular note is calcium binding to the citrated anticoagulant in blood products. This can inactivate the anticoagulant and promote the formation of clots in donor blood (7). For this reason, **lactated Ringer's solution is contraindicated as a diluent for blood transfusions** (7).

NORMOSOL OR PLASMA-LYTE

Features

The major feature of these solutions is the added buffer capacity, which gives them a pH that is equivalent to that of plasma. An additional feature is the addition of magnesium, which may provide some benefit in light of the high incidence of magnesium depletion in hospitalized patients (see Chapter 42).

Disadvantages

Magnesium administration can promote hypermagnesemia in renal insufficiency and can counteract compensatory vasoconstriction and promote hypotension in low flow states.

DEXTROSE SOLUTIONS

Dextrose is a common additive in intravenous solutions, for reasons that are unclear. A 5% dextrose-in-water solution is not an effective volume expander, as shown in Figure 15.1. The use of 5% dextrose solutions was originally intended to supply nonprotein calories and thus provide a protein-sparing effect. However, total enteral and parenteral nutrition is now the standard of care for providing daily energy requirements, and the use of 5% dextrose solutions to provide calories is obsolete.

Features

A 5% dextrose solution (50 g dextrose per liter) provides 170 kcal per liter (3.4 kcal/g dextrose).

Disadvantages

The addition of dextrose to intravenous fluids increases osmolarity (50 g of dextrose adds 278 mosm to an intravenous fluid) and creates a hypertonic infusion when 5% dextrose is added to lactated Ringer's solution (525 mOsm/L) or isotonic saline (560 mOsm/L). If glucose use is impaired (as is common in critically ill patients), the infused glucose accumulates and creates an undesirable osmotic force that can promote cell dehydration.

Other undesirable effects of glucose infusions in critically ill patients include enhanced CO_2 production (which can be a burden in ventilator-dependent patients) (8), enhanced lactate production (9,10), and aggravation of ischemic brain injury (11).

Lactate Production

The proportion of a glucose load that contributes to lactate formation can increase from 5% in healthy subjects to 85% in critically ill patients (9). This can produce an increase in circulating lactate levels, even when infusing 5% dextrose solutions. This is demonstrated in Figure 15.2. In this case, patients undergoing abdominal aortic aneurysm surgery were given either a Ringer's solution or a 5% dextrose solution intraoperatively to maintain normal cardiac filling pressures. As shown, the 5% dextrose infusions were associated with a 125% increase in arterial lactate levels (from 1.85 to 4.15 mmol/L). Thus, in patients with circulatory compromise, abnormal glucose metabolism can transform glucose from a source of useful energy to a source of toxin production. The deleterious metabolic effects of glucose infusions are discussed again in Chapter 17 (on resuscitation of cardiac arrest) and in Chapter 48 (on parenteral nutrition).

The disadvantages noted above, when combined with a lack of doc-

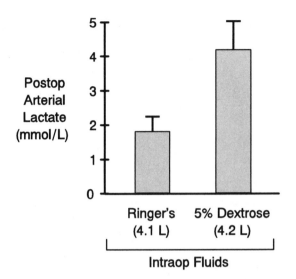

Figure 15.2. The influence of intravenous fluid therapy with and without dextrose on blood lactate levels in patients undergoing abdominal aortic aneurysm surgery. Each column represents data (mean and standard deviation) from 10 patients. Total intraoperative volumes for each fluid are indicated in parentheses. (From Degoute CS et al. Intraoperative glucose infusion and blood lactate: endocrine metabolic relationships during abdominal aortic surgery. Anesthesiology 1989;17:355–361.)

umented benefit, favor the recommendation that the **routine use of 5% dextrose infusions be abandoned in critically ill patients.**

COLLOID FLUIDS

As mentioned earlier, colloids are large molecules that do not pass across diffusional barriers as readily as crystalloids. Colloid fluids infused into the vascular space therefore have a greater tendency to stay put and enhance the plasma volume than do crystalloid fluids. This is illustrated in Figure 15.1. The colloid fluid in this case is 5% albumin, and as demonstrated, the plasma expansion with this colloid fluid is nearly twice that produced by an equivalent volume of isotonic saline (500 mL versus 275 mL, respectively). This is the principal benefit of colloid fluid resuscitation: more effective resuscitation of plasma volume than that produced by crystalloid fluids. The potency of colloid fluids as plasma volume expanders can differ with individual fluids, as shown in Table 15.3. Much of this potency is related to the colloid osmotic pressure exerted by each fluid.

COLLOID OSMOTIC PRESSURE

Large solute molecules that do not move freely across barriers separating fluid compartments create a force that draws water into the

TABLE 15.3. CHARACTERISTICS OF INTRAVENOUS COLLOID FLUIDS*				
Fluid	Average Molecular Weight[†] (daltons)	Oncotic Pressure	Plasma Volume Expansion[‡]	Serum Half-Life
5% Albumin	69,000	20 mm Hg	0.7–1.3	16 hr
25% Albumin	69,000	70 mm Hg	4.0–5.0	16 hr
6% Hetastarch	69,000	30 mm Hg	1.0–1.3	17 days
10% Pentastarch	120,000	40 mm Hg	1.5	10 hr
10% Dextran-40	26,000	40 mm Hg	1.0–1.5	6 hr
6% Dextran-70	41,000	40 mm Hg	0.8	12 hr

* All data from References 1–4.
† Arithmetic mean of the weight of all molecules.
‡ Ratio of increase in plasma volume to volume infused.

large solute compartment. This force opposes the hydrostatic pressure (which favors the movement of water out of a fluid compartment) and is called the colloid osmotic pressure (COP) or oncotic pressure. The COP of the commercially available colloid fluids is shown in Table 15.3. As would be expected, the ability of each fluid to expand the plasma volume is directly related to the COP; that is, the higher the COP, the greater the volume expansion. If the COP of a colloid fluid is greater than the COP of plasma (i.e., greater than 25 mm Hg), the plasma volume expansion exceeds the infused volume. This is demonstrated in Table 15.3 by the 25% albumin solution, which has a COP of 70 mm Hg and a plasma volume expansion that is 4 to 5 times the infused volume.

ALBUMIN

Albumin is a transport protein that is responsible for 75% of the oncotic pressure of plasma (1,12–14). Heat-treated preparations of human serum albumin are commercially available in a 5% solution (50 g/L) and a 25% solution (250 g/L) in an isotonic saline diluent. The 25% solution is given in small volumes (50 to 100 mL) and because the accompanying sodium load is small, 25% albumin is also called salt-poor albumin.

Features

A 5% albumin solution (50 g/L or 5 g/dL) has a COP of 20 mm Hg and thus is similar in oncotic activity to plasma. Approximately half of the infused volume of 5% albumin stays in the vascular space, as shown in Figure 15.1. The oncotic effects of albumin last 12 to 18 hours (1,4).

The 25% albumin solution has a COP of 70 mm Hg and expands the plasma volume by 4 to 5 times the volume infused. Thus, infusion of 100 mL of 25% albumin can increase the plasma volume 400 to 500 mL (1). This plasma volume expansion occurs at the expense of the interstitial fluid volume, so **25% albumin should not be used for volume resuscitation in hypovolemia.** It is intended for shifting fluid from the interstitial space to the vascular space in hypoproteinemic conditions, although the wisdom of this application is questionable (2).

Disadvantages

Because albumin preparations are heat-treated, **there is no risk of viral transmission (including human immunodeficiency virus).** Allergic reactions are rare, and although coagulopathies can occur, most are dilutional and not accompanied by bleeding (1,4).

HETASTARCH

Hetastarch is a synthetic colloid available as a 6% solution in isotonic saline. It contains amylopectin molecules that vary in size from a few hundred to over a million daltons. The average molecular weight of the starch molecules is equivalent to that of albumin, and the colloid effects are equivalent to those of 5% albumin (1,4). The main advantage of hetastarch over albumin is its lower cost.

Features

Hetastarch is slightly more potent than 5% albumin as a colloid. It has a higher COP than 5% albumin (30 versus 20 mm Hg, respectively) and causes a greater plasma volume expansion (up to 30% greater than the infused volume). It also has a long elimination half-life (17 days), but this is misleading because the oncotic effects of hetastarch disappear within 24 hours (1).

Disadvantages

Hetastarch molecules are constantly cleaved by amylase enzymes in the bloodstream before their clearance by the kidneys. Serum amylase levels are often elevated (2 to 3 times above normal levels) for the first few days after hetastarch infusion, and return to normal at 5 to 7 days after fluid therapy (15). This hyperamylasemia should not be mistaken for early pancreatitis. Serum lipase levels remain normal, which is an important distinguishing feature (15).

Anaphylactic reactions to hetastarch are decidedly rare (incidence as low as 0.0004%) (15). Laboratory test coagulopathy (prolonged partial thromboplastin time from an interaction with Factor VIII) can occur, but is not accompanied by bleeding (15,16). Coagulopathy claims have dogged hetastarch for years, without evidence of hetastarch-induced bleeding (1,15).

PENTASTARCH

Pentastarch is a low-molecular-weight-derivative of hetastarch that is available as a 10% solution in isotonic saline. Although it is not currently approved for clinical use in the United States, there is considerable evidence indicating that pentastarch is an effective and safe plasma volume expander (1,17,18).

Features

Pentastarch contains smaller but more numerous starch molecules than hetastarch, and thus has a higher colloid osmotic pressure (see Table 15.3). It is more effective as a volume expander than hetastarch, and can increase plasma volume by 1.5 times the infusion volume (1). The oncotic effects dissipate after 12 hours (1). Pentastarch shows less of a tendency to interact with coagulation proteins than hetastarch, but the significance of this tendency is unclear.

THE DEXTRANS

The dextrans are glucose polymers produced by a bacterium (*Leuconostoc*) incubated in a sucrose medium. First introduced in the 1940s, these colloids are not popular (at least in the United States) because of the perceived risk of adverse reactions. The two most common dextran preparations are 10% dextran-40 and 6% dextran-70, both diluted in isotonic saline.

Features

Both dextran preparations are hyperoncotic to plasma (COP = 40 mm Hg). Dextran-40 causes a larger increase in plasma volume than dextran-70, but the effects last only a few hours. Dextran-70 is the preferred preparation because of its prolonged action (1).

Disadvantages

Dextrans produce a dose-related bleeding tendency by inhibiting platelet aggregation, reducing activation of Factor VIII, and promoting fibrinolysis (15). The hemostatic defects are minimized by limiting the daily dextran dose to 20 mL/kg (15).

Anaphylactic reactions were originally reported in as many as 5% of patients receiving dextran infusions. However, this has improved considerably in the last 20 years because of improvements in antigen detection and desensitization and improvements in preparation purity. The current incidence of anaphylaxis is 0.032% (15).

Dextrans coat the surface of red blood cells and can interfere with the ability to cross-match blood. Red cell preparations must be washed to eliminate this problem. Dextrans also increase the erythrocyte sedimentation rate as a result of their interactions with red blood cells (15).

Finally, dextrans have been implicated as a cause of acute renal failure (15,18). The proposed mechanism is a hyperoncotic state with reduced filtration pressure. However, this mechanism is unproven, and renal failure occurs only rarely in association with dextran infusions.

COLLOID–CRYSTALLOID CONUNDRUM

There is considerable disagreement about the most appropriate fluid for volume resuscitation in critically ill patients. The following is a brief description of the issues involved in the colloid–crystalloid debate.

CRYSTALLOID ORIGINS

Because crystalloid fluids fill primarily the interstitial space, these fluids are not useful for filling the vascular space. The early popularity of crystalloid fluid resuscitation in hypovolemia stems from two observations (described in Chapter 14) made about 40 years ago. The first is the response to mild hemorrhage, which involves a shift of fluid from the interstitial space to the vascular space (19). The second observation stems from studies in an animal model of hemorrhagic shock, where survival was much improved if a crystalloid fluid was given along with reinfusion of the shed blood volume (20). The combination of these two observations has been interpreted as indicating that the major consequence of hemorrhage is an interstitial fluid deficit, and that replacement of interstitial fluid with crystalloid fluids is important for survival.

COLLOID PERFORMANCE

The interstitial fluid deficit is predominant only when blood loss is mild (less than 15% of the blood volume), and in this situation, no volume resuscitation is necessary (because the body is capable of fully compensating for the loss of blood volume). When blood loss is more severe, the priority is to keep the vascular space filled and thereby support the cardiac output. Because colloid fluids are about three times more potent than crystalloid fluids for increasing vascular volume and supporting the cardiac output (as shown in Figures 14.5 and 15.1), **colloid fluids are more effective than crystalloid fluids for volume resuscitation** in moderate to severe blood loss. Crystalloid resuscitation can achieve the same endpoint as colloid resuscitation, but larger volumes of crystalloid fluid (about three times the volume of colloid fluids) must be used. This latter approach is less efficient, yet it is the one favored by crystalloid users.

SURVIVAL

Despite the superiority of colloid fluids for expanding plasma volume, **colloid fluid resuscitation does not confer a higher survival rate** in patients with hypovolemic shock (1,4,21,22). This lack of improved outcomes is a major rallying point for crystalloid users, but it does not negate the fact that colloid fluids are more effective for maintaining blood volume in patients who are actively bleeding.

EXPENSE

The biggest disadvantage of colloid resuscitation is the higher cost of colloid fluids. Table 15.4 shows a cost comparison for colloid and crystalloid fluids. Using equivalent volumes of 250 mL for colloid fluids and 1000 mL for crystalloid fluids, the cost of colloid resuscitation is three times as high (if hetastarch is used) to six times as high (if albumin is used) than volume resuscitation with isotonic saline.

EDEMA

The risk of edema has been used to discredit each type of fluid. Because crystalloid fluids distribute primarily in the interstitial space, edema is an expected feature of crystalloid fluid resuscitation. However, edema is also a risk with colloid fluid resuscitation. This is particularly true with albumin-containing fluids; even though albumin is the principal oncotic force in plasma, over half of the albumin in the human body is in the interstitial fluid (12,13). Therefore, a large proportion of infused albumin eventually finds its way into the interstitial

TABLE 15.4. RELATIVE COST OF INTRAVENOUS FLUIDS			
Fluid	**Manufacturer**	**Unit Size**	**AWP***
Crystalloid Fluids			
0.9% NaCl	Abbot HP	1000 mL	$10.35
5% Dextrose	Abbot HP	1000 mL	$11.35
Lactated Ringer's	Abbot HP	1000 mL	$11.55
Normosol-R	Abbot HP	1000 mL	$28.03
Colloid Fluids			
5% Albumin	Red Cross	250 mL	$65.00
25% Albumin	Red Cross	50 mL	$65.00
6% Hetastarch	Abbot HP	500 mL	$65.31
10% Dextran-40	Baxter	500 mL	$99.43
6% Dextran-70	Baxter	500 mL	$73.45

* Average wholesale prices in the 1996 Drug Topics Redbook. Montvale, NJ: Medical Economics Co., 1996.

fluid and promotes edema. Furthermore, this egress of albumin from the bloodstream is magnified when capillary permeability is disrupted, which is a common occurrence in critically ill patients. Despite this risk, troublesome edema (e.g., pulmonary edema) is not common with either type of fluid resuscitation when capillary hydrostatic pressure is not excessive (23).

HOLE-IN-THE-BUCKET ANALOGY

The following analogy helped me resolve the colloid–crystalloid conundrum. Assume that the goal is to recreate the performance of crystalloid and colloid fluids in expanding the plasma volume by filling a bucket. Because the volume of crystalloid fluids needed to expand the plasma volume (fill the bucket) is three times larger than the volume of colloid fluid that fills the bucket, holes will need to be punched in the bucket while it is filled with crystalloid fluids (to allow the extra fluid to escape). Therefore, the question is this: If the goal is to fill a bucket with fluid, do you want to punch holes in the bucket (and make the bucket more difficult to fill)? Seen in this light, it is more efficient to use colloid fluid resuscitation to expand the plasma volume.

HYPERTONIC RESUSCITATION

An interesting approach to volume resuscitation that has stalled in recent years is the use of small-volume hypertonic saline solutions. A 7.5% sodium chloride solution similar to the one described in Table 15.1 is given either in a fixed volume of 250 mL or in a volume of 4 mL/kg. Figure 15.1 shows the expected change in plasma and interstitial fluid produced by administration of 250 mL 7.5% sodium chloride. The volume increments in both fluid compartments are similar to those produced by 1 L of 5% albumin. Thus, hypertonic saline resuscitation can produce equivalent volume expansion to colloid fluids, but at one-fourth the infused volume. Note that the total volume expansion (1235 mL) produced by 7.5% saline is far greater than the infused volume (250 mL). The additional volume comes from intracellular fluid that moves out of cells and into the extracellular space. This movement of intracellular fluid points to one of the feared complications of hypertonic resuscitation: cell dehydration.

WHAT ROLE?

Since the first report of its successful use in 1980, hypertonic saline has been shown repeatedly (but not unanimously) to be safe and effective in the early resuscitation of hypovolemia. However, there is little evidence that hypertonic resuscitation is superior to standard volume resuscitation. Hypertonic resuscitation seems best suited for prehospital resuscitation in cases of trauma, but studies in trauma resuscitation fail to document a clear benefit with this approach in most patients (24,25). Select subgroups of patients (e.g., those with penetrating truncal injuries who required surgery) may benefit from hypertonic resuscitation, but these subgroups are small. Thus, after over 15 years of evaluating this technique, hypertonic resuscitation has few advocates.

REFERENCES

GENERAL WORKS

Kaufman BS, ed. Fluid resuscitation of the critically ill. Critical care clinics. Vol. 8, No. 2. Philadelphia: WB Saunders, 1992.
Weinstein SM. Plumer's principles and practice of intravenous therapy. 5th ed. Philadelphia: Lippincott-Raven, 1993.

REVIEWS

1. Griffel MI, Kaufman BS. Pharmacology of colloids and crystalloids. Crit Care Clin 1992;8:235–254 (118 References).
2. Kaminski MV, Haase TJ. Albumin and colloid osmotic pressure: implications for fluid resuscitation. Crit Care Clin 1992;8:311–322 (13 References).
3. Sutin KM, Ruskin KJ, Kaufman BS. Intravenous fluid therapy in neurologic injury. Crit Care Clin 1992;8:367–408 (181 References).
4. Imm A, Carlson RW. Fluid resuscitation in circulatory shock. Crit Care Clin 1993;9:313–333 (73 References).

CRYSTALLOID & COLLOID FLUIDS

5. Lowery BD, Cloutier CT, Carey LC. Electrolyte solutions in resuscitation in human hemorrhagic shock. Surg Gynecol Obstet 1971;131:273–279.
6. Griffith CA. The family of Ringer's solutions. J Natl Intravenous Ther Assoc 1986;9:480–483.
7. American Association of Blood Banks Technical Manual. 10th ed. Arlington, VA: American Association of Blood Banks, 1990:368.
8. Talpers SS, Romberger DJ, Bunce SB, Pingleton SK. Nutritionally associated increased carbon dioxide production. Chest 1992;102:551–555.
9. Gunther B, Jauch W, Hartl W, et al. Low-dose glucose infusion in patients who have undergone surgery. Arch Surg 1987;122:765–771.
10. DeGoute CS, Ray MJ, Manchon M, et al. Intraoperative glucose infusion and blood lactate: endocrine and metabolic relationships during abdominal aortic surgery. Anesthesiology 1989;71;355–361.
11. Sieber FE, Traystman RJ. Special issues: glucose and the brain. Crit Care Med 1992;20:104–114.

COLLOID FLUIDS

12. Doweiko JP, Nompleggi DJ. Role of albumin in human physiology and pathophysiology. J Parent Enter Nutr 1991;15:207–211.

Colloid and Crystalloid Resuscitation **241**

13. Guthrie RD Jr, Hines C Jr. Use of albumin in the critically ill patient. Am J Gastroenterol 1991;86:255–263.
14. Marik PE. The treatment of hypoalbuminemia in the critically ill patient. Heart Lung 1993;22:166–170.
15. Nearman HS, Herman ML. Toxic effects of colloids in the intensive care unit. Crit Care Clin 1991;7:713–723.
16. Kapiotis S, Quehenberger P, Eichler H-G, et al. Effect of hydroxyethyl starch on the activity of blood coagulation and fibrinolysis in healthy volunteers: comparison with albumin. Crit Care Med 1994;22:606–612.
17. Waxman K, Holness R, Tominaga G et al. Hemodynamic and oxygen transport effects of pentastarch in burn resuscitation. Ann Surg 1989;209:341–345.
18. Strauss RG, Stansfield C, Henriksen RA, et al. Pentastarch may cause fewer effects on coagulation than hetastarch. Transfusion 1988;28:257–261.
19. Drumi W, Polzleitner D, Laggner AN, et al. Dextran-40, acute renal failure, and elevated plasma oncotic pressure. N Engl J Med 1988;318:252–254.

COLLOID-CRYSTALLOID WARS

20. Moore FD. The effects of hemorrhage on body composition. N Engl J Med 1965;273:567–577.
21. Shires T, Carrico J, Lightfoot S. Fluid therapy in hemorrhagic shock. Arch Surg 1964;88:688–693.
22. Bisonni RS, Holtgrave DR, Lawler F, et al. Colloids versus crystalloids in fluid resuscitation: an analysis of randomized controlled trials. J Fam Pract 1991;32:387–390.
23. Schaeffer RC, Reeiewicz RA, Chilton SW, et al. Effects of colloid or crystalloid solutions on edemagenesis in normal and thrombomicroembolized lungs. Crit Care Med 1987;15:1110–1115.

HYPERTONIC RESUSCITATION

24. Mattox KL. Prehospital hypertonic saline-dextran infusion for post-traumatic hypotension: the USA Multicenter Trial. Ann Surg 1991;213:482–486.
25. Vassar MJ, Fischer RP, O'Brien PE, et al. A multicenter trial for resuscitation of injured patients with 7.5% sodium chloride. Arch Surg 1993;128:1003–1013.

chapter

16

ACUTE HEART FAILURES

There's no doubt that the proper functioning of our pipes and pumps does have an immediate urgency well beyond that of almost any of our other bits and pieces.

Steven Vogel

Cardiac pump failure is an ominous sign in the critically ill patient that requires prompt recognition and management. Acute heart failure is not a single entity, but can involve the right or left side of the heart, or can occur during diastole or systole. This chapter uses the principles of cardiac performance provided in Chapter 1 to describe a bedside approach to the varieties of heart failure (1–6). The approach described here requires invasive monitoring with pulmonary artery catheters and centers on the mechanical problem rather than the specific illness. The common causes of acute heart failure in patients in the ICU are indicated in Figure 16.1.

HEMODYNAMIC MANIFESTATIONS

The diagnosis of heart failure begins with recognition of the early signs of heart failure, then identifies the phase of the cardiac cycle and the side of the heart involved.

EARLY RECOGNITION

The serial changes in hemodynamic parameters shown in Figure 16.2 are taken from a patient who developed progressive left heart failure following cardiopulmonary bypass surgery. The sequence of hemodynamic alterations is as follows (the numbers below correspond to the circled numbers in Figure 16.2):

1. The earliest sign of ventricular dysfunction is an increase in pulmonary capillary wedge pressure. The stroke volume is main-

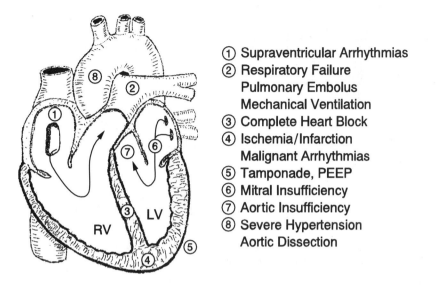

1. Supraventricular Arrhythmias
2. Respiratory Failure
   Pulmonary Embolus
   Mechanical Ventilation
3. Complete Heart Block
4. Ischemia/Infarction
   Malignant Arrhythmias
5. Tamponade, PEEP
6. Mitral Insufficiency
7. Aortic Insufficiency
8. Severe Hypertension
   Aortic Dissection

Figure 16.1. Common causes of acute heart failure in patients in the ICU.

tained at this stage because the ventricle is still preload-responsive (i.e., the Starling curve is still steep).

2. The next stage is marked by a decrease in stroke volume and an increase in heart rate. The tachycardia offsets the reduction in stroke volume, so that the cardiac output remains unchanged.
3. The final stage is characterized by a decrease in cardiac output. The point at which the cardiac output begins to decline marks the transition from compensated to decompensated heart failure. The decompensated phase of heart failure is characterized by peripheral vasoconstriction, which initially maintains peripheral blood flow but eventually causes a further reduction in cardiac output and peripheral flow.

The serial hemodynamic changes shown in Figure 16.2 demonstrate the following important point: **Cardiac output may not be reduced in the early stages of heart failure.** The early recognition of heart failure requires monitoring of the cardiac filling pressures and the ventricular stroke volume.

SYSTOLIC VERSUS DIASTOLIC FAILURE

Heart failure is not synonymous with contractile failure, and 40% of patients with newly diagnosed heart failure have normal systolic function (7–9). The problem in these patients is a decrease in ventricular distensibility, a disorder known as diastolic heart failure. In this type of heart failure, inadequate ventricular filling compromises car-

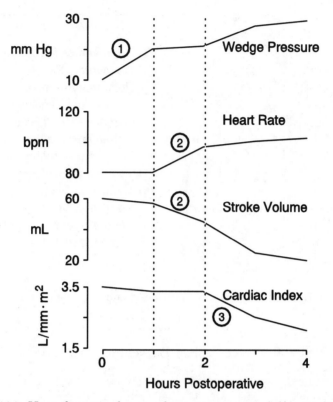

Figure 16.2. Hemodynamic changes during progressive left heart failure in a postoperative patient.

diac output, while the force of ventricular contraction is normal. Common causes of diastolic heart failure in patients in the ICU include ventricular hypertrophy, myocardial ischemia, pericardial effusions, and positive-pressure mechanical ventilation.

The distinction between systolic and diastolic heart failure is important, because what would be appropriate management for one type of heart failure can aggravate the other.

Routine Hemodynamic Monitoring

Routine hemodynamic measurements are incapable of distinguishing diastolic from systolic heart failure (7–9). This is illustrated in Figure 16.3. The curves in this figure are similar to the pressure–volume curves shown in Figure 1.1. The upper curves in the figure are ventricular function curves relating ventricular end-diastolic pressure (EDP) and cardiac stroke volume. These curves demonstrate that heart failure of either type is associated with an increase in EDP and a decrease in stroke volume. The lower set of curves are diastolic pressure–volume curves, and these curves demonstrate that the increase in EDP in heart failure is associated with opposite changes in the end-diastolic volume

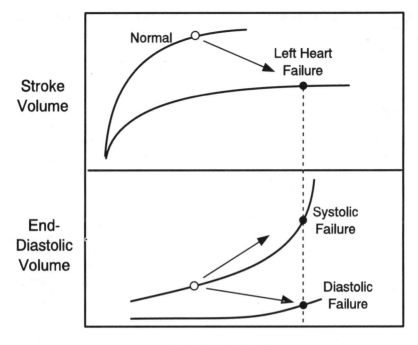

End-Diastolic Pressure

Figure 16.3. Changes in end-diastolic pressure (EDP) and end-diastolic volume (EDV) in systolic and diastolic heart failure. See text for explanation.

(EDV) in the two types of heart failure; that is, the EDV is increased in systolic heart failure and decreased in diastolic heart failure. Therefore, **monitoring cardiac filling pressures as an index of ventricular preload does not allow a distinction between systolic and diastolic heart failure.**

END-DIASTOLIC VOLUME

The end-diastolic volume is thus the best measure for identifying systolic and diastolic heart failure. The EDV can be derived by the following relationship between the stroke volume (SV) and ejection fraction (EF):

$$EDV = SV/EF \qquad (16.1)$$

The ejection fraction of the left ventricle can be measured with radionuclide ventriculography (10), and the ejection fraction of the right ventricle can be measured with a specialized pulmonary artery catheter with a fast-response thermistor, as described in Chapter 12 (see Fig. 12.3). Because bedside radionuclide ventriculography is tedious, and expensive left-ventricular EDV is not a common bedside measurement.

RIGHT VERSUS LEFT HEART FAILURE

Right heart failure (which is predominantly systolic failure) is more prevalent than considered in patients in the ICU (11), and it may be particularly prominent in ventilator-dependent patients. The following measurements can prove useful in identifying right heart failure.

Cardiac Filling Pressures

The relationship between the central venous pressure (CVP) and the pulmonary capillary wedge pressure (PCWP) can sometimes be useful for identifying right heart failure. The following criteria have been proposed for right heart failure (12): **CVP > 15 mm Hg and CVP = PCWP or CVP > PCWP.** Unfortunately, at least one-third of patients with acute right heart failure do not satisfy these criteria (12). One problem is the insensitivity of the CVP; an increase in the CVP is seen only in the later stages of right heart (systolic) failure. Contractile failure of the right ventricle results in an increase in end-diastolic volume, and only when the increase in volume of the right heart is impeded by the pericardium does the end-diastolic pressure (CVP) rise (11).

Another problem with the CVP–PCWP relationship for identifying right heart failure is the interaction between the right and left sides of the heart. This is shown in Figure 16.4. Both ventricles share the same septum, so enlargement of the right ventricle pushes the septum to the left and compromises the left-ventricular chamber. This interaction between right and left ventricles is called interventricular interdependence, and it can confuse the interpretation of ventricular filling pressures. In fact, as indicated by the diastolic pressures in Figure 16.4, **the hemodynamic changes in right heart failure can look much like the hemodynamic changes in pericardial tamponade** (11).

End-Diastolic Volume

The right-ventricular ejection fraction (RVEF) and end-diastolic volume (RVEDV), as determined with pulmonary artery catheters equipped with rapid-response thermistors (see Chapter 12), are the best measures for identifying right heart failure. A decrease in RVEF (normal RVEF is 45 to 50%) and an increase in RVEDV (normal RVEDV is 80 to 140 mL/m^2) is expected in right heart failure (13). The response to volume infusion may be even more diagnostic. In one study, volume infusion resulted in a 30% increase in RVEDV in patients with right-ventricular dysfunction, while in other patients, there was no increase

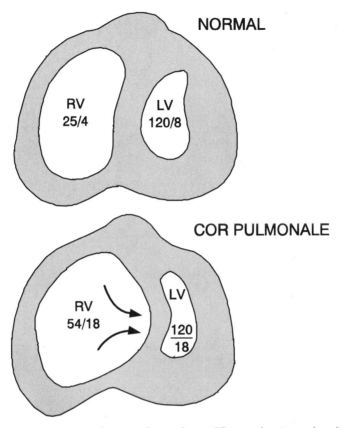

Figure 16.4. Interventricular interdependence. The mechanism whereby right heart failure compromises diastolic filling of the left ventricle and raises the left-ventricular end-diastolic (wedge) pressure. RV = right ventricle, LV = left ventricle.

in RVEDV after a fluid challenge (14). In another study, volume infusion did not result in an increase in cardiac output if the RVEDV was in excess of 140 mL/m^2 (15).

Echocardiography

Cardiac ultrasound can be useful at the bedside for differentiating right from left heart failure. Three findings typical of right heart failure are (*a*) an increase in right-ventricular chamber size, (*b*) segmental wall motion abnormalities on the right, and (*c*) paradoxical motion of the interventricular septum (12).

MANAGEMENT STRATEGIES

The primary goal in managing heart failure is to maintain cardiac output, and the secondary goal is to decrease venous (capillary) pres-

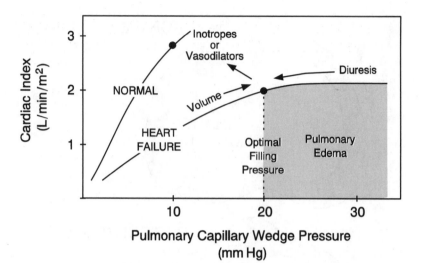

Figure 16.5. Ventricular function curves for the normal and failing left ventricle. Arrows show the expected hemodynamic changes with various interventions in left heart failure.

sure to limit edema formation. The strategies presented here are designed to achieve both of these goals.

LEFT HEART (SYSTOLIC) FAILURE

The approach to left-ventricular (systolic) failure presented here centers on the PCWP). The approach is described graphically in Figure 16.5.

Suboptimal Wedge Pressure

Correction of inadequate filling pressures is the sine qua non of heart failure management. As stated by the cardiovascular physiologist, Carl Wiggers: "It is axiomatic that the heart can pump only as much as it receives."

Condition: Low PCWP
Intervention: Volume infusion to optimal PCWP

The optimal wedge pressure is the highest pressure that augments cardiac output without producing pulmonary edema. This is shown in Figure 16.5 as the highest point on the lower (heart failure) curve that does not enter the hatched pulmonary edema region. The optimal PCWP is determined by the colloid osmotic pressure (COP) of blood (see Chapter 15 for a description of the COP). When the COP is normal (20 to 25 mm Hg), **the optimal PCWP is 20 mm Hg** (16).

TABLE 16.1. PHARMACOTHERAPY OF ACUTE HEART FAILURE[1]		
Drug	**Dose Range**	**Principal Actions**
Amrinone	5–10 μg/kg/min	Positive inotropic effect
		Vasodilator
Dobutamine	3–15 μg/kg/min	Positive inotropic effect
Dopamine	3–10 μg/kg/min	Positive inotropic effect
		Vasodilator
	10–20 μg/kg/min	Vasoconstrictor
Nitroglycerin	1–50 μg/min	Venodilator
	> 50 μg/min	Arterial vasodilator
Nitroprusside	0.3–2 μg/kg/min	Vasodilator

[1] Includes only drugs given by continuous intravenous infusion.

Optimal Wedge Pressure

When the wedge pressure is optimal, therapy is dictated by the blood pressure (BP). The hemodynamic drugs recommended here are those given by continuous IV infusion (1,3–5). These drugs are listed in Table 16.1, along with their appropriate dose ranges. Each of the drugs in this table is described in more detail in Chapter 18.

Condition: Optimal PCWP, low BP
Intervention: Dopamine

Dopamine stimulates both β-receptors (cardio-stimulation and vasodilation) and α-receptors (vasoconstriction). The β effect increases the cardiac output, and the α effect raises the blood pressure. The α effect becomes evident at doses above 5 μg/kg/minute, and vasoconstriction is the predominant effect at doses above 10 μg/kg/minute (1,5).

Condition: Optimal PCWP, normal BP
Intervention: Dobutamine, amrinone

Dobutamine, a synthetic adrenergic agent that does not cause peripheral vasoconstriction, is widely regarded as the **inotropic agent of choice for the acute management of (systolic) heart failure** (17). Amrinone is a phosphodiesterase inhibitor that has both positive inotropic and vasodilator actions. This agent can serve as an effective alternative to dobutamine, or it can be added to dobutamine to enhance the overall effect (5).

Condition: Optimal PCWP, high BP
Intervention: Nitroprusside, nitroglycerin

Nitroprusside is a popular vasodilator in the critical care setting. However, **cyanide accumulation is common during nitroprusside infusions** (see Chapter 18), and the risk of cyanide toxicity should temper the use of nitroprusside. The risk of cyanide toxicity has led the Food and Drug Administration to recommend a **maximum nitroprusside dose rate of 10 μg/minute for no more than 10 minutes.** (For more information about nitroprusside use, see reference 18.) Nitroglycerin is a viable alternative to nitroprusside if administered in dose rates that exceed 50 μg/minute. Other vasodilators that can be given by continuous intravenous infusion, such as labetalol (a combined α–β blocker), esmolol (a short-acting β blocker), and trimethaphan (a ganglionic blocker) can decrease the cardiac output, and thus these agents are more appropriate for treatment of severe hypertension accompanied by an adequate cardiac output.

High Wedge Pressure

If the wedge pressure is high and the patient is at risk for hydrostatic pulmonary edema, the appropriate management is determined by the cardiac output (CO).

Condition: High PCWP, low CO
Intervention: Dobutamine, amrinone

Therapy with dobutamine and amrinone results in significant reductions in wedge pressure (5,19). **Dopamine should be avoided when the wedge pressure is elevated because dopamine constricts pulmonary veins and can increase the wedge pressure further** (19,20). Vasodilators can be detrimental in pulmonary edema because they increase shunt fraction and can aggravate hypoxemia (21).

Condition: High PCWP, normal CO
Intervention: Nitroglycerin, ? furosemide

A normal cardiac output in the face of a high PCWP suggests diastolic heart failure. Aggressive diuresis is not recommended as the first line of therapy in this setting because the high filling pressures help maintain cardiac output. Intravenous nitroglycerin (less than 100 μg/kg/minute) should be useful here because this agent reduces the wedge pressure while also reducing the arterial resistance to maintain cardiac output (21). Sublingual nitroglycerin can be given for immediate results. In the setting of pulmonary edema, nitroglycerin can increase shunt fraction and decrease the arterial P_{O_2}. Therefore, arterial gases should be monitored carefully when using nitroglycerin in pulmonary edema.

Furosemide

Intravenous furosemide is a popular therapy for acute pulmonary edema, and it is usually given with little regard for the effects on cardiac output. However, it is well established that **intravenous furosemide often causes a decrease in cardiac output in patients with acute heart failure** (22–28). To emphasize this point, Table 16.2 shows the hemodynamic effects of intravenous furosemide in acute heart failure from all clinical studies reported from 1970 to 1990 (22–31). A total of 169 subjects are included, and in 7 of 10 studies (involving 113 subjects, or 67% of the total study population) intravenous furosemide caused a significant reduction in cardiac output and/or stroke volume. This effect is the result of a decrease in venous return and an increase

**TABLE 16.2. HEMODYNAMIC EFFECTS OF INTRAVENOUS
FUROSEMIDE IN ACUTE LEFT HEART FAILURE[1]**

Principal Author and Year[2]	No. Subjects	Furosemide Dose (IV)	Acute Hemodynamic Changes		
			LVEDP*	Cardiac Output	Stroke Volume
Davidson, 1971	10	40 mg	− 20%	− 13%*	—
Keily, 1973	9	40 mg	− 28%	− 20%*	—
Mond, 1974	8	40 mg	− 28%	− 14%*	− 17%*
Nelson, 1983a	14	1 mg/kg	− 17%	− 8%*	− 9%*
Nelson, 1983b	22	1 mg/kg	− 16%	− 11%*	− 11%*
Tattersfield, 1974	35	80 mg	− 3%	− 8%	− 16%*
Larsen, 1988	15	40 mg	− 16%	− 4%	− 8%*
Dikshit, 1973	20	0.5–1 mg/kg	− 27%	+ 4%	+ 4%
Biddle, 1979	6	0.5 mg/kg	− 25%	− 6%	− 6%
Nishimura, 1981	30	120 mg	− 28%	− 2%	− 3%

[1] Prepared with the assistance of Satish Reddy, M.D.
[2] For full citations, see references 22–31.
* $p < 0.01$

in systemic vascular resistance. The latter effect is due to the ability of furosemide to stimulate renin release and raise circulating levels of angiotensin, a vasoconstrictor (32). Considering the popularity of lowering angiotensin levels with angiotensin-converting enzyme inhibitors as a therapy in heart failure, the actions of furosemide to promote angiotensin formation seem to be counterproductive. This effect of furosemide should be considered carefully before the knee-jerk response of administering furosemide in acute heart failure is developed.

Because the diuretic effect of furosemide is more closely related to its urinary excretion rate than to its plasma concentration (33), continuous infusion furosemide has been advocated for more effective diuresis in patients with heart failure (33,34). Continuous infusion is usually recommended when more than 80 mg of intravenous furosemide is required to produce the desired diuretic effect. Dose rates range from 2.5 to 160 mg/hr.

LEFT HEART (DIASTOLIC) FAILURE

The optimal treatment for diastolic heart failure is unknown. Diuretic therapy should be avoided, and inotropic therapy should be ineffective. Although vasodilator therapy should carry a high risk of hypotension in diastolic heart failure (because a ventricle with normal systolic function should be unresponsive to changes in afterload), some vasodilator agents (e.g., calcium channel blockers and angiotensin converting enzyme or ACE inhibitors) may also have *lusitropic* actions that enhance myocardial relaxation (7,8). Verapamil has roven effective in idiopathic hypertrophic cardiomyopathies (7,8,35); however, there is evidence that calcium channel blockers do not improve myocardial relaxation in other conditions associated with diastolic heart failure (36). For now, the management of diastolic heart failure is similar to that for systolic heart failure, but careful hemodynamic monitoring is necessary to identify adverse effects in the management of diastolic heart failure.

RIGHT HEART FAILURE

Therapeutic strategies for right heart failure are similar in principle to those just described. The strategies below pertain only to primary right heart failure (e.g., acute myocardial infarction), and not to right heart failure secondary to chronic obstructive lung disease or to left heart failure. The PCWP and RVEDV are used as the focal points of management.

1. If PCWP is below 15 mm Hg, infuse volume until the PCWP or CVP increases by 5 mm Hg or either one reaches 20 mm Hg (12).
2. If the RVEDV is less than 140 mL/m^2, infuse volume until the RVEDV reaches 140 mL/m^2 (15).
3. If PCWP is above 15 mm Hg or the RVEDV is 140 mL/m^2 or higher, infuse dobutamine, beginning at a rate of 5 μg/kg/minute (37,38).
4. In the presence of AV dissociation or complete heart block, institute sequential A-V pacing and avoid ventricular pacing (12).

The response to volume infusion must be carefully monitored in right heart failure because aggressive volume infusion can overdistend the right ventricle and further reduce cardiac output through interventricular interdependence (see Fig. 16.4).

Dobutamine is an effective agent in right heart failure (37,38). Nitroprusside has been used in right heart failure, but it is not as effective as dobutamine (38).

MECHANICAL SUPPORT

A variety of devices are available that provide temporary mechanical support of the failing heart. Most of these devices are used after cardiac surgery, where about 5% of patients require postoperative mechanical assistance to support the cardiac output (39).

INTRAAORTIC BALLOON PUMP (IABP)

Intraaortic balloon counterpulsation has been the standard method of providing mechanical circulatory support for over 25 years (39,40). The IABP consists of a 30-cm polyurethane balloon attached to one end of a large-bore catheter. The device is inserted in the femoral artery at the groin, either percutaneously or via arteriotomy, with the balloon wrapped tightly around the catheter. Once inserted, the catheter is advanced up the aorta until the tip lies just beyond the origin of the left subclavian artery. When in place, the balloon wrapping is released to allow periodic balloon inflations. Correct placement does not require fluoroscopy, and the IABP can be placed successfully at the bedside.

Hemodynamic Effects

The intraaortic balloon is rapidly inflated with helium (35 to 40 mL capacity) at the onset of each diastolic period, when the aortic valve closes. The balloon is then rapidly deflated at the onset of ventricular systole, just before the aortic valve opens. This pattern of balloon inflation and deflation produces two changes in the arterial pressure waveform, as illustrated in Figure 16.6.

1. Inflation of the balloon increases the peak diastolic pressure and displaces blood toward the periphery. The increase in diastolic pressure increases the mean arterial pressure and thereby increases mean blood flow in the periphery. Coronary blood flow should also increase, because the bulk of coronary blood flow occurs during diastole. However, the IABP increases coronary

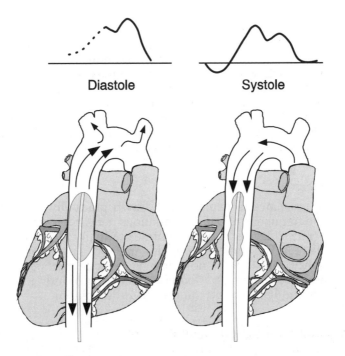

Figure 16.6. The influence of intraaortic balloon counterpulsation on arterial pressure and flow.

flow only in hypotensive patients and does not promote coronary flow in normotensive patients (41).
2. Deflation of the balloon reduces the end-diastolic pressure, which reduces the impedance to flow when the aortic valve opens at the onset of systole. This decreases ventricular afterload and promotes ventricular stroke output.

Indications

The usual indications for the IABP include (a) cardiopulmonary bypass (before and after), (b) cardiac transplantation (before and after), (c) acute myocardial infarction with cardiogenic shock, (d) acute mitral insufficiency, and (e) unstable angina

Almost half of all balloon insertions occur in the immediate postoperative period following cardiopulmonary bypass surgery. The IABP has also gained increasing use as a *bridge* to cardiac transplantation.

Contraindications

The contraindications to the IABP include aortic regurgitation, aortic dissection, and a recently placed (within 12 months) prosthetic graft in the thoracic aorta (40).

Complications

The incidence of complications from the IABP ranges from 15 to 45%, with serious complications reported in 5 to 10% of cases (40). The most common complications are leg ischemia (9 to 22%) and septicemia (1 to 22%). Leg ischemia can occur in the ipsilateral or contralateral leg and can appear either with the device in place or soon after it is removed. When distal pulses disappear while the balloon is in place, removal of the device is often sufficient to restore flow without any further therapy. About 20% of patients require surgical interventions for lower leg vascular complications (42).

Weaning

Balloon assistance is usually withdrawn gradually, by either decreasing the frequency of balloon inflations per cardiac cycle (1:2, 1:3, etc.), or by reducing the inflation volume gradually to 10% of the original volume (40). The choice of weaning method is a matter of individual preference, and there is no evidence that one method is superior to the other. The weaning period is also a matter of individual preference and can range from 60 minutes to 24 hours (40).

VENTRICULAR ASSIST DEVICES

A ventricular assist device (VAD) is a nonpulsatile pump that is placed in parallel with either the right ventricle (RVAD), the left ventricle (LVAD), or both ventricles (BiVAD) (39,43,44). The pump is adjusted to provide a total systemic flow of 2.0 to 3.0 L/min/m². These devices are placed intraoperatively in cases where the IABP fails to provide adequate circulatory support (usually after cardiopulmonary bypass surgery). After 24 hours of operation, attempts to wean pump support are usually initiated by decreasing the pump flow rate until right atrial pressure (RVAD) or left atrial pressure (LVAD) increases to 20 to 25 mm Hg (44). The duration of ventricular support is usually 1 to 4 days, but it can range from a few hours to longer than 10 days (44). Complications occur in over 50% of patients and most often include bleeding or systemic embolism (43,44). Most patients can never be weaned from pump support, but as many as one-third of patients survive the ordeal (44).

CARDIOPULMONARY BYPASS SURGERY

The immediate period following cardiopulmonary bypass surgery is often marked by hemodynamic instability (45). The following are some of the major hemodynamic concerns in the early postoperative period.

CARDIAC TAMPONADE

Cardiac tamponade occurs in 3 to 6% of patients undergoing openheart surgery (46). It often appears in the first few hours after surgery, but can occur at a later time when the pacemaker wires are removed. The pericardium is open after cardiac surgery, and this prevents fluid from accumulating evenly around the heart. The most common cause of tamponade after surgery is a blood clot compressing the right heart.

Clinical Presentation

Cardiac tamponade often has an atypical presentation in the postbypass period (46). **Two typical manifestations of cardiac tamponade may be absent.**

1. Pulsus paradoxus (inspiratory drop in systolic blood pressure of at least 10 mm Hg) can be masked in patients receiving mechanical ventilation. Positive-pressure lung inflation can assist the left ventricle during systole and thereby augment the systolic blood pressure. The increase in systolic pressure produced by positive-pressure mechanical ventilation is called reverse pulsus paradoxus (see Chapter 26).
2. Equalization of diastolic pressures (CVP, pulmonary artery diastolic pressure, PCWP) may not be a feature of cardiac tamponade when a clot is compressing the right atrium. In this situation, the superior vena cava pressure (CVP) can increase while the pulmonary artery and wedge pressures decrease.

Diagnosis

Tamponade is often suspected on clinical grounds when there is a sudden decrease in blood drainage from mediastinal chest tubes followed by a rise in cardiac filling pressures and a progressive decline in cardiac output. The diagnosis is often uncertain (and is a source of much angst in cardiovascular surgeons) and requires repeat thoracotomy for verification and for ligation of bleeding sites. If available, transesophageal echocardiography can be a valuable tool for identifying compression of the right atrium and left-ventricular akinesis (47).

POST-BYPASS HEMODYNAMICS

The rewarming period after cardiopulmonary bypass is associated with a decrease in the compliance of the ventricles (48). The etiology is unclear, but myocardial edema from cooling and reperfusion may play a role. The peripheral vascular resistance can either increase or decrease in the immediate postoperative period. Systolic function is variable but seems to be well maintained in most patients (45). Acute infarction is reported in less than 10% of patients (45).

Management

The decrease in ventricular compliance during the rewarming period causes a decrease in EDV at any given EDP. This means that **a normal wedge pressure in the early postoperative period represents a low EDV.** Therefore, when cardiac output is low and the PCWP is not elevated, volume infusion is indicated until the PCWP is in the range of 20 mm Hg.

Drug therapy can be selected according to the systemic vascular resistance (SVR). The following scheme may be helpful:

SVR	Blood Pressure	Intervention
High	High	Nitroprusside
High	Normal	Dobutamine
High	Low	Dopamine, IABP
Normal	Normal	Dobutamine
Normal	Low	Dopamine, IABP
Low	Normal	Dobutamine
Low	Low	Dopamine, epinephrine

The use of nitroprusside to treat postoperative hypertension carries a particularly high risk of cyanide accumulation after cardiopulmonary bypass surgery because of the depletion of thiosulfate associated with this procedure (see Chapter 18). Nitroglycerin is an effective alternative to nitroprusside (49), and I have been using trimethaphan (a ganglionic blocker) to treat severe hypertension in this situation. For more information on trimethaphan and the other hemodynamic drugs in this chapter, see Chapter 18.

REFERENCES

GENERAL TEXTS

Barnett DB, Pouleur H, Francis GS. Congestive heart failure: pathophysiology and treatment. New York: Marcel Dekker, 1993.

Gaash WH, LeWinter MM. Left ventricular diastolic dysfunction and heart failure. Baltimore: Williams & Wilkins, 1994.

Khan MG, ed. Cardiac drug therapy. 4th ed. Philadelphia: WB Saunders, 1995.

Maccioli GA. Theory and practice of intra-aortic balloon pump therapy. Baltimore: Williams & Wilkins, 1996.

Moreno-Cabral C, Mitchell RS, Miller DC. Manual of postoperative management in adult cardiac surgery. Baltimore: Williams & Wilkins, 1988.

REVIEWS

1. Lollgen H, Drexler H. Use of inotropes in the critical care setting. Crit Care Med 1990;18:S56–S60 (32 References).
2. Smith TW, Braunwald E, Kelly RA. The management of heart failure. In: Braunwald E, ed. Heart disease. A textbook of cardiovascular medicine. 4th ed. Philadelphia: WB Saunders, 1992;464–519 (600 References).
3. Alpert J, Becker JA. Mechanisms and management of cardiogenic shock. Crit Care Clin 1993;9:205–218 (32 References).
4. Snell RJ, Calvin JE. Cardiogenic shock: pathophysiology, management and treatment. In: Edwards JD, Shoemaker WC, Vincent J-L, eds. Oxygen transport: principles and practice. Philadelphia: WB Saunders, 1993;246-273 (99 References).
5. Zaloga GP, Prielipp RC, Butterworth JF, Royster RL. Pharmacologic cardiovascular support. Crit Care Clin 1993;9:335–362 (192 References).
6. Wilson RF. Trauma in patients with pre-existing cardiac disease. Crit Care Clin 1994;10:461–506 (163 References).

DIASTOLIC HEART FAILURE

7. Bonow RO, Udelson JE. Left ventricular diastolic dysfunction as a cause of congestive heart failure. Ann Intern Med 1992;117:502–510.
8. Goldsmith S, Dick C. Differentiating systolic from diastolic heart failure: pathophysiologic and therapeutic considerations. Am J Med 1993;95:645–655.
9. Gaasch WH. Diagnosis and treatment of heart failure based on left ventricular systolic or diastolic dysfunction. JAMA 1994;271:1276–1280.
10. Clements IP, Sinak LJ, Gibbons RJ, et al. Determination of diastolic function by radionuclide ventriculography. Mayo Clin Proc 1990;65:1007–1019.

RIGHT HEART FAILURE

11. Hurford WE, Zapol WM. The right ventricle and critical illness: a review of anatomy, physiology, and clinical evaluation of its function. Intensive Care Med 1988;14:448–457.
12. Isner JM. Right ventricular myocardial infarction. JAMA 1988;259:712–718.
13. Robotham JL, Takala M, Berman M, et al. Ejection fraction revisisted. Anesthesiology 1991;74:172–183.

14. Boldt J, Kling D, Moosdorf R, Hempelmann G. Influence of acute volume loading on right ventricular function after cardiopulmonary bypass. Crit Care Med 1989;17:518–521.
15. Reuse C, Vincent JL, Pinsky MR. Measurement of right ventricular volumes during fluid challenge. Chest 1990;98:1450–1454.

MANAGEMENT STRATEGIES

16. Franciosa JA. Optimal left heart filling pressure during nitroprusside infusion for congestive heart failure. Am J Med 1983;74:457–464.
17. Chatterjee K, ed. Dobutamine. A ten year review. New York: NCM Publishers, 1989.
18. Robin ED, McCauley R. Nitroprusside-related cyanide poisoning. Time (long past due) for urgent, effective interventions. Chest 1992;102:1842–1845.
19. Teboul J-L. Therapy: effects of vasoactive drugs. In: Edwards JD, Shoemaker WC, Vincent J-L, eds. Oxygen transport. Principles and practice. Philadelphia: WB Saunders, 1993;193–208.
20. Gardaz JP, McFarlane PA, Sykes MK. Mechanisms by which dopamine alters blood flow distribution during lobar collapse in dogs. J Appl Physiol 1986; 60:959–964.
21. Milero RR, Fenwell WH, Young JB, et al. Differential systemic arterial and venous actions and consequent cardiac effects of vasodilator drugs. Prog Cardiovasc Dis 1982;24:353–374.
22. Davidson RM. Hemodynamic effects of furosemide in acute myocardial infarction. Circulation 1971;54(Suppl II):156.
23. Kiely J, Kelly DT, Taylor DR, Pitt B. The role of furosemide in the treatment of left ventricular dysfunction associated with acute myocardial infarction. Circulation 1973;58:581–587.
24. Mond H, Hunt D, Sloman G. Haemodynamic effects of frusemide in patients suspected of having acute myocardial infarction. Br Heart J 1974;36:44–53.
25. Nelson GIC, Ahuja RC, Silke B, et al. Haemodynamic advantages of isosorbide dinitrate over frusemide in acute heart failure following myocardial infarction. Lancet 1983a;i:730–733.
26. Nelson GIC, Ahula RC, Silke B, et al. Haemodynamic effects of frusemide and its influence on repetitive volume loading in acute myocardial infarction. Eur Heart J 1983b;4:706–711.
27. Tattersfield AE, McNicol MW, Sillett RW. Haemodynamic effects of intravenous frusemide in patients with myocardial infarction and left ventricular failure. Clin Sci Molec Med 1974;46:253–264.
28. Larsen FF. Haemodynamic effects of high or low doses of furosemide in acute myocardial infarction. Eur Heart J 1988;9:125–131.
29. Dikshit K, Vyden JK, Forrester JS, et al. Renal and extrarenal hemodynamic effects of furosemide in congestive heart failure after acute myocardial infarction. N Engl J Med 1973;288:1087–1090.
30. Biddle TL, Yu PN. Effect of furosemide on hemodynamics and lung water in acute pulmonary edema secondary to acute myocardial infarction. Am J Cardiol 1979;43:86–90.
31. Nishimura I, Kanbe N. The renal and hemodynamic effects of furosemide in acute myocardial infarction. Crit Care Med 1981;9:829–832.
32. Francis GS, Siegel RM, Goldsmith SR, et al. Acute vasoconstrictor response to intravenous furosemide in patients with chronic congestive heart failure. Ann Intern Med 1986;103:1–6.
33. van Meyel JJM, Smits P, Russell FGM, et al. Diuretic efficiency of furosemide

during continuous administration versus bolus injection in healthy volunteers. Clin Pharmacol Ther 1992;51:440–444.

34. Martin SJ, Danzinger LH. Continuous infusion of loop diuretics in the critically ill: a review of the literature. Crit Care Med 1994;22:1323–1329.
35. Tamborini G, Pepi M, Susini G, et al. Reversal of cardiogenic shock and severe mitral regurgitation through verapamil in hypertensive hypertrophic cardiomyopathy. Chest 1993;104:319–324.
36. Nishimura R, Schwartz RS, Holmes DR, Tajik J. Failure of calcium channel blockers to improve ventricular relaxation in humans. J Am Coll Cardiol 1993; 21:182–188.
37. Vincent RL, Reuse C, Kahn RJ. Effects on right ventricular function of a change from dopamine to dobutamine in critically ill patients. Crit Care Med 1988; 16:659–662.
38. Dell'Italia LJ, Starling MR, Blumhardt R, et al. Comparative effects of volume loading, dobutamine and nitroprusside in patients with predominant right ventricular infarction. Circulation 1986;72:1327–1335.

MECHANICAL SUPPORT

39. Golding LAR. Postcardiotomy mechanical support. Semin Thorac Cardiovasc Surg 1991;3:29–32.
40. Kantrowitz A, Cordona RR, Freed PS. Percutaneous intra-aortic balloon counterpulsation. Crit Care Clin 1992;8:819–837.
41. Williams DO, Korr KS, Gewirtz H, Most AS. The effect of intra-aortic balloon counterpulsation on regional myocardial blood flow and oxygen consumption in the presence of coronary artery stenosis with unstable angina. Circulation 1982;3:593–597.
42. Mackenzie DJ, Wagner WH, Kulber DA, et al. Vascular complications of the intra- aortic balloon pump. Am J Surg 1992;164:517–521.
43. Killen DA, Piehler JM, Borkon AM, et al. Bio-Medicus ventricular assist device for salvage of cardiac surgical patients. Ann Thorac Surg 1991;52:230–235.
44. Lee WA, Gillinov AM, Cameron DE, et al. Centrifugal ventricular assist device for support of the failing heart after cardiac surgery. Crit Care Med 1993;21: 1186–1191.

CARDIOPULMONARY BYPASS SURGERY

45. Marino PL, Sink JD. Cardiac performance and systemic oxygen transport after cardiopulmonary bypass surgery. In Salmasi A-M, Iskandrian AS, eds. Cardiac output and regional flow in health and disease. Dordrecht, The Netherlands: Kluwer Academic Publishers, 1993;195–212.
46. D'Cruz IA, Callaghan WE. Atypical cardiac tamponade. Clinical and echocardiographic features. Internal Med Specialist 1988;9:68–78.
47. Khoury AF, Afridi I, Quinones MA, et al. Transesophageal echocardiography in critically ill patients: feasibility, safety, and impact on management. Am Heart J 1994;127:1363–1371.
48. Ivanov J, Weisel RD, Mickelborough LL, et al. Rewarming hypovolemia after aorto-coronary bypass surgery. Crit Care Med 1984;12:1049–1054.
49. Flaherty JT, Magee PA, Gardner TL, et al. Comparison of intravenous nitroglycerin and sodium nitroprusside for treatment of acute hypertension developing after coronary artery bypass surgery. Circulation 1982;65:1072–1077.

17

CARDIAC ARREST

Medicine cannot, except over a short period, increase the population of the world.
                                                                    Bertrand Russell

In 1960, an article was published in the *Journal of the American Medical Association* that became the single most influential study in twentieth-century medicine. The article, titled "Closed-Chest Cardiac Massage," presented five cases of acute cardiopulmonary arrest, which are summarized in Table 17.1. Although recovery in each case can be attributed to other interventions (e.g., intubation and cardioversion), the conclusion of the report stated, "Closed-chest cardiac massage has been proved to be effective in cases of cardiac arrest" (1). This report represents the birth of what is known today as cardiopulmonary resuscitation (CPR). As shown in Figure 17.1, CPR is far from successful as a life-saving intervention (2). Yet despite this poor performance, CPR not only is a universally accepted practice, but is considered a human right.

This chapter describes the mechanical and pharmacologic interventions involved in the management of cardiac arrest. Also included are recommendations for clinical monitoring during CPR and some concerns in the early postresuscitation period. A more detailed description of this topic is available in the American Heart Association guidelines for basic and advanced cardiac life support (see Suggested Readings at the end of the chapter).

BASIC LIFE SUPPORT

The ABCs of basic life support are Airway, Breathing, and Circulation. Clearing the airway is achieved by maneuvers such as the Heimlich maneuver that relieve airway obstruction. Breathing is achieved

TABLE 17.1. SUMMARY OF ORIGINAL REPORT ON CLOSED-CHEST CARDIAC MASSAGE	
Case	Description
1	35-year-old female undergoing cholecystectomy. Difficult intubation while paralyzed, and lost pulses. Recovered when intubated.
2	9-year-old boy undergoing mastoidectomy. In recovery room, respirations stopped, but still had pulses. Given mouth-to-mouth resuscitation and recovered.
3	80-year-old woman in operating room for thyroidectomy. After induction and paralysis, lost pulses. Given neosynephrine, with return of pulses. Time of closed chest cardiac massage = 2 min.
4	12-year-old boy in operating room for removal of warts. Under general anesthesia, developed irregular pulse and lost pulse. After closed chest cardiac massage for 1 min, pulse returned.
5	45-year-old male in emergency room with chest pain and subsequent ventricular fibrillation arrest. Successfully cardioverted.
Concluding statement: "Closed-chest cardiac massage has been proved to be effective in cases of cardiac arrest."	
Kouwenhoven WB et al. Closed-chest cardiac massage. JAMA 1960;173: 1064–1067.	

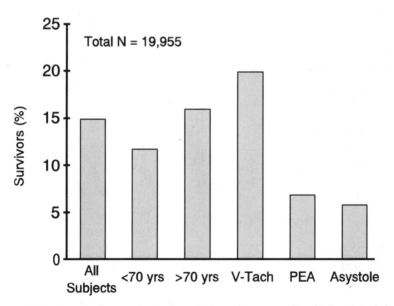

Figure 17.1. Survival rates for in-hospital cardiac arrest in all clinical reports published over a 30-year period from 1960 to 1990. Cases are grouped according to age and initial cardiac rhythm. Total number (N) of subjects involved is shown in the upper left corner of the graph. *PEA* = pulseless electrical activity, *V-Tach* = ventricular tachycardia. (Data from Schneider AP II et al. In-hospital cardiopulmonary resuscitation: a 30-year review. J Am Board Fam Pract 1993;6:91–101.)

by mouth-to-mouth resuscitation. Circulation involves closed-chest cardiac massage. Circulation is the heart of basic life support, and it is performed as follows:

CHEST COMPRESSIONS

1. Place the heel of one hand on the lower half of the patient's sternum so that the long axis of the hand runs perpendicular to the long axis of the sternum. Place the other hand, palm down, on top of the sternal hand, and interlace the fingers while keeping them off the chest.
2. Lock the elbows so that both arms are kept straight, and, with the shoulders positioned directly above the point of contact, depress the sternum by 1.5 to 2 inches at a rate of 80 to 100 times per minute. The duration of chest compression should take up half of the total compression–release cycle. The traditional ratio of chest compressions to lung inflations is 5:1.
3. If Steps 1 and 2 do not produce a palpable carotid or femoral pulse, increase the force of chest compressions.

Problems

The weak link in CPR is the inability of chest compressions to achieve adequate flow to the vital organs. In the original report in 1960, the ability to achieve a palpable pulse with chest compressions was mistakenly interpreted as indicating that chest compression could achieve adequate systemic blood flow. The problem is illustrated in Figure 17.2. The pressure tracings in this figure are taken from a patient

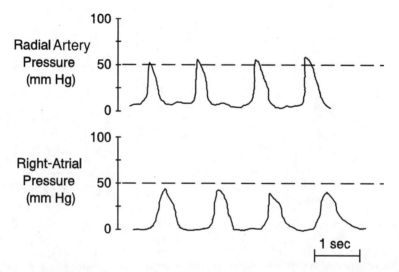

Figure 17.2. The influence of chest compressions on arterial and venous (right-atrial) pressure tracings in an adult patient with asystolic cardiac arrest. Note that the difference in arterial and venous (peak) pressures is negligible.

who received standard CPR with rhythmic chest compressions performed as just described. Note that similar pressures were achieved in the radial artery and the right atrium (the right-atrial pressure was recorded through a central venous catheter). Therefore, even though the chest compressions produced a systolic blood pressure slightly greater than 50 mm Hg, the arteriovenous pressure *difference*, which is the principal determinant of systemic and regional blood flow, is negligible. This is why **blood flow in both systemic and regional (e.g., coronary) circulations is less than one-quarter of prearrest levels during closed-chest compressions** (4–6). It also explains why CPR has had such a poor success rate. (If the original investigators had evaluated a venous pressure tracing during chest compressions, we may have been spared many of the false claims about CPR that predominate today.)

Coronary Perfusion Pressure

The difference between aortic pressure and right-atrial pressure, called coronary perfusion pressure (CPP), is the pressure gradient that drives coronary blood flow. Studies of CPR outcomes in humans show that a CPP of at least 15 mm Hg is necessary for a satisfactory outcome (7).

ACTIVE COMPRESSION–DECOMPRESSION CPR

In 1990, a case was reported where a cardiac arrest patient was resuscitated with a toilet plunger applied to the anterior chest wall (8). This led to the development of a plunger device that, when applied over the sternum, produces alternating chest compression and decompression. Although this device can produce higher cardiac outputs than standard chest compressions (9), clinical trials with this device have not resulted in higher survival rates in either out-of-hospital or in-hospital cardiac arrests (10,11).

OPEN-CHEST CARDIAC MASSAGE

Emergency thoracotomy with direct cardiac massage can achieve normal and even supranormal rates of blood flow during CPR (3,4,6). Unfortunately, the role of open-chest cardiac massage is limited by the reluctance to perform this procedure on cardiac arrest patients.

ADVANCED LIFE SUPPORT

Advanced life support (also called advanced cardiac life support, ACLS) includes maneuvers such as airway intubation, mechanical ventilation, and adjunctive measures (e.g., electric shock and drug administration) to enhance cardiac performance and promote blood flow.

The following description focuses on the adjunctive measures used to promote cardiac output during CPR (intubation and mechanical ventilation are presented in Chapters 26–29).

ACLS ALGORITHMS

The flow diagrams in Tables 17.2, 17.3, and 17.4 show the most recent recommendations of the American Heart Association for the management of cardiac arrest due to ventricular fibrillation and pulseless ventricular tachycardia (Table 17.2); pulseless electrical activity (PEA), which is the new term for electromechanical dissociation (Table 17.3); and ventricular asystole (Table 17.4). The following is a brief description of the resuscitative measures included in these diagrams.

DEFIBRILLATION

Direct-current cardioversion is the single most effective resuscitative measure for improving survival in cardiac arrest (2–6). In patients with ventricular tachycardia and ventricular fibrillation, the time from cardiac arrest to defibrillation is the most important factor in determining outcomes. The influence of treatment delays on survival is shown in Figure 17.3 (12). The data in this figure are taken from a study of 1667 cardiac arrest patients with ventricular fibrillation. Note that survival decreases linearly with increasing time to defibrillation. Survival decreased from 40% to less than 10% when defibrillation was delayed 15 minutes (from 5 to 20 minutes after arrest). These results emphasize the importance of avoiding delays in initiating defibrillation.

Dosage
The strength of defibrillation is usually expressed in units of energy (joules) rather than units of electric current (amperes). **The recommended energy for three successive defibrillations (if necessary) is 200 J, then 300 J, then 360 J.** If the initial three defibrillation attempts are unsuccessful, the drugs listed in Table 17.2 (e.g., epinephrine and lidocaine) are administered and the sequence of cardioversions is repeated. This pattern of defibrillations–drugs–defibrillations is the basic management strategy for ventricular tachycardia and fibrillation.

ROUTES OF DRUG ADMINISTRATION

Central versus Peripheral Veins
The initial site of venous cannulation for CPR should be the external jugular vein or the veins in the antecubital fossa (because these sites do not interfere with chest compressions and endotracheal intubation).

TABLE 17.2. ACLS ALGORITHM FOR VENTRICULAR FIBRILLATION AND PULSELESS VENTRICULAR TACHYCARDIA

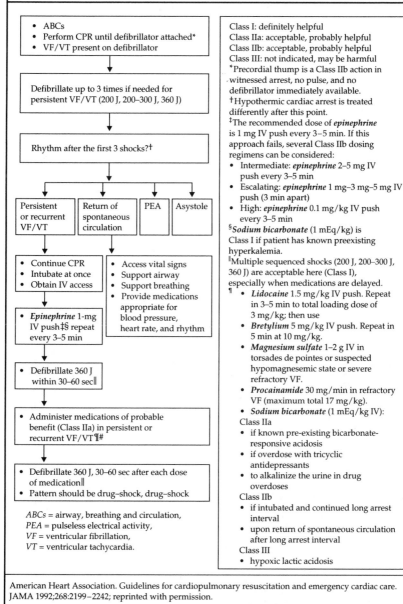

- ABCs
- Perform CPR until defibrillator attached*
- VF/VT present on defibrillator

↓

Defibrillate up to 3 times if needed for persistent VF/VT (200 J, 200–300 J, 360 J)

↓

Rhythm after the first 3 shocks?†

↓

| Persistent or recurrent VF/VT | Return of spontaneous circulation | PEA | Asystole |

Persistent or recurrent VF/VT:
- Continue CPR
- Intubate at once
- Obtain IV access

↓

- *Epinephrine* 1-mg IV push‡§ repeat every 3–5 min

↓

- Defibrillate 360 J within 30–60 sec‖

↓

- Administer medications of probable benefit (Class IIa) in persistent or recurrent VF/VT¶#

↓

- Defibrillate 360 J, 30–60 sec after each dose of medication‖
- Pattern should be drug–shock, drug–shock

Return of spontaneous circulation:
- Access vital signs
- Support airway
- Support breathing
- Provide medications appropriate for blood pressure, heart rate, and rhythm

ABCs = airway, breathing and circulation,
PEA = pulseless electrical activity,
VF = ventricular fibrillation,
VT = ventricular tachycardia.

Class I: definitely helpful
Class IIa: acceptable, probably helpful
Class IIb: acceptable, probably helpful
Class III: not indicated, may be harmful
*Precordial thump is a Class IIb action in witnessed arrest, no pulse, and no defibrillator immediately available.
†Hypothermic cardiac arrest is treated differently after this point.
‡The recommended dose of *epinephrine* is 1 mg IV push every 3–5 min. If this approach fails, several Class IIb dosing regimens can be considered:
- Intermediate: *epinephrine* 2–5 mg IV push every 3–5 min
- Escalating: *epinephrine* 1 mg–3 mg–5 mg IV push (3 min apart)
- High: *epinephrine* 0.1 mg/kg IV push every 3–5 min
§*Sodium bicarbonate* (1 mEq/kg) is Class I if patient has known preexisting hyperkalemia.
‖Multiple sequenced shocks (200 J, 200–300 J, 360 J) are acceptable here (Class I), especially when medications are delayed.
¶
- *Lidocaine* 1.5 mg/kg IV push. Repeat in 3–5 min to total loading dose of 3 mg/kg; then use
- *Bretylium* 5 mg/kg IV push. Repeat in 5 min at 10 mg/kg.
- *Magnesium sulfate* 1–2 g IV in torsades de pointes or suspected hypomagnesemic state or severe refractory VF.
- *Procainamide* 30 mg/min in refractory VF (maximum total 17 mg/kg).
- *Sodium bicarbonate* (1 mEq/kg IV):
Class IIa
- if known pre-existing bicarbonate-responsive acidosis
- if overdose with tricyclic antidepressants
- to alkalinize the urine in drug overdoses
Class IIb
- if intubated and continued long arrest interval
- upon return of spontaneous circulation after long arrest interval
Class III
- hypoxic lactic acidosis

American Heart Association. Guidelines for cardiopulmonary resuscitation and emergency cardiac care. JAMA 1992;268:2199–2242; reprinted with permission.

TABLE 17.3. ACLS ALGORITHM FOR PULSELESS ELECTRICAL ACTIVITY (PEA)

PEA includes
- Electromechanical dissociation (EMD)
- Pseudo-EMD
- Idioventricular rhythms
- Ventricular escape rhythms
- Bradyasystolic rhythms
- Postdefibrillation idioventricular rhythms

- Continue CPR
- Intubate at once
- Obtain IV access
- Assess blood flow using Doppler ultrasound

↓

Consider possible causes
(Parentheses = possible therapies and treatments)
- Hypovolemia (volume infusion)
- Hypoxia (ventilation)
- Cardiac tamponade (pericardiocentesis)
- Tension pneumothorax (needle decompression)
- Hypothermia
- Massive pulmonary embolism (surgery, *thrombolytics*)
- Drug overdoses such as tricyclics, digitalis, β-Blockers, calcium channel blockers
- Hyperkalemia*
- Acidosis†
- Massive acute myocardial infarction

↓

- *Epinephrine* 1 mg IV push, *† repeat every 3–5 min

↓

- If absolute bradycardia (< 60 beats/min) or relative bradycardia, give *atropine* 1 mg IV
- Repeat every 3–5 min up to a total of 0.04 mg/kg§

Class I: definitely helpful
Class IIa: acceptable, probably helpful
Class IIb: acceptable, possibly helpful
Class III: not indicated, may be harmful
Sodium bicarbonate 1 mEq/kg in Class I if patient has known preexisting hyperkalemia.
†*Sodium bicarbonate* 1 mEq/kg:
Class IIa
- if known preexisting bicarbonate-responsive acidosis
- if overdose with tricyclic antidepressants
- to alkalinize the urine in drug overdoses
Class IIb
- if intubated and long arrest interval
- upon return of spontaneous circulation after long arrest interval
Class III
- hypoxic lactic acidosis
‡The recommended dose of *epinephrine* is 1 mg IV push every 3–5 min.
If this approach fails, several Class IIb dosing regimens can be considered.
- Intermediate: *epinephrine* 2–5 mg IV push every 3–5 min
- Escalating: *epinephrine* 1 mg–3 mg–5 mg IV push (3 min apart)
- High: *epinephrine* 0.1 mg/kg IV push every 3–5 min
§Shorter *atropine* dosing intervals are possibly helpful in cardiac arrest (Class IIb).

American Heart Association. Guidelines for cardiopulmonary resuscitation and emergency cardiac care. JAMA 1992;268: 2199–2242; reprinted with permission.

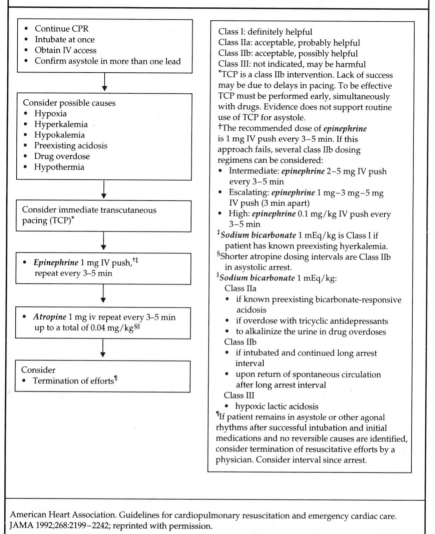

TABLE 17.4. ACLS ALGORITHM FOR MANAGEMENT OF ASYSTOLE

- Continue CPR
- Intubate at once
- Obtain IV access
- Confirm asystole in more than one lead

↓

Consider possible causes
- Hypoxia
- Hyperkalemia
- Hypokalemia
- Preexisting acidosis
- Drug overdose
- Hypothermia

↓

Consider immediate transcutaneous pacing (TCP)*

↓

- *Epinephrine* 1 mg IV push,†‡ repeat every 3–5 min

↓

- *Atropine* 1 mg iv repeat every 3–5 min up to a total of 0.04 mg/kg§‖

↓

Consider
- Termination of efforts¶

Class I: definitely helpful
Class IIa: acceptable, probably helpful
Class IIb: acceptable, possibly helpful
Class III: not indicated, may be harmful
*TCP is a class IIb intervention. Lack of success may be due to delays in pacing. To be effective TCP must be performed early, simultaneously with drugs. Evidence does not support routine use of TCP for asystole.
†The recommended dose of *epinephrine* is 1 mg IV push every 3–5 min. If this approach fails, several class IIb dosing regimens can be considered:
- Intermediate: *epinephrine* 2–5 mg IV push every 3–5 min
- Escalating: *epinephrine* 1 mg–3 mg–5 mg IV push (3 min apart)
- High: *epinephrine* 0.1 mg/kg IV push every 3–5 min
‡*Sodium bicarbonate* 1 mEq/kg is Class I if patient has known preexisting hyerkalemia.
§Shorter atropine dosing intervals are Class IIb in asystolic arrest.
‖*Sodium bicarbonate* 1 mEq/kg:
  Class IIa
  - if known preexisting bicarbonate-responsive acidosis
  - if overdose with tricyclic antidepressants
  - to alkalinize the urine in drug overdoses
  Class IIb
  - if intubated and continued long arrest interval
  - upon return of spontaneous circulation after long arrest interval
  Class III
  - hypoxic lactic acidosis
¶If patient remains in asystole or other agonal rhythms after successful intubation and initial medications and no reversible causes are identified, consider termination of resuscitative efforts by a physician. Consider interval since arrest.

American Heart Association. Guidelines for cardiopulmonary resuscitation and emergency cardiac care. JAMA 1992;268:2199–2242; reprinted with permission.

Drug administration through peripheral veins should always be bolus injection, followed by a 20-mL saline flush (3). If spontaneous circulation does not return after the initial drug injection, central venous cannulation should be performed for subsequent drug administration (3). This latter maneuver reduces the circulation time for drug distribution by at least 2 minutes (3).

Endobronchial Drug Administration

When venous access is not readily available and an endotracheal tube is in place, certain drugs can be injected through the endotracheal

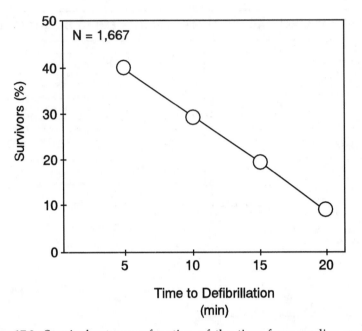

Figure 17.3. Survival rate as a function of the time from cardiac arrest to defibrillation in patients with ventricular fibrillation. The number (N) of subjects studied is shown in the upper left corner of the graph. (Data from Larsen MP et al. Predicting survival from out-of-hospital cardiac arrest: a graphic model. Ann Emerg Med 1993;22:1652.)

tube (13). **The drugs that can be given via the endobronchial route are atropine, epinephrine, and lidocaine.** The endobronchial dose is twice the recommended intravenous dose for each drug (3). Epinephrine seems to be less effective when given via the endobronchial route, and more than twice the recommended intravenous dose of epinephrine may be necessary to produce the desired result when the drug is given endobronchially (14). All drugs injected into the airways should be diluted in 10 mL saline or sterile water, and the injection should be made through a long catheter (such as a 20-cm central venous catheter) whose tip extends beyond the tip of the endotracheal tube. Drugs should not be injected directly into the endotracheal tube. Chest compressions should be discontinued while the drug is injected into the upper airways, and the injection should be followed with a few manual lung inflations. This maneuver is effective in promoting drug absorption from the lung (13).

EPINEPHRINE

Intravenous epinephrine is a mainstay in ACLS and is indicated for pulseless ventricular tachycardiac and ventricular fibrillation, electromechanical dissociation, and ventricular asystole. The rationale for epinephrine administration is to promote systemic vasoconstriction and thereby direct blood flow to the coronary and cerebral circulations.

Dosage

The standard dose of epinephrine in ACLS protocols is 1 mg (10 mL of a 1:10,000 solution), repeated every 3 to 5 minutes if necessary. The optimal dose of epinephrine in CPR may actually be much higher, particularly in larger patients. In animal studies, the optimal hemodynamic dose of epinephrine is 0.045 to 2.0 mg/kg (3), which is considerably higher than the standard epinephrine dose recommended in human ACLS protocols. However, two clinical studies evaluating high-dose epinephrine (7 mg in one study, 0.2 mg/kg in the other) in CPR show no increase in survival with the high-dose regimens compared with standard-dose regimens (15,16). Despite the lack of evidence for improved outcomes with high-dose epinephrine, the American Heart Association now recommends that **epinephrine doses can be increased to 5 mg if there is no response to an initial 1-mg** dose of the drug (3).

ATROPINE

Atropine is probably one of the least effective drugs in the ACLS armamentarium. It is most effective for the management of bradycardias, but it is also recommended in the management of pulseless electrical activity and ventricular asystole.

Dosage

The recommended dose of atropine for electromechanical dissociation and asystole is 1 mg by intravenous injection, repeated every 3 to 5 minutes if necessary. A total dose of 3 mg (or 0.04 mg/kg) produces complete vagal blockade, so this dose should not be exceeded. Atropine doses that are less than 0.5 mg can have parasympathomimetic effects (i.e., they can promote bradycardia), and thus should be avoided (3).

BICARBONATE

The recommendations for bicarbonate administration in CPR have been revised considerably in recent years because of an accumulation of studies showing little benefit and possible harm associated with bicarbonate administration in metabolic acidoses (17–19). Of note is recent evidence showing that bicarbonate administration in doses recommended for CPR (1 mg/kg) does not result in enhanced vasopressor actions of epinephrine (20).

The current recommendations for bicarbonate therapy in CPR are

TABLE 17.5. RECOMMENDATIONS FOR BICARBONATE ADMINISTRATION	
Class I (beneficial)	• Hyperkalemia
Class IIa (probably beneficial)	• Bicarbonate-responsive acidosis
	• Tricyclic overdose
	• Urinary alkalinization
Class IIb (possibly beneficial)	• Prolonged cardiac arrest
	• Postresuscitation acidosis
Class III (harmful)	• Anaerobic lactic acidosis

shown in Table 17.5. As indicated at the bottom of the table, **bicarbonate is no longer recommended in patients with ischemic lactic acidosis. In fact, it is considered potentially harmful in this condition.** The effects of bicarbonate administration are described in Chapter 37.

CALCIUM

Despite the fact that extracellular calcium enhances the contractile force of cardiac muscle, there is no evidence to indicate that calcium administration during CPR improves cardiac performance. In fact, ischemia promotes the intracellular accumulation of calcium, and this can lead to membrane disruption and uncoupling of oxidative phosphorylation (21). Because of the risk of calcium accumulation and subsequent cell injury during periods of tissue ischemia, the indications for calcium administration during CPR are restricted to cases of acute hyperkalemia, ionized hypocalcemia, and calcium channel blocker overdose.

DEXTROSE INFUSIONS

Although dextrose is a popular additive in intravenous fluids, dextrose administration can have deleterious effects in critically ill patients (22). As mentioned in Chapter 15, dextrose infusions can enhance the production of lactic acid in critically ill patients (see Fig. 15.2). The accumulation of lactic acid can itself promote cell injury, possibly by promoting the formation of toxic oxygen metabolites (23). This may explain why hyperglycemia enlarges infarct size in animal studies of cerebrovascular occlusion (24). The impact of carbohydrate infusions during CPR is not clear. However, the current recommendations from the American Heart Association are that **dextrose infusions are a Class III intervention (harmful) and thus should be avoided** (3).

CLINICAL MONITORING

The number one problem with CPR is the inability of chest compressions to maintain adequate organ blood flow. The number two problem is the inability to monitor the adequacy of organ perfusion during CPR. **The presence of palpable pulses and arterial pressure waves is not an indication of blood flow** (the difference between pressure waves and flow waves is described in Chapter 9). The measurements described in this section can provide a more accurate assessment of organ perfusion than the standard measures used to evaluate the response to CPR.

END-TIDAL CO_2 PRESSURE

The excretion of carbon dioxide in exhaled gas is a function of pulmonary blood flow (cardiac output), and thus the level of CO_2 in exhaled gas changes in direct proportion to changes in cardiac output. The CO_2 pressure (Pco_2) in end-expiratory gas (i.e., the end-tidal Pco_2) is easy to measure at the bedside, and changes in end-tidal Pco_2 can be used as a noninvasive marker of changes in cardiac output (see Chapter 22 for a detailed description of the end-tidal CO_2 measurement and its applications). End-tidal Pco_2 has been used to monitor the cardiac output in hypovolemia (see Fig. 14.1) and during cardiopulmonary resuscitation (25–27).

Prognostic Value

A progressive rise in end-tidal Pco_2 during CPR indicates that the resuscitation effort is successful in promoting cardiac output. As such, **a steady rise in end-tidal Pco_2 during CPR is more likely to be associated with a successful outcome than a persistently low end-tidal Pco_2.** The correlation between survival and end-tidal Pco_2 during CPR is shown in Figure 17.4. The data in this figure are from a study of

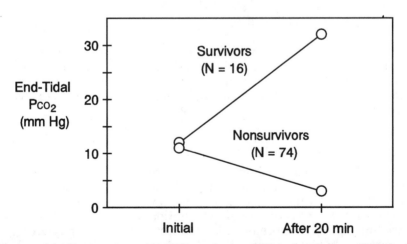

Figure 17.4. Changes in end-tidal Pco_2 during CPR in survivors and nonsurvivors of cardiac arrest associated with pulseless electrical activity. Open circles represent the mean values for each group. (Data from Wayne MA et al. Use of end-tidal carbon dioxide to predict outcome in prehospital cardiac arrest. Ann Emerg Med 1995;25:762–767.)

90 cardiac arrest patients with PEA (27). The initial end-tidal P_{CO_2} measurement, obtained at the onset of CPR, is very low (11 to 12 mm Hg, compared to a normal end-tidal P_{CO_2} of 40 to 45 mm Hg), and is similar in survivors and nonsurvivors. However, in the survivors, the end-tidal P_{CO_2} increased considerably (from 12 to 31 mm Hg) after 20 minutes of CPR, whereas in the nonsurvivors the end-tidal P_{CO_2} decreased further (from 10.9 to 3.9 mm Hg). These results are supported by the results of another study where CPR that failed to raise the end-tidal P_{CO_2} above 10 mm Hg was universally unsuccessful (26).

The tendency of the end-tidal P_{CO_2} to rise during CPR can thus be a valuable prognostic marker. **When end-tidal P_{CO_2} does not rise above 10 mm Hg after a resuscitation time of 15 to 20 minutes, the resuscitative effort is unlikely to be successful.**

VENOUS BLOOD GASES

The common practice of monitoring arterial blood gases during CPR should be abandoned in favor of monitoring *venous* blood gases. The rationale for this switch is the greater propensity for venous blood to represent the oxygenation and acid–base status of peripheral tissues (28,29). The tendency for arterial blood gases to provide misleading information during CPR is demonstrated by the observation that arterial blood can show a respiratory alkalosis while venous blood shows a metabolic acidosis during CPR (28,29).

The superiority of venous blood gases for monitoring tissue events during CPR (or in any low-flow state) has been ignored for over a decade, resulting in suboptimal care for cardiac arrest patients.

HOW LONG TO RESUSCITATE

There is little doubt that CPR is inappropriately prolonged in a significant percentage of resuscitative efforts. The goal of prolonged CPR is to increase the chance for survival, but this is not a desirable goal if the survivor is mentally impaired, as is often the case in survivors of prolonged CPR.

Ischemic Time and Neurologic Recovery

The risk of functional impairment in any of the major organs is directly related to the duration of the ischemic insult. The ischemic time following cardiac arrest includes the time from onset of the arrest to onset of CPR (arrest time) and the duration of the resuscitative effort (CPR time). The influence of these two ischemic times on neurologic recovery is shown in Figure 17.5. The data in this figure are taken from a multicenter study of patients who did not regain consciousness in the first hour following successful CPR (30). If the arrest time was less than 6 minutes and the CPR time did not exceed 30 minutes, half of the survivors had a satisfactory neurologic recovery. However if

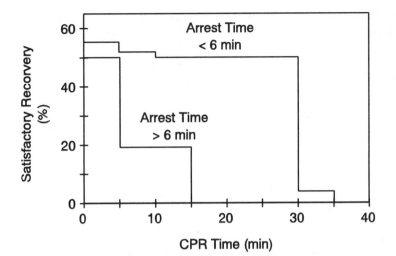

Figure 17.5. Time sequence plots showing the incidence of satisfactory neurologic recovery as a function of both the duration of the resuscitative effort (CPR time) and the time from cardiac arrest to CPR (arrest time). The study group included 262 survivors of cardiac arrest who did not regain consciousness in the first hour after CPR. (From Abramson NS et al. Neurologic recovery after cardiac arrest: effect of duration of ischemia. Crit Care Med 1985; 13:930–931.)

the arrest time exceeded 6 minutes, more than 15 minutes of CPR always produced neurologic impairment in the survivors. Thus, **in witnessed cardiac arrest** (when arrest time can be accurately determined), **CPR can be continued for 30 minutes if the arrest time is less than 6 minutes, but if the arrest time is longer than 6 minutes, CPR should be terminated after 15 minutes.**

POSTRESUSCITATION CONCERNS

When CPR is successful in restoring spontaneous circulation, two concerns deserve attention in the early postresuscitation period. The first is the potential for continued and progressive multiorgan damage (i.e., postresuscitation injury). The second is the likelihood of neurologic recovery in patients who do not regain consciousness immediately after CPR.

POSTRESUSCITATION INJURY

The phenomenon of postresuscitation organ damage was described at the end of Chapter 14. This condition is usually seen after prolonged ischemic times, and it is characterized by progressive dysfunction in multiple organs. Other, more familiar terms for this condition are *multiple organ failure* (31) and *multiple organ dysfunction syndrome* (32). This condition is often fatal, and there is no effective therapy at present. Several mechanisms have been proposed for this condition, including persistent vasoconstriction (i.e., the no-reflow phenomenon) and the release of toxins produced during the period of ischemia (i.e., reperfusion injury). (See Chapter 31 for a more detailed description of the multiple organ failure and its management.)

NEUROLOGIC RECOVERY

Neurologic impairment is common in cardiac arrest patients who are successfully resuscitated. Many survivors do not regain consciousness immediately after CPR, and the following are some prognostic factors that help identify patients who are unlikely to awaken or achieve a satisfactory neurologic recovery.

Duration of Coma

Failure to regain consciousness in the first few hours after CPR is not a harbinger of prolonged or permanent neurologic impairment, (33). However, **coma that persists longer than 4 hours after CPR carries a poor prognosis for full neurologic recovery.** The relationship between neurologic recovery and coma that persists longer than 4 hours after CPR is shown in Figure 17.6 (34). Although the recovery rates are low for all points on the graph, there is a linear decline in recovery rate as the duration of coma increases. After 1 day of persistent coma, only 10% of the patients achieved a satisfactory neurologic recovery. The recovery rate drops below 5% when the coma lasts 1 week, and no patient recovers neurologic function when the coma persists for 2 weeks.

The data in Figure 17.6 can be useful for identifying patients who are not likely to benefit from therapeutic interventions (i.e., futile care). It can also be useful for determining the appropriate time to inform close relatives about the patient's prognosis. Three days of persistent coma is my threshold for informing families of the poor prognosis for recovery. The actual time selected for informing families of a poor prognosis is a matter of individual preference. The important point is to keep the family informed and to provide guidance in decisions about future strategies.

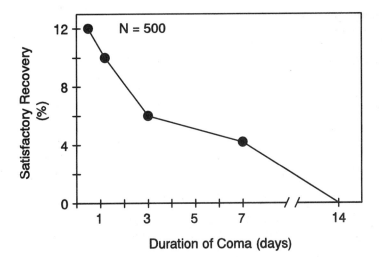

Figure 17.6. Graph showing the relationship between the duration of coma and the incidence of favorable neurologic recovery. The number (N) of subjects studied is indicated at the top of the graph. (Data from Levy DE et al. Prognosis in non-traumatic coma. Ann Intern Med 1981;94:293–301.)

Coma Scores

Scoring systems such as the Glasgow Coma Scale (GCS) can also provide valuable prognostic information. (This scoring method is described in Chapter 50.) A GCS below 5 on the third day of persistent coma is almost always associated with a poor outcome (33).

Pupillary Light Reflex

Several brainstem reflexes can have prognostic value in patients who do not regain consciousness after CPR, but none can match the predictive value of the pupillary light reflex. The importance of this reflex is its negative predictive value (i.e., the ability to identify a poor outcome). **Absence of the pupillary light reflex after one or more days of coma indicates little or no chance for neurologic recovery.** This reflex has no prognostic value in the first 6 hours after CPR because it can be transiently lost and then reappear (35). Finally, the resuscitation drugs atropine and epinephrine can produce pupillary dilation, but these agents do not interfere with the pupillary response to light (33,36).

REFERENCES

GENERAL TEXTS

Baskett PJF. Resuscitation handbook. 2nd ed. London: Mosby Europe, Ltd., 1993.
Cummins RO, ed. Textbook of advanced cardiac life support. Dallas: American Heart Association, 1994.
Paradis NA, Halperin HL, Nowak RM. Cardiac arrest. The science and practice of resuscitation medicine. Baltimore: Williams & Wilkins, 1995.
Parr MJA, Craft TM. Resuscitation: key data. Oxford: Bios Scientific Publishers, Ltd., 1994.

HISTORICAL REPORTS

1. Kouwenhoven WB, Ing, Jude JR, Knickerbocker GG. Closed chest cardiac massage. JAMA 1960;173:1064–1067.
2. Schneider AP II, Nelson DJ, Brown DD. In-hospital cardiopulmonary resuscitation. A 30-year review. J Am Board Fam Pract 1993;6:91–101.

GUIDELINES

3. Emergency Cardiac Care Committee and Subcommittees, American Heart Association. Guidelines for cardiopulmonary resuscitation and emergency cardiac care. JAMA 1992;268:2171–2241.

REVIEWS

4. Weil MH, Gazmuri RJ, Rackow EC. The clinical rationale of cardiac resuscitation. Dis Mon 1990;36:423–468 (195 References).
5. Barton CW, Manning JE. Cardiopulmonary resuscitation. Emerg Med Clin North Am 1995;13:811–830 (101 References).
6. DeBehnke DJ, Swart GL. Cardiac arrest. Emerg Med Clin North Am 1996;14: 57–82 (112 References).

BASIC LIFE SUPPORT

7. Paradis NA, Martin GB, Rivers EP, et al. Coronary perfusion pressure and the return of spontaneous circulation in human cardiopulmonary resuscitation. JAMA 1990;263:1106–1113.
8. Lurie KG, Lindo C, Chin J. CPR: the P stands for plumber's helper. JAMA 1990;264:1661.
9. Orliaguet GA, Carli PA, Rozenberg A, et al. End-tidal carbon dioxide during out-of-hospital cardiac arrest resuscitation: comparison of active compression–decompression and standard CPR. Ann Emerg Med 1995;25:48–51.
10. Lurie KJ, Shultz JJ, Callahan ML, et al. Evaluation of active compression–decompression CPR in victims of out-of-hospital cardiac arrest. JAMA 1994;271: 1405–1411.
11. Tucker KJ, Galli F, Savitt MA, et al. Active compression–decompression resuscitation: effect on resuscitation success after in-hospital cardiac arrest. J Am Coll Cardiol 1994;24:201–209.

ADVANCED LIFE SUPPORT

12. Larsen MP, Eisenberg M, Cummins RO, Hallstrom AP. Predicting survival from out of hospital cardiac arrest: a graphic model. Ann Emerg Med 1993; 22:1652–1658.
13. Aitkenhead AR. Drug administration during CPR: what route? Resuscitation 1991;22:191–195.

14. McCrirrick A, Kestin I. Haemodynamic effects of tracheal compared with intravenous adrenaline. Lancet 1992;340:868–870.
15. Steill IG, Hebert PC, Weitzman BN, et al. High-dose epinephrine in adult cardiac arrest. N Engl J Med 1992;327:1045–1050.
16. Brown CG, Martin DR, Pepe P, et al. A comparison of standard-dose and high-dose epinephrine in cardiac arrest outside the hospital. N Engl J Med 1992;327:1051–1055.
17. Hindman BJ. Sodium bicarbonate in the treatment of subtypes of acute lactic acidosis: physiologic considerations. Anesthesiology 1990;72:1064–1076.
18. Arieff AI. Indications for the use of bicarbonate in patients with metabolic acidosis. Br J Anesth 1991;67:165–177.
19. Ritter JM, Doktor HS, Benjamin N. Paradoxical effect of bicarbonate on cytoplasmic pH. Lancet 1990;335:1243–1246.
20. Bleske BE, Rice TL, Warren EW, et al. The effect of sodium bicarbonate administration on the vasopressor effect of high-dose epinephrine during cardiopulmonary resuscitation in swine. Am J Emerg Med 1993;11:439–443.
21. Rees AP, Valentino VA, Genton E. Pharmacological adjuncts to cardiopulmonary resuscitation. Intern Med 1991;12:22–35.
22. Marino PL, Finnegan MJ. Nutrition support is not beneficial, and can be harmful, in critically ill patients. Crit Care Clin 1996;12:667–676.
23. Sieber FE, Traytsman RJ. Special issues: glucose and the brain. Crit Care Med 1992;20:104–114.
24. de Courten-Meyers G, Meyers RE, Schoolfield L. Hyperglycemia enlarges infarct size in cerebrovascular occlusion in cats. Stroke 1988;19:623–630.

CLINICAL MONITORING

25. Falk JL, Rackow EC, Weil MH. End-tidal carbon dioxide concentration during cardiopulmonary resuscitation. N Engl J Med 1988;318:607–611.
26. Sanders AB, Kern KB, Otto CW, et al. End-tidal carbon dioxide monitoring during cardiopulmonary resuscitation. JAMA 1989;262:1347–1351.
27. Wayne MA, Levine RL, Miller CC. Use of end-tidal carbon dioxide to predict outcome in prehospital cardiac arrest. Ann Emerg Med 1995;25:762–767.
28. Weil MH, Rackow EC, Trevino R. Difference in acid–base state between venous and arterial blood during cardiopulmonary resuscitation. N Engl J Med 1986;315:153–156.
29. Steedman DJ, Robertson CE. Acid–base changes in arterial and central venous blood during cardiopulmonary resuscitation. Arch Emerg Med 1992;9:169–176.

POST-RESUSCITATION CONCERNS

30. Abramson NS, Safar P, Detre KM, et al. Neurologic recovery after cardiac arrest: effect of duration of ischemia. Crit Care Med 1985;13:930–931.
31. Cerra F. Multiple organ failure syndrome. Dis Mon 1992;12:845–878.
32. The ACCP/SCCM Consensus Conference Committee. Definitions for sepsis and organ failure and guidelines for the use of innovative therapies in sepsis. Chest 1992;101:1644–1655.
33. Edgren E, Hedstrand U, Kelsey S, et al. Assessment of neurologic prognosis in comatose survivors of cardiac arrest. Lancet 1994;343:1055–1059.
34. Levy DE, Caronna JJ, Singer BH, et al. Predicting outcome from hypoxic-ischemic coma. JAMA 1985;253:1420–1426.
35. Steen-Hansen JE, Hansen NM, Vaagenes P, Schreiner B. Pupil size and light reactivity during cardiopulmonary resuscitation: a clinical study. Crit Care Med 1988;16:69–70.
36. Goetting MG, Contreras E. Systemic atropine during cardiac arrest does not cause fixed and dilated pupils. Ann Emerg Med 1991;20:55–57.

c h a p t e r

HEMODYNAMIC DRUGS

This chapter contains a brief description of eight pharmaceutical agents given by continuous intravenous infusion to support the circulation. Each agent is listed below in order of presentation. Drugs marked by an asterisk have a dose chart included in the chapter.

1. Amrinone*
2. Dobutamine*
3. Dopamine*
4. Epinephrine
5. Labetalol
6. Nitroglycerin*
7. Nitroprusside*
8. Norepinephrine

INFUSION RATES

Because the drugs in this chapter are administered by continuous infusion, the recommended doses are expressed as dose rates, either in micrograms per minute (μg/min) or micrograms per kilogram body weight per minute (μg/kg/min). To deliver the recommended dose rate, the concentration of the drug in the infusate must be known. The infusion rate (i.e., the rate at which the infusate is delivered) is then determined as the ratio of the dose rate to the drug concentration in the infusate. This is shown in Table 18.1. In this case, the desired dose rate is R μg/min, and the drug concentration in the infusate is C μg/mL, so the ratio R/C derives the infusion rate in mL/min. The infusion rate can be converted to microdrops/minute by multiplying mL/min by 60 (because there are 60 microdrops per mL). The conversion to

278

TABLE 18.1. DETERMINING DRUG INFUSION RATES
If the desired dose rate = R μg/min and the drug concentration in the infusate = C μg/mL, then: $$\text{Infusion rate} = \frac{R}{C} \text{ (mL/min)}$$ $$= \frac{R}{C} \times 60 \text{ (microdrops/min)}$$

microdrops facilitates control of infusion rates when small volumes of fluid are infused. Therefore, all infusion rates included in the drug dosing charts in this chapter are expressed in microdrops/minute. The volumetric equivalent of microdrops/minute is mL/hr (i.e., microdrops/minute $\times$ 60/60 = mL/hr).

AMRINONE

Amrinone is a phosphodiesterase inhibitor that has both positive inotropic and vasodilator actions (1,2). Despite the potential benefit of its combined actions (i.e., greater augmentation of cardiac output with less cardiac work), amrinone has not proven superior to single-action cardiotonic agents such as dobutamine (3,4).

ACTIONS

The combined actions of amrinone produce an increase in cardiac stoke output without an increase in cardiac stroke work (4). The effects of amrinone on cardiac performance are roughly equivalent to those of dobutamine (3–5). However, because amrinone does not stimulate adrenergic receptors, its effects can add to the effects of dobutamine (4). Unlike dobutamine, the actions of amrinone are not attenuated by β-receptor antagonists.

Indications

Amrinone is effective as single-agent therapy in the management of low output states caused by systolic heart failure. However, it is most often used as a second agent that is added to dobutamine in cases of refractory heart failure (3,4).

DRUG ADMINISTRATION

A drug dosing chart for amrinone is shown in Table 18.2. Amrinone is degraded by dextrose and by light. Therefore, amrinone should not be infused in dextrose-containing fluids, and the infusion solution

TABLE 18.2. AMRINONE DOSAGE CHART							
Infusate:	100 mg amrinone in 100 mL diluent (1 mg/mL). *Do not mix amrinone with dextrose.*						
Usual dose:	Initial bolus dose of 0.75 mg/kg; maintenance dose of 5–10 μg/kg/min						
	Weight (kg)						
	40	**50**	**60**	**70**	**80**	**90**	**100**
Initial dose (mg)	30	38	45	53	60	68	75
Dose rate (μg/kg/min)	**microdrops/min (mL/hr)**						
5	12	15	18	21	24	27	30
7	19	21	25	29	34	38	42
10	24	30	36	42	48	54	60

should be protected from light. An initial loading dose is used for amrinone therapy. The usual dose is 0.75 mg/kg but can be as high as 1.5 mg/kg (6). This is followed by a continuous infusion, usually in the range of 5 to 10 μg/kg/min. A dose rate of 10 μg/kg/min will achieve the desired hemodynamic response in over 80% of patients (3).

Incompatabilities

Furosemide should not be injected into intravenous lines carrying amrinone infusions because the drug forms a precipitate when added to amrinone solutions (see Handbook of Injectable Drugs).

ADVERSE EFFECTS

Although the oral form of the drug was discontinued by the FDA because of a high incidence of complications, short-term therapy with intravenous amrinone is relatively free of adverse effects. *Thrombocytopenia* caused by nonimmunogenic platelet destruction was a common side effect of chronic therapy with oral amrinone, but this complication is reported in only 2 to 3% of patients receiving short-term intravenous amrinone (7). The problem resolves when the drug is discontinued, and no cases of abnormal bleeding have been reported. *Hypotension* caused by excessive vasodilation has been a common complication of amrinone therapy in some reports, but it seems to occur mostly in hypovolemic patients (5,7).

Contraindications

Amrinone is contraindicated in patients with hypertrophic cardiomyopathy (7). Thrombocytopenia is not a contraindication to intravenous amrinone, but it is probably wise to avoid the drug if possible in patients with platelet counts below 50,000/mL.

DOBUTAMINE

Dobutamine is a synthetic catecholamine that is generally considered the inotropic drug of choice for the acute management of severe (systolic) heart failure (1,3). It is primarily a β_1-receptor agonist (cardiac stimulation), but it also has mild β-2 effects (vasodilation).

ACTIONS

As demonstrated in Figure 18.1, dobutamine causes a dose-dependent increase in stroke volume (upper graph) accompanied by a decrease in cardiac filling pressures (lower graph). The increase in stroke output is usually accompanied by a proportional decrease in systemic vascular resistance (baroreceptor-mediated), and thus the arterial blood pressure usually remains unchanged. The drug is effective in both right- and left-sided heart failure (8–10).

The inotropic and chronotropic effects of dobutamine can vary widely in critically ill patients (8). This is partly due to variable pharmacokinetics (11) and partly due to variable end-organ responsiveness. Elderly patients are relatively resistant to dobutamine and can have only half the inotropic responsiveness seen in younger patients

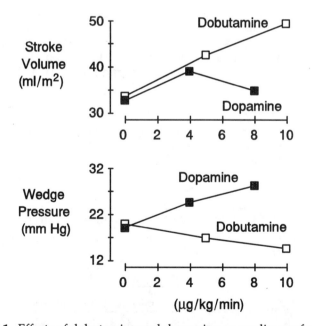

Figure 18.1. Effects of dobutamine and dopamine on cardiac performance in patients with severe heart failure. (Data from Leier CV et al. Comparative systemic and regional hemodynamic effects of dopamine and dobutamine in patients with cardiomyopathic heart failure. Circulation 1978;58:466–475.)

(12). The variable response to dobutamine in critically ill patients emphasizes the need to guide dobutamine therapy by preselected hemodynamic end-points, not by preselected dose rates.

Indications

As mentioned, dobutamine is the preferred inotropic agent for the acute management of low output states due to systolic heart failure. Because dobutamine does not usually raise the arterial blood pressure, it is **not indicated as monotherapy in patients with cardiogenic shock.**

Dobutamine is also used in patients with septic shock and multiple organ failure who may have a normal cardiac output. These conditions are often accompanied by hypermetabolism, and in this situation, a normal cardiac output may be not be adequate for the increased oxygen requirements of hypermetabolism. The goal of dobutamine therapy in these conditions is to drive the cardiac output to supranormal levels (e.g., $> 4.5 \ \text{L/min/m}^2$) to meet the increased oxygen consumption of the hypermetabolic state (13,14). The use of dobutamine to achieve a hyperdynamic state has had an inconsistent effect on survival (see Chapter 31), and thus is not universally accepted.

DRUG ADMINISTRATION

A dobutamine dose chart is shown in Table 18.3. The drug is available in 250-mg vials and is infused in a concentration of 1 mg/mL. The usual dose range is 5 to 15 µg/kg/min, but doses as high as 200 µg/kg/min have been used to achieve a hyperdynamic state in patients with septic shock and multiple organ failure (14).

Incompatibilities

An alkaline pH inactivates catecholamines such as dobutamine (15), and thus sodium bicarbonate or other alkaline solutions should not be administered through intravenous tubing used for dobutamine infusions.

TABLE 18.3. DOBUTAMINE DOSAGE CHART							
Infusate:	250 mg dobutamine in 250 mL diluent (1 mg/mL)						
Usual dose:	5–15 µg/kg/min						
				Weight (kg)			
	40	**50**	**60**	**70**	**80**	**90**	**100**
Dose (µg/kg/min)				**microdrops/min (mL/hr)**			
5	12	15	18	21	24	27	30
10	24	30	36	42	48	54	60
15	36	45	54	63	72	81	90
20	48	60	72	84	96	108	120

ADVERSE EFFECTS

Dobutamine has few serious side effects. As mentioned, tachycardia can develop in some patients. However, malignant tachyarrhythmias are uncommon (7).

Contraindications

Dobutamine is not indicated for the management of heart failure due to diastolic dysfunction and is contraindicated in patients with hypertrophic cardiomyopathy.

DOPAMINE

Dopamine is an endogenous catecholamine that serves as a neurotransmitter. As an exogenous agent, it produces a dose-dependent activation of several types of adrenergic and dopaminergic receptors (10). The overall effect of the drug is determined by the pattern of receptor activation, as described below.

ACTIONS

When given at low dose rates (0.5 to 3 µg/kg/min), dopamine selectively activates dopamine-specific receptors in the renal, mesenteric, and cerebral circulations and increases blood flow in these regions. Dopaminergic activation in the kidneys also produces an increase in urinary sodium and water excretion that is independent of the changes in renal blood flow (16).

At intermediate dose rates (3 to 7.5 µg/kg/min), dopamine stimulates β-receptors in the heart and peripheral circulations, and this produces an increase in cardiac output. The effects of incremental doses of dopamine on cardiac stroke output are shown in Figure 18.1 (upper graph). Note that **the inotropic response to dopamine is modest when compared to dobutamine.**

At high dose rates (> 7.5 µg/kg/min), dopamine produces a dose-dependent activation of α-receptors in the systemic and pulmonary circulations. This results in progressive vasoconstriction, and the resultant increase in ventricular afterload limits the ability of dopamine to augment cardiac output. The loss in cardiac output augmentation at higher doses of dopamine is shown in Figure 18.1 (upper graph).

The effects of dopamine on the pulmonary capillary wedge pressure are shown in Figure 18.1 (lower graph). There is a dose-dependent increase in the wedge pressure, which is independent of the changes in stroke volume in the upper graph. This effect may be the result of vasoconstriction in pulmonary veins. **Dopamine-induced constriction**

of pulmonary veins is an important consideration, because it **invalidates the pulmonary capillary wedge pressure as a measure of left-ventricular filling pressures** (see Chapter 11).

The hemodynamic responses to dopamine are blunted by continued drug administration (10). This tachyphylaxis may be due to dopamine's ability to release norepinephrine from adrenergic nerve terminals. When tachyphylaxis to dopamine develops, discontinuing the drug for a few days (if possible) can restore some of the end-organ responsiveness.

Indications

Dopamine is indicated for the management of cardiogenic shock and any circulatory shock syndrome associated with systemic vasodilation (e.g., septic shock). The drug is particularly valuable for its ability (in intermediate-to-high dose rates) to promote vasoconstriction while preserving the cardiac stroke output. Low-dose dopamine is also used to preserve renal blood flow and to promote urine output in patients with oliguric acute renal failure, or in those at risk for oliguric renal failure. Although dopamine does not improve intrinsic renal function in this situation, it can promote urine output and limit fluid retention (16).

DRUG ADMINISTRATION

A dose chart for dopamine administration is shown in Table 18.4. This chart identifies three dose ranges based on the most prominent clinical response. At low infusion rates of 0.5 to 3 μg/kg/min, natriuresis and diuresis are prominent. As the infusion rate is increased to 4 to 7 μg/kg/min, β-receptor stimulation and augmentation of cardiac output occurs. At dose rates above 8 μg/kg/min, progressive vasoconstriction is the dominant feature.

TABLE 18.4. DOPAMINE DOSAGE CHART								
Infusate:	200 mg dopamine in 250 mL diluent (800 μg/mL)							
		Weight (kg)						
		40	**50**	**60**	**70**	**80**	**90**	**100**
Prominent Effects	**Dose (μg/kg/min)**	**microdrops/min (mL/hr)**						
Diuresis	1	3	4	5	5	6	7	8
natriuresis	3	9	11	14	16	18	20	23
Increase in	5	15	19	23	26	30	34	38
cardiac output	7	21	26	32	37	42	47	53
Vasoconstriction	10	30	38	45	53	60	68	75
	15	45	56	68	79	90	101	113
	20	60	75	90	105	120	135	150

Incompatibilities

The precautions for alkaline fluids mentioned for dobutamine also apply to dopamine.

ADVERSE EFFECTS

Tachyarrhythmias are the most common complication of dopamine administration. Sinus tachycardia is common (8,17) and can occur at β-agonist dose rates (i.e., 5 to 7 μg/kg/min) (8). Malignant tachyarrhythmias (e.g., multifocal ventricular ectopics, ventricular tachycardia) can also occur, but are uncommon.

The most feared complication of dopamine administration is ischemic limb necrosis, which occurs more frequently with dopamine than with any other vasoconstrictor agent (7). Limb necrosis has been reported at dopamine doses as low as 1.5 μg/kg/min (7). Prompt administration of an α-receptor blocking agent such as phentolamine (5 mg as an intravenous bolus, followed by a continuous infusion at 1 to 2 mg/min) is indicated at the earliest signs of limb ischemia. Vasoconstrictor doses of dopamine should not be given through peripheral veins. Extravasation of the drug through a peripheral vein can be treated with a local injection of phentolamine (5 to 10 mg in 15 mL saline) (7).

EPINEPHRINE

Epinephrine is an endogenous catecholamine and the prototype sympathomimetic agent. Because of its potency and risk for adverse effects, epinephrine is used sparingly to support the circulation in conditions other than cardiac arrest.

ACTIONS

Like dopamine, epinephrine is primarily a β-receptor agonist at low doses and an α-receptor agonist at high doses. However, epinephrine is much more potent than dopamine, with an effective dose range that is two-to-three orders of magnitude below the effective dose range for dopamine. As shown in Table 18.5, epinephrine activates β-receptors

| TABLE 18.5. EPINEPHRINE DOSAGE RECOMMENDATIONS ||
Condition	Dose
Aqueous injectate	1:1000 (1.0 mg/mL)
	1:10,000 (0.1 mg/mL)
β-Agonist range	0.005–0.02 μg/kg/min
Vasopressor range	0.01–0.1 μg/kg/min
Anaphylaxis	0.2–0.5 mg SC or IM; repeat in 15 min if needed.
Anaphylactic shock	Add 1 mg epi to 500 mL diluent (2 μg/mL) and infuse at 1 mL/min. Titrate upward to 4 mL/min.

at doses of only 0.005 to 0.02 μg/kg/min. α-Receptor vasoconstriction appears at slightly higher doses, and renal vasoconstriction develops early (7). Dose rates above 0.1 μg/kg/min can produce severe vasoconstriction.

Antiinflammatory Effects

Epinephrine blocks the release of inflammatory mediators by mast cells and basophils in response to an antigenic challenge. This effect may explain the salutary effects of epinephrine in anaphylactic reactions (18).

Metabolic Effects

Epinephrine has several metabolic effects that represent adaptive responses in healthy subjects but can be deleterious in the critically ill patient (7). The metabolic effects that deserve mention include (a) hypermetabolism (calorigenic response), (b) hyperglycemia (enhanced gluconeogenesis and diminished insulin release), (c) an increase in circulating ketoacids (via lipolysis), (d) hyperlactatemia (without ischemia), and (e) a decrease in serum potassium (usually < 1 mEq/L).

Indications

Intravenous epinephrine is indicated for the management of cardiac arrest associated with pulseless ventricular tachycardia and ventricular fibrillation, asystole, and pulseless electrical activity (see Chapter 17). It is also indicated for severe anaphylactic reactions and anaphylactic shock. Because of the narrow therapeutic range and risk of adverse reactions, it is not recommended as a first-line agent for the routine management of low cardiac output or circulatory shock.

DRUG ADMINISTRATION

Epinephrine is available as a 1:1000 solution (1 mg/mL) and can be diluted to create a 1:10,000 solution (0.1 mg/mL). As indicated in Table 18.5, epinephrine is a powerful β agonist, with β-receptor activation at dose rates of only 0.005 to 0.02 μg/kg/min. The safe range for epinephrine infusions is exceeded at dose rates above 0.1 μg/kg/min (8).

The recommended epinephrine doses for anaphylaxis are shown at the bottom of Table 18.5 (18). Epinephrine is the single most effective drug in the management of anaphylaxis, and delays in administering the drug can have adverse consequences (18).

Incompatibilities

Like other catecholamines, epinephrine is inactivated by alkaline solutions.

ADVERSE EFFECTS

Epinephrine is arrhythmogenic, particularly in combination with halothane or electrolyte abnormalities (7). Coronary ischemia can also occur and is not related to dose (7). Although renal vasoconstriction is prominent with epinephrine, ischemic renal failure is seen most often with accidental epinephrine overdose (7). Epinephrine can produce serious hypertension in patients receiving β-receptor antagonists, an effect attributed to unopposed α-receptor stimulation (7).

Calorigenic Effect

Therapeutic doses of epinephrine can produce a 35% increase in resting metabolic rate (19), and the increase in tissue oxygen needs can have adverse consequences in patients with impaired or borderline tissue oxygenation. Dopamine has a similar but less pronounced calorigenic effect (19), whereas dobutamine seems to have little or no effect on the metabolic rate in critically ill patients (20).

LABETALOL

Labetalol is an adrenergic-receptor antagonist that has proven effective in acute management of severe hypertension. Parenteral administration of labetalol can serve as a safer alternative to nitroprusside (21–23).

ACTIONS

Labetalol is a nonselective β-receptor antagonist that also blocks α-receptor–mediated vasoconstriction. The overall effect is a dose-related decrease in systemic vascular resistance and blood pressure, without a reflex tachycardia or increase in cardiac output. Unlike nitroglycerin and nitroprusside, labetalol does not increase intracranial pressure (20).

Indications

Labetalol is indicated for the acute management of severe hypertension associated with a normal or adequate cardiac output. It may be particularly effective in hypertension caused by excess circulating catecholamines, such as the hypertension that occurs in the early postoperative period (23). Because the antihypertensive actions of labetalol are not accompanied by an increase in cardiac output, the drug is particularly useful in the management of aortic dissection (22).

DRUG ADMINISTRATION

Labetalol is available in an aqueous solution (5 mg/mL) that can be given intravenously as a bolus injection or by continuous infusion.

Bolus Therapy

Patients should be placed in the supine position for bolus injections of labetalol to limit the risk of orthostatic hypotension. The initial dose is 20 mg, and repeat doses of 40 mg can be given at 10-minute intervals until the desired antihypertensive effect is achieved. Although the manufacturer recommends a maximum cumulative dose of 300 mg, larger cumulative doses of labetalol have been used without ill effects (23).

Continuous Infusion Therapy

Continuous infusions of labetalol should be preceded by a bolus dose of 20 mg, because the serum half-life of labetalol, which is 6 to 8 hours, indicates that 30 to 40 hours (5 half-lives) may be required to reach steady-state serum drug levels after the start of continuous infusion therapy.

To prepare the infusion solution, 200 mg (40 mL) labetalol is added to 160 mL of diluent for a final drug concentration of 1 mg/mL. The recommended infusion rate is 2 mL/min, which corresponds to a dose rate of 2 mg/min.

ADVERSE EFFECTS

The most notable complications of intravenous labetalol include orthostatic hypotension (αblockade), myocardial depression (β-1 blockade), and bronchospasm (β-2 blockade). Orthostasis should not be a problem in the ICU, because patients are rarely ambulatory or in the upright position. The drug should be avoided in patients with heart failure or asthma.

NITROGLYCERIN

Nitroglycerin is a peculiar chemical because it is both an explosive powder and an effective antianginal agent. It is an organic nitrate (glyceryl trinitrate) that relaxes vascular smooth muscle and produces a generalized vasodilation. This action is mediated by nitric oxide, as shown in Figure 18.2 (24–26).

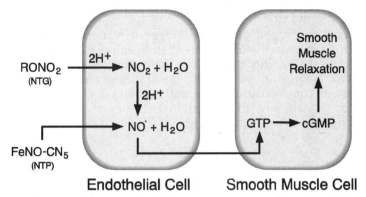

Figure 18.2. The biochemical mechanism for the vasodilator actions of nitroglycerin (NTG) and nitroprusside (NTP). Chemical symbols: nitroprusside (Fe-NO-CN$_5$), organic nitrate (RONO$_2$), nitrite (NO$_2$), nitric oxide (NO), guanosine triphosphate (GTP), cyclic guanosine monophosphate (cGMP).

NITRIC OXIDE

Nitroglycerin binds to the surface of endothelial cells and undergoes two chemical reductions to form nitric oxide (NO). The nitric oxide then moves out of the endothelial cell and into an adjacent smooth muscle cell, where it promotes the formation of cyclic guanosine monophosphate (cGMP), which then promotes muscle relaxation. Vasodilation is a prominent action of nitric oxide, which was known as endothelium-derived relaxing factor before its chemical identification (25,26).

ACTIONS

Nitroglycerin has a dose-dependent vasodilator effect in arteries and veins and is active in the systemic and pulmonary circulations (27). When the drug is given by continuous infusion, venous dilator effects are prominent at low dose rates (< 40 µg/min) and arterial dilator effects predominate at high dose rates (> 200 µg/min). As low-dose infusions are titrated upward, the earliest response is a decrease in cardiac filling pressures (i.e., central venous pressure and wedge pressure) with little or no change in cardiac output. As the dose rate is increased further, the cardiac output begins to rise as a result of progressive arterial vasodilation. Further increases in the dose rate will eventually produce a drop in blood pressure. The hemodynamic responses to intravenous nitroglycerin have a rapid onset and short duration, which permits rapid dose titration.

Antiplatelet Effects

Nitrates can inhibit platelet aggregation via the mechanism proposed for the vasodilator actions (26). Because platelet thrombi are believed to play an important role in the pathogenesis of acute myocardial infarction, the antiplatelet actions of nitroglycerin have been proposed as the mechanism for the antianginal effects of the drug (26). This may explain why the antianginal efficacy of nitroglycerin is not shared by other vasodilator agents.

Indications

Intravenous nitroglycerin can be used to decrease left-ventricular filling pressures (low dose), augment cardiac output (intermediate dose), or lower blood pressure (high dose). It is also useful in relieving anginal chest pain (see Chapter 19).

DRUG ADMINISTRATION

A nitroglycerin dose chart is shown in Table 18.6. The infusion rates in this chart are based on a drug concentration of 400 μg/mL in the infusion solution.

Sorption

Nitroglycerin binds to soft plastics such as polyvinylchloride (PVC), which is a common constituent in plastic bags and infusion tubing. As much as 80% of the drug can be lost by sorption. Glass and hard plastics do not adsorb nitroglycerin, so the problem of adsorption can be eliminated by using glass bottles and stiff polyethylene tubing.

TABLE 18.6. NITROGLYCERIN DOSAGE CHART	
Infusate: 100 mg nitroglycerin in 250 mL diluent (400 μg/mL). *Do not* use PVC infusion system.	
Dose: Start at 5 μg/min. Increase dose rate 5 μg/min every 5 min to desired effect.	
μg/min	microcrops/min
5	1
10	2
25	4
50	8
75	11
100	15
150	23
200	30
250	38
300	45
350	53
400	60

Drug manufacturers often provide specialized infusion sets to deliver nitroglycerin. (For a comprehensive description of nitroglycerin adsorption, see the Handbook on Injectable Drugs, pp 777–781.)

Nitroglycerin infusions should begin at a rate of 5 μg/min. The dose rate is then increased in 5-μg/min increments every 5 minutes until the desired effect is achieved. Although effective dose rates vary, the dose requirement should not exceed 400 μg/min in most patients. High dose requirements (e.g., > 350 μg/min) are often the result of drug loss via adsorption, or nitrate tolerance (see below).

ADVERSE EFFECTS

Nitroglycerin can produce three types of adverse reactions. One is flow related, another is related to oxidant stress, and the final one is related to the way the drug is administered.

Flow-Related Effects

Excessive flow in the cerebral and pulmonary circulations can create complications. Nitroglycerin seems adept at increasing cerebral blood flow (headache is a common complaint), and this can increase intracranial pressure and produce symptomatic intracranial hypertension (28). Because of this effect, nitroglycerin is avoided in patients with increased intracranial pressure. Increases in pulmonary blood flow can become a problem when the augmented flow occurs in areas of the lung that are poorly ventilated. This increases shunt fraction and can lead to hypoxemia. This effect can be prominent in the acute respiratory distress syndrome (29), where much of the lung is poorly ventilated.

Methemoglobinemia

Nitroglycerin metabolism produces inorganic nitrites (see Fig. 18.2), and accumulation of nitrites can result in the oxidation of heme-bound iron in hemoglobin, as shown below.

$$Hb\text{-}Fe(II) + NO_2 + H^+ \rightarrow Hb\text{-}Fe(III) + HONO \qquad (18.1)$$

The oxidation of iron from the Fe(II) to Fe(III) state creates methemoglobin (metHb). Oxidized iron does not carry oxygen effectively, and thus metHb accumulation can impair tissue oxygenation. Clinically significant methemoglobinemia is not a common complication of nitroglycerin therapy and usually occurs only at very high dose rates (28). MetHb accumulation has few specific manifestations other than the characteristic brown discoloration of blood (due to the brown color of metHb). MetHb can be detected by light reflection (oximetry), a technique described in Chapter 22. Pulse oximeters do not reliably detect metHb (30), and the measurement should be performed by more sophisticated oximeters (called co-oximeters) in the clinical laboratory.

MetHb levels above 3% (fraction of total hemoglobin) are abnormal. Levels above 40% can produce tissue ischemia, and levels above 70% are lethal (28). If there is no evidence of tissue hypoxia, discontinuing nitroglycerin is all that is required. If tissue oxygenation is impaired (e.g., lactic acidosis), metHb can be chemically converted back to normal hemoglobin with methylene blue (a reducing agent), 2 mg/kg IV over 10 minutes.

Solvent Toxicity

Nitroglycerin does not readily dissolve in aqueous solutions, and nonpolar solvents such as ethanol and propylene glycol are required to keep the drug in solution. These solvents can accumulate during continuous infusion.

Ethanol intoxication has been reported in association with nitroglycerin infusions (31). Manifestations include a change in mental status and garbled speech. Hypotension can also occur. A blood ethanol level will confirm the diagnosis. *Propylene glycol toxicity* has also been reported (32), and because some commercial nitroglycerin preparations contain 30 to 50% propylene glycol (28), clinical toxicity may be more common than suspected. Toxic manifestations include altered mental status that can progress to coma, metabolic acidosis, and hemolysis. The propylene glycol level in blood confirms the diagnosis.

In patients who develop a change in mental status during prolonged or high-dose nitroglycerin infusions, the serum *osmolal gap* (i.e., the difference between measured and calculated serum osmolality) might be a valuable screening test for possible solvent toxicity. The osmolal gap should be elevated (> 10 mOsm/kg) by the presence of either solvent in the bloodstream. An elevated gap would then prompt more specific assays to identify the toxin.

NITRATE TOLERANCE

Tolerance to the vasodilator and antiplatelet actions of nitroglycerin is more common than suspected and can appear after only 24 hours of continuous drug administration (27). No single mechanism seems to explain this phenomenon. One possible cause is the depletion of reducing agents in the vascular endothelium, which impairs the conversion of nitroglycerin to nitric oxide. This mechanism is supported by the association of nitrate tolerance with decreased nitric oxide production (33). However, the administration of reducing agents (e.g., N-acetylcysteine) does not consistently restore responsiveness in nitrate tolerance. At present, the most effective method for restoring nitroglycerin responsiveness is to discontinue drug administration for at least 6 to 8 hours each day (27).

Sodium Nitroprusside

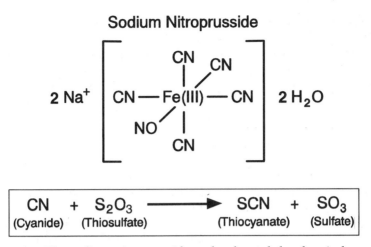

$$2\,Na^+ \quad \left[\begin{array}{c} CN \\ | \\ CN - Fe(III) - CN \\ NO \quad | \\ CN \end{array}\right] \quad 2\,H_2O$$

CN	+	S_2O_3	$\longrightarrow$	SCN	+	SO_3
(Cyanide)		(Thiosulfate)		(Thiocyanate)		(Sulfate)

Figure 18.3. The sodium nitroprusside molecule, and the chemical reaction used to remove free cyanide from the bloodstream.

NITROPRUSSIDE

Nitroprusside is a vasodilator agent that shares many features with nitroglycerin. One of these is the participation of nitric oxide in the vasodilator actions of the drug. The nitroprusside molecule is shown in Figure 18.3. It contains one nitrosyl group (NO), and this is released in the bloodstream as nitric oxide, which then can move into the vessel wall and move along the pathway shown in Table 18.2. As a result of their shared mechanisms of action, nitroprusside and nitroglycerin are classified as *nitrovasodilators* (26).

There is one feature that distinguishes nitroprusside from nitroglycerin: Nitroprusside is a dangerous drug and may be responsible for over 1000 deaths yearly (34). Because the major actions of nitroprusside may be its toxic effects, the adverse effects will be presented first. The description of nitroprusside toxicity in this chapter is brief; Chapter 53 covers this topic in detail.

TOXICOLOGY

The toxic nature of nitroprusside is due to its molecular composition, which is shown in Figure 18.3. The nitroprusside molecule contains five cyanide ions, and almost half of the molecular weight of the parent molecule is cyanide. When nitroprusside disrupts to release nitric oxide and exert its actions, the cyanide is released into the bloodstream. The chemical reaction shown in Figure 18.3 describes how the free cyanide is removed. Sulfur from a donor source combines with the free cyanide and forms thiocyanate (SCN), which is cleared by the kidneys. The sulfur donor for this reaction is thiosulfate.

Cyanide

The capacity of the human body to clear cyanide was grossly overestimated when nitroprusside was first introduced (28). The limiting factor is thiosulfate, which is stored in limited quantities and is easily depleted. The result is early and frequent accumulation of cyanide during nitroprusside infusions. The consequences of this cyanide accumulation is described in Chapter 53.

Thiocyanate

The clearance of thiocyanate by the kidneys is impaired when renal function or renal blood flow is compromised. The accumulation of thiocyanate produces a toxic syndrome that is distinct from cyanide intoxication. Thus, nitroprusside toxicity can be expressed as either cyanide or thiocyanate intoxication. Both of these toxic syndromes are described in Chapter 53.

ACTIONS

Nitroprusside has been favored because the vascular responses are prompt and short lived and this allows for rapid dose titration. Vasodilator effects are often evident at low dose rates (0.5 μg/kg/min), and the sequence of hemodynamic responses is the same as described for nitroglycerin. Blood pressure does not usually decline at dose rates below 1 μg/kg/min. An immediate drop in blood pressure at low dose rates can be a sign of hypovolemia.

Indications

Because of the toxic potential of the drug, nitroprusside should be used only when there is no alternative available. The drug seems best suited for the management of severe hypertension combined with a low cardiac output.

DRUG ADMINISTRATION

A dose chart for nitroprusside is shown in Table 18.7. Note the recommendation to **add thiosulfate to the nitroprusside infusate.** This provides the sulfur needed to detoxify cyanide and should be a mandatory practice. A proportional dose of 500 mg thiosulfate per 50 mg nitroprusside should be used (34). Thiosulfate is provided as sodium thiosulfate (290 mg sodium per gram thiosulfate) and is commercially available as a 10% solution (5 mL = 500 mg thiosulfate).

The FDA recommends starting nitroprusside at a low dose rate (0.2 μg/kg/min) and titrating the dose upward in 5-minute increments (35). The maximum allowable dose rate is 10 μg/kg/min for no longer than 10 minutes.

TABLE 18.7. NITROPRUSSIDE DOSAGE CHART								
Infusate:	50 mg nitroprusside in 100 mL diluent (500 µg/mL)							
	Add 500 mg Thiosulfate							
Initial dose:	0.2 µg/kg/min							
Usual dose:	0.5–2 µg/kg/min (heart failure)							
	2–5 µg/kg/min (hypertension)							
	Weight (kg)							
	40	**50**	**60**	**70**	**80**	**90**	**100**	
Dose (µg/kg/min)	**microdrops/min (mL/hr)**							
0.2	1	1	1	2	2	2	2	
0.5	2	3	4	4	5	5	6	
1	5	6	7	8	10	11	12	
2	10	12	14	17	19	22	24	
3	14	18	22	25	29	32	36	
5	24	30	36	42	48	54	60	

ADVERSE EFFECTS

In addition to cyanide and thiocyanate intoxication, nitroprusside has adverse hemodynamic effects that are identical to those described for nitroglycerin. Nitroprusside increases intracranial pressure, and thus it is not advised for patients with intracranial hypertension. Because hypertensive encephalopathy is associated with a raised intracranial pressure, nitroprusside seems ill-advised for managing hypertensive encephalopathy.

NOREPINEPHRINE

Norepinephrine is an α-receptor agonist that promotes widespread vasoconstriction. As a result of early reports of renal failure from norepinephrine, combined with a general decrease in enthusiasm for vasoconstrictor drugs, norepinephrine is no longer considered a first-line drug for the management of circulatory shock. In cases of hypotension refractory to dopamine, it can be added as a second agent.

There is some renewed interest in norepinephrine because of reports showing that there is less vasoconstriction and even improved organ perfusion in response to norepinephrine in patients with septic shock (36,37). However, it seems foolish to expect that a switch to norepinephrine will improve the clinical outcome in septic shock.

ACTIONS

Norepinephrine produces a dose-dependent increase in systemic vascular resistance. Although the drug can stimulate cardiac β-receptors over a wide range, the cardiac output is increased only at low doses. Over the remainder of the therapeutic dose range, the inotropic response to norepinephrine is overshadowed by the vasoconstrictor response. At high dose rates, the cardiac output decreases in response to the vasoconstriction and increased afterload.

Indications

In cases of septic shock where the desired vasoconstriction is not achieved by a dopamine infusion norepinephrine can be added as a second drug (36).

DRUG ADMINISTRATION

One milligram of norepinephrine is added to a diluent volume of 250 mL (4 μg/mL). The infusion should be begun at 1 μg/min (15 microdrops/min) and titrated to the desired effect. The usual dose rate is 2 to 4 μg/min, with a range of 1 to 12 μg/min. The effective dose of norepinephrine can vary widely, and in clinical reports involving patients with septic shock, the effective norepinephrine dose has varied from 0.7 to 210 μg/min (36).

ADVERSE EFFECTS

The administration of any vasoconstrictor agent carries a risk of hypoperfusion and ischemia involving any tissue bed or vital organ. For any condition that requires vasoconstrictor drugs to maintain a blood pressure, it may be difficult to distinguish adverse drug effects and adverse disease effects. Furthermore, if an adverse drug effect is identified or suspected, there may be little or no room for therapeutic manipulations.

REFERENCES

GENERAL TEXTS

I. Trissel LA (ed). Handbook on injectable drugs. 8th ed. Bethesda: American Society of Hospital Pharmacists, 1994.
II. Kahn MG. Cardiac drug therapy. 4th ed. Philadelphia: W.B. Saunders, Co., 1995.

REVIEWS

1. Zaloga GP, Prielipp RC, Butterworth JF, Royster RL. Pharmacologic cardiovascular support. Crit Care Clin 1993;9:335–362 (192 references).
2. Trujillo MH, Arai K, Bellorin-Font E. Practical guide for drug administration by intravenous infusion in intensive care units. Crit Care Med 1994;22:1049–1063 (80 references).
3. Zaritsky AL. Catecholamines, inotropic medications, and vasopressor agents. In Chenow B, (ed). The pharmacologic approach to the critically ill patient. 3rd ed., Baltimore: Williams & Wilkins, 1994 (224 references).

AMRINONE

4. DiBianco B. Acute positive inotropic intervention: the phosphodiesterase inhibitors. Am Heart J 1991;121:1871–1875.
5. Levy JH, Bailey JM. Amrinone: Its effect on vascular resistance and capacitance in human subjects. Chest 1994;105:62–64.
6. Marcus RH, Raw K, Patel J, et al. Comparison of intravenous amrinone and dobutamine in congestive heart failure due to idiopathic dilated cardiomyopathy. Am J Cardiol 1990;66:1107–1112.
7. Sundram P, Reddy HK, McElroy PA, et al. Myocardial energetics and efficiency in patients with idiopathic cardiomyopathy: Response to dobutamine and amrinone. Am J Cardiol 1990;119:891–898.
8. Butterworth JF, Royster RL, Prielipp RC, et al. Amrinone in cardiac surgical patients with left-ventricular dysfunction. Chest 1993;104:1660–1667.
9. Notterman DA. Inotropic agents. In Blumer JL, Bond R, (eds). Toxic effects of drugs used in the ICU. Crit Care Clin 1991;7:583–614.
10. Scalea TM, Donovan R. Amrinone as an inotrope in managing hypermetabolic surgical stress. J Trauma 1992;32:372–379.

DOBUTAMINE

11. Vincent J-L. Dobutamine in the intensive care setting. In Chatterjee K (ed). Dobutamine. A ten year review. New York: NCM Publishers, 1989:109–121.
12. Klem C, Dasta JF, Reilley TE, Flancbaum LJ. Variability in dobutamine pharmacokinetics in unstable critically ill surgical patients. Crit Care Med 1994; 22:1926–1932.
13. Rich MW, Imburgia M. Inotropic response to dobutamine in elderly patients with decompensated congestive heart failure. Am J Cardiol 1990;65:519–521.
14. Hayes MA, Yau EHS, Timmins AC, et al. Response of critically ill patients to treatment aimed at achieving supranormal oxygen delivery and consumption. Relationship to outcome. Chest 1993;103:886–895.

DOPAMINE

15. Duke GJ, Briedis JH, Weaver RA. Renal support in critically ill patients: Low-dose dopamine or low-dose dobutamine? Crit Care Med 1994;22:1919–1925.
16. Oung CM, English M, Chiu RCJ, Hinchey J. Effects of hypothermia on hemodynamic responses to dopamine and dobutamine. J Trauma 1992;33:671–678.

EPINEPHRINE

17. Hollingsworth HM, Giansiracusa DF, Upchurch KS. Anaphylaxis. J Intensive Care Med 1991;6:55–70.
18. Chiolero R, Flatt J-P, Revelly J-P, Jequier E. Effects of catecholamines on oxygen consumption and oxygen delivery in critically ill patients. Chest 1991;100: 1676–1684.
19. Ronco JJ, Fenwick JC, Wiggs BR, et al. Oxygen consumption is independent of increases in oxygen delivery by dobutamine in septic patients who have normal or increased plasma lactate. Am Rev Respir Dis 1993;147:25–31.

LABETALOL

20. Kaplan NM. Management of hypertensive emergencies. Lancet 1994;344: 1335–1338.
21. DeVault GA Jr. Therapy in hypertensive emergencies: A disease-specific approach. J Crit Illness 1990;6:477–484.

22. Cosentino F, Vidt DG, Orlowski JP, et al. The safety of cumulative doses of labetalol in perioperative hypertension. Clev Clin J Med 1989;56:371–376.

NITROGLYCERIN

23. Anggard E. Nitric oxide: mediator, murderer, and medicine. Lancet 1994;343: 1199–1206.
24. Anderson TJ, Meredith IT, Ganz P, et al. Nitric oxide and nitrovasodilators: similarities, differences and potential interactions. J Am Coll Cardiol 1994;24: 555–566.
25. Stamler JS, Loscalzo J. The antiplatelet effects of organic nitrates and related nitroso compounds in vitro and in vivo and their relevance to cardiovascular disorders. J Am Coll Cardiol 1991;18:1529–1536.
26. Elkayam U. Nitrates in heart failure. Cardiol Clin 1994;12:73–85.
27. Radermacher P, Santak B, Becker H, Falke KJ. Prostaglandin F_1 and nitroglycerin reduce pulmonary capillary pressure but worsen ventilation–perfusion distribution in patients with adult respiratory distress syndrome. Anesthesiology 1989;70:601–606.
28. Curry SC, Arnold-Cappell P. Nitroprusside, nitroglycerin, and angiotensin-converting enzyme inhibitors. In: Blumer JL, Bond GR, (eds). Toxic effects of drugs used in the ICU. Crit Care Clin 1991;7:555–582.
29. Barker SJ, Kemper KK, Hyatt J. Effects of methemoglobinemia on pulse oximetry and mixed venous oximetry. Anesthesiology 1989;70:112–117.
30. Korn SH, Comer JB. Intravenous nitroglycerin and ethanol intoxication. Ann Intern Med 1985;102:274.
31. Demey HE, Daelemans RA, Verpooten GA, et al. Propylene glycol-induced side effects during intravenous nitroglycerin therapy. Intensive Care Med 1988;14:221–226.
32. Husain M, Adrie C, Ichinose F, et al. Exhaled nitric oxide as a marker for organic nitrate tolerance. Circulation 1994;89:2498–2502.

NITROPRUSSIDE

32. Fenichel RR. A quick (high pressure) tour of nitroprusside (NTP). Washington, DC: Food and Drug Administration Center for Drug Evaluation and Research. DHHS, 1990 (April).
33. Robin ED, McCauley R. Nitroprusside-related cyanide poisoning. Time (long past due) for urgent, effective interventions. Chest 1992;102:1842–1845.
34. Hall VA, Guest JM. Sodium nitroprusside-induced cyanide intoxication and prevention with sodium thiosulfate prophylaxis. Am J Crit Care 1992;2:19–27.

NOREPINEPHRINE

36. Dasta JF. Norepinephrine in septic shock: Renewed interest in an old drug. DICP, Ann Pharmacother 1990;24:153–156.
37. Desairs P, Pinaud M, Bugnon D, Tasseau F. Norepinephrine therapy has no deleterious renal effects in human septic shock. Crit Care Med 1989;17: 426–429.

section V
MYOCARDIAL INJURY

We think so because all other people think so;
or because we think we in fact do think so;
or because we were told to think so,
and think we must think so . . .

Rudyard Kipling

chapter

19

EARLY MANAGEMENT OF ACUTE MYOCARDIAL INFARCTION

The management strategies for acute myocardial infarction (MI) shifted focus in the early 1980s, following the discovery that acute (transmural) MI is the direct result of an occlusive thrombosis. The original focus of early management, which included preventing malignant arrhythmias (with lidocaine) and maintaining a satisfactory balance between myocardial oxygen supply and oxygen consumption, was subsequently shifted to the current emphasis on establishing and maintaining reperfusion in the infarct-related artery (1,2). The elements of the reperfusion strategy for acute MI are presented in this chapter. When executed appropriately and promptly, this approach can result in fewer deaths in patients with acute MI.

BACKGROUND

CORONARY THROMBOSIS

A causal relationship between coronary artery thrombosis and acute MI was suggested in the original description of the acute MI syndrome in 1912. However, autopsy studies in the first half of the century showed only sporadic evidence of thrombosis (presumably missing the ones that lysed spontaneously). The first definitive report was an angiographic study published in 1980, which showed that 87% of patients with Q-wave infarctions had complete occlusion of the infarct-related arteries by an obstructing thrombus when studied in the first 4 hours after the onset of symptoms (4). The incidence of complete obstruction was much lower (24%) in patients with non–Q-wave infarctions (4). These results were confirmed in several studies over the next 5 years.

Morphologic studies have identified ruptured atherosclerotic plaques as the nidus for coronary thrombosis (5). The interior of the

301

plaque first undergoes liquefaction necrosis, and the process erodes outward and ruptures into the bloodstream. When blood comes in contact with the thrombogenic lipids, clot formation begins. The trigger for plaque disruption is not known, and the process is independent of the size or age of the plaque (3). The degree of thrombotic obstruction determines the clinical syndrome. Persistent obstruction lasting more than 24 hours results in Q-wave (transmural) infarctions, whereas transient obstruction for 1 to 2 hours results in non–Q-wave (subendocardial) infarctions. Free-floating thrombi attached by a stalk may be the source of unstable angina.

THROMBOLYTIC THERAPY

The evaluation of drugs that stimulate fibrinolysis began immediately after the 1980 discovery of occlusive thrombosis in Q-wave infarctions. Intracoronary installation of fibrinolytic agents resulted in effective clot lysis in 80% of obstructed arteries (6), and one agent (streptokinase) proved equally effective when given intravenously. In 1986, the first clinical trial of intravenous streptokinase in acute MI was completed. Nicknamed GISSI, the study included almost 12,000 subjects, and the results showed fewer deaths in the patients who received thrombolytic therapy (7).

Survival Benefit

The survival benefit of thrombolytic therapy is demonstrated in Table 19.1. Included in this table are the pooled results of nine clinical trials comparing thrombolytic therapy (with different lytic agents) to placebo in patients with acute MI (8).

Lytic therapy given within 12 hours after the onset of chest pain is included in this analysis, and only Q-wave infarctions (identified by ST elevation on the ECG) are represented. Note that the total number of patients studied is close to 60,000. The mortality (1 month after randomization) is lower in the patients given lytic therapy (9.6%) than

TABLE 19.1. SURVIVAL BENEFIT OF LYTIC THERAPY IN NINE CLINICAL TRIALS		
	Placebo	Lytic Therapy
Subjects	29,285	29,315
Deaths	3,357	2,820
Mortality rate	11.5%	9.6%
		Treatment Effect
Absolute reduction in mortality		1.9%
Proportional reduction in mortality		18%
Benefit		1.8% or 18 per 1000
Data from Fibrinolytic Therapy Trialists Collaborative Group (8).		

in the patients given placebo (11.5%). The absolute decrease in mortality rate is 1.9%, with a proportional decrease in mortality of 18% (i.e., 18% of 11.7%). Because the proportional change is a percentage of a percent, the 18% proportional reduction in mortality is equivalent to 1.8% fewer deaths. This can be expressed as a survival benefit of 1.8 lives saved per 100 patients treated (or 18 per 1000). Thus, **for every 1000 patients who received thrombolytic therapy, 18 patients survived because of the therapy.**

Timing

If the average survival benefit in Table 19.1 is analyzed according to the time when thrombolytic therapy was initiated, the result is shown in Figure 19.1. This graph shows the survival benefit of thrombolytic therapy (in lives saved per 1000) in relation to the time elapsed from the onset of chest pain to the initiation of therapy (7). The earlier the thrombolytic therapy is initiated, the greater the survival benefit. **After 12 hours following the onset of chest pain, the survival benefit of thrombolytic therapy is lost.** Over the 12-hour effective treatment period, the decline in survival benefit averages 1.6 lives lost per 1000 patients per hour of delay. In the first 6 hours, the hourly decline in survival (2.6 per 1000) is greater than in the final 6 hours (0.6 per 1000), so treatment delays are four times more costly in the first 6 hours than in the second 6 hours of the effective treatment period.

The time dependence shown in Figure 19.1 illustrates one of the

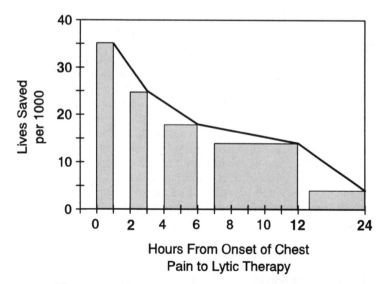

Figure 19.1. The survival benefit (in lives saved per 1000 patients treated) of thrombolytic therapy in relation to the time after the onset of chest pain that therapy is initiated. The height of each column represents the average survival benefit reported over the time period indicated on the horizontal axis. (Data from Fibrinolytic Therapy Trialists Collaborative Group [7].)

most important features of thrombolytic therapy: Time lost is lives lost. This sets the stage for the description that follows of the **initial evaluation** of patients with suspected acute MI where the **goal is to identify candidates for thrombolytic therapy and initiate therapy as quickly as possible.**

THE INITIAL ENCOUNTER

In the initial encounter with patients suspected of having an acute MI, there are four principal tasks:

Relieve the chest pain.
Identify and treat life-threatening conditions.
Initiate thrombolytic therapy in appropriate candidates.
Complete the first three tasks as quickly as possible.

These individual tasks are performed simultaneously, and in no particular order.

RELIEVE CHEST PAIN

If not used before presentation, sublingual nitroglycerin (2 tablets, 3 minutes apart) can be used as an initial attempt to relieve the chest pain. This is usually not successful in chest pain from acute MI (1,2). Persistent chest pain should be treated with morphine instead of intravenous nitroglycerin. This latter intervention is best reserved for patients with hypertension or left-heart failure (1,2). Aggressive use of nitroglycerin via either route is not recommended in right-ventricular infarction because of the risk of hypotension (2).

Morphine is the drug of choice for relieving the chest discomfort in acute MI (1,2). The usual dose is 4 mg by slow intravenous push (e.g., 1 mg/minute), which can be repeated every 5 minutes if necessary. Morphine administration may be followed by a decrease in blood pressure. This is usually the result of a decrease in sympathetic nervous system activity and is not a pathologic process. If the systolic pressure falls to a level of concern (below 100 mm Hg), volume infusion is usually effective in raising the pressure. If hypotension persists and is associated with bradycardia, atropine (0.5 to 1 mg intravenously) may be required (2). *Do not* use pressor agents to reverse the decrease in blood pressure induced by morphine (2).

LIFE-THREATENING CONDITIONS

Masquerading Illness

Do not forget to consider other serious conditions that can produce substernal chest pain, such as **acute aortic dissection,** acute pulmonary embolus, pericarditis, and esophageal rupture. Aortic dissection is described at the end of this chapter.

Complications

About one-quarter of patients with acute MI have evidence of heart failure on initial presentation, and another 3 to 4% are in cardiogenic shock (6). **Thrombolytic therapy has no documented benefit in acute MI accompanied by heart failure or cardiogenic shock** (10), so the presence of either complication excludes a patient from thrombolytic therapy. The management of acute MI accompanied by cardiac pump failure is discussed later in this chapter.

SELECTION CRITERIA FOR LYTIC THERAPY

Patients who are candidates for thrombolytic therapy must be identified as soon as possible after presentation using the eligibility criteria shown in Table 19.2. Unfortunately, only 20% of patients with acute MI receive thrombolytic therapy. An additional 15% are eligible but never receive the therapy.

Indications

Patients are candidates for lytic therapy if they have chest pain for at least 30 minutes but less than 12 hours (as in Figure 19.1) and have a 12-lead ECG that shows ST elevation of 0.1 mm or more in two contiguous leads, or a new left bundle branch block. As mentioned

TABLE 19.2. SELECTION CRITERIA FOR THROMBOLYTIC THERAPY
Indications
• Chest pain for >30 min and <12 hr
• No congestive heart failure or hypotension
• ST elevation (0.1 mm) in 2 contiguous leads, or new left bundle branch block

Absolute Contraindications*	
Acute:	Active internal bleeding
	Blood pressure ≥200/120 mm Hg
	Suspected aortic dissection
Subacute or chronic:	Arteriovenous malformation
	Tumor involving spinal cord or cranial structures
	Hemorrhagic retinopathy
	Pregnancy
In past 2 mo:	Trauma or surgery in the past 2 wk with a risk of bleeding into a closed space
	Spinal or intracranial procedure in the past 8 wk
	Recent head trauma
	Prolonged or traumatic cardiopulmonary resuscitation
Any time in past:	Hemorrhagic stroke
	Allergic reaction to streptokinase

* From National Heart Attack Alert Program Coordinating Committee, 60 Minutes to Treatment Working Group. Ann Emerg Med 1994;23:311–329.

earlier, patients with heart failure or cardiogenic shock are not eligible for thrombolytic therapy.

Contraindications

The absolute contraindications for thrombolytic therapy are listed in Table 19.2. Relative contraindications are not included because the survival benefit from thrombolytic therapy should justify the risks associated with relative contraindications (3). Note that **neither advanced age nor the presence of indwelling vascular catheters** (including central venous pressure and pulmonary artery catheters) **are reasons to exclude a patient from thrombolytic therapy.** Although bleeding complications are more common in the elderly, the survival benefit of thrombolytic therapy is also greater in the elderly (3). Therefore, the enhanced survival cancels the negative effect of enhanced bleeding in the elderly population.

Time to Therapy

Any patient who has all the indications for thrombolytic therapy, and no contraindications, should receive lytic therapy as soon as possible. According to the American Heart Association, **the time from presentation to initiation of thrombolytic therapy should not exceed 1 hour** (2). Longer delays in candidates for thrombolytic therapy will result in unnecessary deaths.

THROMBOLYTIC THERAPY

The thrombolytic agents and dosing regimens for patients with suspected acute MI are included in Table 19.3. In terms of overall clinical

TABLE 19.3. THROMBOLYTIC THERAPY FOR SUSPECTED ACUTE MI			
	Streptokinase	Tissue Plasminogen Activator (TPA)	Anistreplase
Preparation	1.5 million U in 50 mL saline	100 mg in 100 mL diluent (1 mg/mL) *Accelerated Regimen*	Add 5 mL saline to 30 U anistreplase
Dosage	1.5 million U IV over 1 hr	a. 15-mg bolus b. 0.75 mg/kg (to 50 mg) over 30 min c. 0.5 mg/kg (to 35 mg) over 1 hr	30 U IV over 2–5 min
Adverse effects	Hypotension (7%) Fever (25%) Rash, wheezing (5%)	Hypotension (4%)	Same as streptokinase
Cost*	$537.34	$2750.00	$2367.72

* Average wholesale prices in the *1996 Redbook*. Montvale NJ: Medical Economics Co., 1996.

performance, no one thrombolytic agent has proven consistently superior to the others. Therefore, **the important issue in thrombolytic therapy is not which agent to use, but how quickly to use it.**

MECHANISM OF ACTION

All thrombolytic agents promote fibrinolysis by converting plasminogen to plasmin, which breaks fibrin strands into smaller subunits. **Streptokinase** (SK) is a bacterial protein (from streptococci) that acts on plasminogen in the circulating blood and produces a disseminated or systemic lytic state. **Tissue plasminogen activator** (TPA) is the molecular clone of an endogenous fibrinolytic substance with the same name. This agent binds to fibrin in blood clots and converts plasminogen to plasmin locally, in the vicinity of the thrombus. This produces a clot-specific activation of fibrinolysis, with less of a systemic lytic effect. **Anistreplase**, also known as anisolated plasminogen–streptokinase activator complex (APSAC), is a clot-specific version of streptokinase. However, in the dosages needed for clot lysis, this agent also produces a systemic lytic effect.

Lytic Effect

The most rapid lysis is produced by TPA (60 to 70% lysis at 90 minutes), and SK and APSAC are tied for second place (50% lysis at 90 minutes) (9). However, the final lytic effect is the same with all agents (80% lysis at 180 minutes).

BENEFITS AND RISKS

Survival Benefit

All thrombolytic agents improve survival when compared with placebo (Table 19.1). There are three clinical trials comparing survival with different lytic agents. Two trials (GISSI-2 and ISIS-3) show no difference in survival with any of the agents (11,12). The third trial (GUSTO) shows a 1% (absolute) reduction in mortality with TPA given in an accelerated regimen (the same regimen as in Table 19.3) compared to SK (13). Although TPA is being marketed as the best lytic agent based on this 1% difference, it is difficult to take the sum of all megatrials of lytic agents over the last 10 years and identify the superior agent based on a 1% margin in one trial.

Complications

The most feared complication of lytic therapy is intracerebral hemorrhage, which is reported in 0.5 to 1% of cases (8,9). This complication occurs more often with TPA than with the other agents, as documented in three studies (GISSI-2, ISIS-3, and GUSTO-1) (9). Extracranial bleeding that requires blood transfusions occurs in 5 to 15% of patients, regardless of the agent used (9). The risk of bleeding is not related to the extent (systemic versus clot-specific) of the fibrinolysis produced by each agent.

Complications other than bleeding are common with SK, which by virtue of being a bacterial product can act as an antigen (APSAC contains SK, and thus has similar antigenic actions). Common antigen-related reactions are fever (20 to 40%), allergic-type reactions (5%), and the production of neutralizing antibodies (14). The antibody response to SK can persist for up to 8 months (15), so SK should not be readministered for at least 6 months. The antibody response to streptococcal infections (e.g., pharyngitis) can also neutralize SK, so SK should not be used for 6 months after a documented streptococcal infection.

Hypotension of unclear etiology can occur with any of the thrombolytic agents but is more common with SK (14). The hypotension usually resolves when the infusion is stopped, although volume infusion is sometimes necessary. The infusion can be resumed, but the infusion rate should be reduced by 50%.

Cost

A cost comparison for each of the lytic agents is shown at the bottom of Table 19.3. Compared to SK, the additional cost to the patient is $1800 for APSAC and $2200 for TPA. Considering that no individual thrombolytic agent has proven consistently superior to the others, **streptokinase may be the preferred agent by virtue of its reduced cost.**

PREVENTING REOCCLUSION

Initial clot lysis is followed by reocclusion in 15 to 30% of infarct-related arteries. The rate of reocclusion is particularly high with TPA (30%) (8). Agents that inhibit thrombosis (aspirin and heparin) are often added to lytic therapy to help reduce the risk of reocclusion.

Aspirin is used to inhibit platelet aggregation. In one study, aspirin added to the survival benefit of thrombolytic therapy, and also showed a survival benefit independent of lytic therapy (16).

Dosage: 160 mg (chewable tablets) at the time of lytic therapy, then 160 to 325 mg daily.

Heparin is routinely added to lytic therapy with TPA because of the high reocclusion rate with TPA. This regimen should be started in the final hour of the TPA infusion.

Dosage: 5000 U as intravenous bolus, then 1000 U/hour. Check partial thromboplastin time (PTT) in 6 hours (target PTT is 60 to 85 seconds).

The heparin infusion is continued for 24 to 72 hours (1). Heparin does not add to the benefit of aspirin with the other two lytic agents (SK and APSAC), so heparin is not indicated when these lytic agents are used (17).

REPERFUSION INJURY

Clot lysis and reperfusion can itself be a source of injury. One manifestation of reperfusion injury is a form of diastolic dysfunction known as stunned myocardium (18). Oxidant injury has been implicated in this process, and peroxidation of membrane lipids (described in Chapter 3) may be involved. Damage to smooth muscle membranes would lead to calcium influx, and the resulting intracellular calcium accumulation could retard muscle relaxation and produce the myocardial stunning. Although antioxidants have not been effective in preventing reperfusion injury, magnesium may be protective.

THERAPEUTIC OPTIONS

The following therapy can be used with or without thrombolytic therapy. Each agent or class of agents included here has shown a survival benefit in clinical trials, or is recommended by the American Heart Association as a useful intervention (1,2).

β-BLOCKERS

When given within a few hours of onset of acute MI, β-blockers have been shown to reduce infarct size, decrease the incidence of arrhythmias, and improve survival (3,19–21). The combined trials of β-blocker therapy in acute MI (which include a total of 27,000 patients) show an average survival benefit of 13 per 1000 (3).

When to Use

β-Blockers should be used for all patients with acute MI who have no specific contraindication to their use. They are particularly useful for patients who develop a hyperdynamic state with tachycardia and hypertension (e.g., younger patients with anterior MI). **Contraindications** include heart rate below 50 beats/minute, AV block (first-, second-, or third-degree), systolic blood pressure below 100 mm Hg, severe (systolic) heart failure, and reactive airway disease.

Dosing Regimens

The drugs and dosing schedules in Table 19.4 have proven successful in clinical trials of β-blockers in acute MI (19–21). Optimal results are obtained when therapy begins within 4 hours after the onset of chest pain.

TABLE 19.4. β-BLOCKERS IN ACUTE MI	
Agent	**Dosage**
Atenolol	5 mg IV over 5 min × 2 doses.
	Wait 15 min, then
	50 mg p.o. every 12 hr × 2 days, then
	100 mg p.o. daily.
Metoprolol	5 mg IV over 2 min × 3 doses.
	Wait 15 min, then
	50 mg p.o. every 6 hr × 2 days, then
	100 mg p.o. BID.
Timolol	1 mg IV bolus and repeat in 10 min.
	Wait 10 min, then infuse at 0.6 mg/hr × 24 hr.
	Follow with 10 mg p.o. BID.
Dose regimens from References 19–21.	

ANTITHROMBOTIC AGENTS

Aspirin has been shown to improve survival in acute MI independent of thrombolytic therapy (16). Although the evidence of a survival benefit is from a single study, aspirin is universally recommended for patients with suspected acute MI. The dosage is similar to that described for thrombolytic therapy: 160 mg as early as possible after onset of chest pain, followed by 160 to 325 mg daily.

Heparin therapy has been (consistently) inconsistent in improving outcomes in acute MI. However, the American Heart Association continues to recommend full heparinization as a routine measure for all cases of acute transmural MI, presumably to decrease the risk of mural thrombosis (1,2). For dosing information on heparin, see the weight-based heparin dosing nomogram in Chapter 7 (Table 7.4).

NITROGLYCERIN

Intravenous nitroglycerin is effective in relieving anginal chest pain, but the benefits in acute MI have been variable. Clinical trials performed before 1990 (3000 patients) show improved survival, whereas trials performed after 1990 (79,000 patients) show no survival benefit (3).

When to Use

Intravenous nitroglycerin is not recommended for routine use because of the risk of hypotension and lack of survival benefit. It is best used to relieve chest pain or manage hypertension. **Nitroglycerin impairs the lytic actions of TPA** (22), so combined therapy should be avoided.

Dosing Regimen

Chapter 18 has a dose chart for intravenous nitroglycerin (Table 18.6). After 24 hours of continuous infusion, switch to a nitroglycerin patch that delivers 10 mg/day (23). The patch should be removed for 8 to 10 hours during each 24-hour period to prevent nitrate tolerance.

MAGNESIUM

Magnesium has several actions that should be salutary in acute MI: It dilates coronary arteries, inhibits platelet aggregation, suppresses arrhythmias, and can protect against reperfusion injury by blocking the intracellular accumulation of calcium (24,25). In addition, magnesium depletion is common in the setting of acute MI (24), probably as a result of diuretic therapy (which enhances renal magnesium excretion).

Despite its potential benefit, intravenous magnesium has produced conflicting results in clinical trials. In one trial where intravenous magnesium was started within 4 hours after onset of chest pain, there was a survival benefit of 23 per 1000 (26). However, in a larger trial where magnesium was started 8 to 12 hours after onset of chest pain, there was no survival benefit (3). Because lytic therapy was used in both trials, one suggestion is that the earlier use of magnesium was beneficial because it protected against reperfusion injury from the lytic therapy. For now, the discrepancy is not explained.

When to Use

Intravenous magnesium should be used in acute MI associated with hypokalemia, hypocalcemia, and arrhythmias, and in patients receiving daily diuretics without magnesium supplements. Because magnesium depletion is common in MI patients (even with normal serum magnesium levels), routine magnesium infusion seems warranted. **Contraindications** to intravenous magnesium include renal insufficiency, hypotension, severe heart failure, and atrioventricular block.

Dosing Regimen

The dose used in the clinical trials is 2 g $MgSO_4$ intravenously over 5 minutes, then 8 g intravenously by continuous infusion over 24 hours. This dose is designed to double the serum magnesium level. However, in the presence of normal renal function, the extra magnesium is cleared quickly and the hypermagnesemia is transient. A popular dosing regimen is 2 g $MgSO_4$ in 100 mL saline infused over 30 to 60 minutes, which is given routinely on admission to the ICU.

EARLY COMPLICATIONS

ARRHYTHMIAS

The American Heart Association no longer recommends routine prophylaxis for ventricular tachycardia or ventricular fibrillation, or treatment of asymptomatic "warning arrhythmias" (such as a run of six premature ventricular contractions) (1,2). Ventricular ectopic depolarizations are treated only if they are associated with heart failure or hypotension. The recognition and management of arrhythmias are covered in Chapter 20.

PUMP FAILURE

Survival in acute MI declines as ventricular function declines. This is illustrated in the first lytic therapy trial, where mortality rates were 7% for uncomplicated MI, 16% for heart failure, 39% for pulmonary edema, and 70% for cardiogenic shock (6). The management of progressive heart failure and cardiogenic shock in acute MI involves the same measures described in Chapter 16. Two features of the management in acute MI deserve mention.

Angioplasty

Patients with pump failure and ECG evidence of Q-wave infarction (ST elevations) are candidates for angioplasty. A review of 14 reports of angioplasty in cardiogenic shock shows a decrease in mortality from 80 to 44% (10). Angioplasty is therefore appealing in this setting, but unfortunately is not available on an emergency basis in many hospitals.

Limiting Cardiac Work

When cardiac pump failure is accompanied by ischemia, the goal of cardiac support is to augment cardiac output without increasing myocardial oxygen consumption. The influence of cardiac support interventions on myocardial oxygen consumption (Vo_2) can be estimated using the four determinants of myocardial work: preload, contractility, afterload, and heart rate (these four variables also determine myocardial Vo_2). Table 19.5 shows the effects of different cardiac support interventions on the four determinants of myocardial Vo_2, along with the net effect on myocardial Vo_2. Vasodilator therapy is the most beneficial (i.e., it produces the greatest decrease in myocardial Vo_2), whereas dopamine creates the most harm (i.e., produces the greatest increase in myocardial Vo_2). Vasodilators are preferred to dobutamine for treating heart failure, and the intraaortic balloon pump is preferred to dopamine for managing cardiogenic shock. The intraaortic balloon pump is also preferred to dobutamine for managing heart failure ac-

TABLE 19.5. CARDIAC SUPPORT AND MYOCARDIAL OXYGEN CONSUMPTION				
Determinants of Cardiac Performance	Low Cardiac Output		Cardiogenic Shock	
	Dobutamine	Vasodilators	Aortic Balloon	Dopamine
Preload	↓	↓	↓	↑
Contractility	↑↑	—	—	↑
Afterload	↓	↓↓	↓	↑
Heart rate	—	—	—	↑
Myocardial V_{O_2}	—	↓↓↓	↓↓	↑↑↑↑

companied by a borderline or labile blood pressure (see Chapter 16 for more information on the intraaortic balloon pump).

ACUTE AORTIC DISSECTION

Acute aortic dissection involving the ascending aorta is a surgical emergency that produces substernal chest pain that can be confused with pain of cardiac origin.

CLINICAL PRESENTATION

Aortic dissection occurs in all age groups but is three times more common in men. About 75% of subjects have a history of hypertension. Some have connective tissue disorders (e.g., Marfan syndrome).

Chest Pain

Proximal dissection (ascending aorta) typically produces substernal chest pain that can radiate to the neck, jaw, or shoulders. The character of the pain tends to be very sharp, with descriptive terms such as *tearing* or *ripping* that also describe the pathologic process in the aorta. The chest pain tends to remain severe while it is present, but it can also subside spontaneously for hours to days. The disease is not silent during this period, and when the pain returns, it is more severe.

Clinical Findings

The hallmark of this disorder is **aortic insufficiency,** which is present in over 50% of cases of proximal dissection. Proximal dissection can extend into proximal limb vessels (uneven pulses) and coronary arteries (ischemia/infarction) and can rupture into the pericardium (tamponade).

Diagnosis

The chest x ray is usually abnormal, but the diagnosis requires one of several imaging modalities. In order of sensitivity, these include the following (28): (*a*) magnetic resonance imaging (MRI) (sensitivity and specificity 98%), (*b*) transesophageal echocardiography (sensitivity 98%, specificity 77%), (*c*) contrast-enhanced computed tomography (sensitivity 94%, specificity 87%), and (*d*) aortography (sensitivity 88%, specificity 94%). **MRI and transesophageal ultrasound are the most sensitive diagnostic modalities available** (28). Aortography is the least sensitive, but provides valuable information for the operating surgeon.

MANAGEMENT

The appropriate treatment for proximal aortic dissection is immediate surgery (27). Medical management is used to control pain and manage hypertension during the diagnostic evaluation. (Uncomplicated dissections in the descending aorta can often be managed medically.) Because increases in flow rate produce higher shear forces and promote dissection, **the goal of antihypertensive therapy in aortic dissection is to decrease the blood pressure without increasing the cardiac output.** This can be accomplished with the antihypertensive regimens listed in Table 19.6 (29). The traditional regimen for aortic dissection involves a combination of vasodilator therapy with nitroprusside (to decrease blood pressure) and intravenous administration of β-blockers (to prevent the increase in cardiac output that accompanies vasodilator therapy). β-Blockade must be established first, before nitroprusside administration. Single-agent therapy is easier to use, and may be preferred (29). Continuous infusion of the ganglionic blocker trimethaphan camsylate (Arfonad) produces generalized vasodilation while blocking any reflex increase in cardiac output. Effective monotherapy is also possible with labetalol, a combined α- and β-receptor blocker that can be given intravenously as intermittent bolus injections or by continuous infusion. Ganglionic blockade with

TABLE 19.6. TREATING HYPERTENSION IN ACUTE AORTIC DISSECTION	
Agents	**Dose**
Trimethaphan	0.6–6 mg/min
Labetalol	20 mg IV, then
	1–2 mg/min
	or
	20 mg IV, then
	40 mg IV every 10 min
Propranolol and nitroprusside	0.5 mg IV, then
	1 mg IV every 15 min
	0.2–10 μg/kg/min

trimethaphan can be associated with troublesome side effects (such as urinary retention, ileus, constipation, and tachyphylaxis), so **labetalol may be the preferred choice for monotherapy** (except in patients with asthma or atrioventricular block, where labetalol is contraindicated). See Chapter 18 for more information on labetalol.

REFERENCES

REVIEWS

1. Guidelines for the early management of patients with acute myocardial infarction: a report of the American College of Cardiology/American Heart Association Task Force on Assessment of Diagnostic and Therapeutic Cardiovascular Procedures. J Am Coll Cardiol 1990;16:249–292.
2. Cummins RO, ed. Textbook of advanced cardiac life support. Dallas: American Heart Association, 1994:9.1–9.16 (171 References)6.
3. Rogers WJ. Contemporary management of acute myocardial infarction. Am J Med 1995;99:195–206 (62 References).

CORONARY THROMBOSIS

4. DeWood MA, Spores J, Notske R, et al. The prevalence of total coronary occlusion during the early hours of transmural myocardial infarction. N Engl J Med 1980;303:897–902.
5. Davies MJ, Thomas AC. Plaque fissuring: the cause of acute myocardial infarction. Br Heart J 1985;53:363–373.

THROMBOLYTIC THERAPY

6. Anderson HV, Willerson JT. Thrombolysis in acute myocardial infarction. N Engl J Med 1993;329:703–725.
7. Gruppo Italiano per lo Studio della Streptochinasi nell'Infarto Miocardico (GISSI). Effectiveness of intravenous thrombolytic treatment in acute myocardial infarction. Lancet 1986;1:397–401.
8. Fibrinolytic Therapy Trialists Collaborative Group. Indications for fibrinolytic therapy in suspected acute myocardial infarction: collaborative overview of early mortality and major morbidity results from all randomized trials of more than 1000 patients. Lancet 1994;343:311–322.
9. Young GP, Hoffman JR. Thrombolytic therapy. Emerg Med Clin 1995;13:735–759.
10. Bates ER, Topol EJ. Limitations of thrombolytic therapy for acute myocardial infarction complicated by congestive heart failure and cardiogenic shock. J Am Coll Cardiol 1991;18:1077–1084.
11. ISIS-3 (Third International Study of Infarct Survival) Collaborative Group. ISIS-3: a randomized comparison of streptokinase vs. tissue plasminogen activator vs. anistreplase and of aspirin plus heparin vs. aspirin alone among 41,299 cases of suspected acute myocardial infarction. Lancet 1992;339:753–770.
12. Reeder GS, Kopecky SL. Thrombolysis in acute myocardial infarction: t-PA for everyone? Mayo Clin Proc 1994;69:796–799.
13. GUSTO Investigators. An international randomized trial comparing four

thrombolytic strategies for acute myocardial infarction. N Engl J Med 1993; 329:673–682.

14. Guidry JR, Raschke R, Morkunas AR. Anticoagulants and thrombolytics. In: Blumer JL, Bond GR, eds. Toxic effects of drugs in the ICU. Critical care clinics. Vol. 7. Philadelphia: WB Saunders, 1991;533–554.

15. Jalihal S, Morris GK. Antistreptokinase titres after intravenous streptokinase. Lancet 1990;335:184–185.

16. ISIS-2 (Second International Study of Infarct Survival) Collaborative Group. Randomized trial of intravenous streptokinase, oral aspirin, both, or neither among 17,187 cases of suspected acute myocardial infarction: ISIS-2. Lancet 1988;2:349–360.

17. Fuster V. Coronary thrombolysis: a perspective for the practicing physician. N Engl J Med 1993;329:723–725.

18. Reeder GS. Acute myocardial infarction: enhancing the results of reperfusion injury. Mayo Clin Proc 1995;70:1185–1190.

BETA BLOCKERS

19. ISIS-1 (First International Study of Infarct Survival) Collaborative Group. Randomized trial of intravenous atenolol among 16,027 cases of or suspected cases of acute myocardial infarction. Lancet 1986;2:57–66.

20. The MIAMI Trial Research Group. Metoprolol in acute myocardial infarction (MIAMI): a randomized, placebo-controlled international trial. Eur Heart J 1985;6:199–226.

21. The International Collaborative Study Group. Reduction of infarct size with the early use of timolol in acute myocardial infarction. N Engl J Med 1984; 310:9–15.

NITROGLYCERIN

22. Nicolini FA, Ferrini D, Ottani F, et al. Concurrent nitroglycerin therapy impairs tissue-type plasminogen activator–induced thrombolysis in patients with acute myocardial infarction. Am J Cardiol 1994;74:662–666.

23. Gruppo Italiano per lo Studio della Sopravivenza nell'Infarto Miocardico. GISSI-3: effects of lisinopril and transdermal glyceryl trinitrate singly and together on 6-week mortality and ventricular function after acute myocardial infarction. Lancet 1994;343:1115–1122.

24. Heesch CM, Eichhorn EJ. Magnesium in acute myocardial infarction. Ann Emerg Med 1994;24:1154–1160.

25. du Toit EF, Opie L. Modulation of severity of reperfusion stunning in the isolated rat heart by agents altering calcium influx at onset of reperfusion. Circ Res 1992;70:960–967.

26. Woods KL, Fletcher S, Roffe C, Haider Y. Intravenous magnesium sulfate in suspected acute myocardial infarction: results of the second Leicester Intravenous Magnesium Intervention Trial (LIMIT-2). Lancet 1992;339:1553–1558.

27. Crawford ES. The diagnosis and management of aortic dissection. JAMA 1990; 264:2537–2541.

28. Zegel HG, Chmielewski S, Freiman DB. The imaging evaluation of thoracic aortic dissection. Appl Radiol 1995;(June):15–25.

29. Asfoura JY, Vidt DG. Acute aortic dissection. Chest 1991;99:724–729.

c h a p t e r

20

TACHYARRHYTHMIAS

Acute arrhythmias are the gremlins of the ICU because they pop up unexpectedly, create some havoc, and are often gone again in a flash. This chapter describes the acute management of the most common and troublesome rhythm disturbances in the ICU: the tachyarrhythmias.

CLASSIFICATION

Tachycardias (heart rate above 100 beats/minute) can be the result of **increased automaticity** in pacemaker cells (e.g., sinus tachycardias), **triggered activity** (e.g., ectopic impulses), or a process known as **re-entry**, where a triggered impulse encounters a pathway that blocks propagation in the forward direction but allows the impulse to pass in the return (retrograde) direction (1,2). Such retrograde transmission allows a triggered impulse to propagate continually, creating a self-sustaining tachycardia. Re-entry is the most common cause of tachycardias that are clinically significant.

Tachycardias are classified according to the site of impulse generation in relation to the atrioventricular (AV) conduction system (1–3). Supraventricular tachycardias (SVTs) originate above the AV conduction system and have a normal QRS duration. Ventricular tachycardias (VTs) originate below the AV conduction system and have a prolonged QRS duration (more than 0.12 second). As shown in Figure 20.1, both types of tachycardias can be further subdivided by their regularity (i.e., by the regularity of the R–R interval on the ECG).

CLUES FROM THE RHYTHM STRIP

The initial encounter with arrhythmias in the ICU is often the moment the nurse notices an irregularity on a single-lead rhythm strip.

317

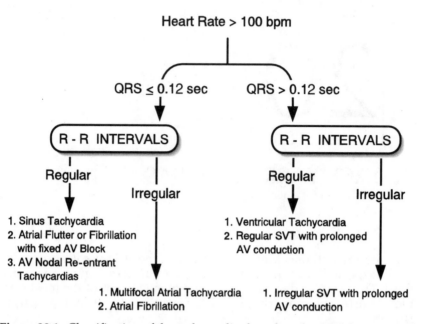

Figure 20.1. Classification of the tachycardias based on the QRS duration and the regularity of the R–R intervals.

If the rhythm strip shows a tachycardia, the major arrhythmias of concern are as follows.

Narrow-Complex Tachycardia

If the QRS duration is 0.12 seconds or less, the arrhythmias to consider include sinus tachycardia, atrial tachycardia, AV nodal tachycardia, atrial flutter, and atrial fibrillation. The following clues may help identify the problem.

Rhythm and Rate

Regular rhythm, rate > 150 bpm	AV nodal re-entrant tachycardia
Regular rhythm, rate = 150 bpm	Possible atrial flutter with 2:1 AV block
Rhythm markedly irregular	Atrial fibrillation or multifocal atrial tachycardia

Atrial Activity

Uniform P waves, fixed P–R interval	Sinus tachycardia
Multiform P waves, variable P–R interval	Multifocal atrial tachycardia
Inverted P waves	AV nodal tachycardia
Sawtooth waves	Atrial flutter
No atrial activity	AV nodal re-entrant tachycardia

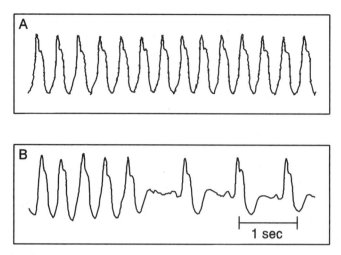

Figure 20.2. An SVT with prolonged AV conduction masquerading as VT. (Tracings courtesy of Dr. Richard M. Greenberg, M.D.)

Wide-Complex Tachycardia

A tachycardia with a prolonged QRS duration is either a VT or an SVT with prolonged AV conduction. The following signs help to differentiate between these two arrhythmias.

Pronounced irregularity	SVT
Fusion beats	VT
AV dissociation	VT

When all R–R intervals are irregular (irregularly irregular rhythm), the problem is either atrial fibrillation or multifocal atrial tachycardia. The presence of fusion beats or AV dissociation before the onset of the tachycardia is evidence of VT. A fusion beat is caused by a ventricular ectopic impulse that merges (fuses) with a normal QRS complex. This results in a QRS complex that is intermediate in morphology between the normal complex and the ectopic impulse. A fusion beat is thus evidence of ventricular ectopic activity.

It may be difficult to distinguish VT from an SVT with prolonged AV conduction, as illustrated in Figure 20.2. In this case, the tracing in the upper panel shows a wide complex tachycardia that looks like VT. However, the tracing in the lower panel reveals that when the arrhythmia converts to a normal sinus rhythm, the QRS duration remains prolonged. This indicates that the tachycardia is an SVT superimposed on a bundle branch block.

SINUS TACHYCARDIA

Increased automaticity in the pacemaker cells of the sinoatrial node produces a regular, narrow-complex tachycardia with a gradual onset and rate of 100 to 140 beats/minute. The ECG shows uniform P waves and a fixed P–R interval. Sinus tachycardia can also be the result of re-entry into the sinus node. This variant sinus tachycardia has an abrupt onset, but is otherwise indistinguishable from the increased automaticity type of sinus tachycardia (2).

MANAGEMENT

Sinus tachycardia is usually a response to a systemic or noncardiac condition and is often an adaptive response (as in exercise). It is usually well tolerated (cardiac filling is usually not compromised until the heart rate rises above 180 beats/minute) (4) and does not require primary treatment. **The primary goal of management is to identify and treat the associated condition.** Potential sources of sinus tachycardia in the ICU are hypoxemia, sepsis, hypovolemia, and adrenergic drugs.

The main indication for slowing a sinus tachycardia is the presence of myocardial ischemia or infarction. In this situation, β-receptor antagonists can be used to slow the heart rate. Because these agents also depress ventricular function, they are not recommended for sinus tachycardias associated with systolic heart failure. The use of β-blockers in myocardial ischemia and infarction is described in Chapter 19 (see Table 19.4).

ATRIAL FLUTTER AND FIBRILLATION

With the possible exception of sinus tachycardia, the most common tachycardia in ICU patients is atrial fibrillation. Atrial flutter is an uncommon and transient arrhythmia that often turns into atrial fibrillation. Atrial flutter and fibrillation are both abbreviated as AF in this chapter.

PREVALENCE

There are an estimated 2.2 million adults in the United States with AF (5). Most are elderly (median age 75 years) and have either valvular heart disease, coronary artery disease, or dilated cardiomyopathy. Contrary to popular perception, few have hyperactive thyroid disease (6). Additional predisposing factors in the ICU include recent cardiac surgery (particularly valvular surgery), resectional lung surgery, and acute myocardial infarction.

POSTOPERATIVE AF

About 30% of patients undergoing cardiopulmonary bypass surgery develop AF in the second to fourth postoperative day (7). Patients treated with β-blocker drugs before surgery, and those undergoing valvular surgery, are at highest risk. The etiology is unclear, but the delayed onset suggests electrolyte (magnesium, potassium) shifts. These arrhythmias are more of a nuisance than a life-threatening complication, but they often prolong the hospital stay by a few days. β-Blockers are popular agents for the prevention and treatment of postoperative AF.

ADVERSE CONSEQUENCES

The loss of atrial contraction in AF, plus the decrease in diastolic filling time that accompanies the tachycardia, both impair cardiac filling. Contraction of the atria is responsible for 25% of the ventricular end-diastolic volume (preload) in the normal heart (4), and this contribution is lost when the ventricle becomes noncompliant and resists diastolic filling. The loss of the atrial component of cardiac filling is well tolerated in the normal heart, but it can significantly impair cardiac performance in the noncompliant (e.g., hypertrophied) heart.

The other notable complication of AF is mural thrombosis in the left atrium and cerebral embolic stroke. Atrial thrombosis can be demonstrated in 15% of patients who have AF for longer than 3 days (5), and 4 to 5% of patients with chronic AF suffer an embolic stroke each year without warfarin anticoagulation (5). Although it is possible for a mural thrombus to appear within 3 days after the onset of AF (5), the thromboembolism associated with AF is usually a subacute or chronic complication, and is not discussed here. (For an informative description of thromboembolism in AF, see Reference 5.)

MONITORING AND MANAGEMENT GOALS

The acute management of AF is usually aimed at decreasing the ventricular rate rather than conversion to a normal sinus rhythm. In other words, the management is designed for rate control rather than rhythm control. The **goals of rate control** should include all of the following:

Normal stroke volume
Absence of a pulse deficit
Ventricular rate below 100 beats/minute

Because of the direct relationship between preload and ventricular stroke output (see Fig. 1.2), the stroke volume is the single best parameter to follow for determining the impact of AF on cardiac performance. If invasive hemodynamic monitoring is not available, then the next best parameter to monitor is the **pulse deficit** (i.e., the **difference between the precordial heart rate and the pulse rate in a peripheral artery)**. The presence of a pulse deficit in AF indicates that cardiac stroke output is significantly impaired, so disappearance of a pulse deficit should be a goal of rate-control management in AF. The most commonly monitored parameter is the heart rate, which should be kept within the normal range (less than 100 beats/minute).

TABLE 20.1. DIRECT-CURRENT CARDIOVERSION	

Indications:
  1. Hypotension or impaired vital organ function
  2. Ventricular rate >150 beats/min
Premedication:
  Give a sedative (e.g., diazepam or midazolam) with or without an
  analgesic (e.g., morphine or fentanyl).
Synchronization:
  Synchronized shocks are not necessary.

Tachycardia	Energy of Sequential Shocks (J)
SVT and atrial flutter	50, 100, 200, 300, 360
VT and atrial fibrillation	100, 200, 300, 360
Polymorphic VT	200, 200–300, 360

Adapted from the ACLS guidelines in Reference 1 for patients not in cardiac arrest.

ELECTRICAL CARDIOVERSION

Recommendations for direct-current (DC) cardioversion, taken from the most recent advanced cardiac life support (ACLS) guidelines, are summarized in Table 20.1 (1). Electrical cardioversion should be reserved for cases where blood flow to the major organs is impaired (such as hypotension or a change in mental status). Although shocks are normally synchronized to the R wave of the QRS complex (to prevent shocks from being delivered during the vulnerable period of ventricular repolarization) synchronization has no proven benefit, and can delay the delivery of the DC countershocks (1). Thus, unsynchronized shocks are not only acceptable, they may be preferred when immediate cardioversion is desirable. The strength of DC shocks is expressed in joules (J), which is a unit of energy (see Appendix 1). The recommended strength of the shocks for different arrhythmias is shown in Table 20.1. The energy of the initial shock should be 100 J for atrial fibrillation and 50 J for atrial flutter (flutter is easier to convert). If these initial shocks are not successful, then successive shocks of increasing strength are delivered, if necessary, using the energy sequences shown in Table 20.1. At these energy levels, DC cardioversion should be successful in 90% of patients with recent-onset AF.

ALTERNATIVE STRATEGY

DC cardioversion can be a very distressing and painful experience for patients who are awake and aware. In the patient who is hypotensive but awake, blood flow is adequate for at least one vital organ, so immediate cardioversion is not necessary. In this situation, volume infusion can be used in an attempt to raise the blood pressure and obviate electrical cardioversion. As long as the central venous and wedge pressures are below 20 mm Hg, infuse 100-mL aliquots of 5% albumin or 6% hetastarch until the systolic blood pressure rises above 100 mm Hg. If this is successful, proceed with the conventional (pharmacologic) management of AF. Colloid fluids are preferred here because they provide more rapid expansion of the intravascular volume than crystalloid fluids (see Chapter 15).

PHARMACOTHERAPY

The pharmacologic agents listed in Table 20.2 have all proven successful in the acute management of AF. Only one of the agents (procai-

TABLE 20.2. ACUTE PHARMACOTHERAPY OF ATRIAL FIBRILLATION		
Agent	**Intravenous Dosing**	**Comments**
Digoxin	0.75 mg over 5 min, then 0.25 mg every 4 hr × 2 doses.	Not used for rapid rate control (may take 9–10 hr).
Diltiazem	0.25 mg/kg over 2 min, then 0.35 mg/kg 15 min later if needed. Can infuse at 10–15 mg/hr.	The preferred agent for patients with systolic heart failure.
Esmolol	Load with 0.5 mg/kg then infuse at 50–300 μg/kg/min. (See text for full dosing information).	Ultra–short-acting β-blocker. Drawbacks are hypotension and tedious dosing.
Magnesium	2 g MgSO$_4$ (in 50 mL saline) over 15 min, then 6 g MgSO$_4$ (in 500 mL saline) over 6 hr.	Safe and effective in preliminary reports. Probable mechanism is calcium channel blockade.
Metoprolol	5 mg over 2 min. Repeat every 5 min if needed to total dose of 15 mg.	Cardioselective β-blocker. Has been used safely in nonasthmatic chronic obstructive pulmonary disease.
Procainamide	Load with 10 mg/kg at a maximum rate of 25 mg/min, then infuse at 1–6 mg/min.	For cardioversion, not rate control. Transiently enhances AV conduction, and thus is used with agents that prolong AV conduction.
Verapamil	0.075 mg/kg over 2 min, then 0.15 mg/kg in 15 min if needed. Can infuse at 5 μg/kg/min.	Provides effective rate control, but its use is limited by side effects (cardiac depression and hypotension).
From References 8–20.		

namide) is capable of converting AF to a normal sinus rhythm. The remainder act by slowing the ventricular rate.

Verapamil

Intravenous verapamil, a calcium channel blocker, provides effective rate control in 70% of patients with rapid AF (2).

Dosage: 0.075 mg/kg intravenously over 2 minutes. If no response after 10 minutes, give a second dose of 0.15 mg/kg.

The response is evident within minutes after drug injection, and the effect lasts up to 1 hour (2). Because the response is short-lived, the effective dose of verapamil should be followed by continuous infusion (5 to 20 mg/hour) (9,10). Verapamil is metabolized in the liver, and the dosage should be reduced 50% in patients with hepatic insufficiency.

The major drawbacks with verapamil are hypotension (due to vasodilator actions) and worsening systolic heart failure (due to the negative inotropic actions) (10). The risk of hypotension is reduced by pretreatment with intravenous calcium (11).

Calcium pretreatment: Give 10 mL of 10% calcium *gluconate* intravenously over 5 minutes, just before verapamil.

This regimen provides 90 mg of elemental calcium. Calcium is also available as **10% calcium chloride,** but this salt **contains three times more elemental calcium than 10% calcium gluconate** (i.e., 10 mL of 10% calcium chloride provides 270 mg of elemental calcium). Therefore, do not ask for an "amp of calcium"—specify the gluconate salt.

The drug interactions involving verapamil are included in Table 20.3. Verapamil increases serum digoxin levels (mechanism not clear), so it is wise to monitor serum digoxin levels when instituting therapy with verapamil. Verapamil can also precipitate cardiovascular collapse when given in combination with β-blockers, and combined therapy is contraindicated. Other contraindications to verapamil infusion include second- or third-degree AV block, systolic heart failure, hypotension, and Wolf–Parkinson–White (WPW) syndrome (2). The problem in the WPW syndrome is the tendency for verapamil (and all agents that prolong AV conduction) to paradoxically increase the ventricular rate in AF.

Diltiazem

Another calcium channel blocker, diltiazem, provides the same rapid and effective rate control in AF as verapamil. However, diltiazem produces less myocardial depression than verapamil (12). For this reason, **diltiazem is the preferred agent for patients with (systolic) heart failure.** The dosage shown here (and in Table 20.2) has been used safely in patients with moderate to severe heart failure (13).

Dosage: 0.25 mg/kg intravenously over 2 minutes. If no response after 10 minutes, give a second dose of 0.35 mg/kg.

TABLE 20.3. ANTIARRHYTHMIC DRUG INTERACTIONS			
Primary Drug	Interfering Drugs	Mechanism	Action
Adenosine	Dipyridamole	Blocks adenosine uptake and metabolism	Reduce adenosine dose by 50%.
	Theophylline	Antagonizes adenosine actions	Avoid combined therapy.
β-blockers	Calcium antagonists	Additive cardiodepressant effects	Avoid combined therapy.
Digoxin	Diltiazem Quinidine Verapamil	Increased serum digoxin levels (mechanism unclear)	Monitor serum digoxin levels.
Lidocaine	β-blockers Cimetidine	Reduced hepatic clearance	Reduce lidocaine dose by 50%.
	Barbiturates Phenytoin Rifampin	Enhanced hepatic clearance	Use high range of recommended lidocaine doses.
Metoprolol	Verapamil	Reduced hepatic clearance	Avoid combined therapy.
Procainamide	Cimetidine	Reduced renal clearance	Avoid combined therapy.

Like those of verapamil, diltiazem's effects are short-lived, so the effective dose should be followed by a continuous infusion of the drug (10 to 15 mg/hour) (12,13).

β-Receptor Antagonists

β-Blockers are used for rate control in AF when it is accompanied by hyperadrenergic states (such as acute MI and after cardiac surgery). The cardioselective β-blockers (which preferentially block β-1 receptors) have largely replaced the nonselective blockers such as propranolol. Table 20.2 includes two cardioselective agents: esmolol and metoprolol. **Esmolol** (Brevibloc) has received much attention because it is an ultra–short-acting agent (serum half-life of 9 minutes) that can be titrated rapidly (14). However, as demonstrated in the recommended dosing regimen here, therapy with esmolol can be a tedious process.

Esmolol dosing regimen: Start with a 30-second loading dose of 0.5 mg/kg and follow with continuous infusion at 50 μg/kg/minute for 4 minutes. If the rate is not adequately controlled, repeat the loading dose and increase the infusion to 100 μg/kg/minute for another 4 minutes. If the rate is still not controlled, increase the dosing rate in increments of 50 mg/kg/minute every 4 minutes to a maximum dosing rate of 300 μg/kg/minute. Each increase in dosing rate should be preceded by a loading dose of 0.5 mg/kg (15).

Of the β-blockers, metoprolol (Lopressor) is much more convenient to use. **Combined therapy with β-blockers and calcium channel**

blockers should be avoided, because this combination can produce severe cardiac depression (see Table 20.3) (8).

Magnesium

Intravenous magnesium has proven safe and effective for rate control in AF (16,17) and for prophylaxis of postoperative AF (18).

Dosage: 2 g $MgSO_4$ over 5 to 15 minutes. Then infuse 6 g $MgSO_4$ in 500 mL saline over 6 hours (1 g/hour).

Although the clinical experience with magnesium in AF is limited, there is reason to believe that magnesium will be a valuable intervention for AF in the ICU. First, magnesium is a calcium channel blocker, and other agents with a similar action (i.e., verapamil and diltiazem) provide effective rate control in AF. Second, magnesium is a necessary cofactor for the proper function of the membrane pump for sodium and potassium. Because this pump maintains a hyperpolarized state in cells, magnesium could act as an antiarrhythmic agent by virtue of its ability to stabilize excitable cell membranes. Third, because magnesium deficiency is common in ICU patients (see Chapter 42), magnesium infusion could reduce the ventricular rate in AF by correcting an underlying magnesium deficiency.

Digoxin

Digoxin is a popular agent for chronic rate control in AF, but because of a delayed onset of action, **digoxin is not indicated for the acute management of AF.** The delayed action of intravenous digoxin is illustrated in Figure 20.3. This figure is taken from a study of patients who presented to the emergency room with recent-onset AF and were randomized to receive either intravenous diltiazem (same dosage as in Table 20.2) or intravenous digoxin (0.5 mg in two divided doses over 30 minutes) (19). As demonstrated, the patients who received diltiazem showed adequate rate control (i.e., a heart rate below 100 beats/minute) by 15 minutes after the onset of drug therapy, whereas the patients who received digoxin were not adequately controlled after 3 hours.

Procainamide

The goal of intravenous procainamide therapy is not to control the ventricular rate, but to convert AF to a normal sinus rhythm.

Dosage: 10 mg/kg intravenously at a maximum rate of 25 mg/minute. Follow with a continuous infusion at 1 to 6 mg/minute (20).

Half of a procainamide dose is cleared unchanged by the kidneys, and 15% is first converted in plasma to an active metabolite, to N-acetyl procainamide (NAPA), which is then cleared by the kidneys.

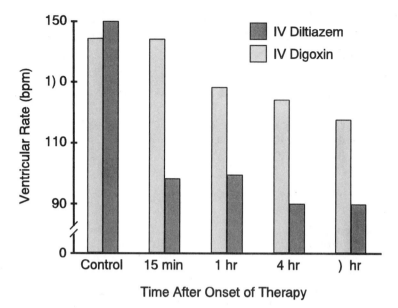

Figure 20.3. Acute rate control of AF with IV diltiazem (dose same as in Table 20.2) and IV digoxin (0.5 mg in two divided doses over 6 hours). Height of the vertical columns indicates the mean heart rate for all patients in each treatment group. (Data from Schreck DM et al. Emergency treatment of atrial fibrillation and flutter: comparison of IV digoxin versus IV diltiazem. Ann Emerg Med 1995;25:127.)

The dosage of procainamide should be reduced by 50% in elderly patients and in patients with renal dysfunction, and the dosage should be reduced by 25% in heart failure (20).

Procainamide transiently facilitates AV conduction, so the drug should be given in combination with an agent that blocks AV conduction. Because procainamide has negative inotropic actions, digitalis is favored over calcium blockers or β-blockers to provide the AV block. Procainamide also prolongs the Q–T interval, and can be proarrhythmic in patients with a prolonged Q–T interval. For this reason, procainamide is **contraindicated in patients with prolonged Q–T interval.** The drug should also be avoided in patients with renal failure.

WOLF–PARKINSON–WHITE SYNDROME

Patients with WPW syndrome (short P–R interval and Δ waves before the QRS) have an accessory, re-entrant pathway in the AV node that predisposes them to recurrent tachycardias (both narrow complex and wide complex), including atrial fibrillation. Agents that block AV conduction and slow the rate in conventional AF, such as digoxin and verapamil, can paradoxically accelerate the ventricular rate (by blocking the wrong pathway) in the AF associated with WPW syndrome. In patients with a history of WPW syndrome who develop AF, calcium channel blockers and digoxin are contraindicated, and the treatment of choice is electrical cardioversion or procainamide infusion.

ATRIAL AND JUNCTIONAL TACHYCARDIAS

Some atrial tachycardias are caused by ectopic foci, but most are the result of re-entry through the AV node. The following arrhythmias are commonly encountered in the ICU.

MULTIFOCAL ATRIAL TACHYCARDIA

Multifocal atrial tachycardia (MAT) is characterized by multiple P wave morphologies and a variable P–R interval (21). The ventricular rate is highly irregular, and MAT is easily confused with atrial fibrillation when atrial activity is not clearly displayed on a single-lead rhythm strip. MAT is most often seen in patients with chronic lung disease and has also been linked to theophylline therapy (22). Other predisposing conditions include hypokalemia, magnesium deficiency, acute pulmonary embolism, acute MI, and congestive heart failure (1,2,21).

Acute Management

MAT can be a difficult arrhythmia to manage. In patients with severe lung disease, aggravating conditions, such as hypoxemia, should be corrected. Then proceed as follows.

1. **Discontinue ongoing therapy with theophylline.** In one study, this maneuver resulted in conversion to sinus rhythm in half the patients with MAT (22).
2. In the absence of contraindications to magnesium therapy, give **intravenous magnesium** using the dosing regimen in Table 20.2 (23). In addition to its antiarrhythmic actions, magnesium also dilates pulmonary arteries (which might help in patients with MAT secondary to chronic obstructive pulmonary disease, COPD).
3. If the serum potassium is low, give intravenous magnesium first (2 g MgSO$_4$ in 50 mL saline over 15 minutes), then infuse 40 mg potassium over 1 hour. The magnesium pretreatment is often necessary for correcting the hypokalemia (see Chapter 42).
4. If the above measures are ineffective, consider therapy with verapamil or metoprolol (see dosages in Table 20.2). If the patient has a history of reactive airway disease, verapamil (which is a mild bronchodilator) is preferred to β-blockers. If the patient has COPD without reactive airways, selective β-1 receptor antagonists such as metoprolol can be used safely. **Metoprolol has been**

reported to convert MAT to sinus rhythm in 70 to 100% of cases (2).

AV NODAL RE-ENTRANT TACHYCARDIA

Re-entry of impulses through the AV node (triggered by an ectopic pulse) is the most common cause of narrow-complex tachycardias with a regular rate (other than sinus tachycardia). These tachycardias are also known as paroxysmal SVTs, and are characterized by an abrupt onset and the absence of identifiable atrial activity (P waves hidden in the QRS complex). These tachycardias are faster than a sinus tachycardia, with rates usually between 140 and 220 beats/minute.

Acute Management

Maneuvers aimed at increasing vagal tone were once popular for AV nodal re-entrant tachycardia (AVNRT). However, most of these maneuvers are ineffective, and some (such as eyeball compression) are downright dangerous. The standard approach for terminating AVNRT is to administer drugs that block the re-entrant pathway in the AV node. The most effective agents for this purpose are the calcium channel blockers, (verapamil and diltiazem), and adenosine. These agents are equally effective for terminating AVNRT, but adenosine has less cardiovascular depressant effect than the calcium antagonists. The salient features of adenosine administration are presented in Table 20.4.

Adenosine (Adenocard)

Adenosine is an endogenous substance that dilates coronary arteries, slows the sinus rate, prolongs AV conduction, and blocks the positive inotropic actions of catecholamines (24). When given by rapid intravenous injection, **adenosine terminates AVNRT in 90 to 100% of cases** (24–26). However, because adenosine is an ultra–short-acting agent (effects last 1 or 2 minutes), the cardiac depressant actions of adenosine are too short-lived to produce significant myocardial depression (24–26). For this reason, adenosine is **the drug of choice for terminating AVNRT in patients with heart failure.**

The intravenous dosing recommendations for adenosine are included in Table 20.4. Note that **the dosage of adenosine should be reduced by 50% when the drug is injected through a central venous (CVP) catheter** instead of a peripheral vein (27). This recommendation is based on reports of ventricular asystole when adenosine in standard doses is given through CVP catheters (27).

The drug interactions with adenosine are shown in Table 20.3. Note that theophylline antagonizes the actions of adenosine by blocking adenosine receptors. As a result, therapeutic doses of **adenosine may not be effective in patients receiving theophylline,** so combined therapy with adenosine and theophylline is not advised.

TABLE 20.4. INTRAVENOUS ADENOSINE FOR SVT	
Indications:	Termination of AV nodal re-entrant tachycardia, particularly in patients with • Heart failure • Hypotension • Ongoing therapy with calcium channel blockers or β-blockers • WPW syndrome
Contraindications:	Asthma, AV block
Dose:	For delivery via peripheral veins, 1. Give 6 mg by rapid IV injection and flush with saline. 2. After 2 min, give a second dose of 12 mg if necessary. 3. The 12 mg dose can be repeated once.
Dose Adjustments:	Decrease dose by 50% for • Injection into superior vena cava • Patients receiving calcium blockers, β-blockers, or dipyridamole
Response:	Onset of action <30 sec. Effects last 1–2 min.
Side Effects:	Facial flushing (50%) Sinus bradycardia, AV block (50%) Dyspnea (35%) Anginal-type chest pain (20%) Nausea, headache, dizziness (5–10%)
From References 24–27.	

Side effects are common after adenosine injection, and the most common ones are listed in Table 20.4 (along with the incidence of each in parentheses) (26). Fortunately, these side effects are short-lived. The anginal-type chest pain is often a source of concern, but is not the result of myocardial ischemia. Adenosine also provokes bronchoconstriction in asthmatic subjects (28,29), and the drug is **contraindicated in patients with asthma.**

VENTRICULAR TACHYCARDIA

The identity of a wide (QRS) complex tachycardia is easily confused on a single-lead ECG recording, as demonstrated in Figure 20.2. Although it is possible to differentiate between VT and SVT using a 12-lead ECG (30), this type of detailed analysis is more suited to the cardiac electrophysiology lab than the ICU. As stated in the most recent ACLS guidelines, "Faced with urgent care of an ill patient, the physician should ignore detailed criteria for ECG analysis and attend to the patient" (1). In fact, detailed ECG criteria may not be necessary, because as many as 95% of wide complex tachycardias in patients with underlying cardiac disease represent VT (31). Because most patients in the ICU have cardiac disease, **a wide complex tachycardia in an ICU patient should be treated as probable VT.**

ACUTE MANAGEMENT

The acute management of probable ventricular tachycardia should proceed as follows (1,32). This approach is outlined in Table 20.5.

1. If there is evidence of hemodynamic compromise, initiate DC cardioversion *immediately* with an initial shock of 100 J, followed by repetitive shocks of 200, 300, and 360 J, if necessary (see Table 20.1).
2. If there is no evidence of hemodynamic compromise, administer **lidocaine** at the dosages shown in Table 20.5. If bolus doses of lidocaine are successful in terminating the arrhythmia, start a continuous infusion at 2 to 4 mg/minute. Prolonged infusions of lidocaine can cause an excitatory neurotoxic syndrome, particularly in elderly patients and in those receiving β-blockers or ci-

TABLE 20.5. STAGED APPROACH TO VENTRICULAR TACHYCARDIA		
Stage	**Intervention**	**Recommended Dose**
Stage 1	DC cardioversion	• Use shock sequence shown in Table 20.1.
Stage 2	Lidocaine	• 1–1.5 mg/kg as bolus injection. • Wait 5 min, then give second dose of 0.5–0.75 mg/kg if necessary. • Follow effective dose with continuous infusion at 2–4 mg/min.
Stage 3: Q–Tc < 0.44 sec	Procainamide	• Infuse at 25 mg/min until conversion or until total dose of 17 mg/kg. • Stop infusion temporarily for hypotension or a 50% increase in QRS duration.
Stage 3: Q–Tc > 0.44 sec	Magnesium	• 2 g MgSO₄ IV over 1 min. • Repeat in 10 min if no response. • Follow effective dose with continuous infusion of MgSO₄ at 1 g/hr × 6 hr.
Stage 4	Bretylium	• 5–10 mg/kg IV over 10 min. • If effective, follow with continuous infusion at 1–2 mg/hr.
From References 1, 32.		

metidine (see Table 20.3). Therefore, lidocaine infusion should not be continued beyond 6 to 12 hours.

3. If there is no response to lidocaine, check the Q–T interval on a recent ECG recording. The Q–T interval is usually measured in lead II, and is corrected for the heart rate as follows: Corrected Q–T (Q–Tc) = measured Q–T divided by the square root of the R–R interval. A Q–Tc > 0.44 second is considered abnormal (33). **If the Q–T interval is normal (Q–Tc < 0.44 second), administer procainamide.** As indicated in Table 20.5, procainamide is not given as a bolus injection, but is infused slowly at a rate of 25 mg/minute. As a result, the response to procainamide can be delayed (up to 15 minutes after the onset of drug administration). The procainamide infusion should be continued until cardioversion, or until the cumulative dose reaches a maximum of 17 mg/kg (1 to 1.5 g) (34). If the QRS duration increases by more than 50%, or if hypotension develops, the infusion should be stopped temporarily.

Procainamide is an appealing agent for wide complex tachycardias because the drug can convert both VT and SVT. As mentioned earlier, the drug is contraindicated in patients with a prolonged Q–T interval (can be proarrhythmic).

If the Q–T interval is prolonged (Q–Tc > 0.44 second), intravenous magnesium is recommended (except in the presence of renal failure). Magnesium not only is effective in suppressing ventricular arrhythmias, but can be effective in VT refractory to lidocaine (35). Because a prolonged Q–T interval can be the result of magnesium depletion, magnesium infusions may be particularly effective in patients with a prolonged Q–T interval.

The ACLS guidelines recommend **bretylium** for VT that is refractory to lidocaine (1). However, bretylium has not proven more effective in suppressing VT than lidocaine (32). In addition, bretylium can cause profound hypotension (the drug was originally developed as an antihypertensive agent). The lack of improved efficacy, along with the potential for serious toxicity, suggests that the recommendations for bretylium in VT must be re-examined.

Precipitating Factors

Cardioversion of VT (either electrical or pharmacologic) should be followed by a search for precipitating conditions. The standard approach should include an ECG (ischemia), arterial blood gases (hypoxemia and alkalosis), serum electrolytes (hypokalemia, hypocalcemia, hypomagnesemia), and serum levels of select drugs (e.g., digitalis and theophylline).

TORSADE DE POINTES

Torsade de pointes ("twisting around the points") is a polymorphic VT characterized by phasic changes in the amplitude and polarity of

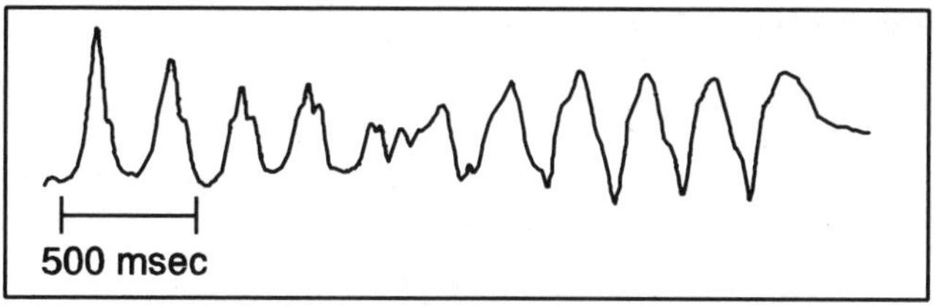

Figure 20.4. Torsade de pointes, which means "twisting around (the isoelectric) points." (Tracing courtesy of Dr. Richard M. Greenberg, M.D.)

the ventricular complexes (Fig. 20.4). This arrhythmia is often, but not always, associated with a prolonged Q–T interval (36). A variety of drugs and electrolyte deficiencies can predispose to this arrhythmia. Predisposing drugs include antiarrhythmic agents (quinidine, procainamide), antimicrobial agents (erythromycin, pentamidine), and psychotropic agents (haloperidol, phenothiazines). Predisposing electrolyte disorders include calcium, magnesium, and potassium deficiency.

Management

The management of this arrhythmia is guided by the Q–T interval.

When the Q–T interval is prolonged, the arrhythmia is often resistant to traditional antiarrhythmic agents. The treatment of choice is temporary ventricular pacing to increase the heart rate (100 to 120 beats/minute) and thereby shorten the Q–T interval.

When the Q–T interval is normal, traditional antiarrhythmic therapy (e.g., with lidocaine or procainamide) is usually effective.

After this arrhythmia is terminated, potentially offending drugs should be discontinued and electrolyte deficiencies should be corrected.

REFERENCES

GENERAL TEXTS

Podrid PJ, Kowey PR, eds. Handbook of cardiac arrhythmia. Baltimore: Williams & Wilkins, 1996.

REVIEWS

1. Emergency Cardiac Care Committee and Subcommittees, American Heart Association. Guidelines for cardiopulmonary resuscitation and emergency cardiac care. JAMA 1992;268:2199–2241 (430 References).
2. Collier WW, Holt SE, Wellford LA. Narrow complex tachycardias. Emerg Med Clin North Am 1995;13:925–954 (99 References).
3. Dellbridge TR, Yealy DM. Wide complex tachycardia. Emerg Med Clin North Am 1995;13:903–924 (69 References).

ATRIAL FLUTTER AND FIBRILLATION

4. Guyton AC. The relationship of cardiac output and arterial pressure control. Circulation 1981;64:1079–1088.
5. Blackshear JL, Kopecky SL, Litin SC, et al. Management of atrial fibrillation in adults: prevention of thromboembolism and symptomatic treatment. Mayo Clin Proc 1996;71:150–160.
6. Siebers MJ, Drinka PJ, Vergauwen C. Hyperthyroidism as a cause of atrial fibrillation in long-term care. Arch Intern Med 1992;152:2063–2064.
7. Creswell LL, Schuessler RB, Rosenbloom M, Cox JL. Hazards of postoperative atrial arrhythmias. Ann Thorac Surg 1993;56:539–549.
8. Kuhn M, Schriger DL. Verapamil administration to patients with contraindications: is it associated with adverse outcomes? Ann Emerg Med 1991;20:1094–1099.
9. Edwards JD, Kishen R. Significance and management of intractable supraventricular arrhythmias in critically ill patients. Crit Care Med 1986;14:280–282.
10. Iberti TJ, Benjamin E, Paluch TA, et al. Use of constant-infusion verapamil for the treatment of postoperative supraventricular tachycardia. Crit Care Med 1986;14:283–284.
11. Dolan DL. Intravenous calcium before verapamil to prevent hypotension. Ann Emerg Med 1991;20:588–589.
12. Ellenbogen KA, Dias VC, Plumb VJ, et al. A placebo-controlled trial of continuous intravenous diltiazem infusion for 24-hour heart rate control during atrial fibrillation and atrial flutter: a multicenter study. J Am Coll Cardiol 1991;18:891–897.
13. Goldenberg IF, Lewis WR, Dias VC, et al. Intravenous diltiazem for the treatment of patients with atrial fibrillation or flutter and moderate to severe congestive heart failure. Am J Cardiol 1994;74:884–889.
14. Gray RJ. Managing critically ill patients with esmolol. An ultra-short-acting β-adrenergic blocker. Chest 1988;93:398–404.
15. Brevibloc (esmolol HCL) Dosage Chart. Pharmaceutical Products Division. Ohmeda, Inc., Liberty Corner, NJ: 1993.
16. Brodsky MA, Orlov MV, Capparelli EV, et al. Magnesium therapy in acute-onset atrial fibrillation. Am J Cardiol 1994;73:1227–1229.
17. Hays JV, Gilman JK, Rubal BJ. Effect of magnesium sulfate on ventricular rate control in atrial fibrillation. Ann Emerg Med 1994;24:61–64.
18. Fanning WJ, Thomas CS Jr, Roach A, et al. Prophylaxis of atrial fibrillation with magnesium sulfate after coronary artery bypass grafting. Ann Thorac Surg 1991;52:529–533.
19. Schreck DM, Rivera AR, Zacharias D. Emergency treatment of atrial fibrillation and atrial flutter: comparison of IV digoxin versus IV diltiazem. Ann Emerg Med 1995;25:127 (abstract).
20. Marcus FI, Opie LH. Antiarrhythmic drugs. In: Opie LH, ed. Drugs for the heart. 4th ed. Philadelphia: WB Saunders, 1995;207–246.

ATRIAL & JUNCTIONAL TACHYCARDIAS

21. Kastor J. Multifocal atrial tachycardia. N Engl J Med 1990;322:1713–1720.
22. Levine J, Michael J, Guanieri T. Multifocal atrial tachycardia: a toxic effect of theophylline. Lancet 1985;1:1–16.
23. Iseri LT, Fairshter RD, Hardeman JL, Brodsky MA. Magnesium and potassium therapy in multifocal atrial tachycardia. Am Heart J 1985;312:21–26.
24. Shen W-K, Kurachi Y. Mechanisms of adenosine-mediated actions on cellular and clinical cardiac electrophysiology. Mayo Clin Proc 1995;70:274–291.

25. Rankin AC, Brooks R, Ruskin JM, McGovern BA. Adenosine and the treatment of supraventricular tachycardia. Am J Med 1992;92:655–664.
26. Chronister C. Clinical management of supraventricular tachycardia with adenosine. Am J Crit Care 1993;2:41–47.
27. McCollam PL, Uber W, Van Bakel AB. Adenosine-related ventricular asystole. Ann Intern Med 1993;118:315–316.
28. Cushley MJ, Tattersfield AE, Holgate ST. Adenosine-induced bronchoconstriction in asthma. Am Rev Respir Dis 1984;129:380–384.
29. Bjorck T, Gustafsson LE, Dahlen S-E. Isolated bronchi from asthmatics are hyperresponsive to adenosine, which apparently acts indirectly by liberation of leukotrienes and histamine. Am Rev Respir Dis 1992;145:1087–1091.

VENTRICULAR TACHYCARDIA

30. Brugada P, Brugada J, Mont L, et al. A new approach to the differential diagnosis of a regular tachycardia with a wide QRS complex. Circulation 1991;83: 1649–1659.
31. Akhtar M, Shenasa M, Jazayeri M, et al. Wide QRS complex tachycardia. Ann Intern Med 1988;109:905–912.
32. Slovis CM, Wrenn KD. The technique of managing ventricular tachycardia. J Crit Illness 1993;8:731–741.
33. Garson A Jr. How to measure the QT interval: what is normal? Am J Cardiol 1993;72:14B–16B.
34. Sharma AD, Purves P, Yee R, et al. Hemodynamic effects of intravenous procainamide during ventricular tachycardia. Am Heart J 1990;119:1034–1041.
35. Roden D. Magnesium treatment of ventricular arrhythmias. Am J Cardiol 1989;63:43G–46G.
36. Vukmir RB. Torsades de pointes: a review. Am J Emerg Med 1991;9:250–262.

section VI
ACUTE RESPIRATORY FAILURE

Respiration is but slow combustion, . . . and from this point of view, animals which breathe are really combustible bodies which burn and are consumed.

Antoine Lavoisier

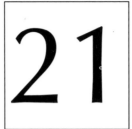

c h a p t e r

21

HYPOXEMIA AND HYPERCAPNIA

There is a distinct fondness for arterial blood gas analysis in ICU patients. In fact, arterial blood gases are the most commonly performed laboratory test in ICU patients (1,2); and with the advent of bedside methods for measuring blood gases (*point of patient care* laboratory testing) (3) and continuous in vivo blood gas monitoring (4), it is likely that blood gas measurements in days to come will be even more inundating. This chapter focuses on what to do when the arterial blood gas shows a low Po_2 or a high Pco_2.

PULMONARY GAS EXCHANGE

The adequacy of gas exchange in the lungs is determined by the balance between pulmonary ventilation and capillary blood flow (5–8). This balance is commonly expressed as the ventilation–perfusion (V/Q) ratio. The influence of V/Q ratios on pulmonary gas exchange can be described using a schematic alveolar–capillary unit, as shown in Figure 21.1. The upper panel shows a perfect match between ventilation and perfusion; that is, a V/Q ratio of 1.0. This is the reference point for defining the abnormal patterns of gas exchange.

DEAD SPACE VENTILATION

A V/Q ratio above 1.0 (Fig. 21.1, middle panel) describes the condition where ventilation is excessive relative to capillary blood flow. The excess ventilation, known as dead space ventilation, does not participate in gas exchange with the blood. There are two types of dead space ventilation.

Anatomic dead space is the gas in the large conducting airways that does not come in contact with capillaries. Approximately 50% of the anatomic dead space is in the pharynx.

Physiologic dead space is the alveolar gas that does not equilibrate

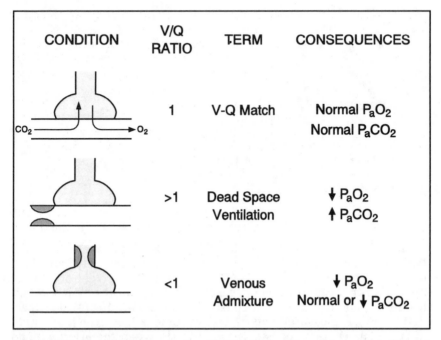

CONDITION	V/Q RATIO	TERM	CONSEQUENCES
$CO_2 \longrightarrow O_2$	1	V-Q Match	Normal P_aO_2 Normal P_aCO_2
	>1	Dead Space Ventilation	↓ P_aO_2 ↑ P_aCO_2
	<1	Venous Admixture	↓ P_aO_2 Normal or ↓ P_aCO_2

Figure 21.1. Ventilation–perfusion (V/Q) relationships and associated blood gas abnormalities.

fully with capillary blood. This represents excess *alveolar* ventilation relative to capillary blood flow. In normal subjects, dead space ventilation (Vd) accounts for 20 to 30% of the total ventilation (Vt); that is, Vd/Vt = 0.2 to 0.3 (5,7). An increase in Vd/Vt results in both hypoxemia and hypercapnia (analogous to what would happen if you held your breath). The hypercapnia usually appears when the Vd/Vt rises above 0.5 (7).

Pathophysiology

Dead space ventilation increases when the alveolar–capillary interface is destroyed (e.g., emphysema), when blood flow is reduced (e.g., heart failure, pulmonary embolism), or when alveoli are overdistended by positive-pressure ventilation.

INTRAPULMONARY SHUNT

A V/Q ratio below 1.0 (Fig. 21.1, lower panel) describes the condition where capillary blood flow is excessive relative to ventilation. The excess blood flow, known as intrapulmonary shunt, does not participate in pulmonary gas exchange. There are two types of intrapulmonary shunt.

True shunt indicates the total absence of exchange between capillary blood and alveolar gas (V/Q = zero), and is equivalent to an anatomic shunt between the right and left sides of the heart.

Venous admixture represents the capillary flow that does not equilibrate completely with alveolar gas (V̇/Q above zero but less than 1.0). As the venous admixture increases, the V/Q imbalance approaches true shunt conditions (V/Q = 0).

The fraction of the cardiac output that represents intrapulmonary shunt is known as the shunt fraction. In normal subjects, intrapulmonary shunt flow (Qs) represents less than 10% of the total cardiac output (Qt); that is, the shunt fraction (Qs/Qt) is less than 10% (5,6,8).

Pathophysiology

Intrapulmonary shunt fraction increases when the small airways are occluded (e.g., asthma, chronic bronchitis), when alveoli are filled with fluid (e.g., pulmonary edema, pneumonia) or when alveoli collapse (e.g., atelectasis), and when capillary flow is excessive (e.g., nonembolized regions of lung in pulmonary embolism).

Arterial Blood Gases

The influence of shunt fraction on arterial oxygen and carbon dioxide tensions (P_{AO_2}, Pa_{CO_2}, respectively) is shown in Figure 21.2. The P_{AO_2} falls progressively as shunt fraction increases, but the Pa_{CO_2} re-

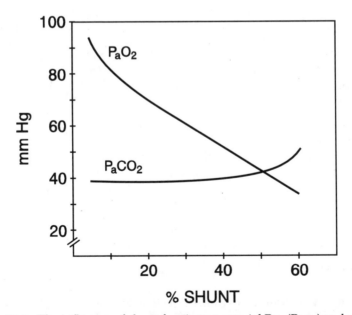

Figure 21.2. The influence of shunt fraction on arterial Po_2 (P_{AO_2}) and arterial Pco_2 (Pa_{CO_2}). (From D'Alonzo GE, Dantzger DR. Med Clin North Am 1983; 67:557–571.)

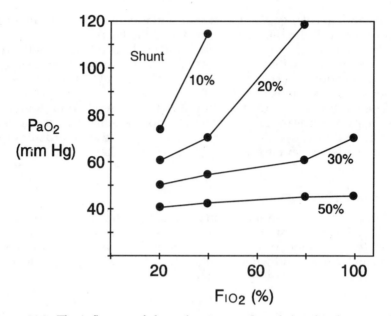

Figure 21.3. The influence of shunt fraction on the relationship between the inspired oxygen (F_{IO_2}) and the arterial P_{O_2} (P_{AO_2}). (From D'Alonzo GE, Dantzger DR. Med Clin North Am 1983;67:557–571.)

mains constant until the shunt fraction exceeds 50% (8). The P_{aCO_2} is often below normal in patients with increased intrapulmonary shunt as a result of hyperventilation from the disease process (e.g., pneumonia) or from the accompanying hypoxemia.

The shunt fraction also determines the influence of inspired oxygen on the arterial P_{O_2}. This is shown in Figure 21.3 (8). As intrapulmonary shunt increases from 10 to 50%, the increase in fractional concentration of inspired oxygen (F_{IO_2}) produces less of an increment in the arterial P_{O_2}. When the shunt fraction exceeds 50%, the P_{AO_2} is independent of changes in F_{IO_2}. This latter condition mimics the behavior of a true (anatomic) shunt.

The diminished influence of inspired oxygen on arterial P_{O_2} as shunt fractions rises has important implications for limiting the risk of pulmonary oxygen toxicity. That is, in conditions associated with a high shunt fraction (e.g., acute respiratory distress syndrome), the F_{IO_2} can often be reduced to levels considered nontoxic (i.e., F_{IO_2} below 50%) without further compromising arterial oxygenation.

QUANTITATIVE DETERMINATIONS

The following determinations can be used to identify and quantitate ventilation–perfusion abnormalities. As will be demonstrated, these determinations can prove useful in both the diagnosis and management of respiratory failure.

DEAD SPACE (VD/VT)

The determination of dead space ventilation (Vd/Vt) is based on the difference between the P_{CO_2} in exhaled gas and the P_{CO_2} in end-capillary (arterial) blood. In the normal lung, the capillary blood equilibrates fully with alveolar gas, and the exhaled P_{CO_2} (P_{ECO_2}) is roughly equivalent to the arterial P_{CO_2} (P_{aCO_2}). As dead space ventilation (Vd/Vt) increases, the P_{ECO_2} falls below the P_{aCO_2}. The Bohr equation shown below (derived by Cristian Bohr, father of Neils Bohr) is based on this principle.

$$Vd/Vt = \frac{P_{aCO_2} - P_{ECO_2}}{P_{aCO_2}} \qquad (21.1)$$

Thus, as the exhaled P_{CO_2} decreases relative to the arterial P_{CO_2}, the calculated Vd/Vt rises. The P_{ECO_2} is measured by collecting expired gas in a large collection bag and using an infrared CO_2 analyzer to measure the P_{CO_2} in a sample of the gas. This is usually done on request by the respiratory therapy department.

SHUNT FRACTION (QS/QT)

The shunt fraction (Qs/Qt) is not as easily determined as the Vd/Vt. The Qs/Qt is derived by the relationship between the O_2 content in arterial blood (C_{aO_2}), mixed venous blood (C_{vO_2}), and pulmonary capillary blood (C_{cO_2}).

$$Qs/Qt = \frac{C_{cO_2} - C_{aO_2}}{C_{cO_2} - C_{vO_2}} \qquad (21.2)$$

The problem here is the inability to measure the capillary O_2 content (C_{cO_2}) directly. As a result, pure oxygen breathing has been recommended (to produce 100% oxyhemoglobin saturation in pulmonary capillary blood) for the shunt calculation. However in this situation, Qs/Qt measures only true shunt.

THE A-a P_{O_2} GRADIENT

The P_{O_2} difference between alveolar gas and arterial blood (A-a p_{O_2} gradient) is used as an indirect measure of ventilation–perfusion abnormalities (9–11,13). The A-a p_{O_2} gradient is determined with the alveolar gas equation shown below.

$$P_{AO_2} = P_{IO_2} - (P_{aCO_2}/RQ) \qquad (21.3)$$

This equation describes the relationship between the alveolar P_{O_2} (P_{AO_2}), the P_{O_2} in inspired gas (P_{IO_2}), the alveolar (arterial) P_{CO_2}, and the respiratory quotient (RQ). The latter variable defines the proportional exchange of O_2 and CO_2 across the alveolar–capillary interface; that is, $RQ = \dot{V}_{CO_2}/\dot{V}_{O_2}$. The P_{IO_2} is a function of the fractional concentration of inspired oxygen (F_{IO_2}), the barometric pressure (P_B), and the partial pressure of water vapor (P_{H_2O}) in humidified gas; that is, $P_{IO_2} = F_{IO_2}(P_B - P_{H_2O})$. The P_{H_2O} is 47 mm Hg at body temperature.

In a healthy subject breathing room air at sea level, where $F_{IO_2} = 0.21$, $P_B = 760$ mm Hg, $P_{H_2O} = 47$ mm Hg, $P_{AO_2} = 90$ mm Hg, $P_{aCO_2} = 40$ mm Hg, and $RQ = 0.8$:

$$
\begin{aligned}
P_{AO_2} &= F_{IO_2}(P_B - P_{H_2O}) - (P_{aCO_2}/RQ) \\
&= 0.21(760 - 47) - (40/0.8) \qquad\qquad (21.4) \\
&= 100 \text{ mm Hg}
\end{aligned}
$$

Because the arterial P_{O_2} is 90 mm Hg, the A-a p_{O_2} gradient in this example is 10 mm Hg. This represents an idealized rather than normal A-a p_{O_2} gradient, because the A-a p_{O_2} gradient varies with age and with the concentration of inspired oxygen.

Influence of Age

As shown in Table 21.1, the normal A-a p_{O_2} gradient rises steadily with advancing age (10). Assuming that most patients in an adult ICU are 40 years of age or older, a normal A-a p_{O_2} gradient in an ICU patient's breathing room air may be as high as 25 mm Hg. However, few ICU patients breathe room air, and as demonstrated next, the normal A-a p_{O_2} gradient is increased during supplemental oxygen breathing.

Influence of Inspired Oxygen

The influence of inspired oxygen on the A-a p_{O_2} gradient is shown in Figure 21.4 (11). The A-a p_{O_2} gradient increases from 15 to 60 mm Hg as the F_{IO_2} increases from room air to pure oxygen. According to this relationship, **the normal A-a p_{O_2} gradient increases 5 to 7 mm**

TABLE 21.1. NORMAL ARTERIAL BLOOD GASES			
Age (years)	P_{aO_2} (mm Hg)	P_{aCO_2} (mm Hg)	A-a P_{O_2} (mm Hg)
20	84–95	33–47	4–17
30	81–92	34–47	7–21
40	78–90	34–47	10–24
50	75–87	34–47	14–27
60	72–84	34–47	17–31
70	70–81	34–47	21–34
80	67–79	34–47	25–38

All values pertain to room air breathing at sea level.
From the Intermountain Thoracic Society Manual of Uniform Laboratory Procedures. Salt Lake City, 1984;44–45.

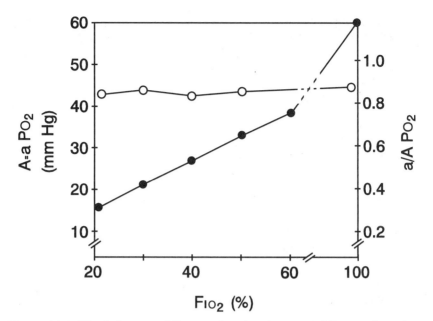

Figure 21.4. The influence of F_{IO_2} on the alveolar-arterial P_{O_2} gradient (A-a p_{O_2}) and the arterial-alveolar P_{O_2} ratio (a/A P_{O_2}) in normal subjects. (From Gilbert R, Kreighley JF. Am Rev Respir Dis 1974;109:142–145.)

Hg for every 10% increase in F_{IO_2}. This effect is presumably caused by the loss of regional hypoxic vasoconstriction in the lungs. Hypoxic vasoconstriction in poorly ventilated lung regions can serve to maintain V/Q balance by diverting blood to more adequately ventilated lung regions. Loss of this regional hypoxic vasoconstriction during supplemental oxygen breathing increases blood flow in poorly ventilated lung regions. This increases the intrapulmonary shunt fraction and thereby increases the A-a p_{O_2} gradient.

Positive-Pressure Ventilation

Positive-pressure mechanical ventilation elevates the pressure in the airways above the ambient barometric pressure. Therefore, when determining the A-a p_{O_2} gradient in a ventilator-dependent patient, the mean airway pressure should be added to the barometric pressure (12). In the example presented previously, a mean airway pressure of 30 cm H_2O would increase the A-a p_{O_2} gradient from 10 to 16 mm Hg (a 60% increase in the A-a p_{O_2} gradient). Although this correction is necessary for optimal accuracy in determining the A-a p_{O_2} gradient, the clinical significance is unproven.

THE a/A P_{O_2} RATIO

Unlike the A-a p_{O_2} gradient, the a/A P_{O_2} ratio is relatively unaffected by the F_{IO_2}. This is demonstrated in Figure 21.4 (11). The independence of the a/A Po_2 gradient in relation to the Fio_2 is explained by the equation below.

$$a/A \ Po_2 = 1 - (A-a \ po_2)/P_{AO_2} \qquad (21.5)$$

Because the alveolar Po_2 is in both the numerator and denominator of the equation, the influence of Fio_2 on the P_{AO_2} is eliminated. Thus, the a/A Po_2 ratio is a mathematical manipulation that eliminates the influence of Fio_2 on the A-a gradient. The normal a/A Po_2 ratios during room air and pure oxygen breathing are shown below (11).

Fio_2	Normal a/A Po_2
0.21	0.74 to 0.77
1.0	0.80 to 0.82

THE Pao_2/Fio_2 RATIO

Another simple determination that can correlate with shunt fraction is the ratio of arterial Po_2 to Fio_2. The following correlations have been reported (13).

Pao_2/Fio_2	Qs/Qt
< 200	> 20%
> 200	< 20%

The major limitation of the P_{AO_2}/Fio_2 ratio is the variability of the Fio_2 in patients receiving oxygen via nasal prongs or face mask (see Chapter 23). This limitation also applies to the A-a po_2 gradient.

BLOOD GAS VARIABILITY

The very first step in the approach to managing hypoxemia and hypercapnia is defining what constitutes an abnormal change in the arterial Po_2 and Pco_2. The information in Table 21.2 is relevant to this issue. The data in this table are from a study of 26 clinically stable, ventilator-dependent trauma victims who each had a series of four arterial blood gas measurements performed over a 1-hour period (14). The variability in the arterial Po_2 and Pco_2 for all patients is presented

TABLE 21.2. SPONTANEOUS BLOOD GAS VARIABILITY		
Variation	**Pao_2**	**$Paco_2$**
Mean	13 mm Hg	2.5 mm Hg
95th Percentile	±18 mm Hg	±4 mm Hg
Range	2–37 mm Hg	0–12 mm Hg

Represents variation over a 1-hour period in 26 ventilator-dependent trauma victims who were clinically stable.
From Hess D, Agarwal NN. J Clin Monitor 1992;8:111.

in the table. The arterial Po_2 varied by as much as 36 mm Hg, whereas the arterial Pco_2 varied by as much as 12 mm Hg. This variability is similar to that reported in another study involving patients in a medical ICU (15).

The variability in measured blood gas variables shown in Table 21.2 highlights the following two important points.

1. **Routine monitoring of arterial blood gases** (without a change in the clinical condition of the patient) is not warranted and often yields misleading information.
2. **A change in arterial Po_2 and Pco_2 on routine blood gas analysis is not necessarily abnormal** if the clinical condition of the patient has not changed. This should be considered before a lengthy and time-consuming search for something that may not be found is initiated.

HYPOXEMIA

When a blood gas showing a significant reduction in the arterial Po_2 is encountered, there are three principal disorders to consider (5,8,16,17). These are shown in Table 21.3, along with the measurements that will help identify each disorder. Note that one of the causes of hypoxemia is an imbalance between oxygen delivery and oxygen uptake in the systemic circulation (Do_2/Vo_2 imbalance). In this situation, the peripheral O_2 extraction is increased (due to a low O_2 delivery or an increased O_2 uptake) and the mixed venous Po_2 is reduced. The relationship between the mixed venous Po_2 and the arterial Po_2 is described below.

MIXED VENOUS Po_2

The oxygen in arterial blood represents the sum of the oxygen in mixed venous (pulmonary artery) blood and the oxygen added from alveolar gas. When gas exchange is normal, the Po_2 in alveolar gas is the major determinant of the arterial Po_2. However when gas exchange is impaired, the contribution of the alveolar Po_2 declines and the contribution of the mixed venous Po_2 rises (17). If gas exchange declines to zero, the venous Po_2 is the sole determinant of the arterial Po_2.

TABLE 21.3. EVALUATION OF HYPOXEMIA		
Disorder	A-a Po_2	Pvo_2
Hypoventilation	Normal	Normal
Pulmonary disorder	Increased	Normal
Do_2/Vo_2 imbalance	Increased	Decreased

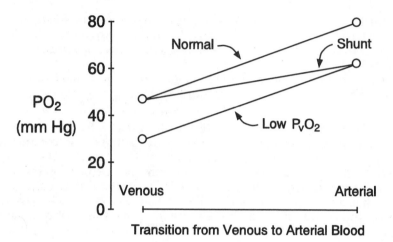

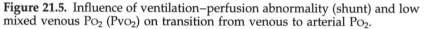

Transition from Venous to Arterial Blood

Figure 21.5. Influence of ventilation–perfusion abnormality (shunt) and low mixed venous Po_2 (Pvo_2) on transition from venous to arterial Po_2.

The diagram in Figure 21.5 illustrates how hypoxemia can result from either a gas exchange abnormality or a low mixed venous Po_2. The graph shows the transition from venous Po_2 to arterial Po_2 in normal, increased shunt fraction, and low venous Po_2 conditions. The slope of the transition curve is determined by the efficiency of oxygen exchange from alveoli to capillary blood. Abnormal gas exchange therefore reduces the slope of the curve, as indicated by the curve for increased intrapulmonary shunt. When the mixed venous Po_2 is reduced and the slope of the transition curve is normal (i.e., normal gas exchange), the arterial Po_2 is decreased to the same degree as seen when intrapulmonary shunt is increased. This illustrates how a low mixed venous Po_2 can be the source of decreased arterial Po_2.

Shunt Fraction

The influence of the mixed venous Po_2 on the arterial Po_2 is determined by the degree of intrapulmonary shunt. In the normal lung, decreases in venous Po_2 have relatively little effect on the arterial Po_2. However, as shunt fraction increases, changes in venous Po_2 begin to affect the arterial Po_2. If shunt fraction is increased to 100%, the venous Po_2 is the sole determinant of the arterial Po_2. Thus, **in pulmonary conditions associated with a high shunt fraction**, such as pulmonary edema or pneumonia, **the mixed venous Po_2 is an important consideration in the evaluation of hypoxemia** (5,8,17).

DIAGNOSTIC EVALUATION

The search for the source of hypoxemia in the individual patient can proceed according to the flow diagram in Figure 21.6. This approach

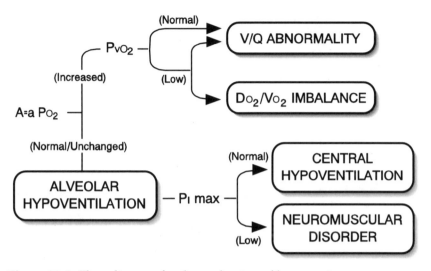

Figure 21.6. Flow diagram for the evaluation of hypoxemia.

requires a measurement of the Po_2 in superior vena cava or pulmonary artery blood, and thus it applies only to patients who have indwelling central venous or pulmonary artery catheters.

Step 1: A-a Po_2 Gradient

The first step in the approach involves a determination of the A-a po_2 gradient. After correcting for age and Fio_2, the A-a po_2 gradient can be interpreted as follows:

> *Normal A-a po_2:* Indicates a generalized hypoventilation disorder rather than a cardiopulmonary disorder. In this situation, the most likely problems are drug-induced respiratory depression and neuromuscular weakness. The latter condition can be uncovered by measuring the maximum inspiratory pressure (Pimax). This measurement is described in the upcoming section on hypercapnia.
>
> *Increased A-a po_2:* Indicates a V/Q abnormality (cardiopulmonary disorder) and/or a systemic Do_2/Vo_2 imbalance. When the A-a po_2 gradient is increased, a mixed venous Po_2 (or central venous Po_2) is needed to identify a systemic Do_2/Vo_2 imbalance.

Step 2: Mixed Venous Po_2

When the A-a gradient is increased, obtain a blood sample from the distal port of a pulmonary artery catheter or from a central venous catheter (superior vena cava blood). The Po_2 in either blood sample can be interpreted as follows:

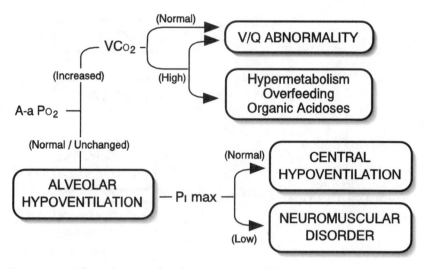

Figure 21.7. Flow diagram for the evaluation of hypercapnia.

Normal venous P_{O_2}: Indicates that the problem is solely a V/Q abnormality in the lungs. If the venous P_{O_2} is 40 mm Hg or higher, then the lungs may be the source of the hypoxemia. If a chest x-ray examination is unrevealing, an acute pulmonary embolism should be considered. *Low venous* P_{O_2}: Indicates a systemic D_{O_2}/V_{O_2} imbalance (i.e., a low D_{O_2} or a high V_{O_2}). A mixed venous P_{O_2} below 40 mm Hg indicates either a decreased rate of oxygen delivery (anemia, low cardiac output) or an increased rate of oxygen consumption (hypermetabolism).

Thus, the approach outlined above and shown in Figure 21.7 uses three variables (A-a p_{O_2} gradient, $P_{I}max$, and $P_{V_{O_2}}$) to pinpoint the source of hypoxemia. Although this approach does not identify the disease process, it helps focus the search for the responsible illness.

HYPERCAPNIA

The evaluation of hypercapnia (Pa_{CO_2} above 46 mm Hg) proceeds in a very similar fashion to the hypoxemia evaluation. Before beginning the evaluation, the increase in arterial P_{CO_2} must not be a compensatory response to metabolic alkalosis (see Chapter 36). If this is not the case, then proceed as described below.

CAUSES OF HYPERCAPNIA

The carbon dioxide level in arterial blood (Pa_{CO_2}) is directly proportional to the rate of CO_2 production by oxidative metabolism (V_{CO_2}) and inversely proportional to the rate of CO_2 elimination by alveolar ventilation (VA) (5,18). Therefore, $Paco_2 = k \times (Vco_2/VA)$, where k is the proportionality constant. Alveolar ventilation is the fraction of the total expired ventilation (VE) that is not dead space ventilation (Vd/Vt); that is, $VA = VE (1 - Vd/Vt)$. Therefore, the above relationship can be rewritten as follows:

$$Paco_2 = k \times [Vco_2/VE (1 - Vd/Vt)] \tag{21.6}$$

This equation identifies **three major sources of hypercapnia:** (*a*) increased CO_2 production (Vco_2), (*b*) hypoventilation (VE), and (*c*) increased dead space ventilation (Vd/Vt).

Increased CO_2 production (e.g., from hypermetabolism) is normally accompanied by an increase in minute ventilation. The ventilatory response serves to eliminate the excess CO_2 and maintain a constant arterial Pco_2. Therefore, excess CO_2 production does not normally cause hypercapnia. However when CO_2 excretion is impaired by an increase in dead space ventilation, an increase in CO_2 production can result in an increase in the arterial Pco_2. Thus, increased CO_2 production is an important factor in promoting hypercapnia only in patients with underlying lung disease.

DIAGNOSTIC EVALUATION

The bedside evaluation of hypercapnia is strikingly similar to the evaluation of hypoxemia. The flow diagram for the evaluation is shown in Figure 21.7 (note the similarities between Figures 21.6 and 21.7). As was the case with hypoxemia, the evaluation begins with the A-a po_2 gradient (19). An increased A-a gradient indicates an increase in dead space ventilation (i.e., a pulmonary disorder), possibly complicated by an increase in CO_2 production. A normal or unchanged A-a po_2 gradient indicates that the problem is alveolar hypoventilation.

CO_2 Production

The rate of CO_2 production (Vco_2) can be measured at the bedside with specialized *metabolic carts* that are normally used to perform nutritional assessments. These instruments use infrared light to measure the CO_2 in expired gas (much like the end-tidal CO_2 monitors described in Chapter 22), and they provide a measure of total CO_2 excreted per minute. In steady-state conditions, the rate of CO_2 excretion is equivalent to the Vco_2. The **normal Vco_2 is 90 to 130 L/minute/m²**, which is roughly 80% of the Vo_2 (see Table 2.4). An increased Vco_2 is evidence for one of the following abnormalities: generalized hypermetabolism, overfeeding (excess calories, or organic acidoses.

Overfeeding, or the provision of calories in excess of daily needs, is a recognized cause of hypercapnia in patients with severe lung disease and acute respiratory failure (20). Nutrition-associated hypercapnia has been reported predominantly in ventilator-dependent patients and can delay weaning from mechanical ventilation (22). Thus, overfeeding should be considered as a possible cause of CO_2 retention in any patient in the ICU with respiratory impairment, and particularly in patients who require mechanical ventilation. This possibility can be investigated by asking the nutrition support team to measure the V_{CO_2} at the bedside.

ALVEOLAR HYPOVENTILATION

The causes of alveolar hypoventilation that are most likely to be encountered in the ICU are listed in Table 21.4. The most common causes in the ICU are drug-induced respiratory depression and neuromuscular weakness.

Respiratory Muscle Weakness

Possible causes of neuromuscular weakness in patients in the ICU include shock, multiorgan failure, prolonged neuromuscular blockade, electrolyte abnormalities, and cardiac surgery (phrenic nerve injury). Critical illness itself may damage peripheral nerves and produce a syndrome known as critical illness polyneuropathy (21) that can be associated with profound generalized weakness and delayed weaning from mechanical ventilation. This and other sources of neuromuscular weakness in patients in the ICU are described in Chapter 51.

The standard measurement for evaluating respiratory muscle strength is the maximum inspiratory pressure (PImax), which is obtained by having the patient make a maximum inspiratory effort from functional residual capacity (FRC) against a closed valve. The normal PImax depends on both age and sex, and it can vary widely in individual patients. However, most healthy adults have a PImax above 80 cm H_2O (22). **Carbon dioxide retention develops when the PImax falls to less than 40% of normal values** (23).

Central Hypoventilation Syndromes

Hypoventilation without evidence of respiratory muscle weakness indicates possible drug-induced respiratory depression. Opiates (and

TABLE 21.4. ALVEOLAR HYPOVENTILATION IN THE ICU	
Brainstem depression	1. Drugs (e.g., opiates)
	2. Obesity
Neuropathic disorders	1. Critical illness polyneuropathy
	2. Phrenic nerve injury (cardiac surgery)
	3. Shock/multiorgan failure
	4. Myasthenia/Guillain-Barré
Myopathic disorders	1. Prolonged paralysis
	2. Hypophosphatemia
	3. Magnesium depletion
	4. Low cardiac output (diaphragm)

benzodiazepine in the elderly) are the most likely offenders. Hypoventilation without apparent cause in an obese patient may be the result of a chronic and poorly understood disorder known as obesity-hypoventilation syndrome (OHS). Hypoventilation without apparent cause in a lean patient, known as primary alveolar hypoventilation, is rare.

REFERENCES

GENERAL TEXTS

Grippi MA , ed. Pulmonary pathophysiology. Philadelphia: JB Lippincott, 1995.

Sutton JR, Coates G, Remmers JE, eds. Hypoxia: the adaptations. Philadelphia: BC Decker, 1990.

West JB. Ventilation/blood flow and gas exchange. 5th ed. Philadelphia: JB Lippincott, 1990.

Zander R, Mertzlufft F, eds. The oxygen status of arterial blood. Basel, Switzerland: S. Karger Publishers, 1991.

INTRODUCTION

1. Raffin TA. Indications for blood gas analysis. Ann Intern Med 1986;105: 390–398.
2. Maukkassa FF, Rutledge R, Fakhry SM, et al. ABGs and arterial lines: the relationship to unnecessarily drawn arterial blood gas samples. J Trauma 1990; 30:1087–1095.
3. Shapiro BA, Mahutte CK, Cane RD, Gilmour IJ. Clinical performance of an arterial blood gas monitor. Crit Care Med 1993;21:487–494.
4. Zimmerman JL, Dellinger RP. Initial evaluation of a new intra-arterial blood gas system in humans. Crit Care Med 1993;21:495–500.

PULMONARY GAS EXCHANGE

5. Dantzger DR. Pulmonary gas exchange. In: Dantzger DR, ed. Cardiopulmonary critical care. 2nd ed. Philadelphia: WB Saunders, 1991;25–43.
6. Lanken PN. Ventilation-perfusion relationships. In: Grippi MA, ed. Pulmonary pathophysiology. Philadelphia: JB Lippincott, 1995;195–210.
7. Buohuys A. Respiratory dead space. In: Fenn WO, Rahn H, eds. Handbook of physiology: respiration. Bethesda: American Physiological Society, 1964; 699–714.
8. D'Alonzo GE, Dantzger DR. Mechanisms of abnormal gas exchange. Med Clin North Am 1983;67:557–571.

QUANTITATIVE DETERMINATIONS

9. Tobin MJ. Respiratory monitoring during mechanical ventilation. Crit Care Clin 1990;6:679–709.
10. Harris EA, Kenyon AM, Nisbet HD, et al. The normal alveolar-arterial oxygen tension gradient in man. Clin Sci 1974;46:89–104.

11. Gilbert R, Kreighley JF. The arterial/alveolar oxygen tension ratio. An index of gas exchange applicable to varying inspired oxygen concentrations. Am Rev Resp Dis 1974;109:142–145.
12. Carroll GC. Misapplication of the alveolar gas equation. N Engl J Med 1985; 312:586.
13. Covelli HD, Nessan VJ, Tuttle WK. Oxygen derived variables in acute respiratory failure. Crit Care Med 1983;11:646–649.

BLOOD GAS VARIABILITY

14. Hess D, Agarwal NN. Variability of blood gases, pulse oximeter saturation, and end-tidal carbon dioxide pressure in stable, mechanically ventilated trauma patients. J Clin Monit 1992;8:111–115.
15. Sasse SA, Chen P, Mahutte CK. Variability of arterial blood gas values over time in stable medical ICU patients. Chest 1994;106:187–193.

HYPOXEMIA

16. Kreimeier U, Mesmer K. The differential diagnosis of arterial hypoxemia. In: Zander R, Mertzlufft F, eds. The oxygen status of arterial blood. Basel, Switzerland: S. Karger Publishers, 1991;196–202.
17. Rossaint R, Hahn S-M, Pappert D, et al. Influence of mixed venous Po_2 and inspired oxygen fraction on intrapulmonary shunt in patients with severe ARDS. J Appl Physiol. 1995;78:1531–1536.

HYPERCAPNIA

18. Weinberger SE, Schwartzstein RM, Weiss JW. Hypercapnia. N Engl J Med 1989;321:1223–1230.
19. Gray BA, Blalock JM. Interpretation of the alveolar-arterial oxygen difference in patients with hypercapnia. Am Rev Respir Dis 1991;143:4–8.
20. Talpers SS, Romberger DJ, Bunce SB, Pingleton SK. Nutritionally associated increased carbon dioxide production. Chest 1992;102:551–555.
21. Wijdicks EFM, Litchy WJ, Harrison BA, Gracey DR. The clinical spectrum of critical illness polyneuropathy. Mayo Clin Proc 1994;69:955–959.
22. Bruschi C, Cerveri I, Zoia MC, et al. Reference values for maximum respiratory mouth pressures: A population-based study. Am Rev Respir Dis 1992;146: 790–793.
23. Baydur A. Respiratory muscle strength and control of ventilation in patients with neuromuscular disease. Chest 1991;99:330–338.

chapter

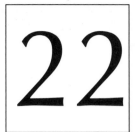

OXIMETRY AND CAPNOGRAPHY

The noninvasive detection of arterial blood gases using optical and colorimetric techniques (1–6) is the most significant advance in critical care monitoring in the last quarter-century. This chapter describes the techniques that have become an integral part of daily patient care in the ICU. Despite their routine use, surveys indicate that 95% of staff physicians and staff nurses working in ICUs have little or no understanding of how these techniques work (7).

DEFINITIONS

All atoms and molecules reflect specific wavelengths of light (this is the source of color in the lighted world). Spectrophotometry is an optical detection method that uses the light reflection properties of molecules to measure the concentration of chemical species in a gaseous or liquid environment. When spectrophotometry is applied to the detection of oxygenated and deoxygenated hemoglobin, the method is known as oximetry. The optical detection of carbon dioxide is known as capnometry. The term *capnography* refers to the optically recorded pattern of CO_2 excretion in single-breath exhalations.

OXIMETRY

Hemoglobin (like all proteins) changes its structural configuration when it participates in a chemical reaction, and each of the configurations has a different pattern of light reflection. The patterns of light reflection associated with oxygenated hemoglobin (HbO_2) and deoxygenated hemoglobin (Hb) are shown in Figure 22.1. At wavelengths of 660 nanometers (nm), which corresponds to the red region of the light spectrum, oxygenated hemoglobin (HbO_2) reflects light more effectively than deoxygenated hemoglobin (Hb). (This explains why oxygenated blood is more intensely red than deoxygenated blood.)

355

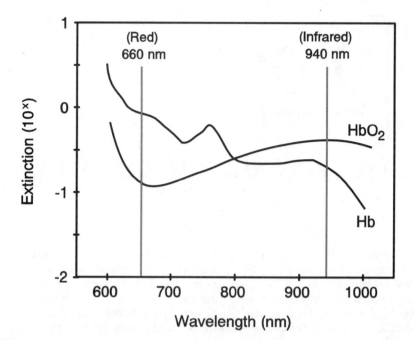

Figure 22.1. The pattern of light reflection by oxygenated hemoglobin (HbO_2) and deoxygenated hemoglobin (Hb). The vertical lines represent the two wavelengths of light (660 nm and 940 nm) used by pulse oximeters. (From the Ohmeda Biox 3700 Pulse Oximeter Operating and Maintenance Manual. Louisville, CO: BOC Health Care, 1988;1–2.)

This relationship is reversed at 940 nm (the infrared spectrum), where Hb reflects light more effectively than HbO_2. Thus, when both wavelengths of light are passed through a sample of blood, the intensity of light transmission at 660 nm is primarily a function of the concentration of HbO_2 in the sample, whereas the transmission at 940 nm is determined primarily by the concentration of Hb. The concentrations of HbO_2 and Hb are expressed in relative terms, that is, as the fraction of hemoglobin that is in the oxygenated form. This is known as the percent oxyhemoglobin saturation (% saturation), and is derived as follows:

$$\% \text{ Saturation} = (HbO_2/HbO_2 + Hb) \times 100 \qquad (22.1)$$

Limitations

The use of two wavelengths of light to derive the fractional concentration of HbO_2 is based on the assumption that other forms of hemoglobin such as methemoglobin (metHb) and carboxyhemoglobin (COHb) have a negligible contribution to the total hemoglobin pool. In most situations, less than 5% of hemoglobin is present as COHb and metHb (3,4,6), so the assumption is valid. However, in conditions associated with an increase in COHb (e.g., smoke inhalation) or metHb (e.g., high-dose nitroglycerin), the exclusion of these forms of hemoglobin leads to falsely high estimates of the prevalence of HbO_2 (% saturation).

TYPES OF OXIMETRY

Oximetry can be performed both in vivo and in vitro. There are two in vivo techniques. One uses probes placed on the surface of the skin to measure the O_2 saturation in the underlying blood vessels. The other uses a pulmonary artery catheter to measure the O_2 saturation in mixed venous (pulmonary artery) blood.

Ear Oximetry

Oximeters capable of continuous, on-line monitoring of arterial oxygen saturation (Sao_2) at the bedside were introduced in the 1960s. The original devices were placed on the earlobes. The oximeter probe consisted of a phototransmitter situated on one side of the earlobe that emitted red and infrared light waves, and a photodetector situated on the opposite skin surface to record light transmission through the intervening tissue. These early oximeters suffered from two major limitations. First, the transmission of light was affected by factors other than hemoglobin, such as earlobe thickness and skin pigments. The second problem was the inability to differentiate between hemoglobin in arteries and veins.

Pulse Oximetry

The problems encountered with the early ear oximeters were largely eliminated with the introduction of pulse oximetry in the mid-1970s. The principle of pulse oximetry is illustrated in Figure 22.2 (3–6). Arterial pulsations are associated with changes in blood volume that produce phasic changes in the intensity of transmitted light. The photodetectors in pulse oximeters are designed to sense only light of alternating intensity (analogous to AC amplifiers, which process only alternating-current electrical impulses). This eliminates errors created by light reflection in nonpulsatile structures such as extravascular tissues and (nonpulsating) veins.

Co-Oximeters

In vitro oximetry is performed with instruments called co-oximeters that transmit four wavelengths of light through a blood sample. These devices are capable of detecting methemoglobin and carboxyhemoglobin (in addition to Hb and HbO_2), but do not provide the continuous monitoring available with pulse oximeters.

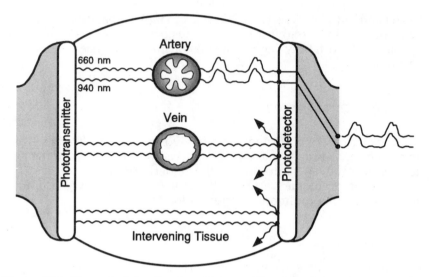

Figure 22.2. The principle of pulse oximetry. The photodetector senses only light of alternating intensity (analogous to an AC amplifier).

Mixed Venous Oximetry

The O_2 saturation in mixed venous (pulmonary artery) blood can be measured continuously with specialized pulmonary artery catheters that emit red and infrared light from the catheter tip and record the light reflected back from the hemoglobin in circulating erythrocytes. This technique is called *reflectance* spectrophotometry, whereas pulse oximeters and co-oximeters use *transmission* spectrophotometry.

PULSE OXIMETRY

As mentioned previously, **pulse oximeters record light transmission through pulsating arteries only.** Like the early ear oximeters, pulse oximeters use two wavelengths of light, one in the red spectrum (660 nm) and the other in the infrared spectrum (940 nm). Pulse oximetry probes are usually placed on the fingers.

Accuracy

At clinically acceptable levels of arterial oxygenation (Sao_2 above 70%), the O_2 saturation recorded by pulse oximeters (Spo_2) differs by less than 3% from the actual Sao_2 (measured by co-oximeters) (3–6). Spo_2 also shows a high degree of precision (consistency of repeated measurements). This is demonstrated in Table 22.1, which shows the spontaneous variation in Spo_2 over a 1-hour period in ventilator-dependent patients who appeared clinically stable (8). The variation in

TABLE 22.1. VARIABILITY IN OXIMETRY AND CAPNOMETRY RECORDINGS			
Study Parameters	Spo_2*	Svo_2**	Petco_2*
Time period	60 min	120 min	60 min
Mean variation	1%	6%	2 mm Hg
95th percentile	±2%	—	±3 mm Hg
Range of variation	0–5%	1–19%	0–7 mm Hg

Clinically stable patients. 95% of the measurements were obtained during mechanical ventilation.
* From Hess D, Agarwal NN (8).
** From Noll ML et al. (21).

Spo_2 was 2% or less in 95% of cases, indicating that there is little random variability (or random error) in pulse oximeter recordings.

COMMON CONCERNS ABOUT Spo_2

A number of conditions are cited as sources of erroneous pulse oximetry recordings, and some of these are listed in Table 22.2.

Dyshemoglobinemias

As mentioned, oximeters that use two wavelengths of light are not reliable when hemoglobin forms other than HbO_2 and Hb are elevated. Carboxyhemoglobin (COHb) reflects as much red light as HbO_2, which explains the cherry red color of blood in carbon monoxide intoxication. Pulse oximeters therefore record COHb as HbO_2, and Spo_2 then overestimates the actual Sao_2 (3,4,6). The same error occurs with high levels of methemoglobin (metHb): Spo_2 rarely falls below 85% in methemoglobinemia despite much lower levels of Sao_2 (6). Thus, **pulse oxime-**

TABLE 22.2. ACCURACY OF PULSE OXIMETRY RECORDING (Spo_2)		
Condition	Accuracy of Spo_2	Reference
$\text{Sao}_2 > 70\%$	98% correlation between Spo_2 and Sao_2.	6
Dyshemoglobinemia • COHb • metHb	Spo_2 unreliable (spuriously high).	6
Hypotension	Spo_2 accurate down to blood pressure of 30 mm Hg.	9
Anemia	Spo_2 accurate down to Hb of 3 g/dL.	11
Skin pigmentation • Melanin • Bilirubin	Spo_2 usually accurate, but occasional false reductions with very dark skin.	12
Fingernail polish	Blue or black hues can cause 3–5% false reduction in Spo_2.	13

try should not be used when methemoglobinemia or carbon monoxide intoxication is suspected. Accurate measurements of COHb, metHb, and Sao_2 are provided only by four-wavelength co-oximeters.

Hypotension

Although pulse oximetry is based on the presence of pulsatile blood flow, Spo_2 is an accurate reflection of Sao_2 down to blood pressures as low as 30 mm Hg (9). Damped pulsations also do not affect the accuracy of fingertip Spo_2 recordings when the radial artery is cannulated (10).

Anemia

In the absence of hypoxemia, pulse oximetry is accurate down to hemoglobin levels as low as 2 to 3 g/dL (11). With lesser degrees of anemia (Hb between 2.5 and 9 g/dL), Spo_2 underestimates Sao_2 by only 0.5% (11).

Pigments

Skin pigmentation (bilirubin or melanin) usually does not affect the accuracy of pulse oximetry. However, Spo_2 can be spuriously low in patients with very dark skin (12). Fingernail polish containing blue and black colors can result in spurious decreases of 3 to 5% in Spo_2 (6,13). Onychomycosis (a fungal infection of the fingernails) can result in a similar 3- to 5% decrease in Spo_2 relative to Sao_2 (14). The largest pigment effect is produced by methylene blue, which can produce a 65% decrease in Spo_2 when injected intravenously (6). Because methylene blue is used to treat methemoglobinemia (see Chapter 18), this is another reason to avoid pulse oximetry in patients with methemoglobinemia.

WHEN TO USE PULSE OXIMETRY

Pulse oximetry offers several advantages over conventional arterial blood gases for monitoring arterial O_2 saturation:

More accurate determination of arterial O_2 saturation (15)
Superior detection of hypoxemic episodes (6)
Noninvasive, less involved
Less morbidity, greater patient satisfaction
Less expensive (16)

Pulse oximetry is thus superior to blood gases in every aspect of performance. In fact, Sao_2 from arterial blood gases is not a measured variable, but rather is derived from a nomogram, and this derived parameter has been shown to be much less accurate than the measurement provided by pulse oximetry (15). The value of pulse oximetry has been recognized by the American Society of Anesthesiologists in a formal statement recommending pulse oximetry as a routine measure during and immediately after general anesthesia (17,18). A similar recommendation seems warranted **for all patients receiving supplemental oxygen in the ICU.**

Detection of Hypoxemia

At least 15 clinical studies attest to the superiority of pulse oximetry over periodic blood gas measurements for detecting episodes of significant hypoxemia in critically ill patients (6). However, these studies also reveal that **the enhanced detection of hypoxemic episodes with pulse oximetry has no impact on either morbidity or mortality** (6). This is not the fault of pulse oximetry, but may be the fault of those who continually emphasize the largely undocumented dangers of hypoxemia (discussed in more detail in Chapter 24).

Limitation

One limitation of pulse oximetry that deserves mention is the insensitivity of the Sa_{O_2} for detecting abnormalities in pulmonary gas exchange (19). This is explained by the shape of the oxyhemoglobin dissociation curve. When Sa_{O_2} exceeds 90% (arterial oxygen pressure [Pa_{O_2}] above 60 mm Hg), the curve is flat, and large changes in Pa_{O_2} are associated with small changes in Sa_{O_2}. Thus, Sa_{O_2} is not a sensitive marker of changes in pulmonary gas exchange in the range where Sa_{O_2} is usually maintained.

MIXED VENOUS OXIMETRY

The continuous measurement of O_2 saturation in mixed venous (pulmonary artery) blood is performed with specialized PA catheters (manufactured by Baxter Health Care, Santa Ana, CA and Abbot Critical Care, North Chicago, IL) equipped with fiberoptic bundles that can transmit light to and from the catheter tip. The optical detection of mixed venous O_2 saturation (Sv_{O_2}) is performed by reflection spectrophotometry. Wavelengths of light similar to those used in pulse oximetry are passed along fiberoptic bundles in the PA catheter and out from the catheter tip. The light beam is transmitted through the circulating blood, and the light that comes in contact with hemoglobin in the circulating erythrocytes is reflected back to the catheter tip. This light is then transmitted back through the catheter to a photodetector and microprocessor that record the average Sv_{O_2} at 5-second intervals.

Reliability

Sv_{O_2} measured by PA catheters is within 1.5% of the Sv_{O_2} measured by co-oximeters (the latter being the gold standard) (20). Although accuracy seems acceptable, Svo_2 can vary considerably without a change in hemodynamic status. The spontaneous variability of Svo_2 is shown in Table 22.1. The average variation over a 2-hour period is 6%, but it can be as high as 19% (21). For practical purposes, **a greater than 5% variation in Svo_2 that persists for longer than 10 minutes is considered a significant change** (22). Svo_2 is normally between 65 and 75% (21).

Clinical Uses

Svo_2 is a marker of the balance between (whole body) O_2 delivery and O_2 consumption; that is, $Svo_2 = Do_2/Vo_2$. If Do_2 and Vo_2 are broken down into their component parts (see Chapter 2), the determinants of Svo_2 can be expressed as follows:

$$Svo_2 = (Q/Vo_2) \times Hb \times Sao_2 \qquad (22.2)$$

(where Q is cardiac output and Hb is the hemoglobin concentration in whole blood). Thus, Svo_2 varies in the same direction with changes in cardiac output, hemoglobin, and arterial O_2 saturation, and varies in the opposite direction to changes in Vo_2. A change in Svo_2 thus signals a change in any one or more of the four variables in the Svo_2 equation. Identifying the culprit then requires the appropriate measurements.

Thus, **continuous monitoring of Svo_2 provides a general screening method for monitoring a group of four variables (Q, Hb, Sao_2, and Vo_2).** A change in the Svo_2 cannot be interpreted in isolation, but should serve as a trigger to perform other measurements to identify the problem.

Dual Oximetry

The predictive value of Svo_2 can be increased by adding the Spo_2 (Sao_2) measurement provided by pulse oximetry. This creates a continuous measure of whole body O_2 extraction (i.e., $Sao_2 - Svo_2$), known as dual oximetry (23). The Svo_2 equation can be rearranged as follows to define the determinants of whole body O_2 extraction:

$$Sao_2 - Svo_2 = Vo_2/Q \times Hb \qquad (22.3)$$

Thus, Sao_2–Svo_2 changes in the same direction as the changes in the metabolic rate (Vo_2), and changes in the opposite direction to the changes in cardiac output and hemoglobin. This is the basis for the interpretations shown in Table 22.3. For more on O_2 extraction, see Chapters 2 and 11.

COLORIMETRIC CO_2 DETECTOR

The colorimetric detection of CO_2 in exhaled gas with a disposable device, such as the one shown in Figure 22.3, has become a standard

TABLE 22.3. DUAL OXIMETRY	
(Sao_2–Svo_2)	Interpretation
20–30%	Normal range
30–50	Low cardiac output
	Anemia
	Hypermetabolism
>50–60	High risk of dysoxia
	Transfusion trigger

method for determining the success or failure of endotracheal intubation (24,25). The central ovoid area of the device contains filter paper impregnated with a pH-sensitive indicator that changes color as a function of pH. When exhaled gas passes over the filter paper, the CO_2 in the gas is hydrated by a liquid film on the filter paper, and the resulting pH is detected by a color change. The outer perimeter of the device contains color-coded areas that indicate different concentrations of CO_2. The absence of CO_2 is indicated by a purple color (the color of the "check" area on the device), and a yellow color indicates a CO_2 concentration in excess of 2% (area C on the device). Thus, when the device is attached to an endotracheal tube immediately after intubation, a yellow color in the central area indicates successful tube placement in the upper airways, whereas a purple color indicates that the tube is probably in the esophagus (the *probably* will be explained shortly).

PREDICTIVE VALUE

The accuracy of this colorimetric device for predicting the success of endotracheal intubation is shown in Table 22.4 (24). For patients who are not in cardiac arrest, failure of the central area to turn yellow always indicates that the tube is not in the airways (i.e., sensitivity of

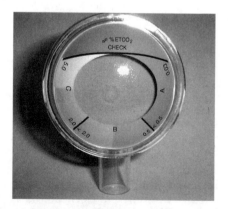

Figure 22.3. A disposable device (Easy Cap, Nellcor Puritan Bennett) for the colorimetric detection of CO_2 in exhaled gas.

TABLE 22.4. PREDICTIVE VALUE OF COLORIMETRIC CO$_2$ DETECTION FOR ENDOTRACHEAL INTUBATION

Clinical Setting	Patients	Sensitivity	Specificity
No cardiac arrest	137	100%	86%
Cardiac arrest	103	72	100
Data from MacLeod BA et al. (24).			

the color change = 100%). However, in the setting of a cardiac arrest, the CO$_2$ in exhaled gas may be too low to produce a yellow color change (the sensitivity is only 72%). Therefore, **for intubations during cardiac arrest, the lack of an appropriate color change (to yellow) does not always indicate improper tube placement.**

According to Table 22.4, a color change to yellow does not always indicate proper endotracheal tube placement. Although gas in the esophagus usually has negligible amounts of CO$_2$ (because it is ambient air that is swallowed), the CO$_2$ in esophageal gas can be elevated following either mouth-to-mouth resuscitation (i.e., exhaled gas insufflation) or the ingestion of carbonated beverages. This CO$_2$ usually clears after a few inflations, so at least 4 inflations should be performed before checking the exhaled CO$_2$.

INFRARED CAPNOMETRY

Infrared light absorption provides a more quantitative measure of exhaled CO$_2$ than colorimetric methods (26,27). Infrared CO$_2$ analyzers can be placed along the expiratory limb of ventilator tubing, as depicted in Figure 22.4. A light-emitting diode generates a steady beam of infrared light that passes across the stream of exhaled gas, and a photodetector on the other side measures the intensity of light that is transmitted. The intensity of light transmission is inversely related to the concentration of CO$_2$ in the intervening gas.

CAPNOGRAM

Infrared CO$_2$ detectors have a rapid response and can measure changes in CO$_2$ during a single exhalation. These changes are recorded as a waveform called a capnogram, which normally appears like the one shown in Figure 22.4. The shape of the normal capnogram has been described as the outline of a snake that has swallowed an elephant (28). The P$_{CO_2}$ at the onset of exhalation is negligible because the gas in the upper airways is first to leave the lungs. As exhalation proceeds, gas from the alveoli begins to contribute to the exhaled gas, and the P$_{CO_2}$ begins to rise steadily. Near the end of exhalation, the P$_{CO_2}$ reaches a plateau and remains there until the onset of inhalation. When gas exchange in the lungs is normal, the P$_{CO_2}$ at the end of exhalation is equivalent to the P$_{CO_2}$ in end-capillary (arterial) blood. The end-expiratory P$_{CO_2}$ is more commonly called end-tidal P$_{CO_2}$ (P$_{ETCO_2}$).

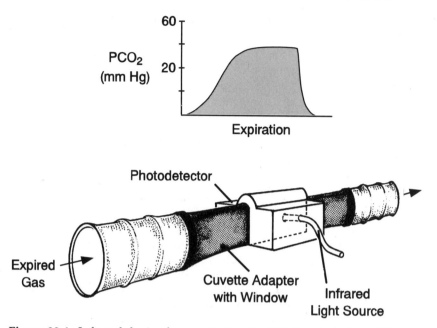

Figure 22.4. Infrared device for monitoring the CO_2 in exhaled gas. The capnogram shows the normal pattern of CO_2 elimination in a single breath.

$Paco_2$ VERSUS $Petco_2$

Normally, the difference between the arterial and end-tidal Pco_2 (called the $Paco_2$–$Petco_2$ gradient) is less than 5 mm Hg (26,27). However, when gas exchange in the lungs is impaired, **$Petco_2$ decreases relative to $Paco_2$**, so the $Paco_2$–$Petco_2$ gradient increases. This occurs in the following conditions:

Increased anatomic dead space

Open ventilator circuit
Shallow breathing

Increased physiologic dead space

Obstructive lung disease
Low cardiac output
Pulmonary embolism
Excessive lung inflation (e.g., PEEP)

Virtually any pulmonary disorder, or any cardiac disorder where cardiac output is reduced, produces an increase in the $Paco_2$–$Petco_2$ gradient. Thus, in patients with cardiopulmonary disease, a blood gas measurement is necessary at the outset to determine the equivalence of $Paco_2$ and $Petco_2$. If there is a $Paco_2$–$Petco_2$ gradient, changes in end-tidal CO_2 can be monitored because in steady-state conditions, changes in $Petco_2$ should be equivalent to changes in $Paco_2$ (i.e., the $Paco_2$–$Petco_2$ gradient will not change). However, any perturbation that affects gas exchange (e.g., changing ventilator settings) can change the $Paco_2$–$Petco_2$ gradient (29), so when a change in gas exchange is suspected, another blood gas is needed to determine the P_{aCO_2}–P_{ETCO_2} gradient.

P_{ETCO_2} Higher Than P_{aCO_2}

Although uncommon, end-tidal CO_2 can be higher than arterial P_{CO_2} in the following conditions (27,30):

Excessive CO_2 production, plus

Low inspired volume
High cardiac output

High inspired O_2 (CO_2 displaced from Hb)

NONINTUBATED PATIENTS

Although usually reserved for intubated patients, end-tidal CO_2 monitoring is possible in nonintubated patients as well (31–33). Nasal prongs adapted for end-tidal CO_2 monitoring are commercially available (Datascope Corp., Paramus, NJ: Salter Labs, Arvin, CA), and Figure 22.5 shows how to modify a nasal cannula for exhaled CO_2 monitoring (31). The trick is to occlude the tubing between the two nasal prongs (either with a cotton ball inserted through one of the nasal prongs or with a small screw clamp). This allows one nasal prong to be used for oxygen inhalation while the other nasal prong is used to transmit exhaled gas. A 14-gauge intravascular catheter (2 inches long) is inserted into the exhalation side of the nasal prong apparatus to transmit gas to the CO_2 detector. A sidestream CO_2 detector (i.e., one that applies suction to draw gas from the tubing) is best suited for this application. If one of these is not available, a mainstream CO_2 detector (such as the one shown in Fig. 22.3) can be used with a suction

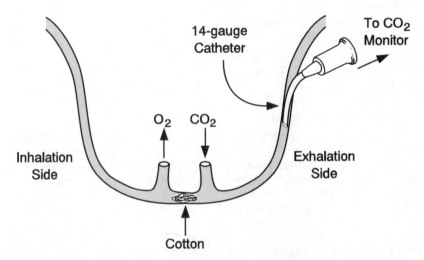

Figure 22.5. Nasal cannula modification for end-tidal CO_2 monitoring.

pump to draw gas samples from the cannula (at 150 mL/minute). The respiratory therapy department should help with this adaptation.

CLINICAL APPLICATIONS

Infrared capnometry has several uses in the ICU. The following are some situations where it can prove valuable.

Cardiac Output Monitor

As mentioned in Chapters 14 and 17, changes in P_{ETCO_2} can be used to monitor changes in cardiac output during volume resuscitation in hypovolemic shock (Fig. 14.1) and during cardiopulmonary resuscitation (Fig. 17.4). The close correlation between changes in P_{ETCO_2} and changes in cardiac output is demonstrated in Figure 22.6 (34).

Because of the ability to monitor trends in cardiac output, end-tidal CO_2 monitoring has several potential applications in the ICU (e.g., monitoring the effects of weaning intraaortic balloon counterpulsation). One of the more important applications is the ability of P_{ETCO_2} to predict the outcome of cardiopulmonary resuscitation (see Chapter 17).

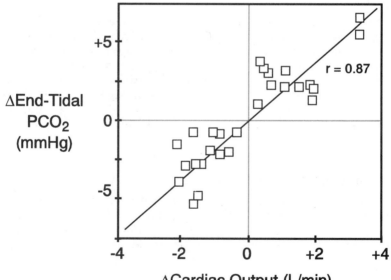

Figure 22.6. Correlation between changes in end-tidal P_{CO_2} and changes in cardiac output. Recordings from nine patients undergoing abdominal aortic aneurysm surgery. Correlation coefficient indicated as *r*. (From Shibutani K et al. Changes in cardiac output affect P_{ETCO_2}, CO_2 transport, and O_2 uptake during unsteady state in humans. J Clin Monit 1992;8:175.)

Ventilator-Related Mishaps

Infrared CO_2 monitors are equipped with alarms that can signal the separation of a patient from the ventilator. In this situation, the ventilator disconnection causes an abrupt drop in exhaled CO_2, causing the alarm to trigger (35). A drop in P_{ETCO_2} can also signal migration of the endotracheal tube into a mainstem bronchus (35).

Early Detection of Nosocomial Disorders

A decrease in P_{ETCO_2} accompanied by an increase in the $P_{aCO_2}-P_{ETCO_2}$ gradient can be an early manifestation of any of the following conditions (26,27):

Acute pulmonary embolism
Atelectasis
Low cardiac output
Pneumonia
Pulmonary edema

An increase in the $P_{aCO_2}-P_{ETCO_2}$ gradient can thus serve as an early warning signal for any of these conditions. This can be particularly valuable in ventilator-dependent patients, who are at risk for nosocomial complications.

Ventilator Weaning

During weaning from mechanical ventilation, end-tidal CO_2 monitoring can serve several purposes (36). In uneventful weaning (e.g., following surgery), it serves as a noninvasive measure of P_{aCO_2}. In difficult or complicated weaning, it can help determine the success or failure of the wean attempt. For example, a progressive rise in P_{ETCO_2} can signal an increased work of breathing (a sign of wean failure), whereas a decline in P_{ETCO_2} with a rising $P_{aCO_2}-P_{ETCO_2}$ gradient can signal respiratory muscle weakness with shallow breathing (another sign of wean failure).

Controlled Hyperventilation

When hyperventilation is used to reduce intracranial pressure in patients with head injuries, monitoring end-tidal CO_2 helps maintain the target P_{aCO_2}. In this setting, the $P_{aCO_2}-P_{ETCO_2}$ gradient must be checked periodically to select the appropriate target P_{ETCO_2}.

REFERENCES

GENERAL TEXTS

Gravenstein JS, Paulus DA, Hayes TJ. Capnography in clinical practice. Boston: Butterworth-Heinemann, 1989.

GENERAL REVIEWS

1. Tobin MJ. Respiratory monitoring. JAMA 1990;264:244–251 (122 references).
2. Clark JS, Votteri B, Ariagno RL, et al. Noninvasive assessment of blood gases. Am Rev Respir Dis 1992;145:220–232 (149 references).

PULSE OXIMETRY: REVIEWS

3. Tremper KK, Barker SJ. Pulse oximetry. Anesthesiology 1989;70:98–108 (59 references).
4. Severinghaus JW, Kelleher JF. Recent developments in pulse oximetry. Anesthesiology 1992;76:1018–1038 (249 references).
5. Council on Scientific Affairs, American Medical Association. The use of pulse oximetry during conscious sedation. JAMA 1993;270:1463–1468 (69 references).
6. Wahr JA, Tremper KK. Noninvasive oxygen monitoring techniques. Crit Care Clin 1995;11:199–217 (110 references).

PULSE OXIMETRY: SELECTED REFERENCES

7. Stoneham MD, Saville GM, Wilson IH. Knowledge about pulse oximetry among medical and nursing staff. Lancet 1994;344:1339–1342.
8. Hess D, Agarwal NN. Variability of blood gases, pulse oximeter saturation, and end-tidal carbon dioxide pressure in stable, mechanically ventilated trauma patients. J Clin Monit 1992;8:111–115.
9. Severinghaus JW, Spellman MJ. Pulse oximeter failure thresholds in hypotension and vasoconstriction. Anesthesiology 1990;73:532–537.
10. Morris RW, Nairn M, Beaudoin M. Does the radial arterial line degrade the performance of a pulse oximeter? Anesth Intensive Care 1990;18:107–109.
11. Jay GD, Hughes L, Renzi FP. Pulse oximetry is accurate in acute anemia from hemorrhage. Ann Emerg Med 1994;24:32–35.
12. Ries AL, Prewitt LM, Johnson JJ. Skin color and ear oximetry. Chest 1989;96:287–290.
13. Rubin AS. Nail polish color can affect pulse oximeter saturation. Anesthesiology 1988;68:825.
14. Ezri T, Szmuk P. Pulse oximeters and onychomycosis. Anesthesiology 1992;76:153–154.
15. Johnson PA, Bihari DJ, Raper RF, et al. A comparison between direct and calculated oxygen saturation in intensive care. Anesth Intensive Care 1993;21:72–75.
16. Roizen MF, Schreider B, Austin W, et al. Pulse oximetry, capnography, and blood gas measurements: reducing cost and improving the quality of care with technology. J Clin Monit 1993;9:237–240.
17. Standards for intra-operative monitoring. Park Ridge, IL: American Society of Anesthesiologists, 1991.
18. Standards for post-anesthesia care. Park Ridge, IL: American Society of Anesthesiologists, 1990.
19. Hutton P, Clutton-Brock T. The benefits and pitfalls of pulse oximetry. Be Med J 1993;307:457–458.

MIXED VENOUS OXIMETRY

20. Armaganidis A, Dhinaut JF, Billard JL, et al. Accuracy assessment for three fiberoptic pulmonary artery catheters for Svo$_2$ monitoring. Intensive Care Med 1994;20:484–488.
21. Noll ML, Fountain RL, Duncan CA, et al. Fluctuation in mixed venous oxygen saturation in critically ill medical patients: a pilot study. Am J Crit Care 1992; 3:102–106.
22. Krafft P, Steltzer H, Heismay M, et al. Mixed venous oxygen saturation in critically ill septic shock patients. Chest 1993;103:900–906.
23. Bongard FS, Leighton TA. Continuous dual oximetry in surgical critical care. Ann Surg 1992;216:60–68.

COLORIMETRIC CO$_2$ DETECTOR

24. MacLeod BA, Heller MB, Gerard J, et al. Verification of endotracheal tube placement with colorimetric end-tidal CO$_2$ detection. Ann Emerg Med 1991; 20:267–270.
25. Deem S, Bishop MJ. Evaluation and management of the difficult airway. Crit Care Clin 1995;11:1–27.

CAPNOGRAPHY: REVIEWS

26. Szaflarski NL, Cohen NH. Use of capnography in critically ill adults. Heart Lung 1991;20:363–374 (45 references).
27. Stock MC. Capnography for adults. Crit Care Clin 1995;11:219–232 (32 references).

CAPNOGRAPHY: SELECTED REFERENCES

28. Gravenstein JS, Paulus DA, Hayes TJ. Capnography in clinical practice. Boston Butterworth-Heinemann, 1989;11.
29. Hoffman RA, Kreiger PB, Kramer MR, et al. End-tidal carbon dioxide in critically ill patients during changes in mechanical ventilation. Am Rev Respir Dis 1989;140:1265–1268.
30. Moorthy SS, Losasso AM, Wilcox J. End-tidal Pco$_2$ greater than Paco$_2$. Crit Care Med 1984;12:534–535.
31. Wright SW. Conscious sedation in the emergency department: the value of capnography and pulse oximetry. Ann Emerg Med 1992;21:551–555.
32. Roy J, McNulty SE, Torjman MC. An improved nasal prong apparatus for end-tidal carbon dioxide monitoring in awake, sedated patients. J Clin Monit 1991;7:249–252.
33. Liu SY, Lee TS, Bongard F. Accuracy of capnography in nonintubated surgical patients. Chest 1992;102:1512–1515.
34. Shibutani K, Shirasaki S, Braatz T, et al. Changes in cardiac output affect PETco$_2$, CO$_2$ transport, and O$_2$ uptake during unsteady state in humans. J Clin Monit 1992;8:175–176.
35. Gandhi SK, Munshi CA, Bardeen-Henschel A. Capnography for detection of endobronchial migration of an endotracheal tube. J Clin Monit 1991;7:35–38.
36. Healey CJ, Fedullo AJ, Swinburne AJ, Wahl GW. Comparison of noninvasive measurements of carbon dioxide tension during weaning from mechanical ventilation. Crit Care Med 1987;15:764–767.

23

ACUTE RESPIRATORY DISTRESS SYNDROME

Physicians think they do a lot for a patient when they give his disease a name.
                                                        Immanuel Kant

The condition described in this chapter is considered to be the leading cause of acute respiratory failure in the United States. It was first described formally in the 1960s and has had several names, including *shock lung, wet lung,* and *leaky-capillary pulmonary edema.* The most popular name is *adult respiratory distress syndrome* (ARDS), recently changed to *acute respiratory distress syndrome* because it is not limited to adults (1). Despite the propensity for naming and renaming this condition over the years, there has been little improvement in the poor clinical outcomes associated with this condition (2). In fact, ARDS is not really a primary disease, but is more of a complication that arises when other diseases produce a severe and progressive form of systemic inflammatory response (3). After finishing this chapter, look at Chapter 31 (Infection, Inflammation, and Multiorgan Injury) and note the similarities between ARDS and the unbridled systemic inflammatory response.

PATHOGENESIS

The first clinical report of ARDS included 12 patients with diffuse infiltrates on chest roentgenogram and hypoxemia that was resistant to supplemental oxygen (4). Seven patients died (mortality 60%), and autopsy findings revealed dense infiltration of the lungs with leukocytes and proteinaceous material. These microscopic findings suggested that ARDS was a diffuse inflammatory injury in the lungs.

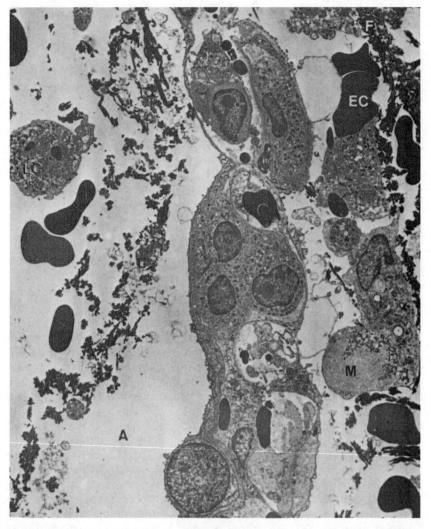

Figure 23.1. Microscopic changes in the lungs in the early stage of ARDS. The vertical column of tissue in the center of the photomicrograph is an inter-alveolar septum. The alveoli (*A*) on either side of the septum contain leuko-cytes (*LC*), erythrocytes (*EC*), pulmonary macrophages (*M*), and strands of fibrin (*F*).

INFLAMMATORY INJURY

The basic pathology of ARDS is a diffuse inflammatory process that involves both lungs. The photomicrograph in Figure 23.1 is from a patient in the early stages of ARDS (less than 24 hours in duration). The alveolar spaces on both sides of the centrally located septum contain erythrocytes, leukocytes, and proteinaceous debris. As the condition progresses, this exudative material accumulates and eventually ob-literates the alveolar airspaces.

The lung consolidation in ARDS is believed to originate from a systemic activation of circulating neutrophils (5). The activated neutrophils become sticky and adhere to the vascular endothelium in the pulmonary capillaries (6). They then release the contents of their cytoplasmic granules (i.e., proteolytic enzymes and toxic oxygen metabolites), and this damages the endothelium and leads to a leaky-capillary type of exudation into the lung parenchyma. Neutrophils and other inflammatory mediators can thus gain access to the lung parenchyma and carry on the inflammatory process. The inflammation then produces the lung injury.

Thus, although ARDS is often referred to as a type of pulmonary edema, **ARDS is an inflammatory process, not an accumulation of watery edema fluid.** This is an important distinction for the diagnosis and management of ARDS.

PREDISPOSING CONDITIONS

Many conditions predispose to ARDS, and the more common ones are indicated on the body map in Figure 23.2. The common feature in these conditions is the activation of neutrophils in the pulmonary or systemic circulation. Thus, the conditions that produce a systemic inflammatory response are the ones that predispose to ARDS. The most common predisposing condition is sepsis, which is a systemic inflammatory response (such as fever or leukocytosis) due to an infection.

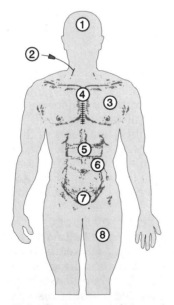

① Intracranial Hypertension
② Blood Products,
   Catheter Sepsis,
   Drugs
③ Pneumonia,
   Pulmonary Contusion
④ Cardiopulmonary Bypass
⑤ Pancreatitis
⑥ Translocation,
   Endotoxemia
⑦ Urosepsis,
   Amniotic Fluid Embolism
⑧ Long Bone Fracture

Figure 23.2. Common conditions that predispose to ARDS.

TABLE 23.1. PREDISPOSING FACTORS AND MORTALITY IN ARDS

High-Risk Condition	Incidence of ARDS (%)	Mortality (%) ARDS	Mortality (%) No ARDS
Sepsis syndrome	41	69	50
Multiple transfusions	36	70	35
Pulmonary contusion	22	49	12
Aspiration of gastric contents	22	48	21
Multiple fractures	11	49	9
Drug overdose	9	35	4
All high-risk conditions	26	62	19

Data from Hudson LD et al. (7).

The distinction between inflammation and infection is an important one because inflammation, not infection, produces the lung injury in ARDS. This distinction becomes important again in Chapters 30 and 31.

The risk of developing ARDS in some high-risk conditions is shown in Table 23.1. The data in this table are from a study of 695 patients with predisposing conditions for ARDS who were admitted to the ICU (7). Overall, one of every four patients developed ARDS (see bottom of the table), and ARDS was most common in those with sepsis syndrome and those given multiple blood transfusions (defined in this study as 15 or more units transfused over 24 hours). Note the negative impact of ARDS on survival. For all patients with high-risk conditions, the mortality rate was tripled (from 19 to 62%) by the appearance of ARDS.

CLINICAL FEATURES

The earliest clinical signs of ARDS include tachypnea and progressive hypoxemia in a patient with a condition that predisposes to ARDS. The hypoxemia is often refractory to supplemental oxygen. The chest roentgenogram can be unrevealing in the first few hours of the illness. However within 24 hours, the chest roentgenogram begins to reveal bilateral pulmonary infiltrates (8). The infiltrates may be more prominent in the peripheral lung fields (9), like the pattern of infiltration in Figure 23.3. Progression to mechanical ventilation often occurs in the first 48 hours of the illness (2).

Experts from Europe and the United States have proposed the clinical criteria for ARDS shown in Table 23.2 (1). The hallmarks of ARDS are diffuse pulmonary infiltrates, refractory hypoxemia (P_{AO_2}/F_{IO_2} less than 200), the presence of a predisposing condition, and no evidence of left-heart failure (wedge pressure less than 18 mm Hg). However, the clinical features of ARDS are shared by other disorders that can cause acute respiratory failure.

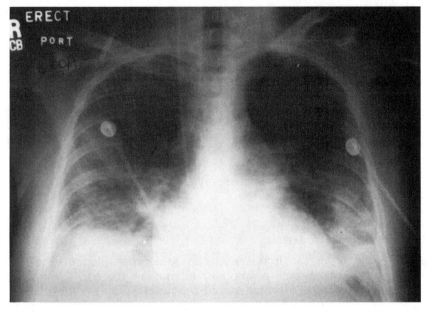

Figure 23.3. Portable chest roentgenogram from a 36-year-old woman who presented with fever and respiratory failure. The patient died two days later. Blood cultures subsequently grew *Escherichia coli.*

DIAGNOSTIC DILEMMAS

The other conditions that can mimic the clinical presentation of ARDS include pneumonia, acute pulmonary embolism, and cardiogenic (hydrostatic) pulmonary edema. The overlapping features of these disorders are shown in Table 23.3.

Physical Examination

The physical findings in ARDS (e.g., fever, tachypnea, and rales) are nonspecific, and can be seen in any of the conditions listed in Table 23.3. Note that fever can be a feature of cardiogenic pulmonary edema

TABLE 23.2. CLINICAL CRITERIA FOR ARDS	
Parameter	**ARDS**
Onset	Acute
Clinical setting	Predisposing condition
Gas exchange	$Pa_{O_2}/Fi_{O_2} < 200$ mm Hg regardless of PEEP level
Chest roentgenogram	Bilateral infiltrates
Wedge pressure	≤ 18 mm Hg
Criteria proposed by the American–European Consensus Conference on ARDS (1).	

TABLE 23.3. OVERLAPPING FEATURES OF ARDS AND OTHER
CAUSES OF ACUTE RESPIRATORY FAILURE

Feature	ARDS	Left-Heart Failure	Pneumonia	Pulmonary Embolism
Fever, leukocytosis	Yes	Possible	Yes	Yes
Bilateral infiltrates	Yes	Yes	Possible	Unlikely
Pleural effusions	Unlikely	Yes	Possible	Possible
Wedge pressure	Normal	High	Normal	Normal
Lung lavage protein	High	Low	High	High

(i.e., edema resulting from an acute myocardial infarction or inflammatory myocarditis).

Severity of Hypoxemia

The severity of the hypoxemia can sometimes help distinguish ARDS from cardiogenic pulmonary edema. In the early stages of ARDS, the hypoxemia is often more pronounced than the chest roentgenogram abnormalities, whereas in the early stages of cardiogenic pulmonary edema, the roentgenogram abnormalities are often more pronounced than the hypoxemia. However, there are exceptions, and severe hypoxemia can occur in cardiogenic pulmonary edema if the mixed venous oxygen pressure (Po_2) is reduced from a low cardiac output (see Figure 21.5).

The Chest Roentgenogram

When a chest roentgenogram shows bilateral pulmonary infiltrates, the principal concern is to differentiate ARDS from cardiogenic pulmonary edema. This can be a difficult task (8). To illustrate the difficulty, compare the chest films in Figures 23.3 and 23.4. Both are from patients with fever and acute respiratory failure, and both show bilateral infiltrates that are more prominent in the peripheral lung fields. Despite the similarities in the chest roentgenograms (and in the clinical presentation), one represents ARDS (Fig. 23.3) and the other represents cardiogenic pulmonary edema (Fig. 23.4). This illustrates why the consensus is that **chest roentgenograms are not reliable for distinguishing ARDS from cardiogenic pulmonary edema** (2,8).

Predisposing Conditions

The presence of high-risk conditions for ARDS may be the best means of distinguishing ARDS from cardiogenic edema. However, many of the conditions that predispose to ARDS also predispose to pneumonia and pulmonary embolism, so the predictive value of these conditions is limited if pneumonia or pulmonary embolism is a consideration.

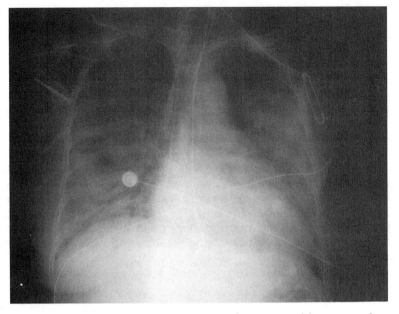

Figure 23.4. Portable chest roentgenogram of a 46-year-old woman who presented with fever and acute respiratory failure. This patient had an acute anterior myocardial infarction with cardiogenic pulmonary edema. The patient survived.

DIAGNOSTIC AIDS

Despite the high prevalence of ARDS, diagnostic recognition can be a problem. The following diagnostic approaches are available.

WEDGE PRESSURE

The standard method of distinguishing ARDS from cardiogenic pulmonary edema is to measure the pulmonary capillary wedge pressure (PCWP) with a pulmonary artery catheter. The PCWP is interpreted as follows (Table 23.2):

PCWP $\leq$ 18 mm Hg = ARDS
PCWP > 18 mm Hg = Cardiogenic pulmonary edema

Wedge versus Hydrostatic Pressure

The use of the wedge pressure to identify ARDS is based on the assumption that PCWP is a measure of pulmonary capillary hydrostatic pressure (P_c). However, PCWP is a measure of left-atrial pressure, and left-atrial pressure cannot be equivalent to pulmonary capillary pressure in the presence of blood flow (see Chapter 11). That is, if the wedge (left-atrial) pressure were equivalent to the pressure in the pulmonary capillaries, there would be no pressure gradient for flow in the pulmonary veins. Thus, PCWP must be lower than P_c.

Estimating Capillary Pressure

P_c can be estimated from PCWP and mean pulmonary artery pressure (Pa) according to the following relationship (from Chapter 11):

$$P_c = PCWP + 0.4 (Pa - PCWP) \tag{23.1}$$

(where 0.4 is the fractional decrease in pressure across the lungs that takes place across the pulmonary veins, as shown in Fig. 11.4). This adjustment produces little difference between P_c and PCWP in normal patients. However, as described in Chapter 11, P_c can be double the PCWP in severe ARDS with pulmonary hypertension. For a more detailed description of the difference between P_c and PCWP, see Chapter 11.

COLLOID OSMOTIC PRESSURE

The value of wedge pressure in distinguishing ARDS from cardiogenic pulmonary edema is limited further because it neglects other factors that govern the tendency for edema formation. These factors are identified by the Starling relationship (10):

$$Q = Kp (Pc - COP) \tag{23.2}$$

where Q is the rate of fluid movement out of the capillaries, Kp is the capillary permeability coefficient, P_c is the capillary hydrostatic pressure, and COP is the colloid osmotic pressure of blood. The colloid osmotic pressure (also called oncotic pressure) is a force created by large plasma proteins that do not move freely across capillaries. This force acts to draw fluid into the vascular space, and therefore opposes the capillary hydrostatic pressure. Most (60% to 80%) of COP is produced by the albumin in plasma; fibrinogen and the immunoglobulins account for the remainder (11,12).

COP Measurement

Plasma COP can be measured with an oncometer (see Reference 11 for a description of how an oncometer works). Normal COP varies with body position (12):

Normal COP (upright): 22–29 mm Hg (mean = 25 mm Hg)
Normal COP (supine): 17–24 mm Hg (mean = 20 mm Hg)

The decrease in COP in the supine position is due to the mobilization of protein-free fluid into the central circulation and takes about 4 hours to develop. Because most patients in the ICU are in the supine position, normal COP is taken as 20 mm Hg in the ICU. The measured COP in patients in the ICU is as low as 10 mm Hg (12). This means that **hydrostatic pulmonary edema can occur when P_c is in the normal range (less than 18 mm Hg) in ICU patients.**

Estimating COP

If an oncometer is not available, COP can be estimated using the total protein (TP) concentration in plasma (11,12):

$$COP = 2.1(TP) = 0.16(TP^2) + 0.009(TP^3) \qquad (23.3)$$

Note that the last two terms of this equation contribute little to the final COP, so they can be eliminated without sacrificing accuracy. Although the reliability of this calculation varies somewhat (6), it should still provide an adequate approximation of COP. One source of error arises when nonprotein colloids (hetastarch or the dextrans) are used as plasma expanders. These colloids dilute the serum proteins and decrease the calculated COP but not the measured COP. Therefore, COP should be measured and not calculated when hetastarch or dextran is used for volume expansion.

Diagnostic Use of COP

The addition of COP should improve the reliability of capillary hydrostatic pressure in identifying cardiogenic (hydrostatic) pulmonary edema. The following rules seem reasonable:

If the adjusted PCWP (P_c) is at least 4 mm Hg less than COP, then hydrostatic pulmonary edema is unlikely.
If the adjusted PCWP (P_c) is more than 4 mm Hg above COP, then hydrostatic pulmonary edema is likely.

BRONCHOALVEOLAR LAVAGE

Bronchoscopy is generally not warranted as a diagnostic tool in ARDS. However, bronchoscopy may be performed occasionally for other reasons in a patient with suspected ARDS (e.g., to identify infection). In this situation, the bronchoscopist can perform a bronchoalveolar lavage for the measurements described below (13). This procedure can be performed safely in patients with ARDS (14).

Neutrophils

In normal subjects, neutrophils make up less than 5% of the cells recovered in lung lavage fluid, whereas in patients with ARDS, as many as 80% of the recovered cells are neutrophils (13). The neutrophil preponderance in lung lavage fluid can help distinguish ARDS from cardiogenic edema (2,13), but may not be helpful if pneumonia is a consideration.

Total Protein

The protein concentration in edema fluid and blood can be used to distinguish watery hydrostatic edema from inflammatory edema. The following criteria have been suggested (15):

Protein (edema/serum) < 0.5 = Hydrostatic edema
Protein (edema/serum) > 0.7 = Inflammatory edema

Once again, this may help distinguish ARDS from cardiogenic edema, but it is of little help if pneumonia is a consideration.

MANAGEMENT STRATEGIES

Because there is no specific therapy that halts the inflammatory lung injury in ARDS, the management of ARDS is usually designed with the following goals in mind: (*a*) preventing iatrogenic lung injury, (*b*) reducing lung water, and (*c*) maintaining tissue oxygenation. These goals can be applied to any patient with acute respiratory failure.

MANAGEMENT FOCUS

Before describing the management of ARDS, it is important to point out that although the bulk of management is focused on the lungs, **only 15 to 40% of deaths in ARDS are caused by respiratory failure** (16–19). The majority of deaths are attributed to multiple organ failure. Age is also an important factor, with mortality being as much as five times higher in patients over 60 years of age (20).

The influence of multiorgan failure on survival in ARDS is shown in Figure 23.5. Included in this graph are the results of a multicenter

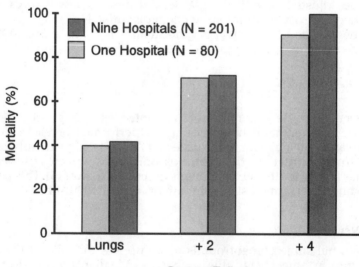

Figure 23.5. Multiorgan failure and survival in ARDS. (Results of the multicenter study from Reference 17. Results of the single center study from Reference 18.)

study (17) and the results of a study conducted at a single hospital (18). Both show a steady rise in mortality as more organs fail in addition to the respiratory failure. This demonstrates that ARDS is often just one part of a multiorgan illness, and it emphasizes the limitations of managements strategies that focus primarily on the lungs.

PREVENTING IATROGENIC INJURY

Ventilator Management

There is now considerable evidence indicating that the large tidal volumes used during conventional mechanical ventilation (10 to 15 mL/kg) can damage the lungs (21,22). The pathologic changes in ARDS are not distributed uniformly throughout the lungs. Rather, there are regions of lung infiltration interspersed with regions where the lung architecture is normal. These normal lung regions (which may make up only 30% of the lung) receive most of the delivered tidal volume. This results in overdistension of normal lung regions, which leads to alveolar rupture, surfactant depletion, and disruption of the alveolar–capillary interface.

Recognition of the risk of lung injury at high inflation volumes and pressures has led to an alternative strategy where **peak inspiratory pressures are kept below 35 cm H_2O by using tidal volumes of 7 to 10 mL/kg** (21,22). According to this strategy, mechanical ventilation is started at inflation volumes of 10 mL/kg. If the resulting peak inspiratory pressure (PIP) is above 35 cm H_2O, the inflation volume is reduced in increments of 2 mL/kg until PIP falls below 35 cm H_2O. When low inflation volumes are used, external positive end-expiratory pressure (PEEP, 5 to 10 cm H_2O) is added to prevent compression atelectasis and to limit phasic collapse of the distal airways (23,24). Inflation volumes of 5 to 8 mL/kg can result in CO_2 retention, but in the absence of adverse effects, the hypercapnia is allowed to continue (permissive hypercapnia) (25). This type of pressure-limited ventilatory support is described again in Chapter 26.

Pulmonary Oxygen Toxicity

The fractional concentration of inspired oxygen (FIO_2) should be kept at 50% or lower to minimize the risk of oxygen toxicity. Arterial oxygen saturation (SaO_2) should be monitored instead of arterial PO_2 because SaO_2 determines the oxygen content in arterial blood. An SaO_2 above 90% should be sufficient to maintain oxygen delivery to peripheral tissues. If the FIO_2 cannot be reduced to below 60%, external PEEP is added to help reduce the FIO_2 to nontoxic levels. Oxygen toxicity is described in Chapter 24.

REDUCING LUNG WATER

The two measures that are advocated for reducing lung water are diuretics and PEEP. Unfortunately, neither measure is likely to be effective in ARDS, as explained below.

Diuretics

Diuretic therapy can reduce lung water by decreasing capillary hydrostatic pressure and increasing colloid osmotic pressure (increased plasma protein concentration). Although this should work in watery hydrostatic edema, the situation is different in ARDS. **The lung infiltration in ARDS is an inflammatory process, and diuretics do not reduce inflammation.** Thus, it is no surprise that diuretics have not been shown to consistently reduce lung water in ARDS (26). Considering the pathology of ARDS, the use of diuretics to reduce lung infiltration in ARDS does not seem warranted as a routine measure (27).

The use of diuretics to minimize or reduce fluid overload seems a more reasonable measure, but only when renal water excretion is impaired (otherwise, the best way to prevent fluid overload is to maintain an adequate cardiac output). Whenever diuretics are used, some form of hemodynamic monitoring must be used to make sure that the diuresis is not adversely affecting cardiac output.

Positive End-Expiratory Pressure

The use of PEEP was popularized in ARDS because of the presumption that lung water could be reduced by this maneuver. However, as demonstrated in Figure 23.6, the application of PEEP does not reduce extravascular lung water in ARDS (28,29). Furthermore, the prophylactic use of PEEP does not reduce the incidence of ARDS in high-risk patients (30). In fact, high levels of PEEP can actually *increase* lung

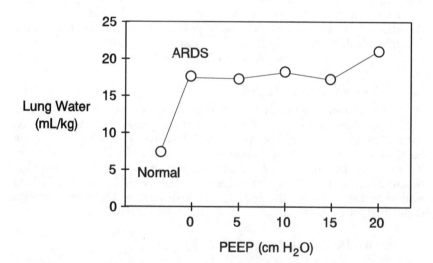

Figure 23.6. Effect of PEEP on extravascular lung water in ARDS. (Adapted from Saul GM et al. Effect of graded administration of PEEP on lung water in noncardiogenic pulmonary edema. Crit Care Med 1982;10:667–669.)

water (31). This latter effect may be the result of alveolar overdistension mentioned earlier, or may be the result of PEEP-induced impairment of lymphatic drainage from the lungs.

Thus, the bulk of evidence indicates that **PEEP is not a therapy for ARDS.** Instead, PEEP is a measure that helps to reduce iatrogenic lung injury by allowing ventilation with low inflation volumes, and by allowing the FIO_2 to be reduced to less toxic levels.

MAINTAINING TISSUE OXYGENATION

The ultimate goal of management in respiratory failure is an adequate level of oxygenation in the vital organs. The evaluation of tissue oxygenation is described in Chapter 13. The best measurements available for evaluating tissue oxygenation at the bedside are systemic oxygen uptake (VO_2), venous lactate level, and gastric intramucosal pH (measured indirectly by gastric tonometry). **Tissue oxygenation is considered to be inadequate if whole body VO_2 is less than 100 mL/minute/m^2, venous lactate is greater than 4 mmol/L, or gastric intramucosal pH is less than 7.32** (Table 13.1). If there is evidence for impaired tissue oxygenation, the sequence of management options shown in Figure 13.4 may be followed. A few points worth mentioning are included below.

Cardiac Filling Pressures

Central venous pressure (CVP) and wedge pressures tend to overestimate cardiac filling volumes during positive-pressure mechanical ventilation, particularly when PEEP is applied. This is partly because of transmission of intrathoracic pressures into the lumen of intrathoracic blood vessels, which increases intravascular pressure without changing transmural pressure (the pressure that determines ventricular stretch and edema formation). Thus, **a normal CVP or wedge pressure does not necessarily indicate normal cardiac filling volumes during positive-pressure mechanical ventilation.** In this setting, CVP and wedge pressure are interpretable only if they are reduced or are less than the level of applied PEEP.

Cardiac Output

If the cardiac output is inadequate (e.g., a cardiac index below 3 L/min/m^2) and the CVP or wedge pressures are not elevated, volume infusion is indicated. Even though ARDS is called leaky-capillary pulmonary edema, the lung infiltration in ARDS is an inflammatory exudate, so volume infusion is not different here from volume infusion in a patient with a pneumonia.

If volume infusion is not indicated, dobutamine is used to augment the cardiac output (see Table 18.3 for a dobutamine dose chart) (26). **Dopamine should be avoided because of its propensity to constrict**

pulmonary veins, which will raise the wedge pressure while reducing the left-ventricular end-diastolic volume (see Fig. 18.1). Vasodilators should also be avoided because of their propensity to increase intra-pulmonary shunt, which can add to the primary gas exchange abnormality in ARDS (vasodilator prostaglandins are the exception).

Blood Transfusions

Transfusion is often recommended to keep the Hb above 10 g/dL, but there is no basis for this recommendation. In fact, given the propensity for blood transfusions to *cause* ARDS (Table 23.1), it seems wise to avoid transfusing blood products in ARDS. **If there is no evidence of inadequate tissue oxygenation, there is no need to correct anemia.**

SPECIFIC THERAPIES

The following therapeutic measures are aimed at reversing the pathologic lung injury in ARDS. Unfortunately, there is little reason for excitement here (32).

Steroids

High-dose steroids have been evaluated for their ability to reduce the inflammatory lung injury in ARDS. Unfortunately, the results do not favor the use of steroids in ARDS, at least not in the early stages of the illness. The following is a brief summary of the available studies.

High-dose methylprednisolone (30 mg/kg intravenously every 6 hours for 4 doses) given to patients within 24 hours of the diagnosis of ARDS has not improved outcome or reduced mortality (33,34). In fact, one study showed a higher mortality associated with steroid therapy in ARDS (34).

High-dose methylprednisolone (same dose as above) given as prophylaxis to patients with sepsis syndrome did not reduce the incidence of ARDS (34).

Secondary infections are increased in patients receiving high-dose methylprednisolone for ARDS (34).

High-dose methylprednisolone (2 to 3 mg/kg/day) given to 25 patients with late ARDS (2 weeks duration) who had evidence of active fibrinoproliferation (leading to irreversible pulmonary fibrosis) resulted in a beneficial response in 21 patients and an 86% survival in the responders (35). This study suggests a possible role for steroids late in the course of ARDS, but corroborative evidence is required.

Surfactant

Aerosolized surfactant (Exosurf, Burroughs Wellcome, and Survanta, Ross Laboratories) has proven effective in improving outcomes in the neonatal form of respiratory distress syndrome, but it has not met with similar success in adults with ARDS (36).

Antioxidants

Considering that oxygen metabolites play an important role in neutrophil-mediated tissue injury (see Chapter 3) and that neutrophil-mediated tissue injury may play an important role in the pathogenesis of ARDS, it is no surprise that there is considerable interest in the possible role of antioxidants as a specific therapy for ARDS. Although nitric oxide can improve oxygenation and reduce pulmonary artery pressures in ARDS, mortality is unchanged (37). There is one report of improved survival in patients with ARDS treated with N-acetylcysteine (a glutathione surrogate described in Chapter 3) (38). However, this study stands alone at present.

REFERENCES

REVIEWS

1. Bernard GR, Artigas A, Brigham KL, et al. The American–European Consensus Conference on ARDS: definitions, mechanisms, relevant outcomes, and clinical trial coordination. Am Rev Respir Crit Care Med 1994;149:818–824.
2. Kollef MH, Schuster DP. The acute respiratory distress syndrome. N Engl J Med 1995;332:27–37 (179 references).
3. Barie PS. Organ-specific support in multiple organ failure: pulmonary support. World J Surg 1995;19:581–591 (140 references).

PATHOGENESIS

4. Petty TL. The acute respiratory distress syndrome. Historical perspective. Chest 1994;105(Suppl):44S–46S.
5. Windsor ACJ, Mullen PG, Fowler AA, Sugerman HJ. Role of the neutrophil in adult respiratory distress syndrome. Br J Surg 1993;80:10–17.
6. Donnelly SC, Haslett C, Dransfield I, et al. Role of selectins in development of adult respiratory distress syndrome. Lancet 1994;344:215–219.
7. Hudson LD, Milberg JA, Anardi D, Maunder RJ. Clinical risks for development of the acute respiratory distress syndrome. Am Rev Respir Crit Care Med 1995;151:293–301.

CLINICAL FEATURES

8. Aberle DR, Brown K. Radiologic considerations in the adult respiratory distress syndrome. Clin Chest Med 1990;11:737–754.
9. Chiles C, Putman CE. Techniques for interpreting pulmonary opacities in the ICU. J Crit Illness 1994;9:198–206.

DIAGNOSTIC AIDS

10. Michel CC. Fluid movement through capillary walls. In: Renkin EM, Michel CC, Geiger SR, eds. The cardiovascular system. Vol. 4. The microcirculation, Part 1. The handbook of physiology. Bethesda, MD: American Physiological Society, 1984;375–410.
11. Sinclair S, Webb AR. Colloid osmotic pressure measurement in critically ill patients. Intensive Care World 1991;8:120–122.
12. Weil MH, Henning RJ. Colloid osmotic pressure. Significance, methods of measurement, and interpretation. In: Weil MH, Henning RJ, eds. Handbook of critical care medicine. Chicago: Year Book, 1979;73–81.
13. Idell S, Cohen AB. Bronchoalveolar lavage in patients with the adult respiratory distress syndrome. Clin Chest Med 1985;6:459–471.
14. Steinberg KP, Mitchell DR, Maunder RJ, et al. Safety of bronchoalveolar lavage in patients with adult respiratory distress syndrome. Am Rev Respir Dis 1993; 148:556–561.
15. Sprung CL, Long WM, Marcial EH, et al. Distribution of proteins in pulmonary edema. The value of fractional concentrations. Am Rev Respir Dis 1987;136: 957–963.

MANAGEMENT FOCUS

16. Montgomery AB, Stager MA, Carrico J, Hudson LD. Causes of mortality in patients with the adult respiratory distress syndrome. Am Rev Respir Dis 1985;132:485–489.
17. Bartlett RH, Morris AH, Fairley B, et al. A prospective study of acute hypoxic respiratory failure. Chest 1986;89:684–689.
18. Gillespie DJ, Marsh HMM, Divertie MB, Meadows JA III. Clinical outcome of respiratory failure in patients requiring prolonged (> 24 hours) mechanical ventilation. Chest 1986;90:364–369.
19. Suchyta MR, Clemmer TP, Elliott CG, et al. The adult respiratory distress syndrome. A report of survival and modifying factors. Chest 1992;101: 1074–1079.
20. Gee M, Gottlieb JE, Albertine KH, et al. Physiology of aging related to outcome in the adult respiratory distress syndrome. J Appl Physiol 1990;69:822–829.

MANAGEMENT

21. Hickling KG. Ventilatory management in ARDS: can it affect outcome? Intensive Care Med 1990;16:219–226.
22. Marini JJ. Pressure-targeted, lung-protective ventilatory support in acute lung injury. Chest 1994;105(Suppl):109S–115S.
23. Gattinoni L, D'Andrea L, Pelosi P, et al. Regional effects and mechanism of positive end-expiratory pressure in early adult respiratory distress syndrome. JAMA 1993;269:2122–2127.
24. Muscedere JG, Mullen JBM, Slutsky AS. Tidal ventilation at low airway pressures can augment lung injury. Am Rev Respir Crit Care Med 1994;149: 1327–1334.
25. Hickling KG, Walsh J, Henderson S, Jackson R. Low mortality rate in adult respiratory distress syndrome using low-volume, pressure-limited ventilation with permissive hypercapnia: a prospective study. Crit Care Med 1994;22: 1568–1578.

26. Broaddus VC, Berthiaume Y, Biondi JW, et al. Hemodynamic management of the adult respiratory distress syndrome. J Intensive Care Med 1987;2:190–213.
27. Hyers Tm. ARDS: the therapeutic dilemma. Chest 1990;97:1025.
28. Saul GM, Feeley TW, Mihm FG. Effect of graded PEEP on lung water in noncardiogenic pulmonary edema. Crit Care Med 1982;10:667–669.
29. Helbert C, Paskanik A, Bredenberg CE. Effect of positive end-expiratory pressure on lung water in pulmonary edema caused by increased membrane permeability. Ann Thorac Surg 1984;36:42–48.
30. Pepe PE, Hudson LD, Carrico J. Early application of positive end-expiratory pressure in patients at risk for the adult respiratory distress syndrome. N Engl J Med 1984;311:281–286.
31. Demling RH, Staub NC, Edmunds LH. Effect of end-expiratory pressure on accumulation of extravascular lung water. J Appl Physiol 1975;38:907–912.
32. Messent M, Griffiths MJD. Pharmacotherapy in lung injury. Thorax 1992;47: 651–656.
33. Bernard GR, Luce JM, Sprung CL, et al. High-dose corticosteroids in patients with adult respiratory distress syndrome. N Engl J Med 1987;317:1565–1570.
34. Bone RC, Fischer CJ Jr, Clemmer TP, et al. Early methylprednisolone treatment for septic syndrome and the adult respiratory distress syndrome. Chest 1987; 92:1032–1036.
35. Meduri GU, Chinn A. Fibrinoproliferation in late adult respiratory distress syndrome. Chest 1994;105(Suppl):127S–129S.
36. Anzueto A, Baughman RP, Guntupalli KK, et al. Aerosolized surfactant in adults with sepsis-induced acute respiratory distress syndrome. N Engl J Med 1996;334:1417–1421.
37. Lunn RJ. Inhaled nitric oxide therapy. Mayo Clin Proc 1995;70:247–255.
38. Suter PM, Domenighetti G, Schaller MD, et al. N-acetylcysteine enhances recovery from acute lung injury in man: a randomized, double-blind, placebo-controlled clinical study. Chest 1994;105:190–194.

chapter

24

OXYGEN INHALATION THERAPY

For as a candle burns out much faster in dephlogisticated than in common air, so we might, as may be said, live out too fast . . . in this pure kind of air.

Joseph Priestley

One of the rare sights in any ICU is a patient who is *not* receiving supplemental oxygen to breathe. Considering the destructive nature of oxygen described in Chapter 3, the tendency to shower ICU patients with oxygen is a risky venture. This chapter begins by examining the indications and goals of supplemental oxygen administration (1). This is followed by a brief description of the different oxygen inhalation devices (2–4). The final section of the chapter is an addendum to Chapter 3 and focuses on the toxic risk of inhaled oxygen.

THE NEED FOR SUPPLEMENTAL OXYGEN

Despite the fact that oxygen inhalation is a therapeutic intervention designed to correct tissue hypoxia, oxygen administration seems to be more of a knee-jerk response to the presence of a life-threatening condition. This is supported by a recent survey showing that over 50% of hospitalized patients were receiving supplemental oxygen without a written order for oxygen therapy (5).

INDICATIONS FOR OXYGEN

Arterial Hypoxemia versus Tissue Hypoxia

Clinical studies reveal a poor correlation between arterial hypoxemia and tissue hypoxia. This is demonstrated in Table 24.1, which shows the arterial P_{O_2} and whole blood lactate level in seven patients with severe hypoxemia (P_{AO_2} below 40 mm Hg) secondary to acute exacerbation of chronic obstructive lung disease (6). If hyperlactatemia

388

TABLE 24.1. SEVERE HYPOXEMIA WITHOUT EVIDENCE OF TISSUE HYPOXIA		
Patient	Arterial P_{O_2} (mm Hg)	Blood Lactate (mmol/L)
1	22	0.90
2	30	0.25
3	32	0.86
4	33	1.57
5	34	2.03
6	37	2.08
7	39	1.12
Data from Reference 6.		

(blood lactate above 4 mmol/L) is used as a marker of tissue hypoxia, there is no evidence of tissue hypoxia in any patient with severe hypoxemia, even at arterial P_{O_2} levels as low as 22 mm Hg. This observation has been corroborated in patients with acute respiratory distress syndrome (7).

The available evidence thus indicates that arterial hypoxemia is not a marker of tissue hypoxia (at least not when using indirect markers of tissue hypoxia). The following statement from the study in Table 24.1 is relevant in this regard: *In the resting patient, even the most severe clinical hypoxemia due to pulmonary insufficiency does not itself lead to generalized tissue anaerobiasis* (6). Remember this statement when giving supplemental oxygen based on measures of arterial oxygenation.

WHAT TO MONITOR

Arterial oxygenation can also be misleading as an endpoint of oxygen inhalation therapy. This point is demonstrated in Figure 24.1. The graphs in this figure show the discrepancy between changes in arterial P_{O_2} and changes in systemic oxygen transport during supplemental oxygen administration (8). Note that arterial P_{O_2} increases from 61 to 83 mm Hg (36% change, $P < 0.01$) while the rate of oxygen transport decreases from 12.8 to 12.1 mL/minute/kg (5% change, not significant). Thus, **an increase in arterial P_{O_2} during oxygen inhalation should not be used as evidence for an increase in tissue oxygen availability** (8,9). This is consistent with the observation that oxygen inhalation does not protect against myocardial ischemia (10).

Oxygen and Systemic Blood Flow

The lack of improvement in systemic oxygen transport during oxygen inhalation is explained by the **tendency for oxygen to reduce systemic blood flow.** There are two mechanisms for this effect. First,

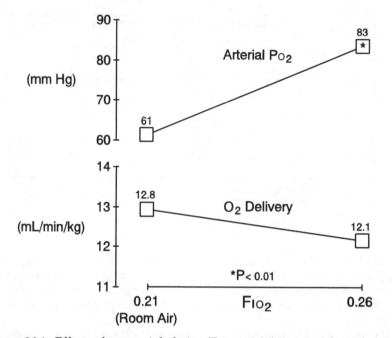

Figure 24.1. Effects of oxygen inhalation (F_{IO_2} = 0.26) on arterial oxygenation and systemic oxygen transport. Points on the graph represent mean values for the group of patients studied. (Data from DeGaute JP et al. Oxygen delivery in acute exacerbation of chronic obstructive pulmonary disease. Effects of controlled oxygen therapy. Am Rev Respir Dis 1981;124:26.)

oxygen acts as a vasoconstrictor in all vascular beds except the pulmonary circulation (where it acts as a vasodilator) (11,12). Second, oxygen inhalation is often associated with a decrease in cardiac output (8,9,13). Although this is caused partly by reversal of the cardiac stimulatory effects of hypoxemia, oxygen also has negative inotropic effects on the heart, and oxygen inhalation can reduce cardiac output in the absence of hypoxemia (13). The tendency for oxygen to reduce cardiac output emphasizes the value of invasive hemodynamic monitoring to evaluate the response to oxygen inhalation.

METHODS OF OXYGEN INHALATION

Oxygen delivery systems are classified as low-flow or high-flow systems. Low-flow delivery systems (nasal prongs, face masks, and masks with reservoir bags) provide a reservoir of oxygen for the patient to inhale. When total ventilation exceeds the capacity of the oxygen reservoir, room air is inhaled. The final concentration of inhaled oxygen (F_{IO_2}) is determined by the size of the oxygen reservoir, the rate at which the reservoir is filled, and the ventilatory demands of the patient. In contrast to the variable F_{IO_2} of the low-flow systems, high-flow oxygen delivery systems provide a constant F_{IO_2}. This is

TABLE 24.2. LOW-FLOW OXYGEN DELIVERY SYSTEMS			
Device	Reservoir Capacity	Oxygen Flow (L/min)	Approximate (F_{IO_2})*
Nasal cannula	50 mL	1	0.21–0.24
		2	0.24–0.28
		3	0.28–0.34
		4	0.34–0.38
		5	0.38–0.42
		6	0.42–0.46
Oxygen face mask	150–250 mL	5–10	0.40–0.60
Mask–reservoir bag:	750–1250 mL		
Partial rebreather		5–7	0.35–0.75
Nonrebreather		5–10	0.40–1.0

* Estimated value based on a tidal volume of 500 mL, a respiratory rate of 20 breaths/min, and an inspiratory:expiratory time ratio of 1:2.
From Shapiro BA et al. (14).

achieved by delivering oxygen at flow rates that exceed the patient's peak inspiratory flow rate, or by using devices that entrain a fixed proportion of room air.

NASAL PRONGS

Nasal prongs deliver a constant flow of oxygen to the nasopharynx and oropharynx, which acts as an oxygen reservoir (average capacity = 50 mL, or about one-third of the anatomic dead space) (2,14). The relationship between the oxygen flow rate and the F_{IO_2} in normal subjects is shown in Table 24.2 (14). As the oxygen flow rate increases from 1 to 6 L/min, the F_{IO_2} increases from 0.24 to 0.46.

It is important to note that the F_{IO_2} values in Table 24.2 pertain only to patients with a normal ventilatory pattern (see footnote). Any variation in the ventilatory pattern will also vary the F_{IO_2}. This effect is illustrated in Figure 24.2 (4). In this example, the respiratory rate is varied from 10 to 40 breaths/minute while the oxygen flow rate through the nasal cannula and the patient's tidal volume are both held constant. A quadrupling of the respiratory rate results in a 48% reduction in F_{IO_2}. This demonstrates the limitations of oxygen delivery through nasal prongs in patients who are breathing rapidly or otherwise have a high minute ventilation.

Advantages and Disadvantages

Nasal prongs are easy to use and well tolerated by most patients. The major disadvantages of nasal prongs are the tendency for the F_{IO_2} to vary as the patient's ventilatory pattern changes and the inability to achieve a high F_{IO_2} in patients with a high ventilatory demand. The continuous flow of oxygen through nasal prongs has been reported

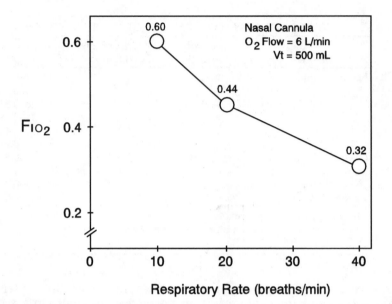

Figure 24.2. The relationship between respiratory rate and F_{IO_2} during oxygen administration at 6 L/minute through a nasal cannula. Assumes a constant tidal volume (Vt) of 500 mL. (Adapted from O'Connor BS, Vender JS. Oxygen therapy. Crit Care Clin 1995;11:67.)

as a cause of spontaneous gastric rupture (15), but this iatrogenic complication is rare.

LOW-FLOW OXYGEN MASKS

Face masks add 100 to 200 mL to the capacity of the oxygen reservoir. These devices fit loosely on the face, which allows room air to be inhaled, if needed. Standard face masks deliver oxygen at flow rates between 5 and 10 L/min. The minimum flow rate of 5 L/min is needed to clear exhaled gas from the mask. Low-flow oxygen masks can achieve a maximum F_{IO_2} of approximately 0.60.

Advantages and Disadvantages
Standard face masks can provide a slightly higher maximum F_{IO_2} than nasal prongs. However, this difference may be small. In general, face masks have the same drawbacks as nasal prongs.

MASKS WITH RESERVOIR BAGS

The addition of a reservoir bag to a standard face mask increases the capacity of the oxygen reservoir by 600 to 1000 mL (depending on the size of the bag). If the reservoir bag is kept inflated, the patient

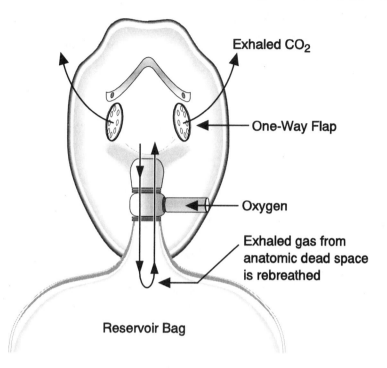

Exhaled CO_2

One-Way Flap

Oxygen

Exhaled gas from
anatomic dead space
is rebreathed

Reservoir Bag

Figure 24.3. Partial rebreathing system. The initial 100 to 150 mL of exhaled gas (anatomic dead space) is returned to the reservoir bag for rebreathing.

will inhale only the gas contained in the bag. There are two types of mask–reservoir bag devices. The one shown in Figure 24.3 is a partial rebreathing system. This device allows the gas exhaled in the initial phase of expiration to return to the reservoir bag. As exhalation proceeds, the expiratory flow rate declines, and when the expiratory flow rate falls below the oxygen flow rate, exhaled gas can no longer return to the reservoir bag. The initial part of expiration contains gas from the upper airways (anatomic dead space), so the gas that is rebreathed is rich in oxygen and largely devoid of CO_2. Partial rebreather devices can achieve a maximum F_{IO_2} of 70 to 80%.

The modified device in Figure 24.4 is a nonrebreathing system. This device has a one-way valve that prevents any exhaled gas from returning to the reservoir bag. Nonrebreather devices permit inhalation of pure oxygen ($F_{IO_2} = 1.0$).

Advantages and Disadvantages

The principal advantage of the reservoir bags is the greater ability to control the composition of inhaled gas. However, because the masks must create a tight seal on the face, it is not possible to feed patients by

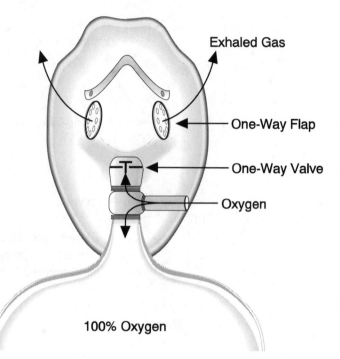

Exhaled Gas

One-Way Flap

One-Way Valve

Oxygen

100% Oxygen

Figure 24.4. Nonrebreathing system. A one-way valve prevents exhaled gas from returning to the reservoir bag.

mouth or nasoenteral tube when these devices are in use. Aerosolized bronchodilator therapy is also not possible with reservoir bag devices.

HIGH-FLOW OXYGEN MASKS

High-flow oxygen inhalation devices provide complete control of the inhaled gas mixture and deliver a constant FIO_2 regardless of changes in ventilatory pattern. The operation of a high-flow oxygen mask is shown in Figure 24.5 (16). Oxygen is delivered to the mask at low flow rates, but at the inlet of the mask, the oxygen is passed through a narrowed orifice, and this creates a high-velocity stream of gas (analogous to the effect created by a nozzle on a garden hose). This high-velocity jet stream generates a shearing force known as viscous drag that pulls room air into the mask. The volume of room air that moves into the mask (which determines the FIO_2) can be varied by varying the size of the openings (called entrainment ports) on the mask. These masks can increase the FIO_2 to a maximum of 0.50. At any given FIO_2, the proportion of inhaled gas provided by entrained room air remains constant; that is, FIO_2 remains fixed regardless of changes in oxygen flow rate or changes in inspiratory flow rate.

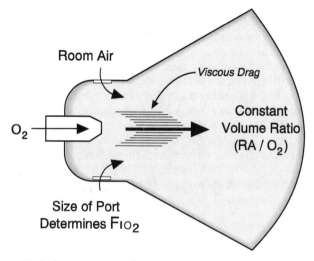

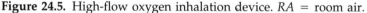

Figure 24.5. High-flow oxygen inhalation device. RA = room air.

Advantages and Disadvantages

The major advantage of high-flow oxygen masks is the ability to deliver a constant F_{IO_2}. This feature is desirable in patients with chronic hypercapnia because an inadvertent increase in F_{IO_2} in these patients can lead to further CO_2 retention. The major drawback with these masks is the inability to deliver high concentrations of inhaled oxygen.

TOXICITY OF INHALED OXYGEN

The damaging effects of oxygen are described in detail in Chapter 3. The oxygen in inhaled gas is an unrelenting threat to the functional integrity of the lungs. Fortunately, the lungs are endowed with a concentrated supply of endogenous antioxidants that protect against the destructive actions of oxygen. However, when these antioxidant defenses are overwhelmed (by too much oxygen or not enough antioxidants), oxygen inhalation can produce widespread damage in the lungs (17).

PULMONARY OXYGEN TOXICITY

Inhalation of pure oxygen can produce a progressive and lethal form of lung injury that is very similar to the acute respiratory distress syndrome (ARDS) described in Chapter 23 (17). This similarity is not surprising because ARDS is the result of inflammatory cell injury, and oxygen metabolites play an important role in the damaging effects of inflammation.

Comparative Physiology

The tendency to develop pulmonary oxygen toxicity varies widely in different species. For example, 5 to 7 days of breathing pure oxygen is fatal in laboratory rats, whereas sea turtles can breathe pure oxygen indefinitely without harm (18). This difference in susceptibility to oxygen toxicity is important because the experimental studies of pulmonary oxygen toxicity have been conducted almost solely in animals. As a result, little is known about the tendency to develop pulmonary oxygen toxicity in humans. In healthy volunteers, inhalation of 100% oxygen for brief periods of time (6 to 12 hours) results in a tracheobronchitis and a decrease in vital capacity (17). The latter effect is considered to be the result of absorption atelectasis, but this is unproven. The longest exposure to 100% oxygen in humans includes 5 patients with irreversible coma (3 to 4 days) and one healthy volunteer (4.5 days) (19,20). In all these cases, prolonged exposure to oxygen resulted in a pulmonary syndrome very much like ARDS.

SAFE VERSUS TOXIC F_{IO_2}

Based on the observation that oxygen inhalation does not reduce the vital capacity when the F_{IO_2} is below 0.60 (17), an F_{IO_2} of 0.60 was established as the threshold F_{IO_2} separating safe from toxic levels of inhaled oxygen. Although this threshold F_{IO_2} was established in healthy adults, it has also been applied to patients in the ICU. The consensus is that **inhalation of a gas mixture with an F_{IO_2} above 0.60 for longer than 48 hours is a toxic exposure to inhaled oxygen.** Therefore, when an F_{IO_2} above 0.60 is required for longer than a few days, other measures should be instituted (such as mechanical ventilation or PEEP) to reduce the F_{IO_2} to less toxic levels.

Antioxidant Depletion

The recommendation of a universal F_{IO_2} threshold separating safe from toxic oxygen inhalation is inappropriate because it neglects the contribution of endogenous antioxidants to the risk of oxygen toxicity. The principal antioxidants are included in Table 3.1. If these antioxidants become depleted, oxygen toxicity is possible at an F_{IO_2} that is much lower than 0.60. Antioxidant depletion may be common in patients in the ICU, particularly during a prolonged ICU stay. This effect is illustrated in Figure 24.6 (21). The antioxidant in this case is selenium, a cofactor for the glutathione peroxidase enzyme (Figure 3.3). In the first week after admission to the ICU, the selenium level (in whole blood) is 37% lower than in the control subjects, and by the fourth week of the ICU stay, the selenium level is about 50% of the control level. Reductions in other antioxidants (glutathione and vitamin E) has also been reported in ICU patients (22,23).

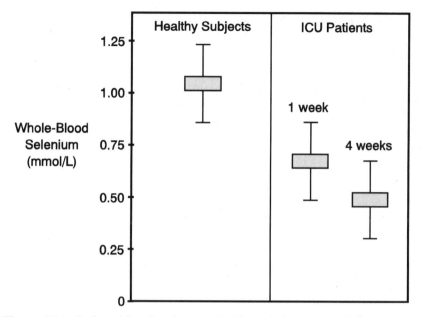

Figure 24.6. Reduced levels of an antioxidant (selenium) in ICU patients. Data (means and standard deviations) from 57 healthy blood donors and 175 consecutive ICU admissions. (From Hawker FH et al. Effects of acute illness on selenium homeostasis. Crit Care Med 1990;18:442.)

Optimal F_{IO_2}

Because antioxidant protection may be defective in ICU patients, the recommendation that an F_{IO_2} below 0.6 is safe does not apply to them. A more reasonable approach is to assume that **any F_{IO_2} above 0.21 (room air) can represent a toxic exposure to oxygen in ICU patients.** Based on this assumption, the optimal F_{IO_2} for safe oxygen inhalation is the lowest tolerable (rather than any) F_{IO_2} below 0.60.

PREVENTIVE MEASURES

The measures presented in Table 24.3 are aimed at reducing the risk of pulmonary oxygen toxicity. These preventive measures are organized according to three goals.

Limit O_2 Inhalation

As stressed repeatedly in this chapter, the routine administration of supplemental oxygen is inappropriate and should be abandoned. The principal indications for oxygen inhalation therapy are listed in Table 24.3. They include clinical evidence of inadequate tissue oxygenation and a high risk of tissue hypoxia. Adherence to these indications

| TABLE 24.3. PREVENTIVE MEASURES FOR OXYGEN TOXICITY ||
Goals	Actions

Limit oxygen inhalation	Use supplemental O_2 only for the following indications:
	 • Arterial hypoxemia that can be harmful:
	     Arterial Po_2 < 55 mm Hg (promote pulmonary
	     hypertension)
	 • Indirect evidence of tissue dysoxia:
	     Whole-body Vo_2 < 100 mL/min/m^2
	     Blood lactate >4 mmol/L
	     Gastric mucosal pH < 7.32
	 • High risk for tissue dysoxia:
	     Cardiac index <2 L/min/m^2
	     Peripheral O_2 extraction >50%
	     Mixed venous O_2 saturation <50%

Limit the Fio_2	• If the Fio_2 is above 0.6 for 48 hr, consider mechanical ventilation or PEEP. • If the Fio_2 is below 0.6 and there are no indications for O_2 inhalation, reduce the Fio_2.

Support antioxidant protection	• Satisfy the RDA for selenium:
	     70 μg/day for men
	     55 μg/day for women
	 • If high risk of O_2 toxicity, evaluate selenium and vitamin E status periodically.

should reduce the risk of oxygen toxicity without creating any added risk of tissue hypoxia.

Limit the Fio_2

The second measure is a corollary of the first and involves using the lowest tolerable Fio_2. First, Fio_2 should not be kept above 0.6 for longer than 48 hours. If the Fio_2 is below 0.6 and there are no indications for supplemental oxygen, Fio_2 should be reduced gradually to the lowest tolerable level. Reduction of the Fio_2 can proceed as long as there is no evidence of (or high risk of) tissue hypoxia.

Limiting supplemental oxygen as described here may not be an easy task; members of the ICU staff who are accustomed to the unregulated use of oxygen may resist. When opposition is encountered, remember to point out that oxygen is a therapy (in fact, oxygen is often classified as a drug), and like all therapies, it is not appropriate if not justified.

Support Antioxidant Protection

Because antioxidant depletion may be common in ICU patients, maintaining the pool of endogenous antioxidants is an important measure for preventing oxygen toxicity. Unfortunately, it is not yet possible to evaluate the capacity for antioxidant protection. However, the measures indicated in Table 24.3 may help maintain the body stores of two endogenous antioxidants: selenium and vitamin E. For more information on the evaluation and administration of these antioxidants, see Chapter 3.

REFERENCES

REVIEWS

1. Fulmer JD, Snider GL. ACCP-NHLBI National Conference on Oxygen Therapy. Chest 1984;86:234–247 (34 references).
2. Kacmarek RM. Supplemental oxygen and other medical gas therapy. In: Pierson DJ, Kacmarek RM, eds. Foundations of respiratory care. New York: Churchill Livingstone, 1992;859–890 (45 references).
3. Carlton TJ, Anthonisen NR. A guide for judicious use of oxygen in critical illness. J Crit Illness 1992;7:1744–1757 (36 references).
4. O'Connor BS, Vender JS. Oxygen therapy. Crit Care Clin 1995;11:67–78 (7 references).

THE NEED FOR SUPPLEMENTAL OXYGEN

5. Small D, Duha A, Wieskopf B, et al. Uses and misuses of oxygen in hospitalized patients. Am J Med 1992;92:591–595.
6. Eldridge FE. Blood lactate and pyruvate in pulmonary insufficiency. N Engl J Med 1966;274:878–883.
7. Lundt T, Koller M, Kofstad J. Severe hypoxemia without evidence of tissue hypoxia in the adult respiratory distress syndrome. Crit Care Med 1984;12:75–76.
8. Corriveau ML, Rosen BJ, Dolan GF. Oxygen transport and oxygen consumption during supplemental oxygen administration in patients with chronic obstructive pulmonary disease. Am J Med 1989;87:633–636.
9. Lejeune P, Mols P, Naeije R, et al. Acute hemodynamic effects of controlled oxygen therapy in decompensated chronic obstructive pulmonary disease. Crit Care Med 1984;12:1032–1035.
10. Kavanaugh PB, Cheng DCH, Sandler AN, et al. Supplemental oxygen does not reduce myocardial ischemia in premedicated patients with critical coronary artery disease. Anesth Analg 1993;76:950–956.
11. Packer M, Lee WH, Medina N, Yushak M. Systemic vasoconstrictor effects of oxygen administration in obliterative pulmonary vascular disorders. Am J Cardiol 1986;57:853–858.
12. Bongard O, Bounameaux H, Fagrell B. Effects of oxygen on skin microcirculation in patients with peripheral arterial occlusive disease. Circulation 1992;86:878–886.
13. Daly WJ, Bondurant S. Effects of oxygen breathing on the heart rate, blood pressure and cardiac index of normal men—resting, with reactive hyperemia, and after atropine. J Clin Invest 1962;41:126–132.

METHODS OF OXYGEN INHALATION

14. Shapiro BA, Kacmarek RM, Cane RD, et al. Clinical application of respiratory care. 4th ed. St. Louis: CV Mosby, 1991;123–134.

15. van der Loos TLJM, Lustermans FAT. Rupture of the normal stomach after therapeutic oxygen administration. Intensive Care Med 1986;12:52–53.
16. Scacci R. Air entrainment masks: jet mixing is how they work. The Bernoulli and Venturi principles is how they don't. Respir Care 1979;24:928–931.

TOXICITY OF INHALED OXYGEN

17. Lodato RF. Oxygen toxicity. Crit Care Clin 1990;6:749–765.
18. Fanburg BL. Oxygen toxicity: why can't a human be more like a turtle? Intensive Care Med 1988;3:134–136.
19. Barber RE, Hamilton WK. Oxygen toxicity in man. N Engl J Med 1970;283:1478–1483.
20. Winter PM, Smith G. The toxicity of oxygen. Anesthesiology 1972;37:210–212.
21. Hawker FH, Stewart PM, Switch PJ. Effects of acute illness on selenium homeostasis. Crit Care Med 1990;18:442–446.
22. Corbucci GG, Gasparetto A, Candiani A, et al. Shock-induced damage to mitochondrial function and some cellular antioxidant mechanisms in humans. Circ Shock 1985;15:15–26.
23. Pincemail J, Bertrand Y, Hanique G, et al. Evaluation of vitamin E deficiency in patients with adult respiratory distress syndrome. Ann N Y Acad Sci 1989;570:498–500.

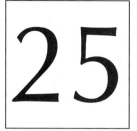

c h a p t e r

25

RESPIRATORY PHARMACOTHERAPY

This chapter focuses on the use of pharmaceutical agents to enhance flow in the conducting airways of the lungs. Three distinct strategies are described. The first involves drugs that increase airway caliber by relaxing bronchial smooth muscle (**bronchodilators**). The second involves drugs that reduce airflow obstruction from inflammation in the walls of the small airways (**corticosteroids**), and the third strategy involves measures that facilitate the removal of obstructing secretions (**mucokinetic therapy**).

BEDSIDE MONITORING

Interventions aimed at enhancing airflow in the lungs must be guided by measurements of airway function. Because ICU patients are not easily transported to the pulmonary function laboratory, these measurements must be obtained at the bedside. The following are three measurements of airway function that are easily performed at the bedside.

PEAK EXPIRATORY FLOW

The *peak expiratory flow rate*, the highest flow achieved during a maximum expiratory effort, is a measurement of the total flow capacity of the airways. The peak expiratory flow is easily measured at the bedside with a hand-held device such as the one in Figure 25.1. The device shown (the MiniWright peak flowmeter) is about 7 inches in length, and weighs only 11 ounces. The patient holds the device in the palm of the hand and inhales as much air as possible (to total lung capacity), then exhales as forcefully as possible into the mouthpiece of the device. The flow of exhaled gas follows a contour like the one illustrated in the figure, with the peak flow occurring early in expiration (when the elastic recoil of the lungs is the highest and the caliber of the airways

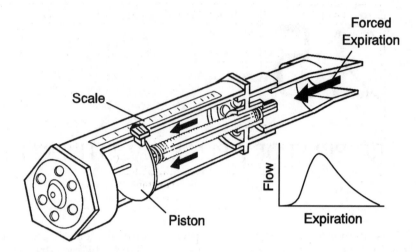

Figure 25.1. A hand-held device for measuring the peak expiratory flow rate (the highest point on the expiratory flow contour).

is the greatest). The flow of exhaled gas displaces a spring-loaded piston in the peak flowmeter, and a pointer attached to the piston records the displacement on a calibrated scale etched on the outer surface of the device. This scale records the displacement as the maximum (peak) flow rate, in liters per minute (L/min). This maneuver is repeated twice, and the highest of the three flows is recorded as the peak expiratory flow at that time (1).

The peak expiratory flow is an effort-dependent parameter and is a reliable index of flow resistance only when the expiratory effort is maximal (and constant). Therefore, it is important to observe the patient during the peak flow measurement to determine whether a maximum effort is being expended. If not, the measurement should be discarded (2-4).

Variability

The peak expiratory flow varies with age, sex, and height, and thus reference tables are needed to interpret the peak flow measurement in individual patients (these tables are included in the Appendix at the end of the text). The influence of sex and age on the peak expiratory flow rate (PEFR) is demonstrated below (5).

	Age (yr)	Normal PEFR
Male (height 70 in)	20	690 L/min
	70	550 L/min
Female (height 65 in)	20	460 L/min
	70	400 L/min

At 20 years of age, the male has a PEFR that is 50% higher than the

TABLE 25.1 PEAK EXPIRATORY FLOW INTERPRETATIONS	
1. Severity of airways obstruction	
PEFR (% predicted)	**Interpretation**
>70	Mild obstruction
50–70	Moderate obstruction
<50	Severe obstruction
<25	CO_2 retention
2. Bronchodilator responsiveness	
PEFR (% increase)	**Interpretation**
>15	Favorable response
<10	Poor response

female, and in both sexes, the PEFR is 15 to 20% slower in the elderly. The PEFR also has a diurnal variation of 10 to 20%, with the nadir in the early morning (6). However, the importance of this diurnal variation in hospitalized patients (where circadian rhythms may be absent) has not been determined.

Clinical Applications

The PEFR can be used to evaluate the severity of airways obstruction (1,7,8) or to determine bronchodilator responsiveness (9). The criteria for these applications are shown in Table 25.1 (1). According to the Expert Panel Report of the National Asthma Education Program (1), the PEFR should be monitored on a regular basis in patients with asthma. The management of acute asthma in the emergency department can be guided by the PEFR as shown in Figure 25.4. The PEFR can also be used to determine the need for bronchodilator therapy. This is accomplished by recording the PEFR just before, and again 20 minutes after, a bronchodilator aerosol treatment (the respiratory therapy department will perform the peak flow measurements on request). If the PEFR increases by 15% or more after the treatment, then therapy with bronchodilator aerosols is justified. This represents a more rational approach to bronchodilator therapy than the current practice of ordering bronchodilator aerosol treatments routinely for all hospitalized patients with obstructive airways disease.

PEAK INSPIRATORY PRESSURE

Aerosol bronchodilator treatments are given routinely to ventilator-dependent patients, often without documented need or benefit. One method of assessing bronchodilator responsiveness during mechanical ventilation is to monitor changes in the peak inspiratory pressure (PIP) measured in the endotracheal tube at the end of lung inflation. This pressure is determined by the inflation volume, the distensibility (compliance) of the lungs, and the resistance to flow in the endotracheal tube and airways. If a bronchodilator treatment has effectively decreased airways resistance, the PIP should also decrease. Therefore, assuming all other variables are constant, a decrease in PIP after an aerosol bronchodilator treatment can be used as evidence for bronchodilator responsiveness (9). The PIP is described in more detail in Chapter 26.

AUTO-PEEP

When flow in the airways is reduced, exhaled gas does not escape completely from the lungs, and the gas that is trapped in the distal airspaces creates a positive pressure at the end of expiration. This positive end-expiratory pressure (PEEP) is known as intrinsic PEEP or *auto-PEEP*, and it is an indirect measure of the severity of airways obstruction. (This phenomenon is an expression of the hyperinflation that occurs in obstructive airways disease.) Thus, in the presence of auto-PEEP, a favorable response to a bronchodilator treatment should be accompanied by a decrease in the level of auto-PEEP. The measurement of auto-PEEP is described in Chapter 28.

β-RECEPTOR AGONISTS

The most effective bronchodilators are pharmaceutical agents that stimulate β-adrenergic receptors in bronchial smooth muscle (β-2 subtype) and promote smooth muscle relaxation. These β-receptor agonists are most effective and least toxic when they are given as an aerosol that is inhaled (1–4,10). The drugs and dose recommendations for β-agonist aerosol treatments are shown in Table 25.2. All treatments in this table should be considered equivalent in efficacy and toxicity.

TABLE 25.2 AEROSOL THERAPY WITH β-RECEPTOR AGONISTS

β-Receptor Agonist	Nebulizer		Metered-Dose Inhaler	
	Formulation	Dose	Metered Dose	Treatment
Albuterol	0.5% solution (5 mg/mL)	2.5 mg	0.09 mg	2–3 sprays
Isoetharine	1% solution (10 mg/mL)	5.0 mg	0.34 mg	2–3 sprays
Metaproterenol	5% solution (50 mg/mL)	15 mg	0.65 mg	2–3 sprays

Dosing frequency varies according to the clinical situation.

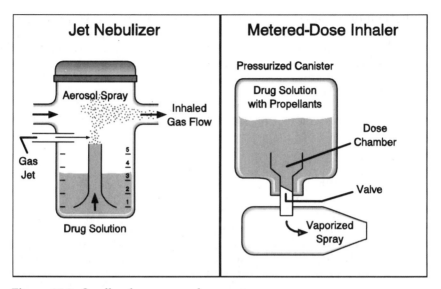

Figure 25.2. Small-volume aerosol generators.

AEROSOL THERAPY

There are two devices used to generate bronchodilator aerosols, and each is depicted schematically in Figure 25.2 (see reference 2 for a detailed description of aerosol generators).

Jet Nebulizer

The jet nebulizer operates on the same principle as the high-flow oxygen mask shown in Figure 24.5. One end of a narrow capillary tube is submerged in the drug solution, and a rapidly flowing stream of gas is passed over the other end of the tube. This gas jet creates a viscous drag that draws the drug solution up the capillary tube, and when the solution reaches the gas jet, it is pulverized to form the aerosol spray, which is then carried to the patient with the inspiratory gas flow. Small-volume jet nebulizers use a reservoir volume of 3 to 6 mL (drug solution plus saline diluent) and can completely aerosolize the reservoir volume in less than 10 minutes.

Metered-Dose Inhaler

The metered-dose inhaler operates in much the same way as a hair spray canister. This device has a pressurized canister that contains a drug solution with a boiling point below room temperature. When the canister is squeezed between the thumb and fingers, a valve opens that releases a fixed volume of the drug solution. The liquid immediately vaporizes when it emerges from the cannister, and a liquid propellant in the solution creates a high-velocity spray. The spray emerging from the canister can have a velocity in excess of 30 meters per second (over 60 miles per hour) (11). Because of the high velocity of the emerging spray, when a metered-dose inhaled is placed in the mouth, most of the aerosol spray impacts on the posterior wall of the oropharynx and is not inhaled. This *inertial impaction* is reduced somewhat by using a spacer device to increase the distance between the canister and mouth (this reduces the velocity of the spray reaching the mouth).

Nebulizer versus Metered-Dose Inhaler

As indicated in Table 25.2, the therapeutic dose delivered by metered-dose inhalers (usually 2 or 3 sprays) is only a fraction of the dose delivered by nebulized aerosols. Yet despite this dose difference, the bronchodilator response to metered dose inhalers and nebulized aerosols is often indistinguishable. This is demonstrated in Figure 25.3. In this case, patients with severe asthma (PEFR less than 50% predicted) were given albuterol aerosol treatments with a hand-held nebulizer (2.5 mg albuterol per treatment) or metered-dose inhaler (4 puffs or 0.36 mg albuterol per treatment) (12). After two treatments with each type of aerosol therapy, the increase in peak expiratory flow is equivalent. Thus, despite an almost tenfold difference in total drug dose (5 mg via nebulizer versus 0.7 mg via metered-dose inhaler), the bronchodilator response to each type of aerosol therapy is the same.

Equivalent bronchodilator responses to nebulizer and metered-dose aerosols have been documented in both spontaneously breathing and

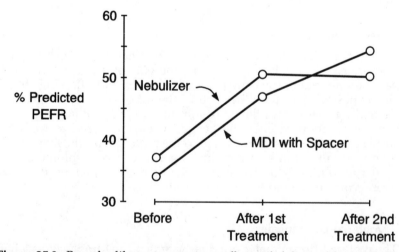

Figure 25.3. Bronchodilator responses to albuterol delivered by a nebulizer (2.5 mg per treatment) and a metered-dose inhaler (*MDI*) (0.4 mg per treatment) in patients with acute exacerbation of asthma. Each point represents the mean value for all patients in each treatment group. *PEFR* = peak expiratory flow rate. (Data from Idris AH, et al. Emergency department treatment of severe asthma. Chest 1993;103:665–672.)

ventilator-dependent patients (2,12–14). The likely reason for this is that very little of the drug dose (less than 10%) is deposited in the lungs with either type of aerosol therapy (most of the dose is lost via condensation on the equipment). Because drug therapy with a metered-dose inhaler is less expensive and less labor-intensive than nebulizer treatments, there has been a general trend to adopt metered-dose inhalers for bronchodilator treatments in hospitalized patients. At one hospital, the annual savings from such a change were estimated at $83,000 for the hospital and $300,000 for the patients (15).

Ventilator-Dependent Patients

Although nebulizers have been the standard aerosol generator for ventilator-dependent patients, metered-dose inhalers have also been used to deliver bronchodilator aerosols during mechanical ventilation (see reference 2 for examples of how to connect the metered-dose inhaler to the ventilator circuit). The best results are obtained when the aerosol spray from the metered-dose inhaler is passed through a narrow-gauge catheter extending beyond the tip of the tracheal tube (16). The following steps achieve optimal delivery with either type of aerosol therapy (13,17): (a) turn the humidifier off, (b) decrease the inspiratory flow rate, and (c) increase inspiratory time.

MANAGEMENT OF ACUTE ASTHMA

Inhaled β agonists are the drugs of choice for the initial management of patients with asthma. The initial management of patients with acute exacerbation of asthma can be organized as shown in Figure 25.4. Treatment begins with a series of β-agonist aerosol treatments given at 20-minute intervals. Each treatment can be given by nebulizer or metered-dose inhaler, and each treatment is followed by a peak flow measurement. If a satisfactory response is not obtained after three aerosol treatments (which covers a 1-hour period), a corticosteroid is administered, and subsequent aerosol treatments can be given at 1-hour intervals until a satisfactory response is achieved. After the patient has stabilized, the β-agonist aerosol treatments are given every 6 hours.

SIDE EFFECTS

The most commonly reported side effects of β-agonist aerosol therapy are **tachycardia** (cardiac β receptors), **tremors** (skeletal muscle β receptors), **a decrease in serum potassium** (transcellular potassium shift), and **a decrease in arterial Po_2** (increased intrapulmonary shunt) (18,19). The latter effect is transient (lasting about 30 minutes) and usually is seen during aggressive bronchodilator therapy in acute asthma (18). Other side effects include hyperglycemia and a decrease

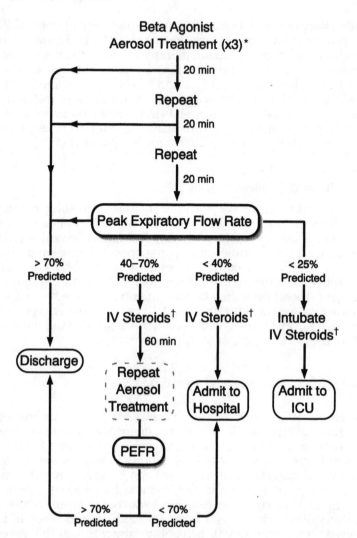

*See Table 25.2 for drugs and dose recommendations.
†Methylprednisolone: 80–125 mg IV push; or hydrocortisone: 2 mg / kg IV push

Figure 25.4. Protocol for the early management of acute asthma in the emergency department. *PEFR* = peak expiratory flow rate. (Adapted from the National Asthma Education Program, Expert Panel Report [1].)

in serum magnesium and serum phosphorous (19). Cardiac ischemia has been reported, but is rare (18).

Hypokalemia

The usual therapeutic doses of inhaled β agonists are associated with only mild decreases in serum potassium (0.5 mEq/L or less) (19).

However, high doses of inhaled β agonists (e.g., 20 mg albuterol) have been used as a treatment for hyperkalemia (20), so aggressive therapy with inhaled β agonists could result in significant hypokalemia.

THEOPHYLLINE

Theophylline has been a popular bronchodilator in the United States for over 50 years, but the drug has little value in the acute care setting (21). **Theophylline is less effective and more likely to produce undesirable side effects than the β-agonist aerosols** (1,22,23). This is reiterated in the statements shown in Table 25.3, which are taken from the National Asthma Education Program (1). As shown in Figure 25.5, theophylline adds little when it is given in combination with β-agonist aerosols for acute asthma (22,23).

Theophylline becomes even more undesirable when you consider the cost of monitoring serum theophylline levels (about $50 per determination). There are an estimated 500,000 hospital admissions annually for asthma (24), and if serum theophylline levels were measured at each admission and discharge, the yearly cost would be $25 million.

DRUG ADMINISTRATION

Although there are no clear indications for theophylline in ICU patients, the drug continues to be used, so I have included some dose recommendations in Table 25.4.

Aminophylline

When theophylline is given intravenously, a solvent must be added to maintain solubility. The solvent is ethylenediamine (also found in shellacs and pesticides), and the theophylline–ethylenediamine preparation is called *aminophylline*. Hypersensitivity reactions to ethylenediamine have been reported (25), and for sensitized patients, there is a solution of theophylline in dextrose available for intravenous use (Travenol Labs).

TABLE 25.3 EXPERT COMMENTARY ON THEOPHYLLINE
• When used alone, intravenous aminophylline is 3 to 4 times less effective in relieving airflow obstruction than repetitive administration of β-agonist bronchodilators
• When used in combination with repetitively administered β-agonist bronchodilators, intravenous aminophylline causes increased adverse side effects without effecting additive bronchodilation.
• It is emphasized that in adults or children treated with repetitive administration of β-agonist bronchodilators, methyxanthines play no significant role in the acute relief of airflow obstruction.
From the National Asthma Education Program, Expert Panel Report (1).

TABLE 25.4 INTRAVENOUS AMINOPHYLLINE DOSING	
Condition	Dose
Loading dose	
No prior treatment	6 mg/kg*
Ongoing treatment	$T_D - T_P/1.6^†$
Rate	<0.2 mg/kg/hr
Continuous dose rate	
Standard	0.5 mg/kg/hr
Low cardiac output	0.2 mg/kg/hr
Smoker	0.8 mg/kg/hr

* Use ideal body weight. In obese subjects, dose may be underestimated.
† T_D and T_P are desired and present serum theophylline levels, respectively.
From Powell JR, et al. Theophylline disposition in acutely ill hospitalized patients. Am Rev Respir Dis 1978;118:229–238.

Drug Doses

The dose regimen in Table 25.4 is meant to achieve a serum theophylline level of approximately 10 mg/L, which is the low end of the therapeutic range. **The therapeutic range for serum theophylline is 10 to 20 mg/L, or 55.5 to 111 μmol/L (1 mg/L = 5.5 μmol/L).** The loading dose in obese patients is usually given according to ideal body weight, but the appropriate dosing weight in obesity is somewhere between ideal and actual body weight (26). Therefore, monitoring serum theophylline levels is very important in obese patients. Note also the marked reduction in theophylline dose for patients with heart failure. Dose adjustments may also be necessary in patients receiving drugs that can alter serum theophylline levels (see Chapter 54 for the drugs that interact with theophylline).

THEOPHYLLINE TOXICITY

Theophylline is the fifth leading cause of (pharmaceutical) drug-induced toxicity, and theophylline toxicity is the fifth leading cause of death from toxic drug exposure (27). One report revealed that physicians' prescribing errors were responsible for 68% of the cases of in-hospital theophylline toxicity (28).

Manifestations

Theophylline toxicity is defined as any serum theophylline level above 20 mg/L. Clinical manifestations of toxicity are present in most patients with serum levels of 20 to 30 mg/L, and in virtually all patients with drug levels above 30 mg/L (29). Common manifestations in mild toxicity include tachycardia, tremors, nausea, diarrhea, and agitation. More severe cases of toxicity are characterized by confusion, hypotension, hypokalemia, and supraventricular tachycardia. The severest cases are characterized by generalized seizures, coma, and ventricular fibrillation. The severity of the clinical manifestations does not always correlate with the degree of elevation in serum theophylline levels (29,30).

Management

The management of theophylline toxicity can be divided into three stages.

Stage 1: The first step is to discontinue drug administration. In mild cases of toxicity, therapy can be restarted at a lower dose.

Stage 2. When the toxic manifestations are more severe (e.g., change in mental status), **oral activated charcoal** is used to enhance theophylline clearance. Charcoal in the lumen of the gastrointestinal (GI) tract can actually speed up theophylline clearance from the bloodstream because the charcoal absorbs some of the drug that circulates back and forth across the GI mucosa (GI dialysis). The dose of charcoal is **20 g every 2 hours, with 75 mL of 70% sorbitol added to every other dose** to facilitate passage of the charcoal (30).

Stage 3: In cases of life-threatening theophylline toxicity (e.g., serious arrhythmias, seizures, or a serum theophylline level above 100 mg/L), **charcoal or resin hemoperfusion** is recommended to enhance theophylline clearance. If these measures are not available, hemodialysis is an effective alternative. Peritoneal dialysis does not enhance theophylline clearance.

More specific measures may be necessary in addition to the measures aimed at removing theophylline. Although seizures are usually not recurrent (29), short-term therapy with anticonvulsants is recommended until serum theophylline is reduced to safe levels. Cardiac arrhythmias can be treated with selective β-1 receptor antagonists (e.g., esmolol) without precipitating bronchospasm (31). Theophylline-induced hypotension may be refractory to conventional vasopressors.

CORTICOSTEROIDS

Corticosteroids have enjoyed a long-standing popularity in the management of asthma that is refractory to bronchodilator therapy. The relative features of the antiinflammatory corticosteroids are shown in Table 25.5.

ASTHMA

Acute asthma is no longer viewed as a purely bronchospastic disorder. The bronchospasm is an early manifestation, but lasts only 30 to

TABLE 25.5 A COMPARISON OF ANTIINFLAMMATORY CORTICOSTEROIDS				
Corticosteroid	Parenteral Form	Equivalent Dose (mg)	Relative Anti-inflammatory Activity*	Relative Sodium Retention*
Hydrocortisone	Solucortef	20	1	20
Prednisone	—	5	3.5	1
Methyprednisolone	Solumedrol	4	5	0.5
Dexamethasone	Decadron	0.75	30–40	0
* From Zeiss CR, Intense pharmacotherapy. Chest 1992;101(Suppl):407S.				

60 minutes. A second episode of airway obstruction occurs 3 to 8 hours later, and is caused by inflammation and edema in the walls of the small airways (32). Thus, bronchodilators should be effective in the early stages of acute asthma, whereas anti-inflammatory corticosteroids should be effective in relieving the obstruction that occurs later in the disorder. The effect of steroids on the delayed obstruction would explain why steroid effects in acute asthma often require 6 to 8 hours to become evident.

Which Agent at What Dose?

As demonstrated in Figure 25.4, acute asthma that is refractory to three successive β-agonist aerosol treatments should be treated with an intravenous corticosteroid. The recommendations of the National Asthma Education Program (1) are methylprednisolone, 80 to 125 mg iv push (then 80 mg iv every 6 to 8 hours), or hydrocortisone, 2 mg/ kg iv push (then 2 mg/kg iv every 4 hours). Although there is no evidence that one corticosteroid is superior to the others for the management of acute asthma, methylprednisolone might be favored over hydrocortisone because of its superior anti-inflammatory activity (Table 25.5). The appropriate dose of corticosteroids is also unknown, but most recommendations favor high-dose regimens. When patients stabilize on intravenous steroids, they can be switched to oral prednisone starting at a daily dose of 60 mg. The oral dose is then tapered as dictated by the clinical situation.

What to Expect

Do not expect miracles. In fact, despite the overwhelming popularity of steroid use in acute asthma, the reported experience with steroid therapy in acute asthma is far from an endorsement of merit. A number of clinical studies have shown *no* benefit with steroid therapy in acute asthma (see references 33–36). These studies provide a more balanced perspective of steroid therapy in acute asthma.

CHRONIC OBSTRUCTIVE PULMONARY DISEASE

Corticosteroids are also popular in the management of patients with severe COPD. However, there is no evidence that corticosteroids are beneficial in COPD (36). Because one of the characteristics of COPD is the lack of airway response to bronchodilators, it is unreasonable to expect an airway response to pharmaceutical manipulation with corticosteroids in COPD.

SIDE EFFECTS

Although chronic steroid therapy is associated with multiple side-effects, short-term administration of steroids (i.e., 1 month or less) is relatively free of adverse reactions.

Mental Status

Acute therapy with high-dose steroids is often accompanied by a sense of euphoria and well-being. Although psychotic reactions are often mentioned as a complication of high-dose steroids (18), this phenomenon is not well documented.

Myopathy

A myopathy has been reported in ventilator-dependent asthmatic patients treated with high-dose steroids and neuromuscular blocking agents (37). Unlike the traditional steroid myopathy, which is characterized by proximal muscle weakness, the myopathy in ventilator-dependent asthmatics involves both proximal and distal muscles, and is often associated with rhabdomyolysis (37). The etiology of this destructive myopathy is unknown, but the combination of steroids and paralyzing drugs is somehow involved. The muscle weakness can be prolonged and can hamper weaning from mechanical ventilation. Once the disorder is suspected, rapid taper of the paralyzing agents and steroids is advised. Fortunately, this disorder is reversible.

MUCOKINETIC THERAPY

The goal of mucokinetic therapy is to facilitate the clearance of respiratory secretions and remove any luminal barriers to airflow (38). This approach is limited primarily to patients who require prolonged mechanical ventilation.

BLAND AEROSOLS

The principal function of aerosols in clinical medicine is to introduce a pharmaceutical agent into the upper airways. Aerosols that do not

TABLE 25.6 MUCOLYTIC THERAPY WITH N-ACETYLCYSTEINE (NAC)	
Aerosol therapy:	• Use 10% NAC solution.
	• Mix 2.5 mL NAC with 2.5 mL saline and place mixture (5 mL) in a small-volume nebulizer for aerosol delivery.
Warning:	• Can provoke coughing and bronchospasm.
Tracheal instillation:	• Use 20% NAC solution
	• Mix 2.0 mL NAC with 2.0 mL saline and inject in 2 mL aliquots.
Warning:	• Can provoke bronchorrhea.

contain a pharmaceutical agent are called *bland aerosols* (38). Most bland aerosols are made up of saline solutions (hypotonic, isotonic, and hypertonic) or distilled water. Bland aerosols are used to induce coughing (hypertonic aerosols) and to liquefy thick and tenacious secretions. The latter practice is common but not justified, as described below.

Sol versus Gel

The respiratory secretions create a blanket that covers the mucosal surface of the airways. This blanket has a hydrophilic region (sol phase) and a hydrophobic region (gel phase). The hydrophilic region faces inward, and helps keep the mucosal surface moist. The hydrophobic region faces the lumen of the airways. This region contains a meshwork of mucoprotein strands (called mucus threads) that is held together by disulfide bridges. This meshwork traps particles and debris in the airways, and the combination of the mucoprotein mesh and the trapped debris is what determines the viscoelastic behavior of the secretions. Because water *cannot* enter the phase of secretions that is responsible for their viscoelastic behavior, the use of bland aerosols to liquefy and disrupt secretions is futile.

MUCOLYTIC THERAPY

The disruption of tenacious secretions is accomplished by disrupting the bonds that link the mucoprotein strands together. Disruption of disulfide bridges between mucoprotein strands is the basis for mucolytic therapy with N-acetylcysteine (Mucomyst) (39), a sulfhydryl-containing tripeptide that is better known as the antidote for acetaminophen overdose (see Fig. 53.1). N-acetylcysteine (NAC) is available in a liquid preparation (10 or 20% solution) that can be given as an aerosol spray, or injected directly into the airways (Table 25.6). Aerosolized

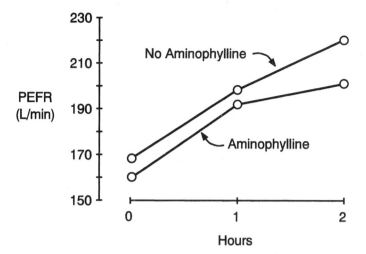

Figure 25.5. Changes in peak expiratory flow rate (*PEFR*) in patients with acute exacerbation of asthma treated with inhaled metaproterenol and intravenous hydrocortisone, with and without intravenous aminophylline. Each point represents the mean value for all patients in each treatment group. (From Wrenn K, et al. Aminophylline therapy for acute bronchospastic disease in the emergency room. Ann Intern Med 1991;115:241–247.)

NAC should be avoided when possible because it is irritating to the airways and can provoke coughing and bronchospasm (particularly in asthmatics) and because it has a disagreeable taste (because of the sulfur content of NAC) and can provoke nausea and vomiting in patients who are not intubated. Direct instillation of NAC into the tracheal tube (two or three times a day) can be used in select patients with problems clearing secretions (I use this approach for postoperative patients who require bronchoscopy to clear obstructing secretions). Excess volumes of intratracheal NAC should be avoided because the solution is hypertonic (even with the saline additive) and can provoke bronchorrhea.

REFERENCES

REVIEWS

1. National Asthma Education Program Expert Panel Report. Guidelines for the diagnosis and management of asthma. Bethesda, MD: U.S. Department of Health and Human Services, Public Health Service. Pub. No. 91-3042, August, 1991.
2. Kacmarek RM. Humidity and aerosol therapy. In: Pierson DJ, Kacmarek RM, eds. Foundations of respiratory care. New York: Churchill Livingstone, 1992; 793–824 (175 references).
3. McFadden ER Jr, Hejal R. Asthma. Lancet 1995;345:1215–1220 (60 references).
4. Manthous CA. Management of severe exacerbations of asthma. Am J Med 1995;99:298–308 (89 references).

BEDSIDE MONITORING

5. Leiner GC. Expiratory peak flow rate. Standard values from normal subjects. Am Rev Respir Dis 1963;88:644.
6. Quackenboss JJ, Lebowitz MD, Kryzyzanowski M. The normal range of diurnal changes in peak expiratory flow rate. Am Rev Respir Dis 1991;143:323–330.
7. Mendoza GR. Peak flow monitoring. J Asthma 1991;28:161–177.
8. Li JTC. Home peak expiratory flow rate monitoring in patients with asthma. Mayo Clin Proc 1995;70:649–656.
9. Gay PC, Rodarte JR, Tayyab M, Hubmayr RD. Evaluation of bronchodilator responsiveness in mechanically ventilated patients. Am Rev Respir Dis 1987; 136:880–885.

BETA-RECEPTOR AGONISTS

10. Salmeron S, Brochard L. Mal H, et al. Nebulized versus intravenous albuterol in hypercapnic acute asthma. Am J Respir Crit Care Med 1994;149:1466–1470.
11. Clarke SW, Newman SP. Differences between pressurized aerosol and stable dust particles. Chest 1981;80(Suppl):907–908.
12. Idris AH, McDermott MF, Raucci JC, et al. Emergency department treatment of severe asthma. Metered-dose inhaler plus holding chamber is equivalent in effectiveness to nebulizer. Chest 1993;103:665–672.
13. Manthous CA, Hall JB. Update on using therapeutic aerosols in mechanically ventilated patients. J Crit Illness 1996;11:457–468.
14. Gay PC, Patel HG, Nelson SB, et al. Metered dose inhalers for bronchodilator delivery in intubated, mechanically ventilated patients. Chest 1991;99:66–71.
15. Bowton DL, Goldsmith WM, Haponik EF. Substitution of metered-dose inhalers for hand-held nebulizers. Chest 1992;101:305–308.
16. Taylor RH, Lerman J. High-efficiency delivery of salbutamol with a metered-dose inhaler in narrow tracheal tubes and catheters. Anesthesiology 1991;74: 360–363.
17. O'Riordan TG, Palmer LB, Smaldone GC. Aerosol deposition in mechanically ventilated patients. Am Rev Respir Crit Care Med 1994;149:214–219.
18. Truwit JD. Toxic effect of bronchodilators. Crit Care Clin 1991;7:639–657.
19. Bodenhamer J, Bergstrom R, Brown D, et al. Frequently nebulized beta-agonists for asthma: effects on serum electrolytes. Ann Emerg Med 1992;21: 1337–1342.
20. Allon M, Dunlay R, Copkney C. Nebulized albuterol for acute hyperkalemia in patients on hemodialysis. Ann Intern Med 1989;110:426–429.

THEOPHYLLINE

21. Johnson ID. Theophylline in the management of airflow obstruction. Difficult drug to use, few clinical indications. Br Med J 1990;300:929–931.
22. Self TH, Abou-Shala N, Burns R, et al. Inhaled albuterol and oral prednisone therapy in hospitalized adult asthmatics. Does aminophylline add any benefit? Chest 1990;98:1317–1321.
23. Rodrigo C, Rodrigo G. Treatment of acute asthma: lack of therapeutic benefit and increase in toxicity from aminophylline given in addition to high dose salbutamol delivered by metered-dose inhaler with spacer. Chest 1994;106: 1071–1076.

24. Weiss KB. Seasonal trends in U.S. asthma hospitalizations and mortality. JAMA 1990;263:2323–2328.
25. Terzian CG, Simon PA. Aminophylline hypersensitivity apparently due to ethylenediamine. Ann Emerg Med 1992;21:312–317.
26. Rizzo A, Mirabella A, Bonanno A. Effect of body weight on the volume of distribution of theophylline. Lung 1988;166:269–276.
27. Litovitz TL. 1992 Annual Report of the American Association of Poison Control Centers Toxic Exposure Surveillance System. Am J Emerg Med 1993;11:494–555.
28. Schiff GD, Hegde HK, LaCloche L, Hryhorczuk DO. Inpatient theophylline toxicity: preventable factors. Ann Intern Med 1991;114:748–752.
29. Sissler CN. Theophylline toxicity: clinical features of 116 consecutive cases. Am J Med 1990;88:567–576.
30. Cooling DS. Theophylline toxicity. J Emerg Med 1993;11:415–425.
31. Seneff M, Scott J, Friedman B, et al. Acute theophylline toxicity and the use of esmolol to reverse cardiovascular instability. Ann Emerg Med 1990;19:671–673.

CORTICOSTEROIDS

32. Kay AB. Asthma and inflammation. J Allergy Clin Immunol 1991;87:893–945.
33. Stein LM, Cole RP. Early administration of corticosteroids in emergency room treatment of asthma. Ann Intern Med 1990;112:822–827.
34. Bowler SD, Mitchell CA, Armstrong JG. Corticosteroids in acute severe asthma: effectiveness of low doses. Thorax 1992;47:584–587.
35. Morrell F, Orriols R, de Gracia J, et al. Controlled trial of intravenous corticosteroids in severe acute asthma. Thorax 1992;47:588–591.
36. Eliasson O, Hoffman J, Trueb D, et al. Corticosteroids in COPD. Chest 1986;89:484–489.
37. Griffin D, Fairman N, Coursin D, et al. Acute myopathy during treatment of status asthmaticus with corticosteroids and steroidal muscle relaxants. Chest 1992;102:510–514.

MUCOKINETIC THERAPY

38. Lebovitz DJ, Reed MD. Clinical pharmacology of mucokinetic drugs. In: Chernow B, ed. The pharmacologic approach to the critically ill patient. 3rd ed. Baltimore: Williams & Wilkins, 1994;605–613.
39. Holdiness MR. Clinical pharmacokinetics of N-acetylcysteine. Clin Pharmacokinet 1991;20:123–134.

MECHANICAL VENTILATION

All who drink of this remedy will recover . . . except those in whom it does not help, who will die. Therefore, it is obvious that it fails only in incurable cases.

Galen

BELONGS TO

DR. SUSANTO

310-386-5955

La Bellasera
HOTEL & SUITES

206 Alexa Court, Paso Robles, California 93446

telephone 805-238-2834   fax 805-238-2826

www.labellasera.com

c h a p t e r

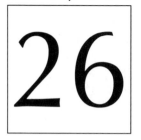

PRINCIPLES OF MECHANICAL VENTILATION

". . . an opening must be attempted in the trunk of the trachea, into which a tube of reed or cane should be put; you will then blow into this, so that the lung may rise again . . . and the heart becomes strong . . . "

Andreas Vesalius (1555)

Vesalius is credited with the first description of positive-pressure ventilation, but it took 400 years to apply his concept to patient care. The occasion was the polio epidemic of 1955, when the demand for assisted ventilation outgrew the supply of negative-pressure tank ventilators (known as *iron lungs*). In Sweden, all medical schools shut down and medical students worked in 8-hour shifts as human ventilators, manually inflating the lungs of afflicted patients. In Boston, the nearby Emerson Company made available a prototype positive-pressure lung inflation device, which was put to use at the Massachusetts General Hospital, and became an instant success. Thus began the era of positive-pressure mechanical ventilation (and the era of intensive care medicine).

CONVENTIONAL MECHANICAL VENTILATION

The first positive-pressure ventilators were designed to inflate the lungs until a preset pressure was reached. This type of *pressure-cycled* ventilation fell out of favor because the inflation volume varied with changes in the mechanical properties of the lungs. In contrast, *volume-cycled* ventilation, which inflates the lungs to a predetermined volume, delivers a constant alveolar volume despite changes in the mechanical properties of the lungs. For this reason, volume-cycled ventilation has become the standard method of positive-pressure mechanical ventilation (1–5).

421

INFLATION PRESSURES

The waveforms produced by volume-cycled ventilation are shown in Figure 26.1. The lungs are inflated at a constant flow rate, and this produces a linear increase in lung volume. The pressure in the proximal airways (P_{prox}) shows an abrupt initial rise, followed by a more gradual rise through the remainder of lung inflation. However, the pressure in the alveoli (P_{ALV}) shows only a gradual rise during lung inflation.

The early, abrupt rise in proximal airway pressure is a reflection of flow resistance in the airways. An increase in airways resistance magnifies the initial rise in proximal airway pressure, while the alveolar pressure at the end of lung inflation remains unchanged. Thus, **when resistance in the airways increases,** higher inflation pressures are needed to deliver the inflation volume, but **the alveoli are not exposed to the higher inflation pressures.** This is not the case when the distensibility (compliance) of the lungs is reduced. In this latter condition, there is an increase in both the proximal airways pressure and the alveolar pressure. Thus, **when lung distensibility (compliance) decreases, the higher inflation pressures** needed to deliver the

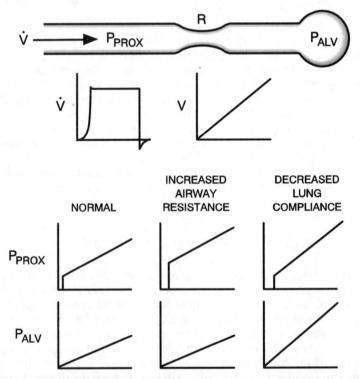

Figure 26.1. Waveforms produced by constant-flow, volume-cycled ventilation. V = inspiratory flow rate, V = inspiratory volume, R = flow resistance in the airways, P_{prox} = proximal airway pressure, P_{ALV} = alveolar pressure.

inflation volume **are readily transmitted to the alveoli.** The increase in alveolar pressure in noncompliant lungs can lead to pressure-induced lung injury (see later in the chapter).

CARDIAC PERFORMANCE

The influence of positive-pressure ventilation on cardiac performance is complex and involves changes in preload and afterload for both the right and left sides of the heart (6). To describe these changes, it is important to review the influence of intrathoracic pressure on transmural pressure, which is the pressure that determines ventricular filling (preload) and the resistance to ventricular emptying (afterload).

TRANSMURAL PRESSURE

The transmission of intrathoracic pressure into the lumen of intrathoracic blood vessels is described briefly in Chapter 11 (see Fig. 11.1). The influence of lung mechanics on this pressure transmission is illustrated in Figure 26.2. The panel on the left shows what happens when a normal lung is inflated with 700 mL from a positive-pressure source. In this situation, the increase in alveolar pressure is completely transmitted into the pulmonary capillaries, and there is no change in transmural pressure (P_{tm}) across the capillaries. However, when the same lung inflation occurs in lungs that are not easily distended (panel on the right), the increase in alveolar pressure is not completely trans-

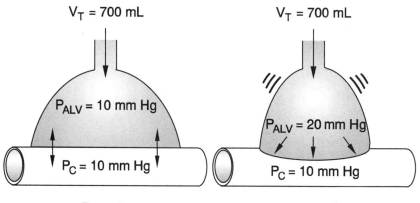

Figure 26.2. Alveolar–capillary units showing the transmission of alveolar pressure (P_{ALV}) to the pulmonary capillaries in normal and noncompliant (stiff) lungs. P_c = capillary hydrostatic pressure, P_{tm} = transmural pressure across the capillary wall, V_T = tidal volume delivered by the ventilator.

mitted into the capillaries and the transmural pressure increases. This increase in transmural pressure acts to compress the capillaries. Therefore, in conditions associated with a decrease in lung compliance (e.g., pulmonary edema, pneumonia), positive-pressure lung inflation tends to compress the heart and intrathoracic blood vessels (7–9). This compression can be beneficial or detrimental, as described below.

Preload

Positive-pressure lung inflation can reduce ventricular filling in several ways, as indicated in Figure 26.3. First, positive intrathoracic pressure decreases the pressure gradient for venous inflow into the thorax. In addition, any increase in positive pressure on the outer surface of the ventricles will reduce ventricular distensibility, and this can reduce ventricular filling during diastole. Finally, compression of pulmonary blood vessels can reduce left ventricular filling by decreasing venous inflow to the left side of the heart, or by impeding right heart ejection. In this latter situation, the right ventricle can dilate and push the interventricular septum toward the left ventricle and reduce left ventricular chamber size. This phenomenon, known as *ventricular interdependence*, is one of the mechanisms whereby right heart failure can impair the performance of the left side of the heart (see Fig. 16.4).

Afterload

Whereas ventricular compression during positive-pressure lung inflation impedes ventricular filling during diastole, this same compression *facilitates* ventricular emptying during systole. This latter effect is

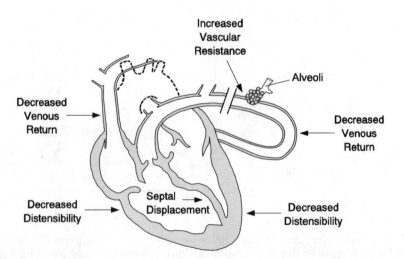

Figure 26.3. The mechanisms whereby positive-pressure mechanical ventilation can decrease ventricular filling (preload).

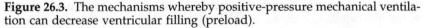

easy to visualize (like a hand squeezing the ventricles during systole) and can also be explained in terms of ventricular afterload. That is, ventricular afterload, or the impedance to ventricular emptying, is a function of the peak systolic *transmural* wall pressure (see Fig. 1.3). Incomplete transmission of positive intrathoracic pressure into the ventricular chambers will decrease the transmural pressure across the ventricles during systole, and this decrease ventricular afterload.

CARDIAC OUTPUT

Positive-pressure lung inflation tends to reduce ventricular filling during diastole but enhances ventricular emptying during systole. When ventricular filling is reduced, cardiac output is similarly reduced. However, *when ventricular filling is not compromised, positive-pressure lung inflation can increase cardiac stroke output.* The increase in stroke volume causes an increase in systolic blood pressure during positive-pressure lung inflation; a phenomenon known as reverse pulsus paradoxus. The favorable influence of positive intrathoracic pressure on cardiac output is one mechanism that explains the beneficial actions of closed chest compressions in cardiac arrest (see Chapter 17).

INDICATIONS FOR MECHANICAL VENTILATION

The decision to intubate and initiate mechanical ventilation has always seemed more complicated than it should be. Instead of the usual lists of clinical and physiologic indications for mechanical ventilation, the following simple rules should suffice.

Rule 1. **The indication for intubation and mechanical ventilation is thinking of it.** There is a tendency to delay intubation and mechanical ventilation as long as possible in the hopes that it will be unnecessary. However, elective intubation carries far fewer dangers than emergent intubation, and thus delays in intubation create unnecessary dangers for the patient. If the patient's condition is severe enough for intubation and mechanical ventilation to be considered, then proceed without delay.

Rule 2. **Intubation is not an act of weakness.** Housestaff tend to apologize on morning rounds when they have intubated a patient during the evening, almost as though the intervention was an act of cowardice. What they must understand is that they will never be faulted for establishing control of the airways.

Rule 3. **Endotracheal tubes are not a disease, and ventilators are not an addiction.** The assumption that "once on a ventilator, always on a ventilator" is a fallacy and should never influence the decision to initiate mechanical ventilation. Endotracheal tubes and ventilators do not create the need for mechanical ventilation; cardiopulmonary and neuromuscular diseases do.

TABLE 26.1. STRATEGIES FOR MECHANICAL VENTILATION		
	Ventilatory Strategies	
Ventilatory Parameter	**Traditional**	**Lung–Protective**
Inflation Volume	10–15 ml/kg	5–10 ml/kg
Mechanical Sighs	Volume: 15–30 ml/kg Rate: 6–12/hr	None
End–Inspiratory Pressure	Peak Pressure < 50 cm H2O	Plateau Pressure < 35 cm H2O
Positive End–Expiratory Pressure (PEEP)	Only when needed to keep the FIO_2 below 0.60	5–15 cm H2O
Arterial Blood Gases	Normal or Usual PaCO2 pH = 7.36–7.44	Hypercapnia allowed pH = 7.20–7.44

VENTILATORY STRATEGIES

Thirty years after positive-pressure mechanical ventilation was introduced on a large scale, it became evident that the traditional methods of assisted ventilation can actually *add* to the underlying cardiopulmonary derangements. This realization has led to a revised strategy for mechanical ventilation (3), which was introduced in Chapter 23 and is outlined in Table 26.1.

LARGE INFLATION VOLUMES

In the early days of positive-pressure mechanical ventilation, large inflation volumes were recommended to prevent alveolar collapse (10), and these large inflation volumes became standard. Thus, **whereas the tidal volume during unassisted ventilation in adults is normally 5 to 7 mL/kg (ideal body weight), the standard inflation volumes during volume-cycled ventilation are 10 to 15 mL/kg** (i.e., at least twice normal). The volume discrepancy is even greater with the addition of mechanical *sighs,* which are 1.5 to two times greater than standard inflation volumes (or 15 to 30 mL/kg) and are delivered 6 to 12 times per hour (Table 26.1).

The large inflation volumes used in conventional mechanical ventilation can reduce cardiac output (8,9). Large inflation volumes can also damage the lungs, as described below.

Ventilator-Induced Lung Injury

In lung diseases that most often require mechanical ventilation (e.g., acute respiratory distress syndrome [ARDS], pneumonia), the pathologic changes are not uniformly distributed throughout the lungs (11). Because inflation volumes are distributed preferentially to regions of normal lung function, inflation volumes tend to overdistend the normal regions of diseased lungs. This tendency to overdistend normal lung regions is exaggerated when large inflation volumes are used.

The **hyperinflation of normal lung regions during mechanical ventilation can produce stress fractures in the walls of alveoli and adjacent pulmonary capillaries** (12,13). The alveolar damage can lead to alveolar rupture, with accumulation of alveolar gas in the pulmonary parenchyma (pulmonary interstitial emphysema), mediastinum (pneumomediastinum), or pleural cavity (pneumothorax). The damage to the pulmonary capillaries can result in a leaky-capillary type of pulmonary edema (14). These complications may be the result of excessive alveolar pressures (barotrauma) or excessive alveolar volumes (volutrauma) (15).

LUNG-PROTECTIVE VENTILATION

Because of the risk of lung injury with large inflation volumes, an alternative approach evolved in recent years where reduced inflation volumes (5 to 10 mL/kg) are advocated (Table 26.1) (3). This strategy also eliminates mechanical sighs and uses positive end-expiratory pressure (PEEP) to prevent collapse of alveoli and small airways (16). The goal is an end-inspiratory plateau pressure that is less than 35 cm H_2O (this pressure is described later in this chapter). Inflation volumes of 8 mL/kg or lower can result in CO_2 retention, which is allowed if no evidence of harm exists. This latter strategy is known as *permissive hypercapnia* (17).

MONITORING LUNG MECHANICS

During spontaneous breathing, the mechanical properties of the lungs (i.e., elastic recoil of the lungs and resistance to flow in the airways) can be monitored with pulmonary function tests. However, these tests are not easily performed during mechanical ventilation. In this setting, the proximal airways pressures can be used to assess pulmonary function (18,19).

PROXIMAL AIRWAY PRESSURES

Positive-pressure mechanical ventilators have a pressure gauge that monitors the proximal airway pressure during each respiratory cycle. The components of this pressure are illustrated in Figure 26.4.

End-Inspiratory Peak Pressure

The peak pressure at the end of inspiration (P_{peak}) is a function of the inflation volume, the flow resistance in the airways, and the elastic recoil force of the lungs and chest wall. At a constant inflation volume, the peak pressure is directly related to airflow resistance and to the elastic recoil force (elastance) of the lungs and chest wall:

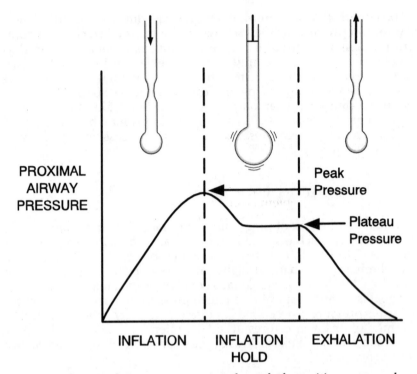

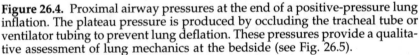

Figure 26.4. Proximal airway pressures at the end of a positive-pressure lung inflation. The plateau pressure is produced by occluding the tracheal tube or ventilator tubing to prevent lung deflation. These pressures provide a qualitative assessment of lung mechanics at the bedside (see Fig. 26.5).

$$P_{peak} \sim \text{Resistance} \times \text{Elastance} \qquad (26.1)$$

Therefore when the inflation volume is constant, an increase in peak inspiratory pressure indicates an increase in either airway resistance or elastance of the lungs and chest wall, or both.

End-Inspiratory Plateau Pressure

The contribution of resistance and elastance to the peak inspiratory pressure can be distinguished by occluding the expiratory tubing at the end of inspiration, as shown in Figure 26.4. When the inflation volume is held in the lungs, the proximal airway pressure decreases initially and then reaches a steady level, which is called the end-inspiratory *plateau pressure*. Because no airflow is present when the plateau pressure is created, the pressure is not a function of flow resistance in the airways. Instead, the plateau pressure ($P_{plateau}$) is directly proportional to the elastance of the lungs and chest wall.

$$P_{plateau} \sim \text{Elastance} \qquad (26.2)$$

Therefore, the difference between end-inspiratory peak and plateau pressures is proportional to the flow resistance in the airways.

$$P_{peak} - P_{plateau} \sim \text{Airflow resistance} \qquad (26.3)$$

Practical Applications

The flow diagram in Figure 26.5 demonstrates how the proximal airways pressures can be applied to patient care. In this case, the pressures are used to evaluate an acute deterioration in respiratory status.

1. If the peak pressure is increased but the plateau pressure is unchanged, the problem is an increase in airways resistance. In this situation, the major concerns are obstruction of the tracheal tube, airway obstruction from secretions, and acute bronchospasm. Therefore, airways suctioning is indicated to clear secretions, followed by an aerosolized bronchodilator treatment if necessary.
2. If the peak and plateau pressures are both increased, the problem is a decrease in distensibility of the lungs and chest wall. In this situation, the major concerns are pneumothorax, lobar atelectasis, acute pulmonary edema, and worsening pneumonia or ARDS. Active contraction of the chest wall and increased abdominal pressure can also decrease the distensibility of the thorax. Finally, a patient with obstructive lung disease who becomes tachypneic can develop auto-PEEP, and this increases the peak and plateau pressures as well (see Chapter 28).
3. If the peak pressure is decreased, the problem may be an air leak in the system (e.g., tubing disconnection, cuff leak). In this situation, the lungs should be manually inflated with an Ambu bag and a cuff leak should be listened for during lung inflation. A decrease in peak pressure can also be due to hyperventilation, when the patient is generating enough of a negative intrathoracic pressure to "pull" air into the lungs.
4. If no change in peak pressure occurs, it does not necessarily mean that there has been no change in lung mechanics. The sensitivity of the proximal airways pressures in detecting changes in lung mechanics is unknown. When the pressures do not change, the evaluation should proceed as it would without the aid of proximal airway pressures.

Bronchodilator Responsiveness

Ventilator-dependent patients often receive aerosolized bronchodilator treatments routinely, without documented need or benefit. The proximal airway pressures provide a more rational approach to the use of bronchodilators in ventilator-dependent patients. If an aerosol bronchodilator treatment does not produce a decrease in peak inspiratory pressures (indicating bronchodilation), there is little justification for continuing the aerosol treatments.

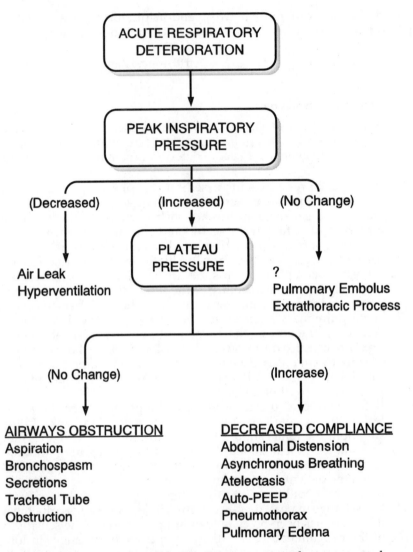

Figure 26.5. The use of proximal airway pressures to evaluate an acute change in ventilatory status at the bedside.

THORACIC COMPLIANCE

The compliance, or distensibility, of the lungs and chest wall (called thoracic compliance) can be determined quantitatively as the ratio of a change in lung volume (i.e., inflation volume) to a change in elastic recoil pressure (i.e., plateau pressure). For a tidal volume (V_T) of 800 mL and a plateau pressure (P_{pl}) of 10 cm H_2O, the static compliance (C_{stat}) of the thorax is as follows:

$$Cstat = V_T/P_{pl}$$

$$= 0.8 \text{ L}/10 \text{ cm H}_2O \qquad (26.4)$$

$$= 0.08 \text{ L/cm H}_2O \text{ (or 80 mL/cm H}_2O)$$

The thoracic compliance in intubated patients with no known lung disease is between 0.05 to 0.08 L/cm H_2O (or 50 to 80 mL/cm H_2O) (18). In patients with stiff lungs, the thoracic compliance is much lower at 0.01 to 0.02 L/cm H_2O (20). Thus, the compliance determination provides an objective measure of the severity of illness in pulmonary disorders associated with a change in lung compliance.

Considerations

The following factors influence the static compliance measurement.

1. **PEEP** increases the plateau pressure. Therefore, the level of PEEP (either externally applied or auto-PEEP) should be subtracted from the plateau pressure for the compliance determination.
2. The **connector tubing** between the ventilator and patient expands during positive-pressure lung inflations, and the volume lost in this expansion reduces the inflation volume reaching the patient. The volume lost is a function of the peak inflation pressure and the inherent compliance of the tubing. The usual compliance of connector tubing is 3 mL/cm H_2O, which means that 3 mL of volume is lost for every 1 cm H_2O increase in inflation pressure. Thus, if the inflation volume from the ventilator is 700 mL and the peak inspiratory pressure is 40 cm H_2O, then (3×40) 120 mL will be lost to expansion of the ventilator tubing and the inflation volume reaching the patient will be $(700 - 120)$ 580 mL. Because of this discrepancy, the predetermined volume setting on the ventilator should not be used as the inflation volume for the compliance calculation. Instead, the exhaled volume, which is usually displayed digitally on the ventilator panel, should be used.
3. Because the proximal airways pressures are transthoracic pressures (i.e., measured relative to atmospheric pressure) and not transpulmonary pressures (i.e., measured relative to intrapleural pressure), the compliance measurement includes the chest wall as well as the lungs. Because contraction of the chest wall muscles can reduce the compliance (distensibility) of the chest wall, the compliance determination should be performed only during passive ventilation. However during passive ventilation, the chest wall can account for 35% of the total thoracic compliance (19, 20).

AIRWAY RESISTANCE

The resistance to airflow during inspiration (R_{insp}) can be determined as the ratio of the pressure gradient needed to overcome airways resistance ($P_{pk} - P_{pl}$) and the inspiratory flow rate (V_{insp}): $R_{insp} = P_{pk} - P_{pl}/V_{insp}$. This resistance represents the summed resistances of the connector tubing, the tracheal tube, and the airways. Because the resistance of the connector tubing and tracheal tube should remain constant (assuming the tracheal tube is clear of secretions), changes in R_{insp} should represent changes in airways resistance.

A sample calculation of inspiratory resistance is shown in Equation 26.5 for an inspiratory flow of 60 L/min (1.0 L/sec), a peak pressure of 20 cm H_2O, and a plateau pressure of 10 cm H_2O.

$$R_{insp} = P_{pk} - P_{pl}/V_{insp}$$

$$= 20 - 10/1 \qquad (26.5)$$

$$= 10 \text{ cm } H_2O/L/sec$$

The minimal flow resistance in large-bore endotracheal tubes is 3 to 7 cm H_2O/L/sec (21), so nonpulmonary resistive elements can contribute a considerable fraction of the total inspiratory resistance.

Limitations

The major limitations of the inspiratory resistance measurement are the contributions of resistive elements not in the lung and the relative insensitivity of the resistance measured during inspiration. Airflow obstruction is usually measured during expiration, when the airways have the greatest tendency to collapse. The distending pressures delivered by the ventilator during lung inflation keep the airways open, and thus the resistance to flow during inspiration does not measure the tendency for the airways to collapse during expiration (19).

REFERENCES

GENERAL TEXTS

Grenvik A, Downs J, Rasanen J, Smith R, eds. Mechanical ventilation and assisted respiration. Contemporary management in critical care. New York: Churchill Livingstone, 1991;1(1).
Hess DR, Kacmarek RM. Essential of mechanical ventilation. New York: McGraw-Hill, 1996.

REVIEWS

1. Slutsky AS (chairman). American College of Chest Physicians' Consensus Conference on Mechanical Ventilation. Chest 1993;104:1833–1859 (158 references).
2. Tobin MJ. Mechanical ventilation. N Engl J Med 1994;330:1056–1061 (58 references).

3. Marini JJ. Pressure-targeted, lung protective ventilatory support in acute lung injury. Chest 1994;105(Suppl):109S–115S (58 references).
4. Gammon RB, Strickland JH Jr, Kennedy KI Jr, Young KR Jr. Mechanical ventilation: a review for the internist. Am J Med 1995;99:553–562.
5. Shapiro BA, Peruzzi WT. Changing practices in ventilator management: a review of the literature and suggested clinical correlations. Surgery 1995;117: 121–133.

CARDIAC PERFORMANCE

6. Pinsky MR. Cardiovascular effects of ventilatory support and withdrawal. Anaesth Analg 1994;79:567–576.
7. Versprille A. The pulmonary circulation during mechanical ventilation. Acta Anesthesiol Scand 1990;34(Suppl):51–62.
8. Venus B, Cohen LE, Smith RA. Hemodynamics and intrathoracic pressure transmission during controlled mechanical ventilation and positive end-expiratory pressure in normal and low compliant lungs. Crit Care Med 1988;16: 686–690.
9. Kiiski R, Takala J, Kari A, Milic-Emili J. Effect of tidal volume on gas exchange and oxygen transport in the adult respiratory distress syndrome. Am Rev Respir Dis 1992;146:1131–1135.

VENTILATORY STRATEGIES

10. Bendixen HH, Egbert LD, Hedley-White J, et al. Respiratory care. St. Louis: Mosby, 1965;137–153.
11. Gattinoni L, Bombino M, Pelosi P, et al. Lung structure and function in different stages of severe adult respiratory distress syndrome. JAMA 1994;271: 1772–1779.
12. Costello ML, Mathieu-Costello OA, West JB. Stress failure of alveolar epithelial cells studied by scanning electron microscopy. Am Rev Respir Dis 1992;145: 1446–1455.
13. Mathieu-Costello OA, West JB. Are pulmonary capillaries susceptible to mechanical stress? Chest 1994;105(Suppl):102S–107S.
14. Timby J, Reed C, Zeilander S, Glauser F. "Mechanical" causes of pulmonary edema. Chest 1990;98:973–979.
15. Bray JC, Cane RD. Mechanical ventilatory support and pulmonary parenchymal injury: positive airway pressure or alveolar hyperinflation? Intensive Crit Care Digest 1993;12:33–36.
16. Muscedere JG, Mullen JBM, Gan K, Slutsky AS. Tidal ventilation at low airway pressures can augment lung injury. Am J Respir Crit Care Med 1994;149: 1327–1334.
17. Bidani A, Tzounakis AE, Cardenas VJ, Zwischenberger JB. Permissive hypercapnia in acute respiratory failure. JAMA 1994;272:957–962.

MONITORING LUNG MECHANICS

18. Tobin MJ. Respiratory monitoring. JAMA 1990;264:244–251.
19. Marini JJ. Lung mechanics determinations at the bedside: instrumentation and clinical application. Respir Care 1990;35:669–696.
20. Katz JA, Zinn SE, Ozanne GM, Fairley BB. Pulmonary, chest wall, and lung–thorax elastances in acute respiratory failure. Chest 1981;80:304–311.
21. Marini JJ. Strategies to minimize breathing effort during mechanical ventilation. Crit Care Clin 1990;6:635–662.

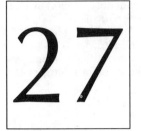

PATTERNS OF ASSISTED VENTILATION

Development in most fields of medicine appears to occur according to sound scientific principles. However, exceptions can be found, and the development of mechanical ventilatory support is one of them.

J. Rasanen

In the half century since positive-pressure ventilation first appeared, at least 15 different methods of assisted breathing have been introduced, each with claims of superiority over the others (1–3). However, these claims usually dissolve in clinical trials. There is a tendency to forget that mechanical ventilation is a support measure, not a therapy for cardiopulmonary disease. To improve outcomes in ventilator-dependent patients, less attention should be paid to the knobs on ventilators, and more attention should be given to the diseases that prompt ventilator dependency.

ASSIST-CONTROL VENTILATION

The standard method of positive-pressure mechanical ventilation involves volume-cycled lung inflation (i.e., each machine breath delivers a preselected inflation volume). The patient can initiate each mechanical breath (assisted ventilation), but when this is not possible, the ventilator provides machine breaths at a preselected rate (controlled ventilation). This pattern is called *assist-control ventilation* (ACV).

VENTILATORY PATTERN

The upper panel in Figure 27.1 shows the changes in airway pressure produced by ACV. The tracing begins with a negative-pressure deflection, followed by a positive-pressure machine breath. The negative

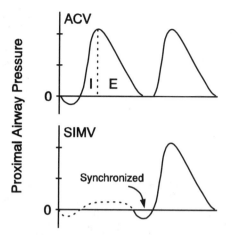

Figure 27.1. Airway pressure patterns in assist-control ventilation (*ACV*) and synchronized intermittent mandatory ventilation (*SIMV*). Spontaneous breaths are indicated by dashed lines, and machine breaths are indicated by solid lines. The mechanical breath in the upper panel indicates the period of lung inflation (*I*) and deflation (*E*).

pressure represents a spontaneous inspiratory effort, which opens a pressure-activated valve that allows the machine breath to be delivered. The second machine breath in the tracing is identical to the first, but it is not preceded by a spontaneous ventilatory effort. The first breath is an example of assisted ventilation, and the second breath is an example of controlled ventilation.

Respiratory Cycle

As mentioned in Chapter 26, conventional volume-cycled ventilation uses large inflation volumes (approximately twice the normal tidal volume during spontaneous breathing). To allow the lungs to empty these large volumes, much more time is allowed for lung deflation than for lung inflation (Fig. 27.1). During conventional volume-cycled ventilation, the I:E ratio (the ratio of inspiratory-to-expiratory duration) is maintained at 1:2 to 1:4 (1–3). This is accomplished by adjusting the inspiratory flow rate (e.g., an increase in the inspiratory flow rate decreases the time for lung inflation and increases the I:E ratio). When the I:E ratio falls below 1:2, the lungs may not empty completely after each inflation. This can result in progressive hyperinflation.

WORK OF BREATHING

A popular misconception about mechanical ventilation is that the diaphragm rests when the ventilator delivers a machine breath. However, the contraction of the diaphragm is dictated by brainstem respiratory neurons that fire in periodic bursts throughout life (4). When the diaphragm contracts and triggers a machine breath, the contraction does not cease, but continues for the duration of the burst activity in the brainstem respiratory neurons. Because the diaphragm is not a voluntary muscle that ceases to contract during assisted machine breaths, **the work of breathing can be considerable during assisted ventilation** (5).

ADVERSE EFFECTS

The undesirable features of ACV occur primarily in patients who are breathing rapidly. In this situation, the increased frequency of machine breaths can lead to overventilation and severe **respiratory alkalosis,** and the decreased time for exhalation can result in **hyperinflation.** Hyperinflation from inadequate lung emptying is accompanied by an intrinsic form of PEEP called auto-PEEP, and this type of PEEP can have the same adverse consequences as externally-applied PEEP (which are described later in the chapter). Hyperinflation and auto-PEEP from excessive positive-pressure ventilation is a source of elec- tromechanical dissociation during CPR (6).

INTERMITTENT MANDATORY VENTILATION

The problems created by rapid breathing during mechanical ventila- tion with ACV led to the introduction of intermittent mandatory venti- lation (IMV). This method, introduced in 1971, was designed to venti- late neonates with respiratory distress syndrome, who typically have respiratory rates in excess of 40 breaths/minute. IMV delivers periodic volume-cycled breaths at a preselected rate, but allows spontaneous breathing between machine breaths (see Fig. 27.1, lower panel). Be- cause each spontaneous breath does not trigger a machine breath, there is a reduced risk of respiratory alkalosis and hyperinflation with IMV.

Shortly after its introduction, IMV was proposed as a valuable method for gradually withdrawing ventilatory support (7). Since then, IMV has become a popular method of weaning patients from mechani- cal ventilation. The description of IMV in this chapter is limited to its use as a mode of ventilation. (The use of IMV in weaning from mechan- ical ventilation is described in Chapter 29.)

BASIC FEATURES

The basic IMV circuit is illustrated in Figure 27.2. The patient is connected to a source of oxygen through two parallel pathways. One pathway contains a volume-cycled ventilator, and the other contains a reservoir bag filled with the desired inspiratory gas mixture. The ventilator delivers machine breaths at a preselected rate and inflation volume. However, a unidirectional valve in the circuit allows the pa- tient to breathe spontaneously from the reservoir bag when a machine breath is not being delivered.

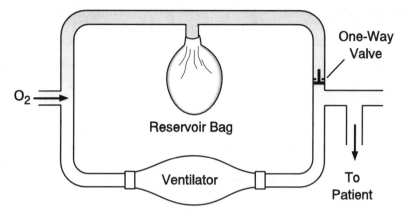

Figure 27.2. Schematic diagram of the circuit used for intermittent mandatory ventilation (IMV).

Ventilatory Pattern

The lower portion of Figure 27.1 shows the pattern of ventilation associated with IMV. The initial negative and positive deflection in the tracing represents a spontaneous breath (dashed line). The second spontaneous breath triggers a machine breath (solid line). This pattern is called *synchronized* IMV because the machine breaths are synchronized to coincide with spontaneous lung inflations. There is also an asynchronous IMV, when machine breaths are delivered at any time during the spontaneous respiratory cycle. This asynchronous pattern is not well tolerated by patients (e.g., the lung inflation can be delivered while the patient is attempting to exhale), and it can produce uneven ventilation. Therefore, the synchronized method of IMV is always favored.

DISADVANTAGES

The principal disadvantages of IMV are an increase in the work of breathing and a tendency for the cardiac output to be reduced.

Work of Breathing

The spontaneous breathing during IMV takes place through a high-resistance circuit (the tracheal tube and ventilator tubing) and requires a valve to be opened. Both of these factors can result in an **increased work of breathing during IMV** (8). In fact, the tendency for less respiratory alkalosis during IMV may be a reflection of an increased work of breathing (which is accompanied by an increase in CO_2 production) and not a decrease in alveolar ventilation (9). The increased work of breathing during IMV could lead to respiratory muscle fatigue, which could then promote further ventilator dependency. To limit the increased work of breathing during IMV, pressure-support can be added during the period of spontaneous breathing (see later for a description of pressure-support).

Cardiac Output

Positive-pressure mechanical ventilation can reduce cardiac output by impeding ventricular filling, and can also increase cardiac output by reducing ventricular afterload (10). In patients with left-ventricular dysfunction, the favorable effects of mechanical ventilation may outweigh the adverse effects (as long as the blood volume is maintained) (9). This may explain why the cardiac output can decrease during IMV in patients with left-ventricular dysfunction (11).

IMV VERSUS ACV

The above descriptions of ACV and IMV suggest the following considerations.

1. In patients who are breathing rapidly during ACV and have evidence of overventilation (respiratory alkalosis) or hyperinflation (auto-PEEP), a switch to IMV should prove beneficial.
2. In patients with evidence of respiratory muscle weakness or with a history of left-ventricular dysfunction, ACV should be favored over IMV.

Otherwise, there is little proven advantage with either mode of ventilation (1,3,12,13), and personal preference largely dictates which mode of ventilation is popular in a particular ICU.

PRESSURE-CONTROLLED VENTILATION

The risk for ventilator-induced lung injury due to large inflation volumes (see Chapter 26) has led to renewed interest in pressure-cycled ventilation. Because peak airway pressures are lower in pressure-cycled than in volume-cycled machine breaths, there is less risk of barotrauma with pressure-cycled ventilation. Pressure-controlled ventilation (PCV) is pressure-cycled breathing that is completed controlled by the ventilator, with no participation by the patient (similar to the control mode of volume-cycled ventilation). The pattern of ventilation produced by PCV is shown in Figure 27.3.

BENEFITS AND RISKS

The major advantage of PCV relates to the inspiratory flow pattern. In volume-cycled breathing, the inspiratory flow rate is constant throughout lung inflation, whereas in pressure-cycled breathing, the inspiratory flow decreases exponentially during lung inflation (to keep the airway pressure at the preselected value). The decreasing inspira-

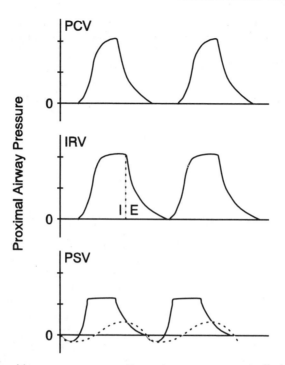

Figure 27.3. Airway pressure patterns in pressure-controlled ventilation (*PCV*), inverse ratio ventilation (*IRV*) and pressure-support ventilation (*PSV*). Spontaneous and machine breaths indicated by dashed and solid lines, respectively.

tory flow pattern reduces peak airway pressures and can improve gas exchange (13,14).

The major disadvantage of PCV is the tendency for inflation volumes to vary with changes in the mechanical properties of the lungs. This is illustrated in Figure 27.4. The inflation volume increases as the

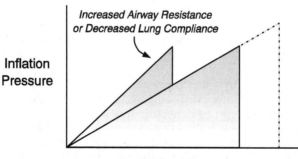

Figure 27.4. The determinants of inflation volume during pressure-cycled ventilation.

peak inflation pressure increases (dashed lines). However, at a constant peak inflation pressure, the inflation volume decreases as the airway resistance increases or the lung compliance decreases. Therefore, any change in lung mechanics during PCV can lead to a change in inflation volumes. Because of the influence of lung mechanics on inflation volumes during PCV, this method of mechanical ventilation seems best suited for patients with neuromuscular disease (and normal lung mechanics).

INVERSE RATIO VENTILATION

When PCV is combined with a prolonged inflation time, the result is *inverse ratio ventilation* (IRV) (15,16). The ventilatory pattern produced by IRV is shown in the middle panel of Figure 27.3. A decrease in inspiratory flow rate is used to prolong the time for lung inflation, and the usual I:E ratio of 1:2 to 1:4 is reversed to a ratio of 2:1. The prolonged inflation time can help prevent alveolar collapse. However, prolonged inflation times also increase the tendency for inadequate emptying of the lungs, which can lead to hyperinflation and auto-PEEP. **The tendency to produce auto-PEEP can lead to a decrease in cardiac output during IRV** (17), and this is the major drawback with IRV. The major indication for IRV is for patients with ARDS who have refractory hypoxemia or hypercapnia during conventional modes of mechanical ventilation (17).

PRESSURE-SUPPORT VENTILATION

Pressure-augmented breathing that allows the patient to determine the inflation volume and respiratory cycle duration is called *pressure-support ventilation* (PSV) (18). This method of ventilation is used to augment spontaneous breathing, not to provide full ventilatory support.

VENTILATORY PATTERN

The ventilatory pattern produced by PSV is shown in the lower panel of Figure 27.3. At the onset of each spontaneous breath, the negative pressure generated by the patient opens a valve that delivers the inspired gas at a preselected pressure (usually 5 to 10 cm H_2O). The patient's inspiratory flow rate is adjusted by the ventilator as needed to keep the inflation pressure constant, and when the patient's inspiratory flow rate falls below 25% of the peak inspiratory flow, the augmented breath is terminated. By recognizing the patient's inherent inspiratory flow rate, **PSV allows the patient to dictate the duration of lung inflation and the inflation volume.** This should result in a more physiologically acceptable method of positive-pressure lung inflation.

CLINICAL USES

PSV can be used to augment inflation volumes during spontaneous breathing or to overcome the resistance of breathing through ventilator circuits. The latter application is the most popular and is used to limit the work of breathing during weaning from mechanical ventilation. The goal of PSV in this setting is not to augment the tidal volume, but merely to provide enough pressure to overcome the resistance created by the tracheal tubes and ventilator tubing. Inflation pressures of 5 to 10 cm H_2O are appropriate for this purpose. PSV has also become popular as a noninvasive method of mechanical ventilation (19). In this situation, PSV is delivered through specialized face masks or nasal masks, using inflation pressures of 20 cm H_2O.

POSITIVE END-EXPIRATORY PRESSURE

Under normal circumstances, the volume of gas inhaled is exhaled completely. As a result, the expiratory airflow ceases by the end of expiration, and the alveolar pressure at end-expiration is equivalent to atmospheric pressure (zero reference point). When the alveolar pressure at end-expiration is above atmospheric pressure, it is referred to as positive end-expiratory pressure (PEEP). There are two ways to create PEEP during mechanical ventilation. One is to add a pressure-limiting device that stops exhalation at a preselected pressure. This is called *extrinsic PEEP*. The other is to ventilate patients at high inflation volumes and rapid rates and promote hyperinflation (20). This is called intrinsic PEEP or *auto-PEEP*. The description of PEEP in this chapter pertains mostly to extrinsic PEEP. Auto-PEEP is described in Chapter 28.

EXTRINSIC PEEP

Extrinsic PEEP is applied by placing a pressure-limiting valve in the expiratory limb of the ventilator circuit. This valve exerts a back pressure, and exhalation proceeds until this back pressure is reached, whereupon flow ceases. A similar effect would be created by placing the distal end of the expiratory tubing under water. The back pressure would then be equivalent to the distance that the tube is submerged. The first time I saw PEEP used, this is how it was done.)

The effect of extrinsic PEEP on the phasic airway pressures is shown in Figure 27.5. Note that the entire pressure waveform is displaced upward by the applied PEEP. This means that PEEP increases not only the end-expiratory pressure, but also the *mean* intrathoracic pressure. This is important in understanding the effects of PEEP on cardiac performance. The effect of PEEP on the proximal airway pressures is an important consideration when using the end-inspiratory peak and plateau pressures to evaluate lung mechanics (see Chapter 26). When doing so, the amount of applied PEEP must be subtracted from the

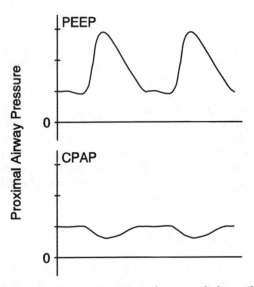

Figure 27.5. Airway pressure patterns in volume-cycled ventilation with positive end-expiratory pressure (*PEEP*), and in spontaneous breathing with continuous positive airway pressure (*CPAP*).

end-inspiratory pressures to determine the actual pressures generated by intrinsic lung mechanics.

THE PHYSIOLOGY OF PEEP

The distal airspaces tend to collapse at the end of expiration, and this tendency is exaggerated when the lungs are stiff (e.g., in ARDS). Alveolar collapse impairs gas exchange and makes the lungs stiffer. PEEP prevents the alveoli from collapsing at the end of expiration and can open alveoli that have already collapsed (21). This improves gas exchange (decreases intrapulmonary shunt) and makes the lungs less stiff (increases lung compliance). The improved gas exchange raises the arterial Po_2, which allows the inspired oxygen (Fio_2) to be reduced to less toxic levels. This latter effect (a decrease to less toxic inhaled O_2 concentrations) is one of the major indications for extrinsic PEEP.

Cardiac Performance

Because PEEP displaces the entire positive-pressure waveform upward, the effects of positive-pressure ventilation on cardiac performance are magnified (see Chapter 26). Thus, the tendency for positive-pressure ventilation to reduce cardiac filling and cardiac output is much greater with PEEP, and this tendency is magnified even further by hypovolemia and cardiac dysfunction. **The tendency for PEEP ventilation to reduce cardiac output is *not* a function of the PEEP level,** but is a function of the PEEP-induced increase in mean intrathoracic pressure. Thus the often-heard proclamation "it's only 5 of PEEP, so the cardiac output should be OK" is meaningless. Low levels of PEEP can be deleterious for the cardiac output if the mean intrathoracic pressure is high.

Oxygen Transport

The tendency for PEEP to reduce the cardiac output is an important consideration, as demonstrated by the determinants of systemic oxygen delivery (Do_2):

$$Do_2 = Q \times 1.3 \times Hb \times Sao_2 \qquad (27.1)$$

Thus, the effect of PEEP on cardiac output (Q) will determine whether a PEEP-induced increase in arterial oxygenation (Sao_2) is associated with a similar increase in systemic oxygenation. This is demonstrated in Figure 27.6. When PEEP does not change the cardiac output, the increase in arterial O_2 saturation is associated with an increase in systemic O_2 delivery. However, when PEEP reduces the cardiac output, the increase in arterial oxygenation is associated with a *decrease* in systemic oxygenation. Thus, the effects of PEEP on systemic oxygenation are determined by the change in cardiac output, not the change in arterial oxygenation. The point at which PEEP best improves systemic oxygen transport is sometimes called *best PEEP*.

The effects of PEEP shown in Figure 27.6 emphasize the following important point: **An increase in arterial oxygenation should never be used as the end-point of PEEP ventilation.** Rather, the cardiac output must be monitored when PEEP is applied. There is a waiting period of at least 15 minutes after PEEP is applied before the effects on cardiac output are fully expressed (22). If the cardiac output is not available, the venous oxygen saturation can be useful. A decrease in venous O_2 saturation after PEEP can be used as evidence for a PEEP-induced decrease in cardiac output.

CLINICAL USES

The following conditions are considered appropriate indications for extrinsic PEEP.

Toxic Level of Inhaled O_2

In patients who require a toxic level of inhaled oxygen (Fio_2 greater than 0.60) to maintain adequate oxygenation, the addition of PEEP can increase arterial and systemic oxygenation, and allow the inhaled oxygen to be reduced to less toxic levels. PEEP is most effective in this regard when the lungs are stiff and the pathologic process is diffuse,

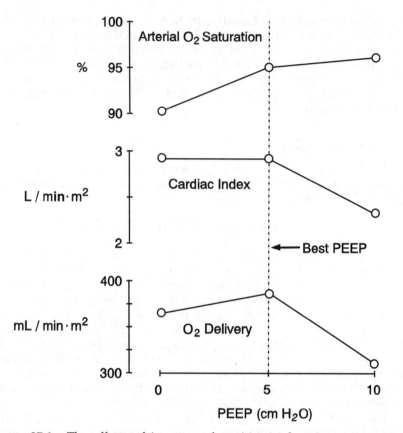

Figure 27.6. The effects of incremental positive end-expiratory pressure (*PEEP*) on arterial and systemic oxygenation in a patient with severe ARDS.

as in ARDS). When lung disease is localized (as in pneumonia), PEEP can overdistend alveoli in normal lung regions and redirect blood back to the diseased areas. In this situation, PEEP can worsen arterial oxygenation (23).

Low-Volume Ventilation

As mentioned in Chapter 26, PEEP is recommended for volume-cycled ventilation with low tidal volumes (5 to 10 mL/kg) (24). The PEEP is meant to prevent repetitive opening and closing of small airways, which is believed to be a source of further lung injury. The level of PEEP should be above the inflection point in the pressure-volume curve (the point of airway closure), but in the absence of such a curve, a PEEP level of 10 cm H_2O may be satisfactory (24).

Obstructive Lung Disease

The small airways tend to collapse at the end of expiration in patients with obstructive lung disease (i.e., asthma and chronic obstructive pulmonary disease). In this situation, extrinsic PEEP can keep the airways open at end-expiration and reduce the tendency for air trapping (25). The use of extrinsic PEEP in obstructive lung disease is discussed in more detail in Chapter 28.

CLINICAL MISUSES

The following uses of PEEP are either inappropriate or unjustified.

Reducing Lung Edema

As described in Chapter 23, PEEP does not reduce lung edema in ARDS (see Fig. 23.6). In fact, **positive intrathoracic pressures can promote water accumulation in the lungs** (26), possibly by impeding lymphatic drainage from the lungs.

Routine PEEP

Because glottic closure at the end of expiration creates low levels of PEEP (physiologic PEEP), the practice of applying PEEP to all intubated patients has become popular. However, there is no evidence that adults produce PEEP from glottic closure (grunting neonates do), and routine PEEP has no documented benefits in intubated patients (26).

Mediastinal Bleeding

The application of PEEP is a common practice for preventing or controlling mediastinal bleeding after cardiopulmonary bypass surgery. This practice is based on a misconception about the effect of PEEP on transmural pressure. Because PEEP is transmitted across the walls of blood vessels, PEEP may not reduce the transmural pressure. Thus, there is no mechanism for PEEP to reduce mediastinal bleeding from intrathoracic blood vessels. This is confirmed by clinical reports showing that PEEP does not reduce postoperative mediastinal bleeding (27).

CONTINUOUS POSITIVE AIRWAYS PRESSURE

Spontaneous breathing in which a positive pressure is maintained throughout the respiratory cycle is called *continuous positive airway pressure* (CPAP). The airway pressure pattern with CPAP is shown in Figure 27.5. Note that the patient does not have to generate a negative airway pressure to receive the inhaled gas. This is made possible by a specialized inhalation valve that opens at a pressure above atmospheric pressure. This eliminates the extra work involved in generating a negative airway pressure to inhale. CPAP should be distinguished from *spontaneous PEEP*. In spontaneous PEEP, a negative airway pressure is required for inhalation. Spontaneous PEEP has been replaced by CPAP because of the reduced work of breathing with CPAP.

CLINICAL USES

The major uses of CPAP are in nonintubated patients. CPAP can be delivered through specialized face masks equipped with adjustable, pressurized valves. CPAP masks have been used successfully to postpone intubation in patients with acute respiratory failure (28). However, these masks must be tight-fitting, and they cannot be removed for the patient to eat. Therefore, they are used only as a temporary measure. Specialized nasal masks may be better tolerated. CPAP delivered through nasal masks (nasal CPAP) has become popular in patients with obstructive sleep-apnea (29). In this situation, the CPAP is used as a stint to prevent upper airway collapse during negative pressure breathing. Nasal CPAP has also been used successfully in patients with acute exacerbation of chronic obstructive lung disease (30).

Airway Pressure Release

A specialized form of CPAP is available in which the positive airway pressure is released temporarily during exhalation, to facilitate exhalation. This method, called *airway pressure release ventilation*, uses higher pressures than conventional CPAP, and has been used as an alternative to mechanical ventilation in patients with acute respiratory failure (31).

REFERENCES

REVIEWS

1. Sassoon CSH, Mahutte K, Light RW. Ventilator modes: old and new. Crit Care Clin 1990;6:605–634 (205 references).
2. Rasanen J. Mechanical ventilatory support: time for appraisal. Int Crit Care Digest 1991;10:3–5 (editorial; 13 references).
3. Slutsky AS. American College of Chest Physicians' Consensus Conference on Mechanical Ventilation. Chest 1993;104:1833–1857 (158 references).

ASSIST-CONTROL VENTILATION

4. Fernandez R, Blanch L, Antigas A. Respiratory center activity during mechanical ventilation. J Crit Care 1991;6:102–111.
5. Marini JJ. Strategies to minimize breathing effort during mechanical ventilation. Crit Care Clin 1990;6:635–661.

6. Rogers RL, Schlichtig R, Miro A, Pinsky M. Auto-PEEP during CPR: an 'occult' cause of electromechanical dissociation. Chest 1991;99:492–493.

INTERMITTENT MANDATORY VENTILATION

7. Downs JB, Klein EF, Desautels D, et al. IMV: a new approach to weaning patients from mechanical ventilation. Chest 1973;64:331–335.
8. Sassoon CSH, Del Rosario N, Fei R, et al. Influence of pressure- and flow-triggered synchronous intermittent mandatory ventilation on inspiratory muscle work. Crit Care Med 1994;22:1933–1941.
9. Hudson LD, Hurlow RS, Craig KC, Pierson DJ. Does intermittent mandatory ventilation correct respiratory alkalosis in patients receiving assisted mechanical ventilation? Am Rev Respir Dis 1985;132:1071–1074.
10. Pinsky MR. Cardiovascular effects of ventilatory support and withdrawal. Anesth Analg 1994;79:567–576.
11. Mathru M et al. Hemodynamic responses to changes in ventilatory patterns in patients with normal and poor left ventricular reserve. Crit Care Med 1982; 10:423–426.
12. Sternberg R, Sahebjami H. Hemodynamic and oxygen transport characteristics of common ventilator modes. Chest 1994;105:1798–1803.

PRESSURE-CONTROLLED VENTILATION

13. Shelledy DC, Rau JL, Thomas-Goodfellow L. A comparison of the effects of assist-control, SIMV, and SIMV with pressure-support on ventilation, oxygen consumption, and ventilatory equivalent. Heart Lung 1995;24:67–75.
14. Rappaport SH, Shipner R, Yoshihara G, et al. Randomized, prospective trial of pressure-limited versus volume controlled ventilation in severe respiratory failure. Crit Care Med 1994;22:22–32.
15. Marcy TW, Marini JJ. Inverse ratio ventilation in ARDS. Rationale and implementation. Chest 1991;100:494–504.
16. Papadakos PJ, Halloran W, Hessney JI, et al. The use of pressure-controlled inverse ratio ventilation in the surgical intensive care unit. J Trauma 1991;31: 1211–1215.
17. Chan K, Abraham E. Effects of inverse ratio ventilation on cardiorespiratory parameters in severe respiratory failure. Chest 1992;102:1556–1561.

PRESSURE-SUPPORT VENTILATION

18. MacIntyre NR. Pressure-support ventilation. In: Grenvik A, Downs J, Rasanen J, Smith R, eds. Mechanical ventilation and assisted respiration. Contemporary management in critical care. New York: Churchill Livingstone, 1991;1:51–62.
19. Brochard L, Mancebo J, Wysocki M, et al. Noninvasive ventilation for acute exacerbations of chronic obstructive pulmonary disease. N Engl J Med 1995; 338:817–822.

POSITIVE END-EXPIRATORY PRESSURE

20. Ligas JR, Mosiehi JR, Epstein MAF. Occult positive end-expiratory pressure with different types of mechanical ventilators. J Crit Care 1990;5:95–100.

21. Ranieri VM, Eissa NT, Corbeil C, et al. Effects of positive end-expiratory pressure on alveolar recruitment and gas exchange in patients with the adult respiratory distress syndrome. Am Rev Respir Dis 1991;144:544–551.
22. Patel M, Singer M. The optimal time for measuring the cardiorespiratory effects of positive end-expiratory pressure. Chest 1993;104:139–142.
23. Hawker FH, Torzillo PJ, Southee AE. PEEP and "reverse mismatch." A case where less PEEP is best. Chest 1991;99:1034–1036.
24. Marini JJ. Pressure-targeted, lung-protective ventilatory support in acute lung injury. Chest 1994;105(Suppl):109S–115S.
25. Pinsky MR. Through the past darkly: ventilatory management of patients with chronic obstructive pulmonary disease. Crit Care Med 1994;22:1714–1717.
26. Petty TL. The use, abuse, and mystique of positive end-expiratory pressure. Am Rev Respir Dis 1988;138:475–478.
27. Zurick AM, Urzua J, Ghattas M, et al. Failure of positive end-expiratory pressure to decrease postoperative bleeding after cardiac surgery. Ann Thorac Surg 1982;34:608–611.

CONTINUOUS POSITIVE AIRWAY PRESSURE

28. Miro AM, Shivaram U, Hertig I. Continuous positive airway pressure in COPD patients in acute hypercapnic respiratory failure. Chest 1993;103:266–268.
29. Takasaki Y, Orr D, Popkin J, et al. Effect of nasal continuous positive airway pressure in sleep apnea in congestive heart failure. Am Rev Respir Dis 1989; 140:1578–1584.
30. de Lucas P, Tarancon C, Puente L, et al. Nasal continuous positive airway pressure in patients with COPD in acute respiratory failure. Chest 1993;104: 1694–1697.
31. Cane R, Peruzzi WT, Shapiro BA. Airway pressure release ventilation in acute respiratory failure. Chest 1991;100:460–463.

THE VENTILATOR-DEPENDENT PATIENT

This chapter describes some of the practices and daily concerns in patients receiving mechanical ventilation. The focus is on practices and complications that are directly related to artificial airways (endotracheal and tracheostomy tubes) and positive-pressure ventilation. The nosocomial illnesses that can appear in ventilator-dependent patients, such as pneumonia and progressive systemic inflammation, are described elsewhere.

ARTIFICIAL AIRWAYS

Positive-pressure mechanical ventilation usually (but not always) requires tracheal intubation, which can be accomplished by translaryngeal (endotracheal) intubation, percutaneous cricothyroidotomy (coniotomy), or tracheotomy (1–3). The tubes used for tracheal intubation in adults are equipped with inflatable balloons that are used to seal the trachea and isolate the airways from the larynx and oral cavity. (Because of the narrow diameter of the trachea in young children, pediatric tracheal tubes do not always have inflatable balloons to create a tracheal seal.) The complications of tracheal intubation are related to the route of intubation and to the airway damage created by the pressurized seal of the trachea. The principal complications of tracheal intubation are shown in Figure 28.1 (2,4,5).

ENDOTRACHEAL INTUBATION

Endotracheal tubes can be inserted through the nose or mouth. The principal features of each insertion route are listed in Table 28.1. The nasal route is often preferred for intubating patients who are awake and cooperative, whereas the oral route is preferred in comatose or

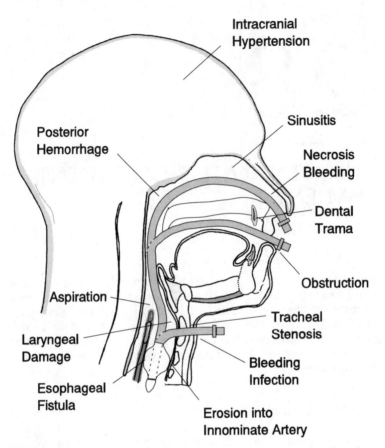

Figure 28.1. Complications of endotracheal intubation (nasal and oral routes) and tracheostomy.

TABLE 28.1. NASAL AND ORAL ROUTES OF ENDOTRACHEAL INTUBATION			
Nasotracheal Intubation		**Orotracheal Intubation**	
Indications	**Complications**	**Indications**	**Complications**
Cervical fractures or cervical halo Mandibular fractures Often preferred in awake and cooperative patients	Epistaxis Esophageal intubation Sinusitis Nasal septal necrosis Bacteremia	Comatose or uncooperative patients When immediate intubation is necessary	Dental trauma Occlusion due to biting down on tubes Increased risk of laryngeal damage

uncooperative patients, or when immediate intubation is necessary (e.g., cardiac arrest). The complications peculiar to nasotracheal intubation include epistaxis and paranasal sinusitis, and necrosis of the nasal mucosa. The complications peculiar to orotracheal intubation include dental trauma and tube occlusion in awake patients (who tend to bite down on the oral tubes). In addition, orotracheal tubes follow an acute angle as they pass from the oropharynx toward the larynx; this angulation creates a torque that can damage the posterior larynx.

Physiologic Implications

The volume of the anatomic dead space in adults is approximately 1 mL/kg, whereas the volume of most endotracheal tubes is 35 to 45 mL (6). Therefore, in the average-sized adult, endotracheal intubation reduces the anatomic dead space by approximately 50%. This, however, has minor clinical significance. The most significant physiologic consequence of tracheal intubation is an increase in the resistance to airflow. As predicted by the Hagen-Poiseuille equation (see Chapter 1), the radius of tracheal tubes has a much greater influence on resistance to airflow than the length of the tubes. Therefore, small-diameter tracheal tubes (both endotracheal tubes and tracheostomy tubes) can cause a significant increase in the work of breathing. This is particularly marked at high flow rates (such as those in patients with respiratory distress) (6). **The diameter of adult tracheal tubes should be no less than 7 mm, and preferably 8 mm, to minimize the extra work of breathing through the tubes when weaning from mechanical ventilation** (6).

Intracranial Pressure

Endotracheal intubation can be accompanied by an increase in intracranial pressure, regardless of the intubation route. The mechanism for this effect is unclear, but it can be blocked by lidocaine. Intravenous **lidocaine (1.5 mg/kg)** produces a more effective blockade than endotracheal lidocaine (7). If intracranial hypertension is a concern, lidocaine is recommended just before endotracheal intubation. **Rapid sequence intubation** with fentanyl (3 to 5 μg/kg) and succinylcholine (1.5 mg/kg IV) can also reduce the intracranial pressure response to endotracheal intubation (4,8). Succinylcholine can increase intracranial pressure, but this response can be blocked by prior administration of vecuronium (0.01 mg/kg) or pancuronium (0.01 mg/kg) (8).

Tracheal Tube Position

In 5 to 10% of endotracheal intubations, the tip of the endotracheal tube is incorrectly positioned in one of the mainstem bronchi (9). Because the right mainstem bronchus runs a straighter course from the trachea, selective intubation of the right lung is most common. The

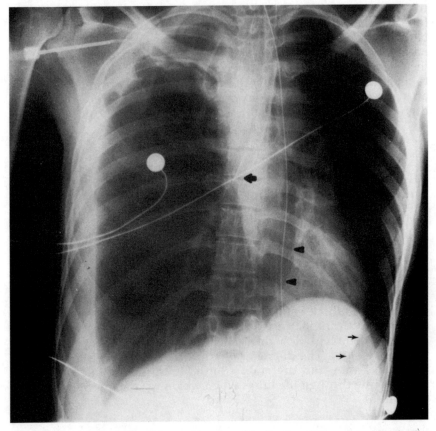

Figure 28.2. Portable chest x-ray film showing the tip of an endotracheal tube in the right mainstem bronchus, with herniation of the right lung into the left hemithorax (*arrowheads*). The thin arrows point to a collection of pleural air at the left lung base.

consequences of right lung intubation are illustrated in Figure 28.2. Note the overinflation of the right lung, with herniation into the left hemithorax (arrowheads). The risk for selective intubation of one lung can be minimized by advancing endotracheal tubes no further than 21 cm from the teeth in women and 23 cm in men (10). Although an established practice, **listening for bilateral breath sounds is not a reliable method for determining endotracheal tube position.** Specifically, the presence of bilateral breath sounds does not rule out either selective lung intubation or esophageal intubation (9,11). Therefore, routine **chest films are required to determine tube position.**

Radiographic Landmarks

Some useful radiographic landmarks for evaluating endotracheal tube position are shown in Table 28.2 (12). The vocal cords are usually

TABLE 28.2. RADIOGRAPHIC EVALUATION OF TRACHEAL INTUBATION	
	Radiographic Location
Anatomic Structures	
Vocal Cords	Usually over the C4–C5 interspace
Carina	Usually over the T4–T5 interspace
Head and Neck Position	
Neutral Position	Inferior border of mandible is over C4–C5
Flexion	Mandible is over T1–T2
Extension	Mandible is above C4
Tracheal Tube Position	
Head in Neutral Position	Tip of the tube should be midway between the vocal cords and carina, or 3–5 cm above the carina.
Head Flexed	Tip of tube will descend 2 cm.
Head Extended	Tip of tube will ascend 2 cm.

From Goodman LR, Putman CE, eds. Critical care imaging. 3rd ed, Philadelphia: WB Saunders, 1992:35–56.

situated at the interspace between the fifth and sixth cervical vertebrae (C5-C6). If not visible, the main carina is usually over the interspace between the fourth and fifth thoracic vertebrae (T4-T5) on a portable chest x-ray film. When the head is in a neutral position, the tip of the tracheal tube should be 3 to 5 cm above the carina, or midway between the carina and vocal cords. The head is in the neutral position when the inferior border of the mandible projects over the lower cervical spine (C5-C6). Note that flexion or extension of the head and neck causes a 2 cm displacement of the tip of the endotracheal tube (12). The total displacement of 4 cm with changes in head position represents about one-third of the length of the trachea.

Sinusitis

Nasotracheal (and nasoenteral) tubes can obstruct the ostia that drain the paranasal sinuses, which can lead to a purulent sinusitis (13,14). The maxillary sinus is almost always involved (see Fig. 30.3). The presence of an air-fluid level by sinus radiography suggests the diagnosis, but confirmation requires aspiration of infected material from the involved sinus. Paranasal sinusitis is an important consideration in the evaluation of fever in intubated patients, and it may be just as common in patients with orotracheal tubes (15). This complication is described in more detail in Chapter 30.

Laryngeal Damage

The risk for laryngeal injury from translaryngeal intubation is the major reason for performing tracheostomies when prolonged intubation is anticipated (1,2). The spectrum of laryngeal damage includes ulceration, granulomas, vocal cord paresis, and laryngeal edema. Some type of laryngeal damage is usually evident after 72 hours of translaryngeal intubation (2), and laryngeal edema is reported in 5% of cases. Fortunately, most cases of laryngeal injury do not result in significant airways obstruction, and the injury resolves within weeks after extubation (16). The problem of laryngeal edema after tracheal decannulation is described in Chapter 29.

TRACHEOSTOMY

Tracheostomy is preferred in patients who require prolonged mechanical ventilation. The advantages of tracheostomy tubes over endotracheal tubes include greater patient comfort and more effective clearing of secretions (17). Tracheostomy patients can also ingest food orally and converse using special tracheal tubes. However, the complications of tracheostomy can overshadow those associated with endotracheal intubation.

Complications

Surgical tracheotomy is accompanied by serious complications in 5% of cases, and the procedure has a reported mortality as high as 2% (compared with a reported mortality of 1:5000 endotracheal intubations) (18). Immediate postoperative complications include pneumothorax (5%), stomal hemorrhage (5%), and accidental decannulation (17,18). The latter complication can be troublesome because the tracheostomy tract closes quickly, and attempts to reinsert the tubes can create false tracts. If a tracheostomy tube has to be reinserted in the first week after surgery, a 12-French suction catheter should be used as a guidewire to reduce the risk for trauma and unsuccessful reintubation.

Tracheal stenosis is the most feared complication of tracheostomy. The stenosis usually occurs at the tracheotomy site and not at the site where the inflated balloon creates the tracheal seal. Stenosis is a late complication that usually appears days to weeks after tracheal decannulation.

When to Perform a Tracheostomy

The optimal time for performing a tracheostomy in patients with prolonged endotracheal intubation is a time-honored controversy. However, the consensus at present seems to favor the following approach. **After 1 week of endotracheal intubation, if little chance for extubation in the ensuing week exists, proceed to tracheostomy** (2,17,18). Because of the increased risk for tracheal stenosis associated with repeated tracheotomy incisions, tracheostomy should not be performed in patients who have had prior tracheostomy until a waiting period of more than 1 week has passed, if possible.

CUFF-RELATED COMPLICATIONS

As mentioned earlier, positive-pressure mechanical ventilation in adults requires tracheal tubes that are equipped with an inflatable balloon (called a cuff) that seals the trachea and prevents gas from escaping back through the larynx. Figure 28.3 shows two tracheostomy tubes with inflated cuffs at their distal ends. The tube on the left has a balloon that is normally deflated and must be inflated by injecting a volume of air into the balloon with an air-filled syringe. The tube on the right has a foam rubber cuff that is normally inflated at atmospheric pressure. This cuff is manually deflated by applying suction from a syringe during insertion of the tube; once the tube is in place, the cuff is allowed to inflate and create the tracheal seal. This cuff design, therefore, allows the trachea to be sealed with minimum risk of pressure-induced injury to the tracheal mucosa.

Aspiration

Contrary to popular belief, **cuff inflation to create a tracheal seal does not prevent aspiration of mouth secretions and tube feedings into the lower airways.** Aspiration of saliva and liquid tube feedings has been documented in more than 50% of ventilator-dependent patients with tracheostomies (19). Furthermore, in over three-fourths of the cases, the aspiration is clinically silent (19). Considering that approximately 1 L of saliva is normally produced each day (the normal rate of saliva production is 0.6 mL/min) and that each *micro*liter of saliva contains approximately 1 billion microorganisms, the danger associated with aspiration of mouth secretions seems considerable (20). This emphasizes the value of routine tracheal suctioning to clear secretions from the airways.

Cuff Leaks

Just as liquid can pass around inflated cuffs and move into the lower airways, gas in the airways can pass around inflated cuffs and move out of the lungs. Cuff leaks are usually detected by sounds generated during lung inflation (created by gas flowing through the vocal cords). When a cuff leak becomes audible, the volume of the leak can be determined by noting the difference between the desired inflation volume and the exhaled volume recorded by the ventilator.

Cuff leaks are rarely due to disruption of the cuff itself (21). The most common cause of cuff leaks is nonuniform contact between the cuff and the tracheal wall. Another source of cuff leaks is faulty function of a one-way valve at the air injection inlet that normally keeps the cuff inflated. These valves can become leaky and allow air to escape from the cuff.

If a cuff leak is suspected, the patient should be separated from the ventilator and the lungs should be manually inflated with an anesthesia bag. If a leak is audible, the cuff should be inflated until the sounds

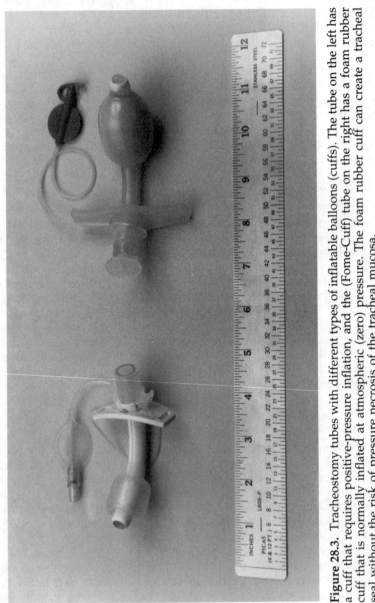

Figure 28.3. Tracheostomy tubes with different types of inflatable balloons (cuffs). The tube on the left has a cuff that requires positive-pressure inflation, and the (Fome-Cuff) tube on the right has a foam rubber cuff that is normally inflated at atmospheric (zero) pressure. The foam rubber cuff can create a tracheal seal without the risk of pressure necrosis of the tracheal mucosa.

disappear, and the resultant cuff pressure should be checked. If the cuff pressure is above 25 cm H_2O, the tracheal tube should be replaced. If the cuff pressure gradually diminishes over time, the one-way valve mentioned earlier may be defective. In this situation, recurrent cuff leaks can be prevented by clamping the cuff inflation tubing to isolate the cuff from the faulty valve.

Tracheal Necrosis

The original tracheal tubes had low-compliance cuffs that promoted pressure-induced tracheal necrosis when inflated. This complication was reduced significantly when larger, more compliant cuffs were introduced in the mid-1970s. The newer cuffs generate lower pressures when inflated, and the larger size of the cuff disperses the cuff pressure over a wider area of the tracheal mucosa. The systolic pressure in the mucosal vessels of the trachea is normally 20 to 25 mm Hg (17), so the goal of cuff inflation is to create a seal at an inflation pressure below 20 cm H_2O. In patients with clinical shock and hypotension, pressure necrosis of the trachea is possible at cuff pressures far below 20 cm H_2O. In this situation, the tracheal tube on the right in Figure 28.3, which creates a tracheal seal at atmospheric (zero) pressure, is my preference.

ALVEOLAR RUPTURE

One of the constant concerns in the ventilator-dependent patient is the risk of alveolar rupture, which occurs in up to one-fourth of patients receiving positive-pressure mechanical ventilation (22). As mentioned in Chapter 26, alveolar rupture can be the result of excessive pressure (barotrauma) or overdistension (volutrauma).

CLINICAL PRESENTATION

Escape of gas from the alveoli can produce a variety of clinical manifestations (23). The alveolar gas can dissect along tissue planes and produce *pulmonary interstitial emphysema*, and can move into the mediastinum and produce *pneumomediastinum*. Mediastinal gas can move into the neck to produce *subcutaneous emphysema*, or can pass below the diaphragm to produce *pneumoperitoneum*. Finally, if the rupture involves the visceral pleura, gas will collect in the pleural space and produce a *pneumothorax*. Each of these entities can occur alone or in combination with the others (22,23).

PNEUMOTHORAX

Radiographic evidence of pneumothorax occurs in 5 to 15% of ventilator-dependent patients (22,23). Risk factors include high inflation pressures and inflation volumes, positive end-expiratory pressure (PEEP), and diffuse lung injury. The highest risk of pneumothorax is in patients with acute respiratory distress syndrome (ARDS), where the incidence of pneumothorax is as high as 60% (23).

Clinical Presentation

Clinical manifestations are either absent, minimal, or nonspecific. The **most valuable clinical sign is subcutaneous emphysema** in the neck and upper thorax, which is pathognomonic of alveolar rupture. Breath sounds are unreliable in ventilator-dependent patients because sounds transmitted from the ventilator tubing can be mistaken for airway sounds.

Radiographic Detection

The radiographic detection of pleural air can be difficult in portable chest films, particularly when the patient is **in the supine position,** when **pleural air does not collect at the lung apex** (23,24). Figure 28.4 illustrates some of the atypical features of pneumothorax in the supine position. The hyperlucent area at the right lung base represents a collection of pleural air that is anterior to the right lung (which is the

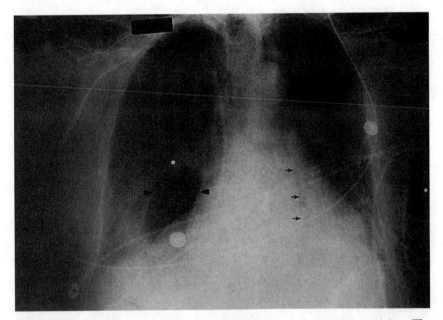

Figure 28.4. Atypical features of pneumothorax in the supine position. The hyperlucent area at the base of the right lung is a collection of pleural air that is anterior to the right lung. In the supine position, this is the highest region of the pleural space. The sharp line demarcating the descending aorta (*thin arrows*) represents air behind the inferior pulmonary ligament.

most superior region of the pleural space in the supine position). A similar collection of pleural air is shown at the left lung base in Figure 28.2. **Basilar and subpulmonic collections of air are characteristic of pneumothorax in the supine position** (24).

Redundant Skin Folds

When the film cartridge used for portable chest x-ray examinations is placed under the patient, the skin on the back can fold over on itself, and the edge of this redundant skin fold creates a radiographic shadow that can be mistaken for a pneumothorax. The radiographic appearance of a redundant skin fold is shown in Figure 28.5. Note that there is a gradual increase in radiodensity that suddenly ends as a wavy line. The increase in density is produced by the skin that is folded back on itself. A pneumothorax would appear as a sharp white line with dark shadows (air) on either side.

When a redundant skin fold is suspected, a repeat chest film should be obtained (it may be wise to alert the x-ray technician to make sure the film cartridge is flush on the patient's back). The shadow should disappear if it is due to a redundant skin fold.

PLEURAL EVACUATION

Evacuation of pleural air is accomplished by inserting a chest tube through the fourth or fifth intercostal space along the mid-axillary line. The tube should be advanced in an anterior and superior direction (because this is where pleural air collects in the supine position). The pleural space is drained of fluid and air using a three-chamber system like the one shown in Figure 28.6 (25).

Collection Chamber

The first bottle in the system collects fluid from the pleural space and allows air to pass through to the next bottle in the series. Because the inlet of this chamber is not in direct contact with the fluid, the pleural fluid that is collected does not impose a back pressure on the pleural space.

Water-Seal Chamber

The second bottle acts as a one-way valve that allows air to escape from the pleural space but prevents air from entering the pleural space. This one-way valve is created by submerging the inlet tube under water. This imposes a back-pressure on the pleural space that is equal to the depth that the tube is submerged. The positive pressure in the pleural space then prevents atmospheric air (at zero pressure) from entering the pleural space. The water thus "seals" the pleural space from the surrounding atmosphere. This water-seal pressure is usually 2 cm H_2O.

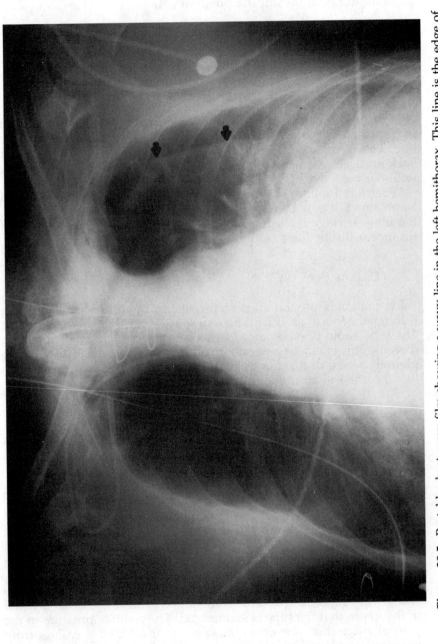

Figure 28.5. Portable chest x-ray film showing a wavy line in the left hemithorax. This line is the edge of a redundant skin fold, not a pneumothorax.

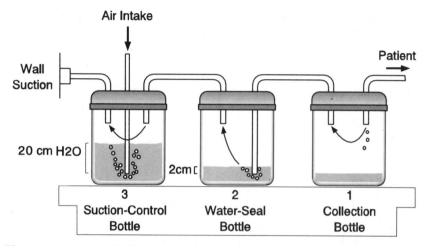

Figure 28.6. A standard pleural drainage system for evacuating air and fluid from the pleural space.

Air that is evacuated from the pleural space passes through the water in the second bottle and creates bubbles. Thus, the presence of bubbles in the water-seal chamber (called bubbling) is used as evidence for a continuing bronchopleural air leak.

Suction-Control Chamber

The third bottle in the system is used to set a maximum limit on the negative suction pressure that is imposed on the pleural space. This maximum pressure is determined by the height of the water column in the air inlet tube. Negative pressure (from wall suction) draws the water down the air inlet tube, and when the negative pressure exceeds the height of the water column, air is entrained from the atmosphere. Therefore, the pressure in the bottle can never become more negative than the height of the water column in the air inlet tube.

Water is added to the suction-control chamber to achieve a water level of 20 cm. The wall suction is then activated and slowly increased until bubbles appear in the water. This bubbling indicates that atmospheric air is being entrained, and thus the maximum negative pressure has been achieved. The continuous bubbling causes water evaporation, so it is imperative that the height of the water in this chamber is checked periodically, and more water is added when necessary.

Why Use Suction?

The practice of using suction to evacuate pleural air is both unnecessary and potentially harmful. Although there is a perception that suction will help the lungs reinflate, the lungs will reinflate without the use of suction. Furthermore, creating a negative pressure in the pleural space also creates a higher transpulmonary pressure (the pressure difference between alveoli and the pleural space), and this increases the rate of the air flowing through the bronchopleural fistula. Thus **applying suction to the pleural space increases bronchopleural air leaks,** and this can keep bronchopleural fistulas patent. If a persistent air leak is present when suction is applied to the pleural space, the suction should be discontinued. Any air that collects in the pleural space will continue to be evacuated when the pleural pressure becomes more positive than the water-seal pressure.

OCCULT PEEP

As mentioned in Chapter 27, mechanical ventilation with high inflation volumes and rapid rates can (and probably often does) produce PEEP as a result of incomplete alveolar emptying during expiration (26–28). The illustration in Figure 28.7 helps explain this phenomenon.

PATHOGENESIS

Under normal circumstances, there is no airflow at the end of expiration, and thus end-expiratory pressure is the same in the alveoli and

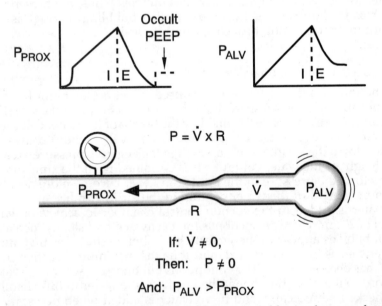

Figure 28.7. The features of intrinsic PEEP produced by inadequate alveolar emptying. The presence of airflow ($\dot{V}$) at end-expiration creates a pressure drop from the alveolus (P_{ALV}) to the proximal airways (P_{prox}). As shown at the top of the figure, the proximal airway pressure returns to zero at end-expiration while the alveolar pressure remains positive; hence the term *occult* PEEP. The upper left panel illustrates the end-expiratory occlusion method for detecting occult PEEP.

proximal airways. On the other hand, when alveolar emptying is incomplete during expiration, airflow is present at the end of expiration, and this creates a pressure drop from the alveoli to the proximal airways at end-expiration. Thus in this situation, alveolar pressure will be positive relative to atmospheric (zero) pressure at end-expiration (i.e., PEEP). As shown in the upper portion of Figure 28.7, the positive alveolar pressure is not evident on the proximal airways pressure tracing, and hence this is an *occult* PEEP (26). Other terms for this pressure are *intrinsic PEEP, auto-PEEP,* and *dynamic hyperinflation* (27). The latter term is usually reserved for PEEP produced by obstructive airways disease (see below).

Predisposing Factors

The factors that predispose to hyperinflation and occult PEEP can be separated into ventilation-associated and disease-associated factors. The ventilatory factors that promote hyperinflation include high inflation volumes, rapid breathing, and a relative decrease in exhalation time relative to inhalation time. The disease-related factor that promotes hyperinflation is airways obstruction (as occurs in asthma and chronic obstructive pulmonary disease [COPD]). All three factors are operative in ventilator-dependent patients with obstructive airways disease. **In patients with asthma and COPD, occult PEEP is probably universal during conventional volume-cycled mechanical ventilation** (27–29). In one study of ventilator-dependent patients with COPD, the level of occult PEEP varied from 2.5 to 15 cm H_2O (27). Occult PEEP may also be common in ventilator-dependent patients with ARDS (30).

CONSEQUENCES

Cardiac Performance

Occult PEEP can have the same effects on cardiac performance as extrinsic PEEP, which are described in Chapter 27. The detrimental effects of occult PEEP on cardiac performance have been implicated as a cause of electromechanical dissociation during cardiopulmonary resuscitation (31).

Alveolar Rupture

Occult PEEP is a manifestation of hyperinflation, and thus there is an increased risk of alveolar rupture (volutrauma) with occult PEEP. Hyperinflation-induced alveolar rupture and pneumothorax are particular concerns in ventilator-dependent asthmatic patients (29).

Thoracic Compliance

Occult PEEP increases the end-inspiratory pressures in the proximal airways (both peak and plateau pressures). When occult PEEP goes undetected, the increase in plateau pressure is misinterpreted as a decrease in the compliance of the lungs and chest wall. Therefore, **failure to consider occult PEEP can result in an underestimation of thoracic compliance** (32). When respiratory compliance is being monitored (see Chapter 27), the level of occult PEEP should be subtracted from the measured plateau pressure and the adjusted plateau pressure should be used for the compliance calculation.

Work of Breathing

Occult PEEP can be accompanied by an increased work of breathing. Two mechanisms are involved. First, the hyperinflation places the lungs on a flatter portion of their pressure-volume curve, so higher pressures are needed to inhale the tidal volume. (To appreciate this effect, take a deep breath, and then try to breathe in further.) The hyperinflation also flattens the diaphragm, and when this occurs, the diaphragm muscle must generate a greater tension to achieve a given change in thoracic pressure. (This effect is predicted by the Law of Laplace: T = Pr.) The increased work of breathing with occult PEEP can impede efforts to wean from mechanical ventilation (see Chapter 29).

MONITORING OCCULT PEEP

Unfortunately, occult PEEP is difficult to monitor, at least in a quantitative manner. The following methods have been used to monitor occult PEEP.

End-Expiratory Occlusion

During controlled ventilation (i.e., when the patient is completely passive), occult PEEP can be uncovered by occluding the expiratory tubing at the end of expiration (32). This maneuver blocks airflow and allows the pressure in the proximal airways to equilibrate with alveolar pressure. Thus, **a sudden rise in proximal airways pressure with end-expiratory occlusion is evidence of occult PEEP** (see the upper left panel in Fig. 28.7). To quantitate the level of occult PEEP, the occlusion must be timed to the very end of expiration. Expiratory flow can persist until the end of expiration, so occlusions performed before end-expiration will overestimate the prevalence and magnitude of occult PEEP. Unfortunately, timing the occlusion to the end of expiration is a difficult task. End-expiratory occlusion becomes more reliable when it is performed electronically, which is anticipated in future models of mechanical ventilators.

Extrinsic PEEP

The application of extrinsic PEEP normally increases the peak inspiratory airway pressure by an equivalent amount. However, in the presence of occult PEEP, the peak inspiratory pressure may not change when extrinsic PEEP is applied (this is explained below). Therefore, **failure of extrinsic PEEP to produce an increase in peak inspiratory airway pressure is evidence of occult PEEP** (33–35). Furthermore, the level of extrinsic PEEP that first produces a rise in peak inspiratory pressures can be taken as the quantitative level of occult PEEP (33).

Management

The methods used to prevent or reduce hyperinflation and occult PEEP are all directed at promoting alveolar emptying during expiration. Ventilator-induced hyperinflation can be minimized by avoiding excessive inflation volumes, and by optimizing the time allowed for exhalation. These measures are described in Chapter 26.

Extrinsic PEEP

When hyperinflation is due to small airway collapse at end-expiration, as occurs in patients with asthma and COPD, the application of extrinsic PEEP can help keep the small airways open at end-expiration. The level of extrinsic PEEP must be enough to counterbalance the pressure causing small airways collapse (the *critical closing pressure*) but should not exceed the level of intrinsic PEEP (so that it does not impair expiratory flow) (34). To accomplish this, the level of extrinsic PEEP should match the level of occult PEEP. The problem then is to obtain an accurate measure of occult PEEP. When this is impossible, an alternative method is to observe the changes in peak inspiratory pressure when extrinsic PEEP is applied. As mentioned earlier, the level of extrinsic PEEP that first causes an increase in peak inspiratory airway pressures can be taken as the level of occult PEEP. Therefore, the extrinsic PEEP can be increased gradually as long as it does not cause an increase in peak inspiratory pressure. When used properly, extrinsic PEEP should reduce the work of breathing created by intrinsic or occult PEEP (35). The clinical significance of this, however, is unclear.

REFERENCES

1. National Association of Medical Directors of Respiratory Care (NAMDRC) Consensus Conference on Artificial Airways in Patients Receiving Mechanical Ventilation. Chest 1989;96:178–180.
2. Gallagher TJ. Endotracheal intubation. Crit Care Clin 1992;8:665–676.
3. Heffner JE. The technique of tracheotomy and cricothyroidotomy. J Crit Illness 1995;10:561–568.
4. Kharasch M, Graff J. Emergency management of the airway. Crit Care Clin 1995;11:53–66.
5. Stauffer JL, Olson DE, Petty TL. Complications and consequences of endotracheal intubation and tracheostomy. 1981;70:65–76.

6. Habib MP. Physiologic implications of artificial airways. Chest 1989;96: 180–184.

7. Hamill JF, Bedford RF, Weaver DC, et al. Lidocaine before endotracheal intubation: intravenous or laryngotracheal? Anesthesiology 1981;55:578–581.

8. Walls RM. Rapid-sequence intubation in head trauma. Ann Emerg Med 1993; 22:1008–1013.

9. Brunel W, Coleman DL, Schwartz DE, et al. Assessment of routine chest roentgenograms and the physical examination to confirm endotracheal tube placement. Chest 1989;96:1043–1045.

10. Owen RL, Cheney FW. Endotracheal intubation: a preventable complication. Anesthesiology 1987;67:255–257.

11. Mizutani AR, Ozaki G, Benumof JL, Scheller ML. Auscultation cannot distinguish esophageal from tracheal passage of tube. J Clin Monit 1991;7:232–236.

12. Goodman LR. Pulmonary support and monitoring apparatus. In: Goodman LR, Putman CE, eds. Critical care imaging. 3rd ed. Philadelphia: WB Saunders, 1992;35–59.

13. Pedersen J, Schurizek BA, Melsen NC, Juhl B. The effect of nasotracheal intubation on the paranasal sinuses. Acta Anesthesiol Scand 1991;35:11–13.

14. Rouby J-J, Laurent P, Gosnach M, et al. Risk factors and clinical relevance of nosocomial maxillary sinusitis in the critically ill. Am J Respir Crit Care Med 1994;150:776–783.

15. Holzapfel L, Chevret S, Madinier G, et al. Influence of long-term oro- or nasotracheal intubation on nosocomial maxillary sinusitis and pneumonia: results of a prospective, randomized clinical trial. Crit Care Med 1993;21:1132–1138.

16. Colice GL. Resolution of laryngeal injury following translaryngeal intubation. Am Rev Respir Dis 1992;145:361–364.

17. Heffner JE, Miller S, Sahn SA. Tracheostomy in the intensive care unit. Parts 1 and 2. Chest 1986;90:269–274, 430–436.

18. Marsh HM, Gillespie DJ, Baumgartner AE. Timing of tracheostomy in the critically ill patient. Chest 1989;96:190–192.

19. Elpern EH, Scott MG, Petro L, Ries MH. Pulmonary aspiration in mechanically ventilated patients with tracheostomies. Chest 1994;105:563–566.

20. Estes RJ, Meduri GU. The pathogenesis of ventilator-associated pneumonia: mechanisms of bacterial transcolonization and airway inoculation. Int Care Med 1995;21:365–383.

21. Kearl RA, Hooper RG. Massive airway leaks: an analysis of the role of endotracheal tubes. Crit Care Med 1993;21:518–521.

ALVEOLAR RUPTURE

22. Gammon RB, Shin MS, Buchalter SE. Pulmonary barotrauma in mechanical ventilation. Chest 1992;102:568–572.

23. Marcy TW. Barotrauma: detection, recognition, and management. Chest 1993; 104:578–584.

24. Tocino IM, Miller MH, Fairfax WR. Distribution of pneumothorax in the supine and semirecumbent critically ill adult. Am J Radiol 1985;144:901–905.

25. Kam AC, O'Brien M, Kam PCA. Pleural drainage systems. Anesthesia 1993; 48:154–161.

OCCULT PEEP

26. Pepe P, Marini JJ. Occult positive end-expiratory pressure in mechanically ventilated patients with airflow obstruction. Am Rev Respir Dis 1982;126: 166–170.

27. Gottfried SB, Rossi A, Milic-Emili J. Dynamic hyperinflation, intrinsic PEEP, and the mechanically ventilated patient. Crit Care Digest 1986;5:30–33.
28. Ligas JR, Mosiehi F, Epstein MAF. Occult positive end-expiratory pressure with different types of mechanical ventilators. J Crit Care 1990;5:95–100.
29. Weiner C. Ventilatory management of respiratory failure in asthma. JAMA 1993;269:2128–2131.
30. Tantucci C, Corbeil C, Chasse M, et al. Flow and volume dependence of respiratory system flow resistance in patients with adult respiratory distress syndrome. Am Rev Respir Dis 1992;145:355–360.
31. Rogers PL, Schlichtig R, Miro A, Pinsky M. Auto-PEEP during CPR. An "occult" cause of electromechanical dissociation. Chest 1991;99:492–493.
32. Tobin MJ. Respiratory monitoring. JAMA 1990;264:244–251.
33. Slutsky AS. Mechanical ventilation. Chest 1993;104:1833–1859.
34. Tobin MJ, Lodato RF. PEEP, auto-PEEP, and waterfalls. Chest 1989;96:449–451.
35. Pinsky MR. Through the past darkly: ventilatory management of pati .ts with chronic obstructive pulmonary disease. Crit Care Med 1994;22:1714–1717.

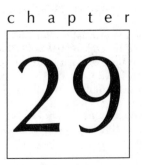

c h a p t e r

29

DISCONTINUING MECHANICAL VENTILATION

Attempts to discontinue mechanical ventilation account for approximately 40% of the time that a patient spends on a ventilator (1). When a ventilator is required because of brainstem respiratory depression (e.g., general anesthesia or a drug overdose), removal of ventilatory assistance is easily accomplished when the patient awakens. However, when a ventilator is required because of cardiopulmonary insufficiency, withdrawing ventilatory support is a more involved and more gradual process. This more gradual withdrawal of mechanical ventilation, commonly known as *weaning*, is the subject of this chapter (2–4).

MISCONCEPTIONS

The practice of weaning from mechanical ventilation has been dominated by a number of misconceptions, which are listed in Table 29.1. Many of these misconceptions are related to the perception that mechanical ventilation weakens the respiratory muscles. Although this may be true for the accessory muscles of respiration, it does not necessarily apply to the diaphragm.

THE DIAPHRAGM

The perceived need for weaning (i.e., gradual withdrawal) is based on the notion that the respiratory muscles become weak during mechanical ventilation, and thus must be strengthened gradually to allow a return to spontaneous breathing. This is what I call the *arm-in-a-cast* approach to weaning. This analogy may be appropriate for the accessory muscles of respiration but not for the diaphragm. That is, as mentioned in Chapter 26, **the diaphragm is not a voluntary muscle**

TABLE 29.1. COMMON MISCONCEPTIONS ABOUT WEANING
• The longer the duration of mechanical ventilation, the more difficult the wean.
• The method of weaning determines the ability to wean.
• Diaphragm weakness is a common cause of failed wean attempts.
• Aggressive nutrition support improves the ability to wean.
• Removal of endotracheal tubes reduces the work of breathing.

that will stop contracting during mechanical ventilation. The contraction of the diaphragm is dictated by the activity of brainstem respiratory neurons, and these neurons continue to fire periodically throughout life. In fact, these neurons *must* continue to fire periodically for life to continue. Thus, the diaphragm contracts periodically throughout life, regardless of the presence or absence of mechanical ventilation. When the diaphragm contracts and triggers a ventilator breath, the contraction does not cease, but continues for the duration of inspiration set by the brainstem respiratory neurons (5).

Therefore, the nature of diaphragm contraction implies that **the diaphragm does not necessarily become weak during mechanical ventilation.** However, other conditions in ventilator-dependent patients in the ICU (e.g., shock, low cardiac output, and hypophosphatemia) could promote diaphragm weakness.

Weaning

Because the diaphragm does not necessarily become weak during mechanical ventilation, the focus on diaphragm weakness as a cause of failure to wean may be misdirected. In fact, in a study we performed, there was no evidence that diaphragm weakness was the cause of failure to wean from mechanical ventilation (6). Failure to document diaphragm weakness as a cause of failure to wean is also noted by others (7).

BEDSIDE WEANING PARAMETERS

The initial step in the wean process is to identify patients who are candidates for weaning. All candidates should have adequate arterial oxygenation at an F_{IO_2} of 0.5 or less and extrinsic positive end-expiratory pressure (PEEP) of 5 cm H_2O or less. Once this condition is satisfied, a number of easily obtained bedside parameters can be used to predict the likelihood of removing the patient from ventilatory support. These parameters are listed in Table 29.2. Although easily obtained, many of the popular bedside weaning parameters have a poor predictive value, particularly when applied to individual patients (8). The poor predictive value of the minute ventilation measurement is shown in Figure 29.1 (8). In this study, the minute ventilation incorrectly predicted the outcome of the wean in 40 to 50% of the patients,

TABLE 29.2. BEDSIDE WEANING PARAMETERS

Parameter	Normal Adult Range	Threshold for Weaning
PaO_2/FiO_2	>400	200
Tidal volume	5–7 mL/kg	5 mL/kg
Respiratory rate	14–18/min	<40/min
Vital capacity	65–75 mL/kg	10 mL/kg
Minute ventilation	5–7 L/min	<10 L/min
	Greater Predictive Value	
Maximum inspiratory	>−90 cm H_2O (F)	−25 cm H_2O
pressure	>−120 cm H_2O (M)	
Rate/tidal volume	<50/min/L	<100/min/L

which is about the predictive value of a coin toss. The most predictive of the bedside parameters are described below.

MAXIMUM INSPIRATORY PRESSURE

The strength of the diaphragm and other muscles of inspiration can be evaluated by having the patient exhale to residual lung volume and then inhale as forcefully as possible against a closed valve (9). The airway pressure generated by this maneuver is called the maximum inspiratory pressure (Pɪmax). Normal men can generate a negative Pɪmax over 100 cm H_2O, whereas women achieve slightly lower levels (Table 29.2). The threshold Pɪmax for predicting a successful wean is 20 to 30 cm H_2O (negative pressure).

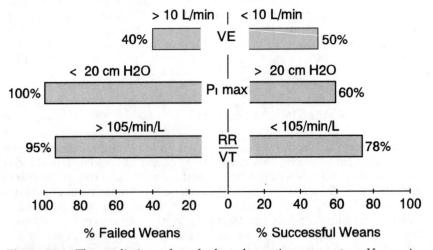

Figure 29.1. The predictive value of selected weaning parameters. V_E = minute ventilation, $Pɪmax$ = maximin inspiratory pressure, RR/V_T = ratio of respiratory rate to tidal volume. (Data from Yang K, Tobin MJ. A prospective study of indexes predicting the outcome of weaning from mechanical ventilation. N Engl J Med 1991;324:1445.)

Predictive Value

The predictive value of the PImax in one large study is shown in Figure 29.1 (8). When the PImax was less than 20 cm H_2O, no patient was successfully weaned. However, 40% of the patients with a PImax above 20 cm H_2O also did not wean. Therefore, a low PImax is valuable for identifying patients who will not wean. However, an acceptable PImax has little value for predicting a successful wean.

FREQUENCY–VOLUME RATIO

Rapid and shallow breathing is common in patients who fail to wean from mechanical ventilation. An index of rapid and shallow breathing is provided by the ratio of respiratory rate to tidal volume (RR/V_T). This ratio is normally less than 50 breaths/minute/L, and is often above 100 breaths/minute/L in patients who do not wean from the ventilator.

Predictive Value

The predictive value of the frequency–volume ratio in one study is shown in Figure 29.1 (8). When the RR/V_T ratio was above 105 breaths/minute/L, 95% of the wean attempts were unsuccessful. However when the RR/V_T ratio was below 105, 80% of the wean attempts were a success. Thus, **the respiratory rate–tidal volume ratio has a high predictive value for identifying patients who will and will not wean.** Unfortunately, this predictive value is not consistently high in all studies (10). Nevertheless, this parameter is one of the most predictive bedside weaning parameters.

METHODS OF WEANING

There are two general approaches to withdrawing ventilator support. One involves periods of spontaneous breathing interspersed with periods of ventilatory support. The other involves a gradual reduction in the fraction of total ventilation contributed by the ventilator. The abrupt withdrawal method is known as *T-piece weaning* because the original breathing apparatus was shaped like the letter *T*. The gradual withdrawal method uses intermittent mandatory ventilation (IMV), a mode of ventilation described in Chapter 27.

T-PIECE WEANING

This method is like an on–off toggle switch that switches between periods on and off the ventilator. The original circuit design for the

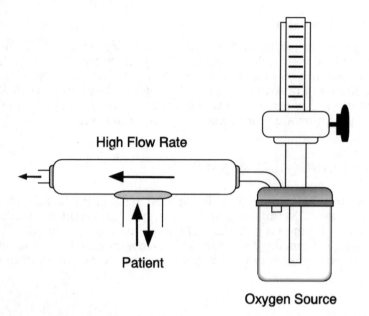

High Flow Rate

Patient

Oxygen Source

Figure 29.2. Diagram of the T-shaped circuit used for spontaneous breathing trials. A continuous flow of gas passes along the horizontal upper arm of the T-circuit, and this prevents the patient from inhaling room air or rebreathing exhaled gas.

spontaneous breathing periods is shown in Figure 29.2 (note the T-shaped arrangement of the tubing). The inhaled gas is delivered at a high flow rate through the upper arm of the apparatus. The high flow rate serves two purposes. First, it prevents the patient from inhaling room air from the exhalation side of the apparatus. Second, it carries the exhaled gas from the patient out of the apparatus, and prevents rebreathing.

Protocols

A variety of protocols are used for T-piece weaning. Each uses a specified period for spontaneous breathing and ventilator support (e.g., 4 hours off, 4 hours on) and gradually increases the time off the ventilator. The method I prefer is to keep the patient off the ventilator as long as tolerated. If spontaneous breathing is tolerated for 24 hours, the wean is considered successful. If the patient fails the T-piece trial, ventilatory support is resumed until the patient appears comfortable, and then another T-piece trial begins and lasts as long as tolerated. With this method, the patient is never placed back on the ventilator as long as spontaneous breathing is tolerated.

Minimum Pressure Support

T-piece breathing trials are now usually conducted while the patient is attached to the ventilator (this allows breath-to-breath monitoring of tidal volume and respiratory rate). The only drawback with this arrangement is the increased resistance to breathing created by the ventilator tubing and the actuator valves in the circuit. To overcome this resistance, pressure-support ventilation (described in Chapter 27) is often used during spontaneous breathing trials. The goal is to provide enough pressure to overcome the resistance of the ventilator circuit without augmenting the patient's spontaneous inflation volumes, so this method is called *minimum pressure-support*.

The minimum pressure needed to overcome resistance in the ventilator circuit can be determined as follows (11):

$$P_{min} = PIFR \times R \qquad (29.1)$$

where PIFR is the peak inspiratory flow rate during spontaneous breathing (measured while the patient breathes spontaneously through the ventilator circuit) and R is the resistance to inspiratory flow during mechanical ventilation. The resistance to flow is derived as descried in Chapter 26; that is, $R = P_{pk} - P_{pl}/\dot{V}_{insp}$, where P_{pk} and P_{pl} are the end-inspiratory peak and plateau pressures, respectively, and $\dot{V}_{insp}$ is the inspiratory flow rate delivered by the ventilator. The minimum pressure derived in this fashion is then used for the periods of spontaneous breathing and is continued until the patient is extubated.

IMV WEANING

IMV provides a predetermined number of machine breaths each minute and allows the patient to breathe spontaneously between the machine breaths (see Fig. 27.1).

IMV can be used to wean ventilatory support by gradually decreasing the number of machine breaths delivered each minute. The time over which this takes place is extremely variable and depends on the condition of the patient and the preferences of the ICU staff. Pressure-support ventilation is often added to assist the spontaneous breathing efforts during IMV, for the same reason as described for T-piece weaning.

The False Security of IMV

There is a tendency to view IMV as safer method of weaning because IMV provides a certain number of backup machine breaths. However, the IMV mode does not adjust to changes in a patient's ventilatory demands (i.e., it is not a closed-loop feedback system). If the minute ventilation of the patient declines, there is no compensation by the ventilator to maintain a constant minute ventilation. Therefore, the patient can crash just as easily during IMV weaning as during a T-piece trial.

The false sense of security with IMV weaning is dangerous because it leads to the perception that patients weaned with IMV can be left unattended more than patients weaned with a T-piece.

WHICH METHOD?

The early experience with weaning suggested that all methods were equivalent. However, more recent studies indicate that daily T-piece trials result in the most rapid weaning from mechanical ventilation (12,13). Furthermore, the superiority of daily T-piece trials seems not to be a function of the method itself, but is rather a result of early recognition of patients capable of spontaneous breathing (13). Remember that the end-point of IMV weaning is a T-piece trial, so the time involved in tapering the machine breaths during an IMV wean is wasted time for patients who are capable of unassisted breathing. This leads to a very important point about weaning: **The important factor in successful weaning is not the method used, but the ability to recognize when a patient is capable of spontaneous unassisted breathing.** Most patients require ventilator assistance because their lungs do not work, and weaning does not improve lung function. When lung function is adequate to support spontaneous breathing, the patient will wean, regardless of the weaning technique used.

COMPLICATING FACTORS

The following factors can make weaning more difficult; attention to these factors is necessary to ensure an optimal attempt at weaning.

DYSPNEA

Anxiety and dyspnea are common during weaning, regardless of the weaning method used (14). Dyspnea itself can be detrimental because it causes rapid breathing, which can produce intrinsic or occult PEEP (see Chapter 28). The best way to avoid or limit anxiety and dyspnea is to provide adequate sedation. Morphine works well for relieving the sense of dyspnea during weaning. For patients with chronic CO_2 retention, haloperidol (which does not depress ventilation) is an appropriate substitute.

CARDIAC OUTPUT

The transition from positive-pressure ventilation to negative-pressure breathing can result in a decrease in cardiac output (caused by an increase in left-ventricular afterload) (15). This decrease can impair weaning, not only by promoting pulmonary congestion, but also by impairing diaphragm function. The diaphragm depends heavily on cardiac output (like the heart, the diaphragm maximally extracts oxygen), and **a drop in cardiac output can decrease the strength of diaphragmatic contractions** (16). Therefore, the cardiac output should be monitored if possible (i.e., with an indwelling pulmonary artery catheter) in patients with cardiac dysfunction. If necessary, dobutamine can be used for temporary support of the cardiac output.

OVERFEEDING

An increase in daily caloric intake results in an increase in metabolic CO_2 production, as illustrated in Figure 29.3 (17). Excess calories therefore result in excess CO_2 production, and this can impair the ability to wean from mechanical ventilation (17,18). For this reason, patients receiving prolonged mechanical ventilation should have their daily energy needs measured with indirect calorimetry (not estimated with conventional formulas) and the daily caloric intake should not exceed daily needs (see Chapter 46).

ELECTROLYTE DEPLETION

Depletion of magnesium and phosphorous can impair respiratory muscle strength (18,19), and deficiencies in these electrolytes should be corrected for optimal weaning.

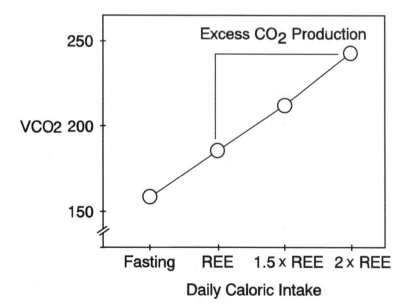

Figure 29.3. The influence of daily caloric intake on metabolic CO_2 production ($\dot{V}_{CO_2}$) in mechanically ventilated patients. REE is the resting energy expenditure (in kcal/24 hours) determined by indirect calorimetry. Each data point represents a mean value for all measurements obtained. (Data from Talpers S, et al. Nutritionally associated increased carbon dioxide production. Chest 1992;102:551.)

THE PROBLEM WEAN

The following problems are common sources of difficulty in discontinuing ventilator support.

RAPID BREATHING

One of the most common problems in weaning is an increase in the respiratory rate. In this situation, the task is to distinguish anxiety from respiratory muscle fatigue or cardiopulmonary insufficiency. The flow diagram in Figure 29.4 shows a simple approach to this problem using the spontaneous tidal volume. Anxiety is accompanied by hyperventilation, where the tidal volume is usually increased, whereas the pathologic causes of wean failure (i.e., muscle fatigue and cardio-

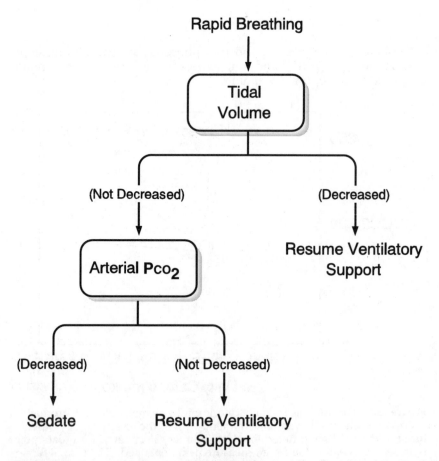

Figure 29.4. An approach to rapid breathing during weaning from mechanical ventilation.

pulmonary disease) usually cause rapid shallow breathing. Therefore, **an increase in tidal volume suggests anxiety, whereas a decrease in tidal volume suggests true wean failure.** When the tidal volume is unchanged or increased, arterial blood gases can further help identify the problem; i.e., a decrease in arterial P_{CO_2} suggests anxiety (hyperventilation), whereas an unchanged or rising arterial P_{CO_2} indicates true wean failure.

ABDOMINAL PARADOX

The respiratory movements of the abdomen can provide information about the functional integrity of the diaphragm (20). When the diaphragm contracts, it descends into the abdomen and increases intraabdominal pressure. This pushes the anterior wall of the abdomen outward. However, when the diaphragm is weak, the negative intrathoracic pressure created by the accessory muscles of respiration pulls the diaphragm upward into the thorax. This decreases the intraabdominal pressure and causes a paradoxical inward displacement of the abdomen during inspiration. This phenomenon is called *abdominal paradox*. Therefore, the appearance of abdominal paradox during weaning is a possible sign of a diaphragmatic weakness.

Predictive Value

Abdominal paradox is a reliable sign of bilateral diaphragm weakness only during quiet breathing. When breathing is labored, contraction of the accessory muscles of inspiration can overcome the contractile force of the diaphragm and pull the diaphragm up into the thorax during inspiration. This results in abdominal paradox in the face of an actively contracting diaphragm. Because quiet breathing may be uncommon during a difficult wean, **the appearance of abdominal paradox during weaning** is not necessarily a sign of diaphragm weakness. However, it is a sign of labored breathing, and **should prompt immediate return to full ventilatory support.**

HYPOXEMIA

The approach to hypoxemia is presented in Chapter 21 (see Fig. 21.6). One potential cause of hypoxemia that deserves mention in this setting is a decrease in cardiac output. The hypoxemia in this case is caused by a decrease in mixed venous oxygen saturation (S_{VO_2}), so S_{VO_2} can be an important measurement in the evaluation of hypoxemia during weaning.

HYPERCAPNIA

The approach to hypercapnia is described in Chapter 21 (see Fig. 21.7). The appearance of hypercapnia is an ominous sign, and should prompt immediate return to full ventilatory support. If the end-tidal P_{CO_2} (P_{ETCO_2}) is being monitored during the wean, the gradient between end-tidal and arterial P_{CO_2} can help identify the problem. An increase in the Pa_{CO_2}– P_{ETCO_2} gradient indicates an increase in dead space ventilation (from a decrease in cardiac output or hyperinflation with intrinsic PEEP), whereas an unchanged gradient suggests respiratory muscle fatigue or enhanced CO_2 production.

TRACHEAL DECANNULATION

When the patient no longer requires ventilator support, the next step is to remove the tracheal tube, if possible. **Successful weaning from mechanical ventilation is *not* synonymous with tracheal decannulation.** When a patient has successfully weaned but is not fully awake, or is unable to clear respiratory secretions, the tracheal tube should be left in place.

WORK OF BREATHING

The cross-sectional area of the glottis (the narrowest portion of the upper airway) is 66 mm^3 in the average-sized adult, whereas the cross-sectional area of an average-sized adult tracheal tube (8 mm internal diameter) is 50 mm^3 (21). The narrower cross-sectional area of the tracheal tube creates an increased resistance to airflow, so the work of breathing should be greater when breathing through tracheal tubes (both endotracheal and tracheostomy tubes). This observation has led to the perception that tracheal decannulation results in a decreased work of breathing. However, as shown in Figure 29.5, tracheal decan-

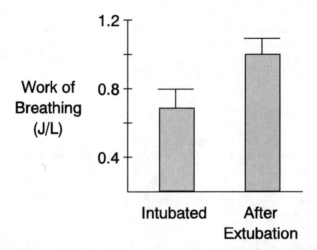

Figure 29.5. The work of breathing in joules/liter (J/L) after removal of endotracheal tubes (size 8). Each column shows the mean and standard error of the mean. (From Nathan SD et al. Prediction of minimal pressure support during weaning from mechanical ventilation. Chest 1993;103:1215.)

nulation is accompanied by an *increased* work of breathing (11). This is presumably the result of laryngeal edema produced by endotracheal tubes. Although this obstruction rarely requires reintubation, the increased work of breathing has implications for the occasional practice of removing tracheal tubes to reduce the work of breathing. That is, **tracheal decannulation should never be performed to reduce the work of breathing.**

ENDOTRACHEAL TUBES

Although some degree of laryngeal edema occurs during more than 90% of endotracheal intubations (22), the incidence of significant upper airway obstruction (i.e., obstruction requiring reintubation) is less than 2% (22,23). The signs of upper airway obstruction following extubation are labored and *stridorous* breathing. Because the obstruction is extrathoracic, the stridorous sounds should occur during inspiration (when the negative pressure of inspiration leads to narrowing in the extrathoracic portion of the upper airways). Inspiratory stridor is a sign of severe obstruction (more than 80%), and should prompt immediate reintubation.

The management of severe upper airway obstruction after extubation includes reintubation followed by tracheostomy. Steroids do not reduce the severity of postextubation laryngeal edema (23). Aerosolized epinephrine (2.5 mL of 1% epinephrine or 2.25% racemic epinephrine) has proven effective in reducing postextubation laryngeal edema in children (24). However, epinephrine treatments should never delay reintubation.

TRACHEOSTOMY TUBES

Removal of tracheostomy tubes is a two-step process. The first step is to replace the cuffed tracheostomy tube with an uncuffed, fenestrated tube of the same size. This tube is then plugged, and the fenestration (hole) in the tube allows the patient to breathe through the normal upper airway route. This is done to identify an upper airway obstruction caused by laryngeal edema. Contrary to popular belief, **tracheostomy may not reduce, and can even aggravate, the laryngeal damage caused by endotracheal intubation** (although the mechanism is unclear) (22). Therefore, evaluation for upper airway obstruction is important before removal of tracheostomy tubes. If there is no evidence of upper airway obstruction after 24 hours of breathing with the tracheostomy tube plugged, then the tube can be removed.

Tracheal stenosis following tracheostomy usually occurs at the site of the tracheal incision, not at the site of cuff inflation. This complication usually becomes evident after the tracheal stoma closes, and is thus a late complication of tracheostomy (usually appearing after the patient leaves the ICU).

REFERENCES

1. Esteban A, Alfa I, Ibanez J, et al. Modes of mechanical ventilation and weaning: a national survey of Spanish hospitals. Chest 1994;106:1188–1193.

REVIEWS

2. Schuster DP. A physiologic approach to initiating, maintaining, and withdrawing mechanical ventilatory support during acute respiratory failure. Am J Med 1990;88:268–278 (148 references).
3. Tobin MJ, Alex CG. Discontinuation of mechanical ventilation. In: Tobin MJ, ed. Principles and practice of mechanical ventilation. New York: McGraw-Hill, 1994;1177–1206.
4. Patel RG, Petrini MF, Norman JR. Strategies for maximizing your chances for weaning success. J Crit Illness 1995;10:411–423.

MISCONCEPTIONS

5. Marini JJ. Strategies to minimize breathing effort during mechanical ventilation. Crit Care Clin 1990;6:635–661.
6. Swartz MA, Marino PL. Diaphragm strength during weaning from mechanical ventilation. Chest 1985;88:736–739.
7. Hubmayr RD, Rehder K. Respiratory muscle failure in critically ill patients. Semin Respir Med 1992;13:14–21.

BEDSIDE WEANING PARAMETERS

8. Yang K, Tobin MJ. A prospective study of indexes predicting the outcome of trials of weaning from mechanical ventilation. N Engl J Med 1991;324:1445–1450.
9. Marini JJ, Smith TC, Lamb V. Estimation of inspiratory muscle strength in mechanically ventilated patients: the measurement of maximal inspiratory pressure. J Crit Care 1986;1:32–38.
10. Lee KH, Hui KP, Chan TB, et al. Rapid shallow breathing (frequency–tidal volume ratio) did not predict extubation outcome. Chest 1994;105:540–543.

METHODS OF WEANING

11. Nathan SD, Ishaaya AM, Koerner SK, et al. Prediction of minimal pressure support during weaning from mechanical ventilation. Chest 1993;103:1215–1219.
12. Esteban A, Frutos F, Tobin MJ, et al. A comparison of four methods of weaning patients from mechanical ventilation. N Engl J Med 1995;332:345–350.
13. Ely W, Baker AM, Dunagen DP, et al. Effect of duration of mechanical ventilation of identifying patients capable of breathing spontaneously. N Engl J Med 1996;335:1864–1869.

COMPLICATING FACTORS

14. Bouley GH, Froman R, Shah H. The experience of dyspnea during weaning. Heart Lung 1992;21:471–476.
15. Pinsky M. Cardiovascular effects of ventilatory support and withdrawal. Anesth Analg 1994;79:567–576.
16. Nishimura Y, Maeda H, Tanaka K, et al. Respiratory muscle strength and hemodynamics in heart failure. Chest 1994;105:355–359.
17. Talpers SS, Romberger DJ, Bunce SB, Pingleton SK. Nutritionally associated increased carbon dioxide production. Chest 1992;102:551–555.
18. Benotti PN, Bistrian B. Metabolic and nutritional aspects of weaning from mechanical ventilation. Crit Care Med 1989;17:181–185.
19. Malloy DW, Dhingra S, Solren F, et al. Hypomagnesemia and respiratory muscle power. Am Rev Respir Dis 1984;129:427–431.

THE PROBLEM WEAN

20. Mier-Jedrzejowicz A, Brophy C, Moxham J, Geen M. Assessment of diaphragm weakness. Am Rev Respir Dis 1988;137:877–883.

TRACHEAL DECANNULATION

21. Kaplan JD, Schuster DP. Physiologic consequences of tracheal intubation. Clin Chest Med 1991;12:425–432.
22. Colice C, Stukel T, Dain B. Laryngeal complications of prolonged intubation. Chest 1989;96:877–884.
23. Gaussorgues P, Boyer F, Piperno D, et al. Do corticosteroids prevent postintubation laryngeal edema? A prospective study of 276 adults. Crit Care Med 1988;16:649–652.
24. Nutman J, Brooks LJ, Deakins K, et al. Racemic versus l-epinephrine aerosol in the treatment of postextubation laryngeal edema: results from a prospective, randomized, double-blind study. Crit Care Med 1994;22:1591–1594.

INFECTIONS AND INFLAMMATORY DISORDERS

Our arsenals for fighting off bacteria are so powerful . . . that we're in more danger from them than from the invaders.

Lewis Thomas

chapter

30

THE FEBRILE PATIENT

Humanity has but three great enemies:
Fever, famine and war.
Of these, by far the greatest,
By far the most terrible, is fever.
                    Sir William Osler

Despite Osler's harsh comments about fever, the appearance of fever in a patient in the ICU may not be a sign of impending disaster. However, it is a sign that requires attention. This chapter presents some of the most likely causes of nosocomial fever (i.e., onset after 48 hours of hospitalization) in patients in the ICU (1–3) and describes some early diagnostic and therapeutic approaches to the febrile patient. The specific concerns in patients who are immunocompromised are presented in Chapter 34.

BODY TEMPERATURE

Two scales (Celsius and Fahrenheit) are used to record body temperature, and the conversion from one scale to the other is shown in Table 30.1. Although readings on the Celsius scale are often called degrees centigrade, this unit is intended for the degrees on a compass, not for temperatures (4). The appropriate term for temperatures on the Celsius scale is degrees Celsius.

NORMAL BODY TEMPERATURE

Despite the fact that the body temperature is one of the most common measurements performed in clinical medicine, there is some disagreement about what the normal body temperature is in healthy adults. The following points illustrate some of the confusion regarding the normal body temperature.

TABLE 30.1. TEMPERATURE CONVERSIONS		
Corresponding Scales		
(°C)	(°F)	Conversion Formulas
100	212	Conversions are based on the corresponding
41	105.8	temperatures at the freezing point of water:
40	104	
39	102.2	$0°$ C $= 32°$ F
38	100.4	and the temperture ranges (from freezing point to
37	98.6	boiling point of water):
36	96.8	
35	95	$100°$ C $= 180°$ F or $5°$ C $= 9°$ F
34	93.2	The above relationships are then combined to derive
33	91.4	the conversion formulas:
32	89.6	
31	87.8	$°$ F $= (9/5°$ C$) + 32$
30	86	$°$ C $= 5/9$ $(°$ F $- 32)$
0	32	

The traditional norm of $37°$ C ($98.6°$ F) is a mean value derived from a study of *axillary* temperatures in 25,000 healthy adults, conducted in the late 19th century (5). A more recent survey of *oral* temperatures in 148 healthy subjects (ages 18 to 40 years) revealed a mean temperature of $36.8°$ C ($98.2°$ F) (6).

Elderly subjects have a mean body temperature that is approximately $0.5°$ C ($0.9°$ F) lower than that of younger adults (5,7).

The normal **body temperature has a diurnal variation,** with the nadir in the early morning (between 4 and 8 a.m.) and the peak in the late afternoon (between 4 and 6 p.m.). The range of diurnal variation varies in individual subjects, with the highest reported range in an individual subject being $1.3°$ C ($2.4°$ F) (6).

In the original 19th-century report, *fever* was defined as an axillary temperature of $38°$ C ($100.4°$ F) or greater at any time of the day (5). In the smaller, more recent survey, fever is defined as an oral temperature of $37.2°$ C ($99°$ F) or greater in the early morning, and $37.8°$ C ($100°$ F) or greater in the late afternoon (6).

The core body temperature is approximately $1.0°$ C ($1.8°$ F) higher than axillary temperatures (8) and $0.5°$ C ($0.9°$ F) higher than oral temperatures (9). The rectal temperature is usually higher than the oral or axillary temperatures, but the relationship is variable and unpredictable (10).

These observations indicate that the normal body temperature is not a single temperature, but rather is a range of temperatures that is influenced by age, time of day, and measurement site.

DEFINITION OF FEVER

The observations just presented illustrate the problem with using a single temperature threshold to define the febrile state. Fever is best defined as a temperature that exceeds the normal daily temperature range for an individual subject. However, **the operational definition**

of fever proposed by a consensus conference on sepsis and inflammation **is a body temperature above 38° C (100.4° F)** (11). Just remember
that this definition has several shortcomings (i.e., it does not take into
account the measurement site, time of the day, or age of the patient),
and its validity is easily questioned.

THE FEBRILE RESPONSE

Fever is an adaptive process where the normal body temperature
is set at a higher level in response to circulating pyrogens (12). This
is distinct from hyperthermia (also called hyperpyrexia), which is not
an adaptive response but represents a condition where the body is
unable to control the core body temperature (13). The following aspects of the febrile response deserve attention.

Fever is a sign of inflammation, not infection. The febrile response is initiated by inflammatory cytokines (e.g., tumor necrosis factor and interleukin 1-B). Therefore, fever is not a specific response to infection, but is a response to whatever incites
the production of inflammatory cytokines. In many instances,
the inciting event is tissue injury, not infection. In fact, **approximately 50% of fevers in patients in the ICU are not the direct
result of infection** (14). The distinction between inflammation
and infection is an important one, not only for the evaluation
of fever, but also for the popular practice of using antimicrobial
agents to treat a fever.

**The severity of the febrile response is not an indication of the
presence or severity of infection** (1,3). High fevers and rigors
can be associated with noninfectious processes (e.g., drug
fever), and minor temperature elevations can accompany life-
threatening infections. Therefore, the clinical presentation
should not dictate the evaluation of fever or the decision to
start antimicrobial therapy.

The usual causes of nosocomial fever in patients in the ICU are
indicated on the body map in Figure 30.1 (1–3). In some instances, the
search for a cause of nosocomial fever is influenced by the clinical
setting. This is the case for postoperative fevers and fevers associated
with specific procedures. These situational fevers are described next.

POSTOPERATIVE FEVER

Surgery is a form of controlled tissue injury (or, in the words of Dr.
John Millili, a surgeon and close friend, surgery is like being hit with
a baseball bat). Because inflammation and fever are the normal response to tissue injury, it is not surprising that infection may be absent
in as many as two-thirds of fevers that occur in the early postoperative
period (15,16). Most noninfectious fevers occur as a single episode.
For the first episode of postoperative fever, a thorough physical examination should be sufficient to identify an underlying infection (16). If
the physical examination is unrevealing, no further clinical evaluation
is necessary.

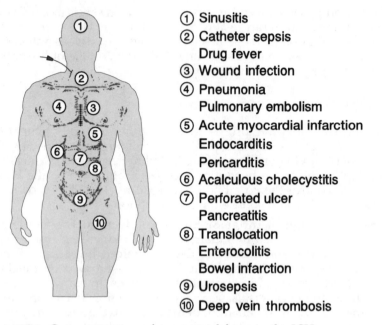

① Sinusitis
② Catheter sepsis
   Drug fever
③ Wound infection
④ Pneumonia
   Pulmonary embolism
⑤ Acute myocardial infarction
   Endocarditis
   Pericarditis
⑥ Acalculous cholecystitis
⑦ Perforated ulcer
   Pancreatitis
⑧ Translocation
   Enterocolitis
   Bowel infarction
⑨ Urosepsis
⑩ Deep vein thrombosis

Figure 30.1. Common causes of nosocomial fever in the ICU.

MALIGNANT HYPERTHERMIA

Malignant hyperthermia is an uncommon disorder that occurs in approximately 1 in 15,000 episodes of general anesthesia and affects approximately 1 in 50,000 adults (17,18). It is an inherited disorder and is characterized by an excessive release of calcium from the sarcoplasmic reticulum in skeletal muscle in response to general anesthetics and muscle relaxants (18).

Clinical features include early-onset muscle rigidity, often appearing in the operating room or postanesthesia recovery area, followed within minutes to hours by fever, hyperpyrexia (i.e., core temperatures above 40° C or 104° F), and depressed consciousness. In 20% of cases, the temperature elevation is not accompanied by observable muscle rigidity (19). The acute syndrome is followed by progression to rhabdomyolysis, myoglobinuric renal failure, and autonomic instability. Mortality is above 80% in untreated cases (18).

Treatment

The mainstay of treatment is the *immediate* administration of the skeletal muscle relaxant **dantrolene.**

Dosing Regimen

Dantrolene should be given in a dose or 1 to 2 mg/kg as an intravenous bolus. This dose should be repeated every 15 minutes if necessary to a total dose of 10 mg/kg. A dose of 1 to 2 mg/kg orally four times a day for 3 days should follow.

Dantrolene works by blocking the release of calcium by the sarcoplasmic reticulum. Early drug administration is necessary to halt the progression to rhabdomyolysis and myoglobinuric renal failure. Therapy with dantrolene has reduced mortality in this disorder to less than 10% (18).

All patients who survive an episode of malignant hyperthermia should be given a Medi-Alert bracelet to prevent further episodes. In addition, because it is a genetic disorder (with an autosomal dominant inheritance pattern), family members should be informed of their genetic predisposition.

WOUND INFECTIONS

Surgical wounds are classified as clean (abdomen and chest unopened), contaminated (abdomen or chest opened), or dirty (direct contact with pus or bowel contents) (20). Most wound infections are uncomplicated (i.e., only the skin and subcutaneous tissues are involved) and the treatment is debridement. Antimicrobial therapy (to cover streptococcus, staphylococcus, and anaerobes) should be reserved for cases of persistent erythema or for evidence of deep tissue involvement (15). In fever that follows median sternotomy, sternal wound infection with spread to the mediastinum is a prominent concern (21). In this situation, sternal instability can be an early sign of infection.

Necrotizing wound infections are produced by Clostridia or β-hemolytic streptococci. Unlike other wound infections, which appear 5 to 7 days after surgery, necrotizing infections are evident in the first few postoperative days. There is often marked edema around the incision, and the skin may have crepitance and fluid-filled bullae. Spread to deeper structures is rapid and produces progressive rhabdomyolysis and myoglobinuric renal failure. Treatment involves extensive debridement and intravenous penicillin. The mortality is high (above 60%) when treatment is delayed.

ATELECTASIS

Atelectasis is considered a common cause of fever in the early postoperative period (15). However, **no correlation exists between the presence of atelectasis and the appearance of postoperative fever** (22). For example, atelectasis is universal after upper abdominal surgery (where the functional residual capacity decreases by 40 to 70% during the first postoperative week) (23), yet fever develops in only 15% of patients following major abdominal surgery (16).

Postoperative atelectasis is a radiographic diagnosis, with linear densities and crowded markings in dependent lung zones. The nonspecific nature of this finding is illustrated in Figure 30.2. The chest film on the left (*arrow pointing down*) shows reduced lung volumes with coalescence of markings at the left lung base. This film might be interpreted as showing atelectasis at the left lung base. However, this film was obtained only minutes after the chest radiograph on the right,

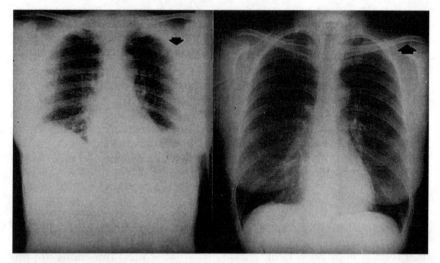

Figure 30.2. The influence of body position on the appearance of the chest radiograph. Both films were obtained within minutes of each other, in the same subject. The arrow pointing upward and downward indicates upright and supine positions, respectively.

using the same subject. The difference between the two radiographs is the body position; the film on the right is in the upright position, whereas the one on the left was obtained in the supine position. Thus, what might be interpreted as atelectasis is merely a consequence of body position. This is an important consideration because most chest radiographs in the early postoperative period are taken with the patient in the supine position.

For these reasons, it is unlikely that atelectasis is an important source of postoperative fever. Because most of the fevers attributed to atelectasis resolve within a day or two, it is likely that these fevers are produced by an inflammatory reaction to the surgical trauma.

THROMBOEMBOLISM

Thromboembolism can produce a fever that lasts for up to 1 week (24). In one autopsy study of postoperative deaths, pulmonary emboli were present in one-third of the patients but were rarely the cause of death (25). This confirms the high risk of thromboembolism in postoperative patients. The risk is highest following orthopedic procedures on the hips and knees and is lowest following cardiopulmonary bypass surgery (26). Thromboembolism can be associated with a normal leg examination in more than half of the cases (27), so the absence of leg swelling and leg tenderness does not rule out the possibility of thromboembolism as a cause of postoperative fever. The approach to suspected thromboembolism is described in Chapter 7.

ABDOMINAL ABSCESSES

Localized collections of infected material in the abdomen can occur with trauma to the abdominal viscera or after laparotomy. Septicemia occurs in approximately 50% of cases (28). Computed tomography of the abdomen can uncover the collection in more than 95% of cases (28). Initial antimicrobial therapy should be directed at Gram-negative enteric pathogens, including anaerobes (e.g., *Bacteroides fragilis*). Definitive treatment requires surgical or percutaneous drainage.

PROCEDURES

Fever associated with the following procedures may be causally linked to the procedure.

HEMODIALYSIS

Febrile reactions during hemodialysis are attributed to endotoxin contamination of the dialysis equipment, but bacteremia occurs on occasion (29). If toxicity is suspected, the dialysis should be stopped, blood cultures should be obtained, and antibiotics should be started immediately. The dialysis need not be stopped if toxicity is not suspected, but blood cultures should always be obtained. Empiric antibiotic therapy should cover both Gram-positive and Gram-negative pathogens. Vancomycin plus aztreonam should suffice pending culture results. Because of their nephrotoxic actions, aminoglycosides should be avoided if there is a chance for recovery of renal function.

ENDOSCOPY

Flexible fiberoptic bronchoscopy is followed by fever in 5% of cases (30). The cause may be release of tumor necrosis factor (an endogenous pyrogen) into the systemic circulation. Pneumonia and bacteremia are rare (30,31). Thus, there is usually no need for blood cultures or empiric antimicrobial therapy for postbronchoscopic fever, unless the patient shows signs of progressive sepsis (e.g., mental status changes or hypotension) or is asplenic (32).

Gastrointestinal endoscopy is also an uncommon source of infection. The highest risk seems to occur with retrograde cholangiopancreatography, which is complicated by infection in 1% of cases (31). Offending organisms are usually enteric pathogens.

BLOOD TRANSFUSION

Febrile reactions occur in as many as 5% of patients receiving blood products. The fever is usually the result of antileukocyte antibodies (not infection), and appears during or shortly after the transfusion. For more information on febrile transfusion reactions, see Chapter 44.

IATROGENIC FEVER

Faulty thermal regulators in water mattresses and aerosol humidifiers can cause fever by transference (33). It takes only a minute to check

---

**TABLE 30.2. GUIDELINES FOR CONFIRMING SUSPECTED
CATHETER SEPSIS**

- Draw 10 mL blood through the catheter and obtain another 10-mL specimen from a distant venipuncture site. Submit both specimens for **quantitative** blood cultures (see Table 5.4).
- If there is erythema or purulence at the insertion site, remove the catheter and use a new venipuncture site for reinsertion.
- If there is no erythema or purulence at the insertion site, change the catheter over a guidewire.
- Submit catheter tips for **semiquantitative** culture (see Table 5.5).

---

the temperature settings on heated mattresses and ventilators, but it can take far longer to explain why such a simple cause of fever was overlooked.

COMMON INFECTIONS

Common infectious sources of fever in patients in the ICU are pneumonia, urinary tract infections, and sepsis from intravascular catheters. These infections are described in detail elsewhere in the book, and are mentioned here only briefly.

PNEUMONIA

Pneumonia is an overdiagnosed cause of nosocomial fever in patients in the ICU. In one study of ventilator-dependent patients with fever and pulmonary infiltrates, pneumonia was the source of fever in only 19% of the patients (34). The diagnosis of pneumonia requires quantitative cultures of deep specimens obtained by bronchoalveolar lavage or bronchoscopic (protected) brush specimens. **Culture of unscreened nasotracheal aspirates is misleading and should be abandoned.** Only nasotracheal aspirates that are screened microscopically (to eliminate upper airway contamination) should be submitted for culture. See Chapter 32 for more information on the diagnosis of pneumonia. The approach to pulmonary infiltrates in the immunocompromised patient is presented in Chapter 34.

UROSEPSIS

Urinary tract infections are responsible for 35 to 45% of nosocomial infections (35). In many cases, the predisposing factor is an indwelling bladder catheter. The diagnostic and therapeutic approach to this problem is presented in Chapter 33.

CATHETER SEPSIS

Infections caused by indwelling vascular catheters should be suspected in any case of unexplained fever when a catheter has been in place for more than 48 hours. Some guidelines for confirming suspected catheter-related sepsis are presented in Table 30.2. For more information on catheter-related sepsis, see Chapter 5.

LESS COMMON INFECTIONS

When the common infections are not evident, the following infections are potential sources of nosocomial fever.

PARANASAL SINUSITIS

Nasogastric and nasotracheal tubes can block the ostia that drain the paranasal sinuses; this can lead to the accumulation of infected secretions in the paranasal sinuses (36,37). The maxillary sinuses are almost always involved, and the resulting acute sinusitis can be an occult source of fever. This complication is reported in 15 to 20% of patients with nasal tubes (36,37). Surprisingly, paranasal sinusitis is also found in patients who are intubated via the oral route and have free nares (36,37).

Diagnosis

Purulent drainage from the nares may be absent, and the diagnosis is suggested by radiographic features of sinusitis (i.e., opacification or air–fluid levels in the involved sinuses). Radiographic detection of sinusitis can be accomplished by conventional radiography, as in Figure 30.3. The maxillary sinuses can be viewed with a single occipito-mental radiograph, called a Waters view, obtained at the bedside (38). Computed tomography is also commonly used (36,37), but seems unnecessary. It is important to emphasize that 30 to 40% of patients with radiographic evidence of sinusitis do not have an infection documented by culture of aspirated material from the involved sinus (36,37). Therefore, **radiographic evidence of sinusitis is not sufficient for the diagnosis of purulent sinusitis.** The diagnosis must be confirmed by sinus puncture and isolation of one or more pathogens by quantitative culture, that is, at least 10^3 colony forming units per milliliter (CFU/mL) (36,37).

Treatment

Responsible pathogens include streptococci, staphylococci (including *Staphylococcus epidermidis*), enteric pathogens, and yeasts (mostly *Candida albicans*) (36,37). Polymicrobial infections are common. Although local irrigation of the sinuses with antimicrobial solutions has been recommended as treatment (37), a brief course of systemic antibiotics seems wise because septicemia is a complication of purulent sinusitis in critically ill patients (unlike outpatients, where septicemia is rare). When a sinus aspirate is purulent or shows organisms on Gram stain, empiric antimicrobial therapy can be started with vancomycin plus aztreonam or an aminoglycoside pending results of sinus cultures and blood cultures. Nasal tubes should also be removed when possible. In cases of recurrent sinusitis, decontamination of the nares with topical antimicrobial paste should be considered (see Chapter 6

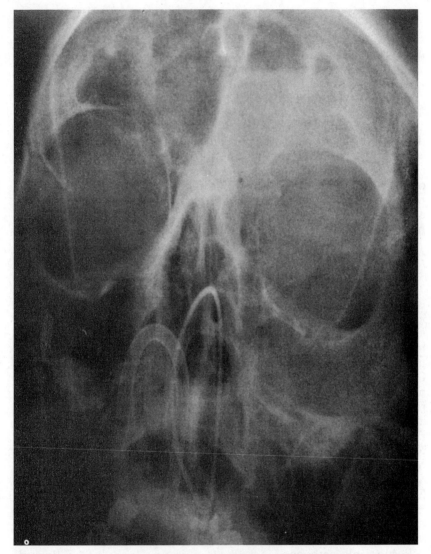

Figure 30.3. Opacification of the left maxillary and frontal sinuses in a patient with nasotracheal and nasogastric tubes. Acute sinusitis was subsequently confirmed by maxillary sinus puncture with isolation of 10^3 CFU/mL *S. epidermidis* on quantitative culture.

for a description of antibiotic paste used for oropharyngeal decontamination).

ACALCULOUS CHOLECYSTITIS

Acalculous cholecystitis is an uncommon but serious disorder reported in up to 1.5% of critically ill patients (39). It is most common in postoperative patients, trauma victims, and patients receiving parenteral nutrition. The inciting event is edema of the cystic duct, which blocks drainage of the gallbladder. The resulting clinical syndrome includes fever (70 to 95% of cases) and right upper quadrant tenderness (60 to 100% of cases) (39). Diagnosis is often possible with right upper quadrant ultrasound. Perforation of the gallbladder can occur within 48 hours after onset. The treatment of choice is cholecystectomy, or percutaneous cholecystostomy in patients who are too ill to undergo surgery. (For more information on this disorder, see Chapter 33.)

PSEUDOMEMBRANOUS ENTEROCOLITIS

Intestinal overgrowth of *Clostridium difficile* is common in patients undergoing antimicrobial therapy, and this can lead to a toxin-mediated enterocolitis characterized by fever and diarrhea (40). The diagnosis requires documentation of *C. difficile* toxin in stool samples or evidence of pseudomembranes on proctosigmoidoscopy. Therapy includes oral or intravenous metronidazole (500 mg every 6 hours) or oral vancomycin (500 mg orally every 6 hours). This disorder is described in more detail in Chapter 33.

OTHER INFECTIONS

Other infections that should be considered in selected patient populations are **endocarditis** (in patients with prosthetic valves), **meningitis** (in neurosurgical patients and those with human immunodeficiency virus infection), and **spontaneous bacterial peritonitis** (in patients with cirrhosis and ascites).

NONINFECTIOUS CAUSES OF FEVER

The following are some noninfectious causes of fever that can be encountered in the ICU.

DRUG FEVER

A variety of pharmacologic agents are capable of causing fever, and some of the likely offenders in the ICU are listed in Table 30.3. The

TABLE 30.3. DRUG-ASSOCIATED FEVER IN THE ICU		
Common Offenders	**Occasional Offenders**	**Clinical Findings***
Amphotericin	Cimetidine	Rigors (53%)
Cephalosporins	Carbamazepine	Myalgias (25%)
Penicillins	Hydralazine	Leukocytosis (22%)
Phenytoin	Rifampin	Eosiniphilia (22%)
Procainamide	Streptokinase	Rash (18%)
Quinidine	Vancomycin	Hypotension (18%)
* From Mackowiak and LeMaistre (41).		

fever can appear as an isolated finding or can be accompanied by the other manifestations listed in the table (41). Note the high incidence of rigors, indicating that drug fever can be mistaken for sepsis. Note also the 18% incidence of hypotension, indicating that **patients with a drug fever can appear to be seriously ill.** Finally, note that evidence of a hypersensitivity reaction (i.e., eosinophilia and rash) is often absent.

The diagnosis of drug fever usually is suggested by excluding all other potential causes of fever. When drug fever is a likely diagnosis, as many drugs as possible should be discontinued and replaced with suitable alternative agents. The fever should disappear in 2 to 3 days if a drug is responsible. The diagnosis can be confirmed by drug rechallenge, which should produce a fever within hours.

Neuroleptic Malignant Syndrome

A variant of malignant hyperthermia that is triggered by neuroleptic agents (e.g., haloperidol) is called the *neuroleptic malignant syndrome* (42). The clinical presentation and management are the same as described for malignant hyperthermia. Haloperidol is a popular sedative in many ICUs, so awareness of this syndrome is important in selected patients (For more information on this syndrome, see Reference 42.)

SYSTEMIC INFLAMMATORY RESPONSE SYNDROME

Evidence of systemic inflammation (i.e., fever and leukocytosis) in the absence of documented infection or other noninfectious source of fever may represent a clinical entity known as the *systemic inflammatory response syndrome* (SIRS). This syndrome can be triggered by traumatic tissue injury or translocation of endotoxin across the bowel mucosa. Evidence of multiorgan dysfunction may be present. This syndrome can lead to progressive multiorgan failure and death (this is described in more detail in Chapter 30).

BOWEL INFARCTION

Mesenteric ischemia and infarction are often accompanied by abdominal pain and tenderness, but these may be masked in patients with altered mental status. Unfortunately, the diagnosis is often difficult because physical findings and laboratory tests are neither sensitive nor specific. Plain radiographs of the abdomen can reveal gas in the bowel wall or portal venous gas, as shown in Figure 30.4. However, radiographic findings are often nonspecific. The diagnosis often requires laparotomy.

OTHER CAUSES

Other noninfectious causes of fever that may be encountered in the ICU are thromboembolism, pancreatitis, and adrenal insufficiency. Each of these disorders is described elsewhere.

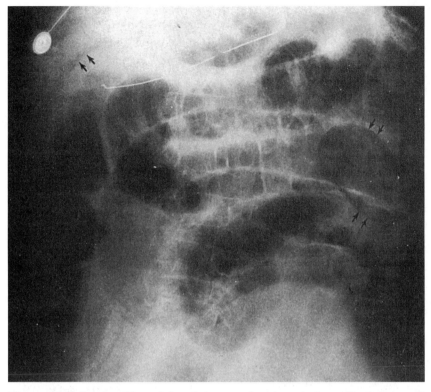

Figure 30.4. Supine film of the abdomen showing air in wall of the small bowel (*outlined by arrows*) and air in the hepatic veins (*arrows in upper left*). The patient died a few hours after this film was obtained.

EARLY MANAGEMENT DECISIONS

BLOOD CULTURES

Blood cultures should be obtained in all cases of nosocomial fever where an infectious source is suspected. In the ICU, this pertains to virtually every nosocomial fever, except those that occur in the early postoperative period. **No more than one set of blood cultures should be obtained from any one venipuncture site** (43). The number of sets of blood cultures (venipuncture sites) is determined by assessment of the likelihood of septicemia in individual cases. A low or moderate probability of bacteremia, such as that expected from a pneumonia or urinary tract infection, merits two sets of cultures. A high probability of bacteremia, as expected in catheter-related sepsis, requires at least three sets of blood cultures. If the patient has received antimicrobial agents, at least four sets of blood cultures are recommended for high-probability septicemia cases (41).

Volume of Blood

The volume of blood cultured is one of the most important factors in determining the yield from blood cultures. As much as **20 to 30 mL per set of blood cultures is recommended as the optimal volume** (41), but the volume ratio of blood to broth (culture medium) should be kept at 1:5 for each culture bottle.

EMPIRIC ANTIMICROBIAL THERAPY

In the absence of an identifiable infection, empiric antibiotic therapy should be reserved for patients with evidence of septic shock (e.g., hypotension or vital organ dysfunction) and patients who are immunocompromised (e.g., those who are neutropenic). The empiric antibiotic therapy of neutropenic patients is presented in Chapter 34. If life-threatening sepsis is suspected in nonimmunocompromised patients, initial therapy with vancomycin and aztreonam provides adequate coverage for most potential offenders pending culture results. Aminoglycosides have no documented benefit over other agents such as aztreonam for covering Gram-negative sepsis in the nonimmunocompromised patient. Considering the potential for nephrotoxicity with aminoglycosides, it seems wise to avoid these agents whenever possible. See Chapter 35 for more information on antimicrobial agents.

ANTIPYRETIC THERAPY

There seems to be general agreement that the inability to mount a fever has adverse consequences in serious infections (44). However, antipyretic therapy is a standard practice in many ICUs. The following are some reasons to avoid antipyretic therapy in the ICU.

Fever as a Host Defense Mechanism

High temperatures inhibit bacterial growth and viral replication. The effect of body temperature on the growth ᴏɪ bacteria in the circulating plasma is illustrated in Figure 30.5. Note that the temperatures used in this study correspond to the normal afebrile and febrile temperatures of the study animals. This clearly demonstrates the benefits of fever as a host defense mechanism. Considering that serious infections are a major source of morbidity and mortality in the ICU, preservation of the febrile response seems desirable to optimize host defenses against microbial invasion.

Cooling Blankets

The common practice of using cooling blankets to suppress fever is contrary to the physiology of fever. That is, the febrile response is an adaptive one that raises the operative range of the body temperature:

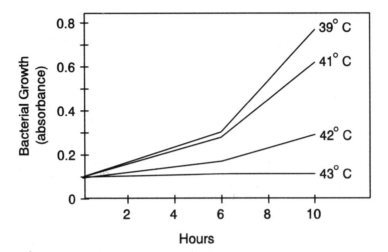

Figure 30.5. The influence of body temperature on the growth of *Pasteurella multocida* in the blood of infected laboratory animals. The temperatures correspond to the normal afebrile and febrile temperatures for the study animals (rabbits). (Data from Kluger M, Rothenburg BA. Fever and reduced iron: their interaction as a host defense response to bacterial infection. Science 1979; 203:374–376.)

The body behaves as if it were responding to a cold environment. Therefore, external cooling will *support* the febrile response, not inhibit it (44). For this reason, **cooling blankets are inappropriate for fever suppression.** External cooling is more appropriate for hyperthermia, where the ability to lower body temperature is impaired.

REFERENCES

GENERAL TEXTS

Mackowiak PA, ed. Fever: basic mechanisms and management. New York: Raven Press, 1991.

REVIEWS

1. Clarke DE, Kimelman J, Raffin TA. The evaluation of fever in the intensive care unit. Chest 1991;100:213–230 (58 references).
2. Holtzclaw BJ. The febrile response in critical care: state of the science. Heart Lung 1992;21:482–501 (71 references).
3. Arbo MJ, Fine MJ, Hanusa BH, et al. Fever of nosocomial origin: etiology, risk factors, and outcomes (32 references).

BODY TEMPERATURE

4. Stimson HF. Celsius versus centigrade: the nomenclature of the temperature scale of science. Science 1962;136:254–255.

5. Wunderlich CA, Sequine E. Medical thermometry and human temperature. New York: William Wood, 1871.
6. Mackowiak PA, Wasserman SS, Levine MM. A critical appraisal of 98.6° F, the upper limit of the normal body temperature, and other legacies of Carl Reinhold August Wunderlich. JAMA 1992;268:1578–1580.
7. Marion GS, McGann KP, Camp DL. Core body temperature in the elderly and factors which influence its measurement. Gerontology 1991;37:225–232.
8. Mellors JW, Horwitz RI, Harvey MR, et al. A simple index to identify occult bacterial infection in adults with acute unexplained fever. Arch Intern Med 1987;147:666–671.
9. Tandberg D, Sklar D. Effect of tachypnea on the estimation of body temperature by an oral thermometer. N Engl J Med 1983;308:945–946.
10. Hirschman JV. Normal body temperature. JAMA 1992;267:414.
11. The ACCP/SCCM Consensus Conference Committee. Definitions for sepsis and organ failure and guidelines for the use of innovative therapies in sepsis. Chest 1992;101:1644–1655.
12. Saper CB, Breder CB. The neurologic basis of fever. N Engl J Med 1994;330: 1880–1886.
13. Simon HB. Hyperthermia. N Engl J Med 1993;329:483–487.
14. Rangel-Frausto MS, Pittet D, Costigan M, et al. The natural history of the systemic inflammatory response syndrome (SIRS). JAMA 1995;273:117–123.

POSTOPERATIVE FEVER

15. Fry DE. Postoperative fever. In: Mackowiak PA, ed. Fever: basic mechanisms and management. New York: Raven Press, 1991;243–254.
Freischlag J, Busuttil RW. The value of postoperative fever evaluation. Surgery 1983;94:358–363.
17. Strazis KP, Fox AW. Malignant hyperthermia: a review of published cases. Anesth Analg 1993;77:297–304.
18. MacLennan DH, Phillips MS. Malignant hyperthermia. Science 1992;256: 789–794.
19. Shannon KM, Bleck TP. How to detect—and manage—catastrophic thermoregulatory disorders. J Crit Illness 1988;3:13–24.
20. Ehrenkranz NJ, Meakins JL. Surgical infections. In: Bennet JV, Brachman PS, eds. Hospital infections. 3rd ed. Boston: Little, Brown, 1992;685–710.
21. Loopp FD, Lytle BW, Cosgrove DM, et al. Sternal wound complications after isolated coronary artery bypass grafting: early and late mortality, morbidity, and cost of care. Ann Thorac Surg 1990;49:179–187.
22. Roberts J, Barnes W, Pennock M, Browne G. Diagnostic accuracy of fever as a measure of postoperative pulmonary complications. Heart Lung 1988;17: 166–169.
23. Meyers JK, Lembeck L, O'Kane H, Baue AE. Changes in functional residual capacity of the lung after operation. Arch Surg 1975;110:576–583.
24. Murray HW, Ellis GC, Blumenthal DS, et al. Fever and pulmonary thromboembolism. Am J Med 1979;67:232–235.
25. Lindblad B, Eriksson A, Bergqvist D. Autopsy-verified pulmonary embolism in a surgical department: analysis of the period from 1951 to 1988. Br J Surg 1991;78:849–852.
26. Deep vein thrombosis. Implications after open heart surgery. Chest 1991;99: 284–288.
27. Weinmann EE, Salzman EW. Deep-vein thrombosis. N Engl J Med 1994;331: 1630–1641.

28. Stilwell M, Caplan ES. The septic multiple-trauma patient. Crit Care Clin 1988; 4:345–373.

PROCEDURES

29. Pollack VE. Adverse effects and pyrogenic reactions during hemodialysis. JAMA 1988;260:2106–2107.
30. Silver MR, Balk RA. Bronchoscopic procedures in the intensive care unit. Crit Care Clin 1995;11:97–109.
31. Spach DH, Silverstein FE, Stamm WE. Transmission of infection by gastrointestinal endoscopy and bronchoscopy. Ann Intern Med 1993;118:117–128.
32. Gillis S, Dann EJ, Berkman N, et al. Fatal *Hemophilus influenzae* septicemia following bronchoscopy in a splenectomized patient. Chest 1993;104: 1607–1609.
33. Gonzalez EB, Suarez L, Magee S. Nosocomial (water bed) fever. Arch Intern Med 1990;150:687 (letter).

INFECTIONS

34. Meduri GU, Mauldin GL, Wunderink RG, et al. Causes of fever and pulmonary densities in patients with clinical manifestations of ventilator-associated pneumonia. Chest 1994;106:221–235.
35. Stamm WE. Nosocomial urinary tract infections. In: Bennet JV, Brachman PS, eds. Hospital infections. 3rd ed. Boston: Little, Brown, 1992;597–610.
36. Holzapfel L, Chevret S, Madinier G, et al. Influence of long-term oro- or nasotracheal intubation on nosocomial maxillary sinusitis and pneumonia: results of a prospective, randomized, clinical trial. Crit Care Med 1993;21:1132–1138.
37. Rouby J-J, Laurent P, Gosnach M, et al. Risk factors and clinical relevance of nosocomial maxillary sinusitis in the critically ill. Am Rev Respir Dis 1994; 150:776–783.
38. Diagnosing sinusitis by x-ray: is a single Waters view adequate? J Gen Intern Med 1992;7:481–485.
39. Walden DT, Urrutia F, Soloway RD. Acute acalculous cholecystitis. J Intensive Care Med 1994;9:235–243.
40. Kelley CP, Pothoulakis C, Lamont JT. *Clostridium difficile* colitis. N Engl J Med 1994;330:257–262.

NONINFECTIOUS SOURCES

41. Mackowiak PA, LeMaistre CF. Drug fever: a critical appraisal of conventional concepts. Ann Intern Med 1987;106:728–733.
42. Prager LM, Millham FH, Stern TA. Neuroleptic malignant syndrome: a review for intensivists. J Intensive Care Med 1994;9:227–234.

EARLY MANAGEMENT DECISIONS

43. Aronson MD, Bor DH. Blood cultures. Ann Intern Med 1987;106:246–253.
44. Styrt B, Sugarman B. Antipyresis and fever. Arch Intern Med 1990;150: 1589–1597.

31

INFECTION, INFLAMMATION, AND MULTIORGAN INJURY

Inflammation is not itself considered to be a disease but a salutary operation . . . but when it cannot accomplish that salutary purpose . . . it does mischief.

John Hunter

Becoming an astute clinician requires avoiding bad habits in clinical reasoning, and one of these bad habits is the tendency to consider signs of inflammation (e.g., fever and leukocytosis) as evidence of infection. As is emphasized repeatedly in this chapter, inflammation and infection are two distinct entities (1). Failure to recognize this distinction can result in errors in the management of two of the most lethal conditions in the ICU: septic shock and multiorgan failure. Errors in management have been identified as a significant source of mortality in multiorgan failure (30% of deaths were attributed to management errors in one report) (2), so equating inflammation and infection can be a lethal error.

THE INFLAMMATORY RESPONSE

The inflammatory response is a complex affair that is initiated by some insult to the host. This insult can be any process capable of injuring the host (e.g., microbial invasion, physical trauma, and burns). The purpose of the inflammatory response is to protect the host from the damaging effects of the insult, as illustrated in Figure 31.1. However, as pointed out by the astute surgeon, John Hunter, over 200 years ago, the inflammatory response can also injure the host. The inflammatory response generates a variety of noxious substances (e.g., proteolytic enzymes and oxygen metabolites) that can damage the tissues of the host (3). This damage is prevented by endogenous substances (e.g., antioxidants) capable of blocking or inactivating the noxious products

502

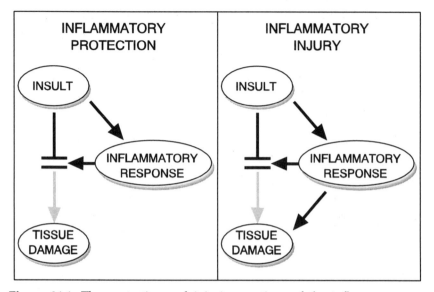

Figure 31.1. The protective and injurious actions of the inflammatory response.

of inflammation. However, when the inflammatory response overwhelms the normal protective mechanisms available to the host, the inflammatory response becomes a source of tissue damage. This is illustrated in the panel on the right in Figure 31.1. When this occurs, the inflammatory response itself becomes an insult to the host, and triggers further inflammation. This creates a chain reaction that leads to widespread and progressive inflammatory injury. The clinical expression of this widespread inflammatory injury is multiple organ dysfunction, which can progress to multiple organ failure (1,4).

CLINICAL SYNDROMES

The relationships between infection, inflammation, and organ injury just described are the basis for a new nomenclature proposed by a Consensus Conference sponsored by the American College of Chest Physicians and the Society of Critical Care Medicine (1). Signs of a systemic inflammatory response (e.g., fever and leukocytosis) are called the *systemic inflammatory response syndrome* (SIRS). When infection is the underlying cause of SIRS, the condition is called *sepsis*. When sepsis is accompanied by dysfunction in one or more vital organs, the condition is called severe sepsis. When severe sepsis is accompanied by hypotension that is refractory to volume infusion, the condition is called *septic shock*. This nomenclature can be summarized as follows:

Fever + Leukocytosis = SIRS
SIRS + Infection = Sepsis
Sepsis + Multiorgan dysfunction = Severe sepsis
Severe sepsis + Refractory hypotension = Septic shock

The major value of this nomenclature is to highlight the distinction between inflammation and infection; that is, signs of inflammation (SIRS) are not evidence of infection.

SYSTEMIC INFLAMMATORY RESPONSE SYNDROME

The diagnosis of SIRS requires the presence of two or more clinical signs of a systemic inflammatory response (1,5,6). These signs are listed in Table 31.1. Because some of the signs (e.g., tachypnea and tachycardia) are common in patients in the ICU, SIRS can be a ubiquitous condition. In one survey of 170 patients in a surgical ICU, 93% of the patients satisfied the criteria for SIRS (5). Infection is identified in only 25 to 50% of patients with SIRS (5,6). The remainder of patients have one of the noninfectious conditions in Table 31.1, and some have no identifiable source. The important message here is that the clinical signs of inflammation should not be assumed to indicate infection.

MULTIPLE ORGAN DYSFUNCTION SYNDROME

The appearance of functional abnormalities in more than one vital organ system in patients with SIRS (with or without infection) is called *multiple organ dysfunction syndrome* (MODS) (1). Several organ systems can be involved, and each is listed in Table 31.2 along with its associated clinical syndrome. The organs most often involved are the lungs, kidneys, cardiovascular system, and central nervous system. Multiorgan dysfunction can progress to multiorgan failure (7,8). The most common organ failure in this setting is the acute respiratory distress syndrome described in Chapter 25.

PATHOGENESIS

As mentioned earlier, **MODS is an inflammatory-mediated injury** that occurs when the host defenses against the inflammatory response are overwhelmed (4). **Infection is not necessary to produce the syndrome.** Activated neutrophils in the circulating blood play an impor-

TABLE 31.1. THE SYSTEMIC INFLAMMATORY RESPONSE SYNDROME	
Clinical Manifestations	**Underlying Causes**
Any two or more of the following:	Any of the following:
Body temperature >38° C or <36° C	Infection
Heart rate >90 bpm	Intestinal endotoxin
Respiratory rate >20	Ischemia
Hyperventilation ($Paco_2$ < 32 mm Hg)	Multiple trauma
WBC >12,000/mm^3 or <4,000 mm^3	Noxious substances
Immature neutrophils >10%	Pancreatitis
	Shock
	Thermal injury
From ACCP/SCCM Consensus Conference on Sepsis and Organ Failure (1).	

TABLE 31.2. MULTIPLE ORGAN DYSFUNCTION SYNDROME (MODS)	
Organ or System Involved	**Clinical Syndrome**
Lungs	Acute respiratory distress syndrome
Kidneys	Acute Tubular Necrosis
Cardiovascular system	Hyperdynamic hypotension
Central nervous system	Metabolic encephalopathy
Peripheral nervous system	Polyneuropathy of critical illness
Coagulation system	Disseminated intravascular coagulation
Gastrointestinal tract	Gastroparesis and intestinal ileus
Liver	Acute noninfectious hepatitis
Adrenal glands	Acute adrenal insufficiency
Skeletal muscle	Rhabdomyolysis
See Appendix for Multiple Organ Dysfunction Scoring System.	

tant role in the inflammatory organ injury (3,9). Specialized adhesion molecules on the surface of endothelial cells and neutrophils promote the adhesion of neutrophils to the endothelium (10). Once adherent, the activated neutrophils can then release the contents of their cytoplasmic granules (which contain proteolytic enzymes and oxygen metabolites) and damage the endothelium (11). The damaged endothelium then permits infiltration of the tissue parenchyma with plasma products and inflammatory mediators; this latter process produces the organ dysfunction. These events are an important consideration in devising strategies for the management of multiorgan failure.

MORTALITY

The **mortality** in MODS **is directly related to the number of organ systems that fail.** This relationship is demonstrated in Figure 23.5 (see Chapter 23). When four or more vital organs have failed, mortality exceeds 80% (7,8). A scoring system (the Multiple Organ Dysfunction Score) has been developed to predict the ICU mortality rate of individual patients with MODS (12) (this scoring system is presented in Appendix 3).

The relationship between organ failures and mortality is not surprising because the chances for survival should diminish as more vital organs fail. In fact, multiorgan failure can be viewed as an expression of the dying process; that is, failure of the vital organs is a necessary feature of death. This may seem a trivial point, but it emphasizes that MODS is not a primary illness but is a manifestation of some other disease process.

SEVERE SEPSIS AND SEPTIC SHOCK

As mentioned earlier, **severe sepsis and septic shock are conditions in which multiorgan dysfunction is the result of infection.** The only difference between the two conditions is the presence of volume-resistant hypotension in septic shock. In surveys of patients in the ICU with SIRS, severe sepsis and septic shock occurred in 18% and 4% of the patients, respectively (5,6). Both these conditions can be present at the initial presentation of SIRS, or can develop days after the onset of SIRS (5,6).

PATHOGENESIS

The spectrum of microorganisms involved in disseminated infections in patients in the ICU are shown in Table 31.3. The most common isolates are Gram-negative enteric pathogens (e.g., *Klebsiella-Enterobacter spp.*, *Pseudomonas aeruginosa*, and *Escherichia coli*), staphylococci (*Staphylococcus epidermidis* and *Staphylococcus aureus*), and *Enterococcus* spp. (13,14). These organisms are also the most common isolates in cases of severe sepsis and septic shock (15). Although Gram-negative septicemia is considered the most common cause of infection-induced multiorgan injury, infection with any microorganism can result in multiorgan damage.

Recent evidence indicates that **the tendency to develop severe sepsis and septic shock** is not a function of the organism involved but rather **is determined by the host response to infection** (14,16–18). That is, the more exaggerated the inflammatory response to infection, the greater the chances of developing multiorgan damage. This correlation is consistent with notion that MODS is a result of inflammatory injury to the vital organs.

HEMODYNAMIC ALTERATIONS

The initial stages of severe sepsis and septic shock are often characterized by hypovolemia (19), either relative (from venous pooling) or absolute (from transudation of fluid). This tends to produce a hypodynamic state (i.e., low cardiac output). When the intravascular volume is adequate, the cardiac output usually is elevated (19,20). However,

TABLE 31.3. NOSOCOMIAL SEPTICEMIA IN CRITICALLY ILL PATIENTS

Organism	Total Isolates (%)	Most Common Source
Gram negative enteric pathogens	38	Pneumonia
Coagulase negative staphylococci	18	Vascular catheters
Staphylococcus aureus	11	Pneumonia
Enterococci	10	Pneumonia
Streptococci	7	Unknown
Anerobic organisms	5	Pneumonia
Candida spp.	5	Vascular catheters
Other	6	Multiple sources

Data from Pittet D et al. (13).

intrinsic cardiac function (systolic and diastolic) is impaired in sepsis (20) and the increase in cardiac output is the result of tachycardia rather than an increase in stroke output. Despite the increase in cardiac output, peripheral blood can be diminished, as demonstrated in Figure 31.2 (21). In fact, contrary to the popular notion that sepsis is a hyperdynamic circulatory condition (i.e., increased blood flow and vasodilation), the hemodynamic changes in advanced stages of sepsis more closely resemble a hypodynamic state (i.e., reduced blood flow and vasoconstriction).

Oxygen Transport

Severe sepsis and septic shock are characterized by **a defect in the peripheral extraction of oxygen** (22). Thus, as peripheral blood flow is reduced, the normal ability to increase peripheral oxygen extraction is impaired, and this results in a decreased oxygen uptake (Vo_2) from the microcirculation. This defect is believed to be the principal cause of impaired tissue oxygenation in septic shock. Hyperlactatemia is a characteristic finding in severe sepsis and septic shock, but this may be the result of impaired pyruvate metabolism (23), not tissue dysoxia (i.e., oxygen-limited energy production). The etiology of sepsis-induced hyperlactatemia is described in Chapter 13 (see Fig. 13.5).

HEMODYNAMIC MANAGEMENT

In light of the tendency for relative and absolute hypovolemia in sepsis, the mainstay of early hemodynamic management is aggressive **volume infusion** (19,24). Because sepsis is often accompanied by hypoalbuminemia (25), initial resuscitation with colloid fluids may be

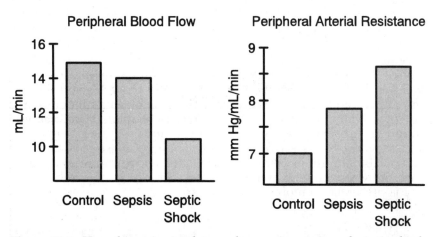

Figure 31.2. Hypodynamic circulatory changes in sepsis and septic shock. (Data from Astiz ME et al. Peripheral vascular tone in sepsis. Chest 1991;99: 1072–1075.)

preferred. The end-point of volume infusion is a right-atrial (central venous) pressure of 8 to 10 mm Hg or a pulmonary capillary wedge pressure of 18 to 20 mm Hg (see Chapter 11).

If hypotension persists despite high-normal cardiac filling pressures, **dopamine** is the hemodynamic drug most often used to raise the blood pressure. The infusion is started at 5 μg/kg/minute and titrated upward (see Chapter 18). However, dopamine can actually impair tissue oxygenation in regional beds such as the splanchnic circulation (26), so gastric intramucosal pH should be monitored (if possible) during dopamine infusions (see Chapter 13 for more information on gastric mucosal pH monitoring).

Oxygen Transport

As in any case of shock, the goal of hemodynamic management should be a normal whole-body oxygen uptake (i.e., V_{O_2} above 100 mL/min/m^2). However, because sepsis is characterized by hypermetabolism and a heightened metabolic oxygen requirement, some have recommended achieving a supranormal level of systemic oxygen delivery (D_{O_2} above 600 mL/min/m^2 V_{O_2} above 170 mL/min/ m^2) in patients with septic shock. Following adequate volume resuscitation, dobutamine is started at 5 μg/kg/minute and titrated upward to achieve the desired end-point. Some studies suggest an improved outcome with this strategy (28), but others do not (29). Furthermore, it is impossible to achieve supranormal levels of systemic oxygen transport in 40 to 50% of patients (28,29), regardless of the dobutamine infusion rate. Therefore, the practice of striving for supranormal levels of systemic oxygen transport is not advised as a general strategy. However, if signs of continuing and progressive organ injury are present at normal levels of D_{O_2} and V_{O_2}, attempts to increase the D_{O_2} and V_{O_2} to supranormal levels with volume infusion and dobutamine are justified.

EMPIRIC ANTIMICROBIAL THERAPY

When sepsis is suspected but not yet documented, empiric antimicrobial therapy should be directed at the common organisms listed in Table 31.3. A combination of **vancomycin** (covers staphylococci, enterococci, and streptococci) **plus aztreonam or an aminoglycoside** (to cover Gram-negative enteric organisms) should suffice, pending culture results. When sepsis of intestinal origin is suspected, coverage for *Bacteroides fragilis* is advised. This can be accomplished by the addition of clindamycin or metronidazole to the above antimicrobial regimen, or by monotherapy with imipenem. Empiric antimicrobial therapy is presented in more detail in Chapter 35.

STEROIDS

In the 1960s, high-dose intravenous steroids emerged as a popular therapy for septic shock. However, steroids have not proven beneficial and may be harmful in patients with severe sepsis and septic shock (30–32). As a result, the Infectious Disease Society of America advises that **steroids should be avoided** in patients with disseminated sepsis and septic shock (33).

NOVEL THERAPIES

Neither hemodynamic nor antimicrobial therapy has had a tremendous impact on reducing the mortality in severe sepsis and septic shock (15,17,28–30). With this in mind and considering that inflammatory tissue injury plays an important role in the pathogenesis of septic shock, newer therapeutic strategies have been directed at the inflammatory response. The following two approaches have received the most attention.

ANTI-INFLAMMATORY ANTIBODIES

Fueled by dreams of a multibillion-dollar industry, drug manufacturers have undertaken enormous (and expensive) efforts to manufacture and use antibodies against various inflammatory mediators in patients with severe sepsis and septic shock. Most of the antibodies have been directed against endotoxin, tumor necrosis factor, or interleukin-1 (17,34–37) because these substances are believed to play an important role in the hemodynamic alterations in sepsis.

Clinical Experience

Large clinical trials have failed to document improved outcomes in patients with severe sepsis and septic shock who were treated with antibodies against endotoxin (35), tumor necrosis factor (36), or interleukin-1 (37). In light of these results and the enormous expense of antibody therapy, little enthusiasm exists for this approach to sepsis at present.

Theoretical Problems

There are two problems with the antibody approach to inflammatory organ injury. First, more than 30 cytokines are involved in the inflammatory response (34), and creating antibodies for many (or all) of these substances is clearly not feasible. Second, as demonstrated in Figure 31.3, inhibiting the inflammatory response can promote tissue injury from infection. The consequences of an inhibited immune response are readily demonstrated in patients who receive chemotherapy. For these two reasons, the future of immunotherapy for inflammatory organ injury is bleak.

ANTIOXIDANT THERAPY

Toxic oxygen metabolites play an important role in the inflammatory response (9,11,38) and may also play an important role in inflam-

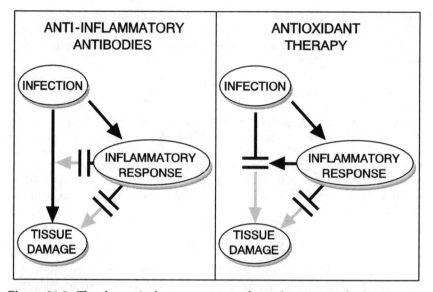

Figure 31.3. The theoretical consequences of novel strategies for limiting inflammatory organ injury. Note that anti-inflammatory (antibody) therapy can be associated with tissue injury, whereas antioxidant therapy is not.

matory-mediated tissue injury (39,40). This latter possibility has led to the consideration of antioxidant therapy as a means of limiting inflammatory organ injury (41,42). In fact, as illustrated in Figure 31.3, antioxidant therapy has an theoretical advantage over anti-inflammatory therapy because antioxidants do not inhibit the inflammatory response, but merely protect the host from it. Another advantage of antioxidant therapy derives from the tendency of oxidation reactions to produce a chain reaction (see Chapter 3), thus creating a self-sustaining source of pathologic tissue injury.

Clinical Experience

Unlike antibody-directed therapy, the clinical experience with antioxidants is extremely limited. Intravenous N-acetylcysteine has shown promising results in improving outcome in acute respiratory distress syndrome (43), but confirmatory studies are needed. Given the theoretical advantages of antioxidants, this should be a fecund area of clinical investigation.

TOXIC SHOCK SYNDROME

Toxic shock syndrome (TSS) is a type of multiorgan dysfunction syndrome caused by colonization or infection with a toxigenic strain of *S. aureus* (43). The responsible organism typically inhabits mucocutaneous regions (such as nasal passages and the vagina), and it releases an exotoxin that is absorbed into the systemic circulation and produces SIRS and MODS. More than 80% of cases of TSS involve tampon use in menstruating females (the tampon may disrupt the vaginal mucosa). Other predisposing conditions are childbirth, pelvic infections, sinusitis, and influenza. Although mucocutaneous colonization or infection predominates, any staphylococcal infection can produce TSS if the strain is toxigenic. In this context, the role of influenza as a predisposing condition for TSS can be explained by the increased risk of staphylococcal pneumonia following influenza (45).

CLINICAL PRESENTATION

The initial presentation of TSS is nonspecific, with fever, headache, and diarrhea predominating. This is followed within 24 to 48 hours by rapid progression to multiorgan dysfunction, often accompanied by a rash (43). The early rash is a **diffuse erythematous rash** that blanches on pressure. Another desquamative rash involving the palms and soles can appear 1 to 2 weeks later, in the convalescent phase of the illness (44). The diagnosis of TSS is based on the clinical presentation and on isolation of a toxigenic strain of *S. aureus* from suspected mucocutaneous regions. Blood cultures are usually sterile.

MANAGEMENT

The management of TSS is very similar to that for septic shock (i.e., volume infusion followed by dopamine for persistent hypotension). Antibiotic therapy has little impact on the acute illness (because disseminated infection is uncommon), but it reduces the recurrence of TSS that can occur in one-third of menstruating patients (44). Vancomycin, nafcillin, or first-generation cephalosporins (e.g., cephalothin) are all effective. In menstruating patients, immediate tampon removal is mandatory. Vaginal douches to clear local toxin are of unproven value. With appropriate management, the mortality in TSS is less than 5% (44).

ANAPHYLAXIS

Anaphylaxis is a form of inflammatory-mediated organ dysfunction that is produced by an abnormal inflammatory response to chemical agents. Common offenders are antimicrobial agents, anesthetics, radiocontrast dyes, nutrients, and insect venoms (46). Radiocontrast dyes are the most common source of serious anaphylactic reactions, with an incidence of 1 in 1000 to 14,000 injections (47). About 10% of these reactions are fatal (47).

CLINICAL PRESENTATION

Anaphylactic reactions vary in presentation and severity. Clinical manifestations appear within minutes to a few hours after exposure to the offending agent. In general, the more severe the reaction, the more rapid the onset of clinical manifestations. Less serious reactions include flushing, erythematous rashes, urticaria, abdominal cramping, and diarrhea. More severe reactions include angioedema, laryngeal edema, bronchospasm, and hypotension. The most life-threatening reaction is a rapid-onset cardiovascular collapse known as *anaphylactic shock*.

MANAGEMENT

The management of anaphylaxis is dictated by the clinical presentation (Table 31.4). For severe reactions, **prompt intervention is the key to a successful outcome.** The following are the common treatment modalities for anaphylaxis.

TABLE 31.4. MANAGEMENT OF ANAPHYLACTIC REACTIONS		
Reaction	**Intervention**	**Regimens**
Uticaria	Histamine H_1 blocker	Diphenhydramine: 50 mg orally every 6 hr
Angioedema	Histamine H_1 blocker	Diphenhydramine: 50 mg intramuscularly or orally every 6 hr
	Sub Q epinephrine	0.3–0.5 mL of a 1:1000 solution (1 mg/mL)
Bronchospasm	Bronchodilators	Inhaled albuterol: 2.5 mL of 0.5% solution IV aminophylline: 5–6 mg/kg load, then 0.2–0.9 mg/kg/hr.
	Sub Q epinephrine	As above
Laryngeal stridor	Aerosolized epinephrine	0.25 mL of 1% solution (10 mg/mL) added to 2 mL isotonic saline
	Intubation	Translaryngeal or cricothyroidotomy
Hypotension	Volume resuscitation	Colloids (5% albumin, 6% hetastarch) may be preferred for initial resuscitation
	IV epinephrine	3–5 mL of 1:10,000 solution (0.1 mg/mL)
Persistent hypotension	Pressor agents	Epinephrine (2–8 μg/min) or Dopamine (5–15 μg/min) or Norepinephrine (2–8 μg/min)
	IV steroids	Hydrocortisone: 100–200 mg intravenously every 4 hr

Histamine blockers have a limited value in the management of anaphylaxis, even though histamine release is believed to play a major role in the pathogenesis of anaphylaxis. Histamine H_1 blockers (such as diphenhydramine) can be used to alleviate the pruritus associated with cutaneous reactions. Histamine H_2 blockers (such as cimetidine) provide no benefit over the H_1 blockers.

Epinephrine is the drug of choice for severe anaphylactic reactions and is capable of blocking inflammatory mediator release from sensitized cells. It is given subcutaneously for most reactions, but can be aerosolized for laryngeal edema or given intravenously for anaphylactic shock (see Table 31.4 for the doses of epinephrine) (48).

Volume infusion is important in hypotension because in disseminated anaphylaxis, fluid loss from the vascular space is rapid and profound. This is one setting where **colloid fluids are preferred to crystalloid fluids** for volume expansion.

Aminophylline is reserved for patients with persistent bronchospasm after epinephrine is administered. This drug may aggravate arrhythmias when given with epinephrine and should be used with caution.

Steroids are used for persistent hypotension, despite little evidence of benefit. Hydrocortisone is favored because of its mineralocorticoid effects, although there is no proven superiority over methylprednisolone.

REFERENCES

CONSENSUS CONFERENCE

1. American College of Chest Physicians/Society of Critical Care Medicine Consensus Conference Committee. Definitions of sepsis and organ failure and guidelines for the use of innovative therapies in sepsis. Chest 1992;101: 1644–1655.

THE SYSTEMIC INFLAMMATORY RESPONSE

2. Pellicane JV, Byrne K, DeMaria EJ. Preventable complications and death from multiple organ failure among geriatric trauma victims. J Trauma 1992;33: 440–444.
3. Fujishima S, Aikawa N. Neutrophil-mediated tissue injury and its modulation. Intensive Care Med 1995;21:277–285.
4. Pinsky MR, Matuschak GM. Multiple systems organ failure: failure of host defense mechanisms. Crit Care Clin 1989;5:199–220.
5. Pittet D, Rangel-Frausto S, Li N, et al. Systemic inflammatory response syndrome, sepsis, severe sepsis, and septic shock: incidence, morbidities and outcomes in surgical ICU patients. Intensive Care Med 1995;21:302–309.
6. Rangel-Frausto MS, Pittet D, Costigan M, et al. Natural history of the systemic inflammatory response syndrome (SIRS). JAMA 1995;273:117–123.

MULTIPLE ORGAN DYSFUNCTION SYNDROME

7. Deitch EA. Multiple organ failure: pathophysiology and potential future therapy. Ann Surg 1992;216:117–133.

8. Beal AL, Cerra FB. Multiple organ failure in the 1990s. Systemic inflammatory response and organ dysfunction. JAMA 1994;271:226–233.

9. Windsor ACJ, Mullen PG, Fowler AA, Sugerman HJ. Role of the neutrophil in the adult respiratory distress syndrome. Br J Surg 1993;80:10–17.

10. Donnelly SC, Haslett C, Dransfield I, et al. Role of selectins in the development of the adult respiratory distress syndrome. Lancet 1994;344:215–219.

11. Rivkind AI, Siegel JH, Littleton M, et al. Neutrophil oxidative burst activation and the pattern of respiratory physiologic abnormalities in the fulminant post-traumatic adult respiratory distress syndrome. Circ Shock 1991;33:48–62.

12. Marshall JC, Cook DJ, Christou NV, et al. Multiple Organ Dysfunction Score: a reliable descriptor of a complex clinical outcome. Crit Care Med 1995;23: 1638–1652.

SEVERE SEPSIS AND SEPTIC SHOCK

13. Pittet D, Tarara D, Wenzel RP. Nosocomial bloodstream infection in critically ill patients. JAMA 1994;271:1598–1601.

14. Dunn DL. Gram-negative bacterial sepsis and sepsis syndrome. Surg Clin North Am 1994;74:621–635.

15. Brun-Buisson C, Doyon F, Carlet J, et al. Incidence, risk factors, and outcome of severe sepsis and septic shock in adults. JAMA 1995;274:968–974.

16. Guillou PJ. Biological variation in the development of sepsis after surgery or trauma. Lancet 1993;342:217–220.

17. Natanson C, Hoffman WD, Suffredini AF, Eichacker PO. Selected treatment strategies for septic shock based on proposed mechanisms of pathogenesis. Ann Intern Med 1994;120:771–783.

18. Parillo JE. Pathogenetic mechanisms of septic shock. N Engl J Med 1993;328: 1471–1477.

19. Rackow EC, Astiz ME. Mechanisms and management of septic shock. Crit Care Clin 1993;9:219–228.

20. Snell RJ, Parillo JE. Cardiovascular dysfunction in septic shock. Chest 1991; 99:1000–1009.

21. Astiz ME, Tilly E, Rackow ED, Weil MH. Peripheral vascular tone in sepsis. Chest 1991;99:1072–1075.

22. Vincent J-L, van der Linden P. Septic shock: particular type of acute circulatory failure. Crit Care Med 1990;18(Suppl):S70–S74.

23. Curtis SE, Cain SM. Regional and systemic oxygen delivery/uptake relations and lactate flux in hyperdynamic, endotoxin-treated dogs. Am Rev Respir Dis 1992;145:348–354.

24. Carcillo JA, Davis AL, Zaritsky A. Role of early fluid resuscitation in pediatric septic shock. JAMA 1991;266:1242–1245.

25. Marik PE. The treatment of hypoalbuminemia in the critically ill patient. Heart Lung 1993;22:166–170.

26. Marik PE, Mohedin M. The contrasting effects of dopamine and norepineph-rine on systemic and splanchnic oxygen utilization in hyperdynamic sepsis. JAMA 1994;272:1354–1357.

27. Yu M, Levy M, Smith P, et al. Effect of maximizing oxygen delivery on morbid-ity and mortality rates in critically ill patients: a prospective, randomized, controlled study. Crit Care Med 1993;21:830–838.

28. Hayes MA, Timmins AC, Yau EHS, et al. Elevation of systemic oxygen delivery in the treatment of critically ill patients. N Engl J Med 1994;330:1717–1722.

29. Gattinoni L, Brazzi L, Pelosi P, et al. A trial of goal-oriented hemodynamic therapy in critically ill patients. N Engl J Med 1995;333:1025–1032.

30. Natanson C, Danner RL, Reilly JM, et al. Antibiotics versus cardiovascular

support in a canine model of human septic shock. Am J Physiol 1990;259: H1440–H1447.

31. Bone RC, Fisher CJ, Clemmer TP. A controlled clinical trial of high-dose methylprednisolone in the treatment of severe sepsis and septic shock. N Engl J Med 1987;317:653–658.

32. VA Systemic Sepsis Cooperative Study Group. Effect of high-dose glucocorticoid therapy on mortality in patients with clinical signs of systemic sepsis. N Engl J Med 1987;317:659–665.

33. McGowan JR Jr, Chesney PJ, Crossley KB, LaForce FM. Guidelines for the use of systemic glucocorticosteroids in the management of selected infections. J Infect Dis 1992;165:1–13.

NOVEL THERAPIES

34. Dinarello CA, Gelfand JA, Wolff SM. Anticytokine strategies in the treatment of the systemic inflammatory response syndrome. JAMA 1993;269:1828–2835.

35. McCloskey RV, Straube RC, Sanders C, et al. Treatment of septic shock with human monoclonal antibody HA-1A. Ann Intern Med 1994;121:1–5.

36. Abraham E, Wunderink R, Silverman H, et al. Efficacy and safety of monoclonal antibody to human tumor necrosis factor alpha in patients with sepsis syndrome. JAMA 1995;273:934–941.

37. Fisher CJ, Dhainaut J-F, Opal SM, et al. Recombinant human interleukin 1 receptor antagonist in the treatment of patients with sepsis syndrome. JAMA 1994;271:1836–1843.

38. Hurst JK, Barrette WC Jr. Leukocyte oxygen activation and microbicidal oxidative toxins. Crit Rev Biochem Molec Biol 1989;24:271–328.

39. Ward PA. Mechanisms of endothelial cell injury. J Lab Clin Med 1991;118: 421–426.

40. Cochrane CG. Cellular injury by oxidants. Am J Med 1991;91(Suppl 3C): 23S–30S.

41. Said SI, Foda HD. Pharmacologic modulation of lung injury. Am Rev Respir Dis 1989;139:1553–1564.

42. Henderson A, Hayes P. Acetylcysteine as a cytoprotective antioxidant in patients with severe sepsis: potential new use for an old drug. Ann Pharmacother 1994;28:1086–1088.

43. Suter PM, Domenighetti G, Schaller MD, et al. N-acetylcysteine enhances recovery from acute lung injury in man: a randomized, double-blind, placebo-controlled clinical study. Chest 1994;105:190–194.

TOXIC SHOCK

44. Ciesielski CA, Broome CV. Toxic shock syndrome: still in the differential. J Crit Illness 1986;1:26–40.

45. Conway EE, Haber RS, Gumprecht J, Singer LP. Toxic shock syndrome following influenza A in a child. Crit Care Med 1991;19:123–125.

ANAPHYLAXIS

46. Hollingsworth HM, Giansiracusa DF, Upchurch KS. Anaphylaxis. J Intensive Care Med 1991;6:55–70.

47. Crnkovich DJ, Carlson RW. Anaphylaxis: an organized approach to management and prevention. J Crit Illness 1993;8:332–246.

48. Fisher M. Treating anaphylaxis with sympathomimetic drugs. Br Med J 1992; 305:1107–1108.

chapter

32

NOSOCOMIAL PNEUMONIA

Everything hinges on the matter of evidence.
Carl Sagan

If nosocomial (hospital-acquired) pneumonia had to be characterized in one word, an appropriate term would be *problematic*. The major
problems in nosocomial pneumonia are determining when it is present
and identifying the responsible pathogen (1–3). For example, although
fever and new pulmonary infiltrates are considered evidence of pneumonia, 50 to 60% of patients with these clinical manifestations do not
have an identifiable lung infection (4,5). As a result of the problem in
identifying pneumonia, the literature on the prevalence, causes, and
consequences of nosocomial pneumonia is confusing. This chapter
summarizes the current knowledge on nosocomial pneumonias in im-
munocompetent patients, with emphasis on the ventilator-dependent
patient in the ICU. The focus here is on the diagnostic methods that
optimize the ability to recognize a parenchymal lung infection and
identify the responsible pathogen. The approach to nosocomial pneumonias in immunocompromised patients is described in Chapter 34.

PATHOGENESIS

Unlike community-acquired pneumonias, in which gram-positive
cocci such as *Streptococcus pneumoniae* are the most common offenders,
the most common isolates in nosocomial pneumonias are gram-negative enteric pathogens. The pathogens responsible for nosocomial
pneumonia in ward patients and ventilator-dependent patients are

TABLE 32.1. MICROBIAL ISOLATES IN NOSOCOMIAL PNEUMONIAS		
Pathogens	Ward Patients (%)	Ventilator Patients (%)
Aerobic gram—negative bacilli	46	83
Pseudomonas sp.	9	30
Acinetobacter sp.	—	19
Escherichia coli	14	8
Klebsiella sp.	14	6
Proteus sp.	11	11
Others	3	4
Streptococcus pneumoniae	31	14
Staphylococcus aureus	26	27
Hemophilus influenza	17	9
Anaerobic orgaisms	35	2
Yeasts and fungi	—	4

All isolates are from blood cultures, empyema fluid, or lower respiratory tract specimens. Adapted from Estes RJ, Meduri GU. Intensive Care Med 1995; 21:365–383.

listed in Table 32.1, along with the frequency that each pathogen is isolated (3). Note that only organisms isolated from blood cultures, empyema fluid, or lower respiratory tract specimens are included in the table.

Nosocomial pneumonias are often polymicrobial, so the percentages listed in the table exceed 100%. In ventilator-dependent patients, the most common isolates are gram-negative enteric pathogens (particularly *Pseudomonas* species) and *Staphylococcus aureus*. As described below, the microbial spectrum in nosocomial pneumonias is a reflection of a change in the resident microflora in the oropharynx.

COLONIZATION OF THE OROPHARYNX

The aspiration of mouth secretions into the upper airways is the inciting event in most cases of pneumonia. **An average of 1 billion bacteria are found in each milliliter of saliva** (6), so aspiration of even *micro*liters of saliva will introduce large numbers of bacteria into the airways. In healthy adults, the resident microflora of the oropharynx is mostly made up of commensal organisms such as anaerobic bacteria and α-hemolytic streptococci. However in hospitalized patients, the oropharynx is often colonized with (aerobic) gram-negative enteric pathogens (3). The prevalence of this colonization in community-based and hospital-based subjects is shown in Figure 32.1. Note that the principal determinant of colonization is the presence and severity of illness and that the environment (i.e., community versus hospital) has no effect. This change in the resident microflora of the oropharynx explains the prevalence of gram-negative pathogens in nosocomial pneumonia.

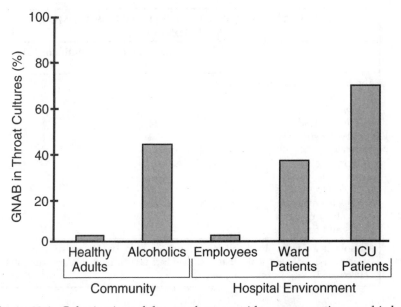

Figure 32.1. Colonization of the oropharynx with gram-negative aerobic bacilli (*GNAB*) in different groups of subjects. (Data from Johanson WG et al.
Changing pharyngeal bacterial flora of hospitalized patients. N Engl J Med
1969;281:1137–1140.)

Bacterial Adherence

The illness-induced change in the microflora of the mouth is due to
a change in the ability of gram-negative organisms to adhere to the
oral mucosa. In healthy volunteers, a substance called fibronectin coats
the epithelial cells in the mouth and prevents gram-negative pathogens
from adhering to the cells. This protective coating is lost in severe
illness, and this allows gram-negative pathogens to bind to the epithelial cells in the oropharynx. This colonization is the basis for the application of antimicrobial paste to the oral mucosa as a method of prophylaxis for nosocomial pneumonia.

GASTRIC COLONIZATION

As described in Chapter 6, the acid pH in the stomach has a bactericidal effect on microorganisms that are swallowed with food or saliva
(see Fig. 6.2), and this action helps maintain a sterile environment in
the upper gastrointestinal tract. When gastric acidity is suppressed
(with antacids, histamine H_2 blockers, hydrogen ion pump inhibitors,
or enteral tube feedings), the bacteria that are swallowed can thrive
and colonize the gastric contents and this provides a reservoir for
bacteria to seed the lungs via regurgitation or translocation (3,7). As
a result, patients who receive gastric acid suppression therapy for prophylaxis of stress ulcer bleeding have an increased risk of nosocomial

pneumonia (8). On the other hand, stress ulcer prophylaxis with sucralfate, which does not decrease gastric pH in most patients, carries a lower risk of nosocomial pneumonia (9). For more information on the risks of gastric acid suppression, see Chapter 6.

CLINICAL PRESENTATION

The clinical manifestations of pneumonia (i.e., fever, new pulmonary infiltrates, tachypnea, and dyspnea) are nonspecific. The Centers for Disease Control and Prevention (CDC) has proposed the following criteria for identifying pneumonia in adults (10).

CDC Criteria for Pneumonia

According to the CDC, a pneumonia is present when the chest x-ray film shows a new or progressive infiltrate, cavitation, or a pleural effusion *and* any of the following occur:

1. A change occurs in character of the sputum.
2. A pathogen is isolated from blood cultures, lung biopsy, or specimens obtained from the distal airways (i.e., bronchial washings or brushings).
3. A virus or viral antigen is isolated in respiratory secretions.
4. There is a diagnostic serum antibody titer (IgM) or a fourfold rise in antibody titers (IgG) in paired serum samples.
5. Histologic evidence of pneumonia exists.

Note that **these criteria do not include sputum gram stains or sputum cultures,** despite the fact that sputum analysis is common in the evaluation of pneumonia.

THE CHEST RADIOGRAPH

Sensitivity

According to the CDC criteria for pneumonia, the presence of a new infiltrate on chest radiograph has a sensitivity of 100% (i.e., always present). However, this is an assumption, and an unlikely one at that. For example, pulmonary edema is not evident on a chest radiograph until extravascular lung water has increased 30 to 50% (11), and this insensitivity is likely to apply to inflammatory infiltration of the lungs as well. The sensitivity of the chest radiograph for parenchymal infiltrates may be further reduced by hyperinflation during mechanical ventilation. Therefore, in the evaluation of nosocomial fever, a clear or unchanged chest radiograph should not be taken as absolute evidence against pneumonia (at least in the early stages of the investigation). If the cause of the fever is not evident on initial evaluation, serial chest films are advised.

Specificity

As mentioned in the introductory paragraph, patients with fever and new pulmonary infiltrates often have no microbial evidence of pneumonia (4,5). In most clinical studies, the presence of new infiltrates on chest radiograph has a specificity of 40 to 60% for the presence of pneumonia (4,5). This means that in 40 to 60% of patients with fever, new pulmonary infiltrates are caused by a process other than a lung infection. The low specificity of the chest radiograph is illustrated by the case shown in Figure 32.2. This chest film was obtained from an elderly patient who presented to the emergency department with fever, obtundation, and acute respiratory failure. No evidence of a lung infection existed in cultures obtained from the lower respiratory

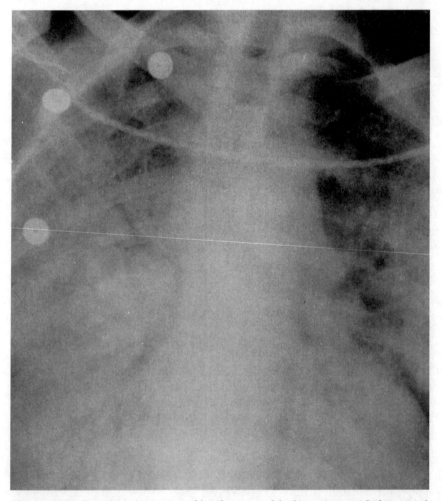

Figure 32.2. Portable chest x-ray film from an elderly patient with fever and acute respiratory failure.

tract (by bronchoscopy). However, the urine culture grew greater than 100,000 colonies of *Escherichia coli,* and the same organism was isolated from blood cultures. Therefore, the chest radiograph in this case represents acute respiratory distress syndrome (ARDS) secondary to urosepsis with gram-negative septicemia.

In some cases, the pattern of lung infiltration can be helpful in identifying a lung infection. For example, the presence of cavitary lesions with air-fluid levels is highly suggestive of a necrotizing lung infection. Another example of a diagnostic pattern on chest x-ray film is shown in Figure 32.3. The chest film in this case shows peripheral infiltrates with a rounded density in the right lower lung field. This pattern is suggestive of septic pulmonary emboli, and subsequent evaluation in this patient revealed evidence of tricuspid valve endocarditis.

In summary, the presence of an infiltrate on chest radiograph should not be regarded as definitive proof of a lung infection, but should prompt further studies aimed at documenting infection and identifying the responsible pathogen.

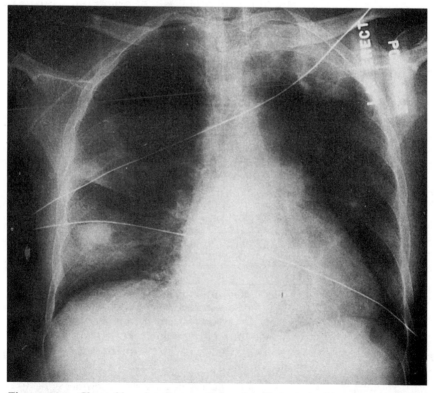

Figure 32.3. Chest film showing peripheral infiltrates and a circular area of dense consolidation in the right lower lung field. The presumptive diagnosis in this case was septic pulmonary emboli, and echocardiography subsequently showed vegetations on the tricuspid valve.

DIAGNOSTIC EVALUATION

The diagnostic evaluation of suspected pneumonia should include cultures of blood, pleural effusions, and specimens obtained from the lower respiratory tract.

EXPECTORATED OR ASPIRATED SECRETIONS

The importance of avoiding bad habits in clinical practice was mentioned in the introduction to Chapter 31. The worst habit to avoid in the evaluation of suspected pneumonia is the practice of **obtaining cultures on nonselected samples of expectorated sputum or tracheal aspirates.** This practice **yields erroneous information in 40 to 60% of cases** (12,13). In other words, the chances of obtaining accurate diagnostic information from (expectorated or aspirated) respiratory secretions is equivalent to the chances of predicting heads or tails on a coin toss. To improve on this bad habit, the specimens must first be screened microscopically to identify their site or origin (i.e., proximal versus distal airways). Some criteria for identifying the origin of respiratory secretions are shown in Table 32.2 (14–17).

Squamous Epithelial Cells

The epithelial cells that line the oral cavity are large, flattened cells with abundant cytoplasm and a small nucleus. The morphologic appearance of these cells is shown in Figure 32.4. The presence of **more than 25 squamous epithelial cells per low-power field (× 100) indicates that the specimen is contaminated with mouth secretions** (15). If evidence of contamination with mouth secretions exists, the specimen should not be submitted for culture.

TABLE 32.2. SPUTUM MORPHOLOGY IN THE EVALUATION OF PNEUMONIA	
Component	**Interpretation**
Squamous epithelial cells	More than 25 epithelial cells per low-power field indicates contamination with mouth secretions.
Macrophages	The presence or one or more macrophage on any power magnification indicates a lower airway specimen.
Elastin fibers	The presence of elastin fibers on a 40% KOH preparation indicates a necrotizing pneumonia.
Neutrophils	More than 25 neutrophils per low-power field indicates infection (tracheobronchitis or pneumonia).
From References 14–17.	

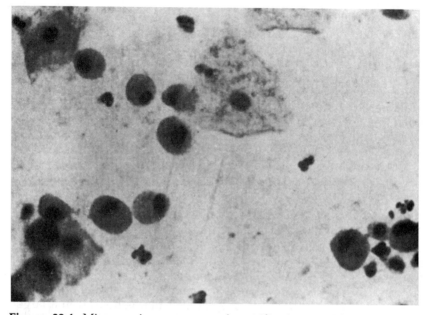

Figure 32.4. Microscopic appearance (magnification ×400) of bronchial brushings from a ventilator-dependent patient. The large, flattened cells are squamous epithelial cells. The oval cells with eccentric nuclei are macrophages. The smallest cells are neutrophils.

Lung Macrophages

Lung macrophages are large, oval-shaped cells with a granular cytoplasm and a small, eccentric nucleus (Fig. 32.4). The size of the nucleus in a macrophage is roughly the same size as a neutrophil. Although macrophages can inhabit the airways (16), the predominant home of the lung macrophage is the distal airspaces. Therefore, **the presence of macrophages indicates that the specimen is from the lower respiratory tract.** As such, a sputum sample or tracheal aspirate that contains even one macrophage can be considered suitable for culture.

Elastin Fibers

In necrotizing lung infections, elastin fibers from the lung parenchyma can be recovered in expectorated or aspirated airway secretions. These elastin fibers are filamentous strands that can be visualized by placing a drop of 40% potassium hydroxide on a sputum smear and placing a cover slip over the smear (17). When low-power magnification is used, elastin fibers are seen as clumps of interlacing filaments. The presence of these elastin strands indicates not only that the specimen is from the distal airspaces, but also that ongoing lung necrosis is present.

Neutrophils

Abundant neutrophils in expectorated or aspirated lung secretions indicate probable infection, but they do not localize the site of the infection (i.e., tracheobronchitis versus pneumonia). The term *abundant* deserves emphasis here because neutrophils can make up 20% of the cells recovered from a routine mouthwash (16). **More than 25 neutrophils per low-power field (× 100) can be used as evidence of infection** (14). However, this is not to be taken as evidence of pneumonia. To mark the location of an infection, the criteria listed in Table 32.2 must be used.

PROTECTED SPECIMEN BRUSHING (PSB)

Bronchoscopic aspirates and brushings tend to produce false-positive cultures because the channel through which the specimens are obtained often picks up contaminants as the bronchoscope is passed through the upper respiratory tract (18). To eliminate the problem of contamination, a specialized brush device similar to the one shown in Figure 32.5 has been developed for collecting specimens from the lower airways. The brush sits in a catheter that is housed in a larger outer cannula that is plugged at the distal end. When the entire device is advanced through the bronchoscope, the seal on the outer catheter protects the brush from contamination with upper airways secretions. When the device is passed out of the bronchoscope and into the lower airways, the inner catheter is advanced until it knocks off the distal occluding plug of the outer catheter (this plug is made of gelatin or some other dissolvable material). The brush is then advanced farther into the lower airways to collect the specimen. After the brushing is

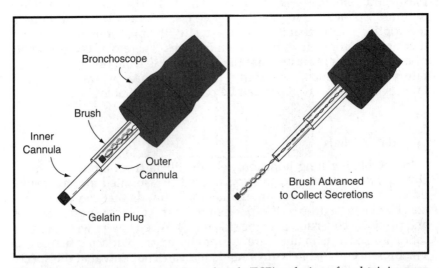

Figure 32.5. The protected specimen brush (PSB) technique for obtaining uncontaminated lower airways secretions.

obtained, the brush is retracted into the inner cannula, the inner cannula is retracted into the outer cannula, and the entire device is retracted through the bronchoscope.

Processing the Specimen

Once the device is withdrawn from the bronchoscope, the brush is placed in 1 mL of transport medium. The 1-mL mixture of diluent and brush specimen is then cultured *quantitatively*, and growth of 10^3 colonies (per mL) or higher is used as a positive culture result (3,19,20). This threshold corresponds to a bacterial density of 10^5 to 10^6 colonies per mL in undiluted secretions (3). The relevant volumes and bacterial counts for PSB cultures are shown in Table 32.2.

Diagnostic Value

The diagnostic yield from quantitative PSB cultures is strongly influenced by the presence of ongoing antibiotic therapy (3,19,20). This is illustrated in Figure 32.6 (20). In this study, the incidence of false-

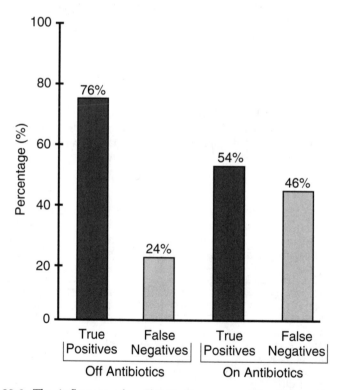

Figure 32.6. The influence of antibiotic therapy on the diagnostic yield of protected specimen brush cultures. All cultures are quantitative, with a threshold of 10^3 cfu/mL for a positive result. (From Meduri GU, Chastre J. The standardization of bronchoscopic techniques for ventilator-associated pneumonia. Chest 1993;102(Suppl):557S–564S.)

negative PSB cultures increased from 24 to 46% when the PSB was obtained during ongoing antibiotic therapy. Because of the increased incidence of false-negative PSB cultures during antibiotic therapy, **the PSB technique is not recommended for patients receiving antibiotic therapy.** Therefore, in cases of suspected pneumonia, PSB cultures should be obtained before empiric antimicrobial therapy is instituted.

BRONCHOALVEOLAR LAVAGE

Bronchoalveolar lavage (BAL) is performed by wedging the bronchoscope in a distal airway and lavaging the wedged lung segment with isotonic saline. A specialized dual catheter device with a plugged tip (similar in design to the catheter in Figure 32.5) is also available. When this catheter is used, the technique is called *protected BAL* (3). A minimum lavage volume of 120 mL is recommended for adequate sampling of the lavaged lung segment (20), but smaller volumes are also used (when lavage volumes of 10 to 20 mL are used, the technique is called mini-BAL). Only 25% or less of the volume instilled will be returned via aspiration, which is then submitted for quantitative culture, as is done for PSB specimens. However for BAL, the threshold for a positive culture is 10^4 colonies per mL (3). The BAL threshold is 10 times higher than the PSB threshold, but both thresholds correspond to the same bacterial count in undiluted secretions (Table 32.3).

Diagnostic Value

The sensitivity and specificity of BAL cultures ranges from 70 to 100% (3). Similar to PSB cultures, the diagnostic yield from BAL cultures is markedly reduced by ongoing antibiotic therapy (21). Therefore like PSB, BAL is not recommended as a high yield procedure in patients receiving antibiotic therapy.

PARAPNEUMONIC EFFUSIONS

Pleural effusions are present in up to 50% of bacterial pneumonias (22), and these *parapneumonic* effusions should be evaluated when possible. If the effusion is loculated (i.e., it does not move with change in body position), bedside ultrasound can be used to mark the location

TABLE 32.3. QUANTITATIVE CULTURES OR PROTECTED SPECIMEN BRUSHINGS (PSB) AND BRONCHOALVEOLAR LAVAGE (BAL)		
	PSB	**BAL**
Volume of secretions	0.01–0.001 mL	≥ 1 mL
Volume of diluent	1 mL	10–100 mL
Threshold for a positive culture result	10^3 colonies/mL	10^4 colonies/mL
Corresponding concentration in secretions	10^5–10^6 colonies/mL	10^5–10^6 colonies/mL

Adapted from Griffin JJ, Meduri GU. New approaches to the diagnosis of nosocomial pneumonia. Med Clin North Am 1994;78:1091–1122.

TABLE 32.4. MANAGEMENT OF PARAPNEUMONIC EFFUSIONS		
	Immediate Draininage?	
Clinical Finding	Yes	No
Air–fluid level	X	
Hydropneumothorax	X	
Grossly purulent fluid	X	
Pleural fluid pH:		
<7.0	X	
>7.2		X
Pleural fluid glucose:		
<40 mg/dL	X	
>40 mg/mL		X

and depth of the fluid. In addition to Gram's stain and culture, the pleural fluid glucose concentration and pH should be measured. Classification of the fluid as a transudate or exudate (by pleural fluid protein and LDH levels) is unnecessary because this does not reliably identify infected versus sterile effusions.

Indications for Drainage

The indications for immediate drainage of parapneumonic effusions are listed in Table 32.4. The radiographic criteria for drainage include the presence of an air–fluid level in the effusion, or a hydropneumothorax (both are signs of a bronchopleural fistula). Chemical criteria for drainage include a pleural fluid glucose concentration below 40 g/dL (2.4 μmol/L) or a pleural fluid pH below 7.0 (22). If a patient with a parapneumonic effusion improves clinically on antibiotics, there is little need for further evaluation or drainage of the effusion.

ANTIMICROBIAL THERAPY

EARLY ANTIBIOTIC THERAPY

Early antibiotic therapy is guided by microscopic inspection of lower respiratory tract secretions and parapneumonic effusions. Some initial antibiotic regimens based on the results of the Gram's stain are shown in Table 32.5. These regimens are meant for the initial 24 to 48 hours of therapy, pending culture results.

Gram-Negative Bacilli

When gram-negative bacilli are the sole or predominant organisms, the likely pathogens are the enteric pathogens listed in Table 32.1. The principal concern is to provide adequate coverage for *Pseudomonas* species. Combination antibiotic therapy has been shown to reduce mortality compared with monotherapy in patients with bacteremic *Pseudomonas* pneumonias (23), and thus combination therapy is advo-

---

TABLE 32.5. EARLY ANTIMICROBIAL THERAPY OF NOSOCOMIAL PNEUMONIA IN NONIMMUNOCOMPROMISED PATIENTS

Gram's Stain[a]	Antibiotic Regimen[b]	Comments
Gram-Negative Bacilli:		
Single Morphology	Aminglycoside plus an antipseudomonal penicillin or ceftazidime	Provides double coverage for *Pseudomonas* sp.
Multiple Morphologies	Aminglycoside plus cefuroxime or TMP–SMZ[3]	Multiple morphologies may indicate *Mycoplasma pneumoniae.*
Gram-Positive Cocci	Vancomycin	Covers all possible gram-positive pathogens, including methicillin-resistant staphylococci and penicillin-resistant streptococci.
Mixed Flora	Imipenem	Mixed flora may indicate anaerobic or polymicrobial aerobic pathogens.

[a] Pertains to secretions from the lower respiratory tract or parapneumonic effusions.
[b] See Chapter 35 for antibiotic dose recommendations.
[c] TMP–SMZ = trimethoprim–sulfamethoxazole.

cated for suspected *Pseudomonas* pneumonias. Suitable regimens include an aminoglycoside plus an antipseudomonal penicillin (carbenicillin or ticarcillin) or ceftazidime.

When gram-negative bacilli show multiple morphologies, the organisms may represent *Hemophilus influenza*. Because of the rising incidence of ampicillin-resistant *H. influenza* isolates, early coverage for this organism is best achieved with trimethoprim–sulfamethoxazole or cefuroxime (24).

Gram-Positive Cocci

When gram-positive cocci are the predominant organism of Gram's stain, the most likely pathogens are *Streptococcus* and *Staphylococcus* species. Vancomycin is the favored agent in this situation, particularly if there is a risk of methicillin-resistant staphylococci or penicillin-resistant streptococci (25). Although vancomycin-resistant enterococci are becoming more prevalent (see Chapter 35), enterococci are not common offenders in nosocomial pneumonia (3).

Mixed Flora

The presence of mixed flora, with no one predominant organism, is characteristic of anaerobic infections, but might also represent a polymicrobial aerobic infection. In both situations, monotherapy with imipenem will cover most of the potential offenders (the exceptions being methicillin-resistant staphylococci and some strains of *Pseudomonas* species). Combination therapy with aztreonam or an aminoglycoside (for Enterobacteriaceae) plus metronidazole or clindamycin (for anaerobic coverage) also provides adequate broad-spectrum coverage. Anaerobic organisms will *not* grow on routine cultures of respiratory secretions, so a sterile culture report does not eliminate the possibility of an anaerobic infection.

ANTIBIOTIC PROPHYLAXIS

A seemingly effective yet neglected approach to nosocomial pneumonia involves the topical application of an antimicrobial paste to the oral mucosa to prevent colonization of the oropharynx with pathogenic organisms (26). The preparation most often used is a methylcellulose paste (Orabase, Squibb Pharmaceuticals) containing 2% polymyxin, 2% tobramycin, and 2% amphotericin B, which is applied to the inside of the mouth with a gloved finger every 6 hours (26,27). This measure is part of a larger approach to preventing nosocomial infections known as *selective digestive decontamination* (SDD) (27), which is described at the end of Chapter 6.

The effects of SDD on the incidence of nosocomial pneumonia are shown in Figure 6.3. Considering these results, it seems that this approach to nosocomial pneumonia deserves much more attention that it currently receives.

REFERENCES

CONSENSUS CONFERENCE

1. Meduri GU, Johanson WG, eds. International Consensus Conference: Clinical investigation of ventilator-associated pneumonia. Chest 1992;102(Suppl 1): 551S–588S.

REVIEWS

2. Griffin JG, Meduri GU. New approaches in the diagnosis of nosocomial pneumonia. Surg Clin North Am 1994;78:1091–1122 (141 references).
3. Estes RJ, Meduri GU. The pathogenesis of ventilator-associated pneumonia: I. Mechanisms of bacterial transcolonization and airway inoculation. Intensive Care Med 1995;21:365–383 (93 references).

PATHOGENESIS

4. Meduri GU, Mauldin GL, Wunderink RG, et al. Causes of fever and pulmonary densities in patients with clinical manifestations of ventilator-associated pneumonia. Chest 1994;106:221–235.
5. Bates JH, Campbell D, Barron AL, et al. Microbial etiology of acute pneumonia in hospitalized patients. Chest 1992;101:1005–1012.
6. Higuchi JH, Johanson WG. Colonization and bronchopulmonary infection. Clin Chest Med 1982;3:133–142.

7. Fiddian-Green RG, Baker S. Nosocomial pneumonia in the critically ill: product of aspiration or translocation? Crit Care Med 1991;19:763–769.
8. Cook DJ, Reeve BK, Guyatt GH. Stress ulcer prophylaxis in critically ill patients. JAMA 1996;275:308–314.
9. Driks MR, Craven DE, Celli BR, et al. Nosocomial pneumonia in intubated patients given sucralfate as compared with antacids or histamine type-2 blockers. N Engl J Med 1987;317:1376–1382.

CLINICAL PRESENTATION

10. Garner JS, Jarvis WR, Emori TG, et al. CDC definitions for nosocomial infections, 1988. Am J Infect Control 1988;16:128–140.
11. Pistolesi M, Miniati M, Milne ENC, Giuntini C. Measurement of extravascular lung water. Intensive Care World 1991;8:16–21.

DIAGNOSTIC EVALUATION

12. Berger R, Arango L. Etiologic diagnosis of bacterial nosocomial pneumonia in seriously ill patients. Crit Care Med 1985;13:833–836.
13. Fine M, Orloff J, Rihs JD, et al. Evaluation of housestaff physicians' preparation and interpretation of sputum gram stains for community acquired pneumonia. J Gen Intern Med 1991;6:189–198.
14. Wong LK, Barry AL, Horgan S. Comparison of six different criteria for judging the acceptability of sputum specimens. J Clin Microbiol 1982;16:627–631.
15. Washington JA. Techniques for noninvasive diagnosis of respiratory tract infections. J Crit Illness 1996;11:55–62.
16. Rankin JA, Marcy T, Rochester CL, et al. Human airway macrophages. Am Rev Respir Dis 1992;145:928–933.
17. Salata RA, Lederman MM, Shlaes DM. Diagnosis of nosocomial pneumonia in intubated intensive care unit patients. Am Rev Respir Dis 1987;135:426–432.
18. Ovassapian A, Randel GI. The role of the fiberscope in the critically ill patient. Crit Care Clin 1995;11:29–52.
19. Allen RM, Dunn WF, Limper AH. Diagnosing ventilator-associated pneumonia: the role of bronchoscopy. Mayo Clin Proc 1994;69:962–968.
20. Meduri GU, Chastre J. The standardization of bronchoscopic techniques for ventilator-associated pneumonia. Chest 1992;102(Suppl):557S–564S.
21. Cantral DE, Tape TG, Reed EC, et al. Quantitative culture of bronchoalveolar lavage fluid for the diagnosis of bacterial pneumonia. Am J Med 1993;95:601–607.
22. Light RW, Meyer RD, Sahn SA, et al. Parapneumonic effusions and empyema. Clin Chest Med 1985;6:55–62.

ANTIMICROBIAL THERAPY

23. Hilf M, Yu VL, Sharp J, et al. Antibiotic therapy for *Pseudomonas aeruginosa* bacteremia: outcome correlations in a prospective study of 200 patients. Am J Med 1989;87:540–546.
24. Doern GV. Trends in antimicrobial susceptibility of bacterial pathogens of the respiratory tract. Am J Med 1995;99(Suppl 6B):3–7.
25. Wilhelm MP. Vancomycin. Mayo Clin Proc 1991;66:1165–1170.
26. Rodriguez-Roldan JM, Altuna-Cuesta A, Lopez A, et al. Prevention of nosocomial lung infection in ventilated patients: use of an antimicrobial pharyngeal nonabsorbable paste. Crit Care Med 1990;18:1239–1242.
27. Heyland DK, Cook DJ, Jaeschke R, et al. Selective digestive decontamination: an overview. Chest 1994;105:1221–1229.

c h a p t e r

SEPSIS FROM THE ABDOMEN AND PELVIS

One of the recurring themes in this book is the importance of the gastrointestinal (GI) tract as a source of infection in critically ill patients. This chapter again returns to that theme and describes the infectious risks at both ends of the GI tract, including the neighboring biliary tree. The last section of this chapter describes nosocomial infections in the urinary tract, with emphasis on infections associated with indwelling urethral catheters.

ACALCULOUS CHOLECYSTITIS

Acalculous cholecystitis is a condition that could be described as an ileus of the gallbladder. Although an uncommon condition, it can be fatal if not recognized and treated promptly (1).

PATHOGENESIS

There are a number of conditions that predispose to acalculous cholecystitis, as shown in Table 33.1 (1–3). Most cases occur in association with multiple trauma and abdominal (nonbiliary) surgery. A number of mechanisms may be involved in the pathogenesis of acalculous cholecystitis, including ischemia (e.g., multiple trauma, shock), stasis (e.g., parenteral nutrition), and reflux of pancreatic secretions (e.g., opioid analgesics). In patients with human immunodeficiency virus (HIV) infection, acalculous cholecystitis is most often due to opportunistic infections with cytomegalovirus and *Cryptosporidium* (3).

CLINICAL FEATURES

The clinical manifestations of acalculous cholecystitis include fever, nausea and vomiting, abdominal pain, and right upper quadrant ten-

TABLE 33.1 ACUTE ACALCULOUS CHOLECYSTITIS	
Predisposing Conditions:	
Burns	Opioid analgesia
HIV infection	Parenteral nutrition
Major surgery	Shock
Multiple trauma	
Clinical Presentation:	
Fever (70–95%)	Abdominal pain (60–90%)
Vomiting (35–65%)	RUQ tenderness (60–100%)
Diagnosis:	
Ultrasound: Gallbladder sludge and distension (hydrops)	
Gallbladder wall thickness >3.5 mm	
Subserosal edema (halo sign)	
From References 1–3.	

derness (Table 33.1). Abdominal findings can be minimal or absent, and fever may be the only presenting manifestation. Elevations in serum bilirubin, alkaline phosphatase, and amylase can occur but are variable (1,2).

Diagnosis

An ultrasound of the right upper quadrant often provides diagnostic information. Gallbladder sludge and distension of the gallbladder are common findings but can be nonspecific. More specific findings include a gallbladder wall thickness of at least 3.5 mm and submucosal edema (1,2). If ultrasound visualization is hampered, computed tomography (CT) scanning can provide useful information (1).

Management

Prompt intervention is necessary to prevent progressive distension and **rupture of the gallbladder.** The latter complication **has been reported in 40% of cases when diagnosis and treatment is delayed for 48 hours** or longer after the onset of symptoms (1). The treatment of choice is cholecystectomy. In patients who are too moribund for surgery, percutaneous cholecystostomy is a suitable alternative. Empiric antibiotic therapy should be started when the diagnosis is first confirmed. The combination of vancomycin and imipenem is suitable and covers all intestinal pathogens.

GASTRIC COLONIZATION

The GI tract can become a source of sepsis when overgrowth of pathogenic organisms is present in the bowel lumen. This occurs in the upper GI tract in patients receiving gastric acid suppression therapy and in the lower GI tract in patients receiving antimicrobial therapy (see C. *difficile* colitis later in this chapter).

PATHOGENESIS

Gastric acid suppression and subsequent colonization of the upper GI tract is discussed in Chapter 6. The pathogens that most commonly colonize the stomach are the same pathogens most commonly involved in nosocomial infections (4). This correlation is shown in Figure 33.1. Although it does not prove a causal relationship between gastric colonization and nosocomial infections, it does show that the upper GI tract serves as a reservoir for pathogens that are commonly involved in nosocomial sepsis.

PREVENTIVE MEASURES

The measures aimed at preventing colonization of the upper GI tract are described in Chapter 6. Two basic approaches exist. The first is to avoid the use of agents that suppress gastric acidity (i.e., antacids, histamine H_2 antagonists, and hydrogen ion pump inhibitors). Prophylaxis for stress ulcer bleeding can be accomplished with sucralfate, a cytoprotective agent that does not increase the pH of gastric secre-

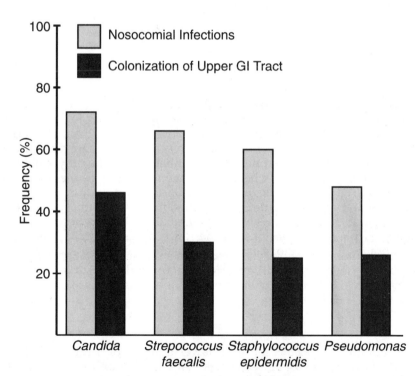

Figure 33.1. The most commonly isolated pathogens in nosocomial infections and colonization of the upper GI tract in patients in the ICU. (Data from Marshall JC, Christou NV, Meakins JL, et al. The gastrointestinal tract: the "undrained abscess" of multiple organ failure. Ann Surg 1993;218:111–119.)

tions. The second measure aimed at preventing colonization of the GI tract is selective digestive decontamination (SDD) with nonabsorbable antibiotics (see Chapter 6 for the antibiotic regimen used in SDD). The success of SDD in reducing the incidence of nosocomial infections is shown in Figure 6.3. Not only do these results demonstrate the efficacy of SDD, but they also provide evidence that the GI tract is indeed an important source of nosocomial sepsis.

Translocation

Another factor that can promote sepsis of GI origin is the tendency for disruption of the bowel mucosa in critically ill patients. This impairs the normal barrier function of the bowel wall, and allows enteric pathogens to gain access to the systemic circulation (see Chapter 6). Two conditions can predispose to microbial translocation across the bowel mucosa: mesenteric hypoperfusion and prolonged bowel rest. Therefore, avoiding these two conditions will help limit the risk of sepsis from the GI tract. Although it is not always possible to avoid mesenteric hypoperfusion, the use of gastric intramucosal pH monitoring (described in Chapter 13) will help maintain mesenteric perfusion in patients with clinical shock. Avoiding prolonged bowel rest to maintain the functional integrity of the GI mucosa is discussed in Chapter 47.

CLOSTRIDIUM DIFFICILE COLITIS

Colonization with pathogenic organisms can also occur in the lower regions of the GI tract. The most troublesome intruder is *Clostridium difficile,* a spore-forming gram-positive anaerobic bacillus that is now the most common cause of nosocomial infections involving the GI tract (5). Although not a prominent bowel inhabitant in healthy subjects, this organism flourishes when the normal microflora of the lower GI tract is altered by antibiotic therapy. *C. difficile* is not an invasive organism, but it elaborates enterotoxins that incite inflammation in the bowel mucosa. Severe cases of mucosal inflammation are accompanied by raised plaque-like lesions on the mucosal surface called pseudomembranes. These lesions are responsible for the term *pseudomembranous colitis,* which is used to describe advanced cases of *C. difficile* enterocolitis.

EPIDEMIOLOGY

Although *C. difficile* is found in fewer than 5% of healthy adults in the community, it can be seen in as many as 40% of hospitalized patients (6). More than half of the patients who harbor *C. difficile* in their stool are asymptomatic (7,8). The organism is found primarily in patients receiving ongoing or recent (within 2 weeks) antibiotic therapy and in patients who are in close proximity to other patients who harbor the organism. C. *difficile* is readily transmitted from patient to patient by contact with contaminated objects (e.g., toilet facilities) and by the hands of hospital personnel (7). Strict adherence to the use of disposable gloves can significantly reduce the nosocomial transmission of C. *difficile* (9).

CLINICAL MANIFESTATIONS

The most common manifestations of symptomatic C. *difficile* infection are fever, abdominal pain, and watery diarrhea. Bloody diarrhea is seen in 5 to 10% of cases (5). Rarely, the enterocolitis can progress to toxic megacolon, which presents with abdominal distension, ileus, and clinical shock. This latter complication can be fatal and requires emergent subtotal colectomy (10).

DIAGNOSTIC TESTS

The diagnosis of C. *difficile* colitis is often based on the results of the laboratory tests listed in Table 33.2. The organism can be cultured from fresh stool samples. However, because growth often requires 48 hours or longer to become evident, cultures do not provide immediate diagnostic information. Rapid confirmation of the presence of C. *difficile* in the stool is possible with a latex agglutination test (11). This test uses latex particles coated with an antibody to C. *difficile* antigens, and when mixed with a stool sample, produces visible clumping when C. *difficile* is present. The most popular diagnostic test is a tissue culture assay for a cytotoxin that is elaborated by C. *difficile*.

The sensitivity and specificity of these laboratory tests are shown in Table 33.2. As is evident, **no single laboratory test is sufficient to confirm or exclude the diagnosis of** C. *difficile* **colitis** (12). Because nontoxigenic strains of **C. *difficile*** can be isolated in the stool of asymptomatic patients (3,6), tests that document the presence of C. *difficile* in stool (i.e., stool culture or latex agglutination test) lack specificity. Furthermore, as many as 30% of patients with presumed C. *difficile* colitis (positive cultures and pseudomembranes) can have a negative cytotoxin assay on a single stool specimen (13,14), so the cytotoxin

TABLE 33.2 LABORATORY TESTS FOR *C. DIFFICILE* ENTEROCOLITIS			
Test	Time to Complete	Sensitivity* (%)	Specificity* (%)
Stool culture	2–7 days	>90	≤80
Latex agglutination test for C. *difficile* antigens	30 minutes	≥70	≤80
Tissue culture assay for C. *difficile* cytotoxin	2–4 days	≥70	≥85
* From references 5–8 and 11–15.			

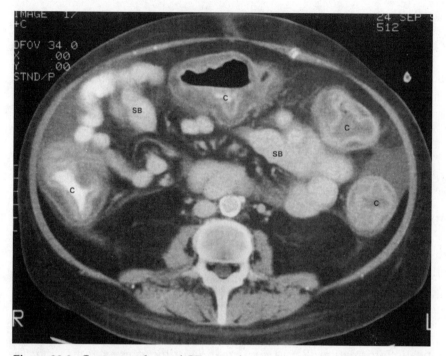

Figure 33.2. Contrast-enhanced CT scan of a patient with *C. difficile* enterocolitis. Note the marked thickening of the wall of the colon (*C*), but not the small bowel (*SB*). The edema fluid produces a low-density stripe between the more radiopaque mucosa and serosa, creating a *target sign*. (From Braley SE et al. Overview of diagnostic imaging in sepsis. New Horiz 1993;1:214–230.)

assay lacks sensitivity. Performing serial stool cytotoxin assays is recommended to improve the sensitivity of the *C. difficile* cytotoxin assay (14). Another approach to optimizing the diagnostic accuracy for *C. difficile* colitis is to combine tests to document both the organism and the cytotoxin in stool (15).

Computed Tomography

When laboratory tests are equivocal or unavailable, CT scanning can provide valuable diagnostic information (16). The characteristic CT findings in *C. difficile* colitis are shown in Figure 33.2. There is marked thickening in the wall of the colon, and the edema fluid in the bowel wall produces a low density stripe between the mucosa and serosa, creating a *target sign*. These signs are highly suggestive of an active inflammatory enterocolitis.

Lower GI Endoscopy

Direct visualization of the lower GI mucosa is a valuable but underused diagnostic test for *C. difficile* colitis. The presence of pseudomembranes on the mucosal surface confirms the diagnosis of C. *difficile* colitis. Colonoscopy is preferred to proctosigmoidoscopy for optimal results.

TREATMENT

The standard treatment for C. *difficile* enterocolitis is to administer antibiotics to eradicate the organism from the stool. The recommended antibiotic regimens are shown below.

1. **Oral vancomycin** (250 to 500 mg every 6 hours for at least 7 days) is the traditional treatment of choice (but may no longer be, as described below). Vancomycin is not absorbed across the bowel mucosa, and thus the drug reaches high levels in the stool. Intravenous vancomycin is ineffective. Despite almost complete eradication of the organism within 1 week of therapy, relapses occur within the first month after therapy in 20% of cases (17).
2. **Oral or intravenous metronidazole** (500 mg every 6 hours for at least 7 days) is as effective as oral vancomycin for eradicating the organism. **Oral metronidazole** has traditionally been considered an alternative to oral vancomycin but **is becoming the preferred therapy to limit the emergence of vancomycin-resistant *enterococci*.** Intravenous metronidazole is reserved for patients who cannot tolerate oral medications.

Although rarely necessary, surgical intervention is required when C. *difficile* colitis is associated with progressive sepsis and multiorgan failure, or signs of peritonitis, despite antibiotic therapy (10). The procedure of choice is subtotal colectomy.

Preventive Therapy

The best method for preventing C. *difficile* colitis is to limit the use of antibiotics, particularly clindamycin (18). Another preventive measure is the oral ingestion of the yeast *Saccharomyces boulardii* (which is normally found on lychee fruits). This organism produces a protease that destroys the receptor site for the C. difficile enterotoxin, and thus colonization of the lower GI tract with this organism can prevent the inflammatory response to toxigenic strains of C. *difficile*. One gram of a lyophilized yeast preparation given orally each day can produce a 50% decrease in the incidence of antibiotic-associated diarrhea (19). Despite its efficacy, this approach has not gained popularity in the United States.

ABDOMINAL ABSCESSES

Abdominal abscesses most often occur as complications of blunt abdominal trauma or abdominal surgery (20,21).

TABLE 33.3. ROUTINE CLINICAL EVALUATION IN 143 PATIENTS WITH INTRA-ABDOMINAL ABSCESSES	
Clinical Finding	Frequency (%)
Physical Examination:	
Localized abdominal tenderness	36
Palpable abdominal mass	7
Chest Films:	
Pleural effusion	33
Basilar atelectasis	12
Abdominal Films:	
Extraluminal air or air–fluid level	13
Mechanical bowel obstruction	4

From Fry D. Noninvasive imaging tests in the diagnosis and treatment of intra-abdominal abscesses in the postoperative patient. Surg Clin North Am 1994; 74:693–709.

CLINICAL FEATURES

Abdominal abscesses are difficult to detect on routine clinical evaluation, and they often present with fever of unclear etiology. The low yield of the routine clinical evaluation is demonstrated in Table 33.3. In this series of 143 patients with abdominal abscesses, localized abdominal tenderness was present in only one-third of cases and a palpable abdominal mass was present in fewer than 10% of cases (21). Although abdominal films taken with the patient in the supine, upright, and lateral decubitus positions are obtained routinely, they provide little useful information.

CT scanning of the abdomen is the single most valuable diagnostic test for suspected intra-abdominal abscess. Sensitivity and specificity for detection of abscesses is 90% or higher (20,21). CT scanning in the early postoperative period can result in false-positive scans because of collections of blood or irrigant solutions in the peritoneal cavity from the operative procedure. For optimal results, CT scanning should be performed after the first postoperative week (when peritoneal fluid collections have resorbed) (21).

MANAGEMENT

Immediate drainage is mandatory for all intra-abdominal abscesses (22). Precise localization with CT scanning allows many abscesses to be drained percutaneously with radiographically directed drainage catheters. Empiric antibiotic therapy should be started while awaiting the culture results from the abscess fluid. Single-drug therapy has been shown to be as effective as multiple drug regimens (23). Popular agents for monotherapy include ampicillin–sulbactam (Unasyn), cefoxitin, and imipenem (23).

UROSEPSIS

Urinary tract infection (UTI) accounts for 30% of all nosocomial infections (24). The single most important predisposing factor is urethral catheterization. Because most patients in the ICU have indwelling urethral catheters, the following description is limited to UTIs in the catheterized patient.

PATHOGENESIS

The presence of an indwelling urethral catheter creates a 4 to 7% risk of developing a UTI *per day* (25). Bacterial migration along the catheter is the presumed mechanism for the link between catheters and UTIs; however, there is more to the puzzle. The remaining question is why bacteria that migrate up the urethra and into the bladder are not washed out of the bladder by the urine flow. The flushing action of urine is a defense mechanism that protects the bladder from retrograde invasion by skin pathogens. This protective action explains why direct injection of bacteria into the bladder will not produce a UTI in a healthy subject (26).

Bacterial Adherence

The missing piece in the UTI puzzle is the adherence of bacteria to the bladder epithelium (27). The epithelial cells of the bladder normally are coated with *Lactobacillus* organisms, as shown in Figure 33.3. These organisms are neither invasive nor virulent, and thus by covering the surface of the bladder epithelium, they prevent more invasive and virulent organisms from attaching to the bladder wall and establishing residence in the bladder. Loss of this protective coating and adherence or urinary pathogens to the bladder mucosa is the final prelude to colonization and infection in the lower urinary tract (27). However, the events that link urethral catheterization to bacterial adherence in the bladder are unknown.

MICROBIOLOGY

The common pathogens responsible for nosocomial UTIs in the United States are listed in Table 33.4. Two surveys from the National Nosocomial Infections Surveillance System are included; one is from the early 1980s (28), and the other is from the early 1990s (29). Note the similarities between the two surveys, indicating that the spectrum of pathogens in nosocomial UTI changed little over the decade separating the two surveys. The predominant pathogens are enteric gram-negative aerobic bacilli, and the most common offender is *Escherichia coli*. Most community-acquired UTIs involve a single pathogen, whereas nosocomial, catheter-associated UTIs can be polymicrobial (particularly with chronic indwelling catheters) (24). Polymicrobial

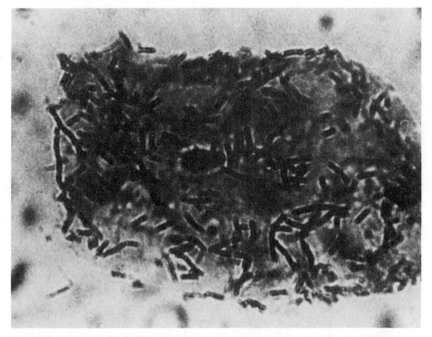

Figure 33.3. Photomicrograph showing *Lactobacillus* organisms blanketing a bladder epithelial cell. (From Sobel JD. Pathogenesis of urinary tract infections: host defenses. Infect Dis Clin North Am 1987;1:751–772.)

growth from urine in the absence of an indwelling urethral catheter is most likely a contaminated specimen.

CLINICAL PRESENTATION

Asymptomatic bacteriuria is not considered an infection in catheterized patients (24), and thus the presence of clinical manifestations is

TABLE 33.4. MICROBIAL ISOLATES IN NOSOCOMIAL UTI		
	Relative Frequency	
Microorganism	1983* (%)	1990–1992† (%)
Escherichia coli	31	25
Enterococcus spp.	15	16
Pseudomonas aeruginosa	13	11
Klebsiella pneumoniae	8	7
Proteus mirabilis	7	5
Candida albicans	5	8
Staphylococcus epidermidis	4	4
Staphylococcus aureus	2	2
* Data from Reference 28. † Data from Reference 29.		

the hallmark of UTI. However, the clinical manifestations are few in number. Fever and leukocytosis (i.e., signs of a systemic inflammatory response) may be the only manifestations of UTI in catheterized patients (the indwelling catheters eliminate complaints of urgency, frequency, and dysuria). Approximately 50% of elderly patients will also develop a change in mental status in association with UTIs (30). Severe cases of urosepsis can be accompanied by multiorgan dysfunction progressing to multiorgan failure (31).

DIAGNOSIS

The diagnosis of UTI is not always straightforward in catheterized patients, particularly in patients with prolonged catheterization (i.e., longer than 4 weeks). Prolonged catheterization is often associated with pyuria and bacteriuria as a baseline condition, and this complicates the use of urine cultures and urine microscopy to identify infection. In this setting, serial changes in the urine are more reliable than evaluation of an isolated urine sample.

Urine Microscopy

Urine microscopy has limited value in the catheterized patient. The usual criteria for pyuria (greater than 10 leukocytes per high-power field) and bacteriuria (2 or more organisms per oil-immersion field) in a spun urine sediment are intended for the evaluation of suspected UTI in outpatients (32), not catheterized patients. As mentioned previously, catheterized patients can have microscopic criteria for a UTI chronically, and thus the criteria have little meaning in these patients. One potential value of urine microscopy is the ability to identify certain microbes on Gram's stain (e.g., gram-positive cocci versus gram-negative rods), which can be used to select early antimicrobial therapy.

Urine Cultures

Urine cultures can also be misleading. The traditional threshold for significant bacteriuria in catheterized patients is 10^5 colony-forming units per mL (cfu/mL). However, colony counts above this threshold can represent colonization, and colony counts as low as 100 cfu/mL can represent infection (24). Microbial growth in a single urine specimen may not be as important as the pattern of growth in serial specimens. However, the time required for the results of serial cultures to become available is too long for the information to be useful in making acute management decisions for suspected urosepsis. In fact, even a single urine culture is of little help in making acute management decisions for the patient with suspected sepsis.

EARLY ANTIBIOTIC THERAPY

Early antibiotic therapy is recommended for patients with suspected UTI who are immunocompromised, have evidence of multiorgan dysfunction, or have a prosthetic or damaged heart valve. As mentioned earlier, the urine Gram's stain can be helpful in selecting the appropriate antibiotic. The following are some suggestions (see also Table 35.1).

Gram-Negative Bacilli

If gram-negative bacilli are the predominant organisms on urine Gram's stain, early antibiotic therapy should include one of the following: a third-generation cephalosporin (e.g., ceftriaxone or ceftazidime), an aminoglycoside (amikacin, gentamicin, or tobramycin), aztreonam, or imipenem. Trimethoprim–sulfamethoxazole is an effective agent for community-based UTIs but is not favored in nosocomial UTIs because of emerging resistance in *E. coli* and *Klebsiella* species (33).

Gram-Positive Cocci

A preponderance of gram-positive cocci on the urine Gram's stain suggests that *enterococcus* is the responsible pathogen (staphylococci are uncommon offenders in nosocomial UTIs). If the patient is not seriously ill, enterococcal UTI can be treated effectively with ciprofloxacin. If the patient is seriously ill or has a prosthetic or damaged heart valve, ampicillin or vancomycin plus gentamicin is the preferred regimen. Ampicillin resistance is reported in 10 to 15% of nosocomial enterococcal infections (34), so vancomycin may be preferred for combination therapy.

CANDIDURIA

The presence of *Candida* in the urine can represent colonization, infection in the urinary tract, or disseminated candidiasis with renal involvement (35,36). Most cases represent colonization of the lower urinary tract, which is a common consequence of antibiotic therapy and prolonged urethral catheterization. Colonization is distinguished from infection by the presence or absence of fever, leukocytosis, and other signs of sepsis. Urine colony counts are unreliable as a discriminatory test.

Local Therapy

Colonization of the urinary tract with *Candida* is not a precursor to disseminated candidiasis, and thus therapy to eradicate the organism is unnecessary. However, when evidence of *Candida* cystitis (i.e., fever, lower abdominal tenderness) exists, bladder irrigation with amphotericin is indicated to eradicate the organism from the urinary tract (35). Amphotericin bladder irrigation is also used in patients who have urine cultures showing 100,000 cfu/mL, although the value of this practice is unproven. Because indwelling urethral catheters prevent retention of the drug solution in the bladder, a continuous infusion technique is used for bladder irrigation. The regimen is as follows:

Continuous bladder irrigation: Add 50 mg amphotericin to 1 L of sterile water (*not* saline) and infuse the solution at 40 mL/ hour using a three-way bladder catheter. Continue the irrigation for 3 to 4 days.

This regimen is effective in eradicating the organism in most cases, unless the candiduria is secondary to disseminated candidiasis. Amphotericin is not absorbed across the bladder mucosa, so there is no risk of systemic toxicity. Once therapy is completed, the urethral catheter should be removed if possible to prevent recurrent colonization.

Disseminated Candidiasis

Although *candida* does not usually disseminate from the urinary tract, disseminated candidiasis can seed the kidneys and produce secondary candiduria. Disseminated candidiasis should be considered when candiduria is associated with signs of progressive sepsis, multiorgan dysfunction, or clinical shock. The diagnosis can be elusive because **blood cultures are sterile in more than 50% of cases** of disseminated candidiasis (36). *Candida* infiltration of the retina can produce an endophthalmitis, and the lesions in this condition can be pathognomonic for disseminated candidiasis (36). Therefore, a funduscopic examination (by an ophthalmologist) is mandatory when disseminated candidiasis is suspected. If this is unrevealing, evidence of *Candida* at multiple sites should be looked for. Isolation of the organism from three separate sites (e.g., urine, sputum, and vascular catheter) can be used as presumptive evidence of disseminated candidiasis (36).

When disseminated candidiasis is suspected, empiric therapy can begin with intravenous fluconazole (400 mg/day). This antifungal agent may be as effective as amphotericin for treating disseminated *Candida* infections (at least in nonneutropenic patients), while being much less toxic than amphotericin (37). However, if the clinical condition worsens during fluconazole therapy, intravenous amphotericin should be started. (For more information on fluconazole and amphotericin, see Chapter 35.)

REFERENCES

ACALCULOUS CHOLECYSTITIS

1. Walden D, Urrutia F, Soloway RD. Acute acalculous cholecystitis. J Intensive Care Med 1994;9:235–243.
2. Imhof M, Raunest J, Ohmann Ch, Rohrer H-D. Acute acalculous cholecystitis complicating trauma: a prospective sonographic study. World J Surg 1992; 1160–1166.

3. Bonacini M. Hepatobiliary complications in patients with human immunodeficiency virus infection. Am J Med 1992;92:404–411.

GASTRIC COLONIZATION

4. Marshall JC, Christou NV, Meakins JL. The gastrointestinal tract: the "undrained abscess" of multiple organ failure. Ann Surg 1993;218:111–119.
5. Kelly CP, Pothoulakis C, Lamont JT. Clostridium difficile colitis. N Engl J Med 1994;330:257–262.
6. Fekety R, Kim F-H, Brown D, et al. Epidemiology of antibiotic associated colitis. Am J Med 1981;70:906–908.
7. Samore MH, Venkataraman L, DeGirolami, et al. Clinical and molecular epidemiology of sporadic and clustered cases of nosocomial Clostridium difficile diarrhea. Am J Med 1996;100:32–40.
8. Johnson H, Homann SR, Bettin KM, et al. Treatment of asymptomatic Clostridium difficile carriers (fecal excreters) with vancomycin and metronidazole. Ann Intern Med 1992;117:297–302.
9. Johnson S, Gerding DN, Olson MM, et al. Prospective, controlled study of vinyl glove use to interrupt Clostridium difficile nosocomial transmission. Am J Med 1990;88:137–140.
10. Lipsett PA, Samantaray DK, Tam ML, et al. Pseudomembranous colitis: a surgical disease? Surgery 1994;116:491–496.
11. Biddle WL, Harms JL, Greenberger NJ, Miner PB. Evaluation of antibiotic-associated diarrhea with latex agglutination test and cell culture cytotoxicity assay for Clostridium difficile. Am J Gastroenterol 1988;84:279–283.
12. Gerding DN, Brazier JS. Optimal methods for identifying Clostridium difficile infections. Clin Infect Dis 1993;16(Suppl 4):439–442.
13. Gerding DN. Diagnosis of Clostridium difficile-associated disease: patient selection and test perfection. Am J Med 1996;100:485–486.
14. Manabe YC, Vinetz JM, Moore RD, et al. Clostridium difficile colitis: an efficient clinical approach to diagnosis. Ann Intern Med 1995;123:835–840.
15. Gerding DN, Johnson S, Peterson LR, et al. Clostridium difficile-associated diarrhea and colitis. Infect Control Hosp Epidemiol 1995;16:459–477.
16. Fishman EK, Kavuru M, Jones B, et al. Pseudomembranous colitis: CT evaluation of 26 cases. Radiology 1991;180:57–60.
17. Fekety R, Silva J, Kaufmann C, et al. Treatment of antibiotic-associated Clostridium difficile colitis with oral vancomycin: comparison of two dosage regimens. Am J Med 1989;86:15–19.
18. Pear SM, Williamson TH, Bettin KM, et al. Decrease in nosocomial Clostridium difficile associated diarrhea by restricting clindamycin use. Ann Intern Med 1994;120:272–277.
19. Surawicz C. Prevention of antibiotic-associated diarrhea by Saccharomyces boulardii: a prospective study. Gastroenterology 1989;96:981–988.

ABDOMINAL ABSCESSES

20. Mirvis SE, Shanmuganthan K. Trauma radiology: part I. Computerized tomographic imaging of abdominal trauma. J Intensive Care Med 1994;9:151–163.
21. Fry DE. Noninvasive imaging tests in the disgnosis and treatment of intra-abdominal abscesses in the postoperative patient. Surg Clin North Am 1994; 74:693–709.
22. Oglevie SB, Casola G, van Sonnenberg E, et al. Percutaneous abscess drainage:

current applications for critically ill patients. J Intensive Care Med 1994;9: 191–206.

23. Mosdell DM, Morris DM, Voltura A, et al. Antibiotic treatment for surgical peritonitis. Ann Surg 1991;214:543–549.

UROSEPSIS

24. Stamm WE, Hooten TM. Management of urinary tract infection in adults. N Engl J Med 1993;329:1328–1334.
25. Amin M. Antibacterial prophylaxis in urology: a review. Am J Med 1992; 92(Suppl 4A):114–117.
26. Howard RJ. Host defense against infection-Part 1. Curr Probl Surg 1980;27: 267–316.
27. Daifuku R, Stamm WE. Bacterial adherence to bladder uroepithelial cells in catheter-associated urinary tract infection. N Engl J Med 1986;314:1208–1213.
28. Jarvis JR, White JM, Munn VP, et al. Nosocomial infections surveillance, 1983. MMWR 1985;33:14SS.
29. Emori TG, Gaynes RP. An overview of nosocomial infections, including the role of the microbiology laboratory. Clin Microbiol Rev 1993;6:428–442.
30. McCue JD. How to manage urinary tract infections in the elderly. J Crit Illness 1996;11(Suppl):S30–S40.
31. Bone RC, Larson CB. Gram-negative urinary tract infections and the development of SIRS. J Crit Illness 1996;11(Suppl):S20–S29.
32. Bachman JW, Heise RH, Naessens JM, Timmerman MG. A study of various tests to detect asymptomatic urinary tract infections in an obstetric population. JAMA 1993;270:1971–1974.
33. Cockerill FR, Edson RS. Trimethoprim–sulfamethoxazole. Mayo Clin Proc 1991;66:1260–1269.
34. Jenkins SG. Changing spectrum of uropathogens: implications for treating complicated UTIs. J Crit Illness 1996;11(Suppl):S7–S13.

CANDIDURIA

35. Gubbins PO, Piscitelli SC, Danziger LH. Candidal urinary tract infections: a comprehensive review of their diagnosis and management. Pharmacotherapy 1993;13:110–127.
36. British Society for Antimicrobial Chemotherapy Working Party. Management of deep *Candida* infection in surgical and intensive care unit patients. Intensive Care Med 1994;20:522–528.
37. Rex J, Bennett JE, Sugar AM. A randomized trial comparing fluconazole with amphotericin B for the treatment of candidemia in patients without neutropenia. N Engl J Med 1994;331:1325–1330.

c h a p t e r

34

THE IMMUNOCOMPROMISED PATIENT

The care of critically ill patients is a labor-intensive, time-consuming, and mentally exhausting experience, and each of these aspects of critical care reaches its zenith in the care of the immunocompromised patient. This chapter presents some of the major concerns in the care of three different groups of immunocompromised patients: patients with human immunodeficiency virus (HIV) infection, neutropenic patients, and organ transplant recipients. Please understand that this is very fluid area, and the recommendations in this chapter could change at any moment.

INFECTION CONTROL

The practice of infection control involves a number of precautionary measures designed to limit or prevent the transmission of infectious agents between patients and hospital staff. One of the most important goals of infection control is to prevent the transmission of the HIV to those involved in direct patient care (1,2).

HIV TRANSMISSION

Infection with HIV can be transmitted in the body fluids indicated in Table 34.1 (3). In the hospital setting, transmission of HIV occurs via needlestick injuries or by direct contact of mucous membranes with blood from HIV-infected patients. Fortunately, HIV transmission to hospital staff is an uncommon event. As of 1993, only 39 cases of HIV transmission attributed to direct patient care contact had been reported (2).

Needlestick Injuries

A needlestick puncture transfers an average of 1 µL of blood (4). During the viremic stages of HIV infection, there are as many as 5

TABLE 34.1. THE RISK OF HIV TRANSMISSION IN BODY FLUIDS		
Transmission Documented	Transmission Possible	Transmission Not Documented
Blood	Cerebrospinal fluid	Feces
Breast milk	Peritoneal fluid	Saliva
Semen	Pleural fluid	Sputum
Vaginal secretions		Sweat
		Tears
		Urine
From References 1–3.		

infectious particles per μL of blood (3). Therefore, direct contact with less than one-thousandth of a milliliter of blood from an HIV-infected patient can result in transmission of infectious viral particles. In comparison, 1 μL of blood from patients with viral hepatitis can contain as many as one million infectious particles (3), so the risk of transmission of the hepatitis virus via needlestick injuries is far greater than the risk of HIV transmission.

A single needlestick injury with blood from an HIV-infected patient carries a 0.25% risk of HIV transmission (2). This means that for every 10,000 needlestick injuries with HIV-infected blood, 25 cases of HIV transmission occur. There are an estimated 16,000 needlestick exposures to HIV-infected blood each year in the United States (4), which translates to 38 cases of possible HIV transmission annually from accidental needlestick punctures.

Mucous Membrane Exposure

The risk of HIV transmission from direct exposure of broken skin or mucous membranes to contaminated body fluids is lower than the risk of transmission from needlestick injuries. **A single exposure of broken skin or mucous membranes to blood from an HIV-infected patient carries a 0.09% risk of HIV transmission** (2). This means that for every 10,000 mucous membrane exposures to contaminated body fluids, 9 cases of HIV transmission occur.

UNIVERSAL PRECAUTIONS

The discovery that HIV infection is transmitted in blood and body fluids prompted the immediate adoption of blood and body fluid precautions as a universal practice. The resultant guidelines are known as *universal precautions*. The basis of this practice is the assumption that blood and body fluids from all patients are potentially infectious. Therefore, the summary of universal precautions described below is meant for *all* patients (5).

Gloves

Gloves should be worn for procedures that involve direct contact with blood, mucous membranes, and the following body fluids: amniotic fluid, pericardial fluid, peritoneal fluid, pleural fluid, synovial fluid, semen, vaginal secretions, and any body fluid that is contaminated with blood. Gloves are also recommended for the insertion of vascular catheters and for all invasive procedures. Gloves are not required (but are not discouraged) for routine phlebotomy procedures.

Handwashing

Handwashing is recommended after any contact with blood and body fluids, even if gloves have been worn. A simple soap-and-water scrubbing is sufficient, and specialized antimicrobial soaps are unnecessary.

Protective Barriers

The mucous membranes should be protected by barriers such as masks, gowns, facial shields, and protective glasses during any procedure that could generate a spray of blood or body fluids.

Needlestick Precautions

An estimated 800,000 needlestick injuries occur each year (2000 each day) in the United States (4). To prevent these injuries, needles should not be recapped by hand or manipulated by hand in any way (this includes the removal of needles from the hub of a syringe). Used needles should be left attached to the syringe and discarded in special puncture-resistant sharps boxes (which are in every room). If a used needle is recapped, the **one-handed scoop technique** is recommended. Using the hand that grasps the syringe, the needle cap is first scooped up over the needle, and then the tip of the needle cap is pressed against a flat surface to secure the cap firmly to the hub of the needle. This eliminates the risk of puncturing the other hand with the needle. These needlestick precautions are recommended for all used needles, including those used to inject medications into intravenous infusion sets.

Exudative Dermatitis

Any member of the hospital staff who has an exudative or "weeping" dermatitis should not participate in direct patient care or handle patient-care equipment until the problem resolves.

Universal precautions are considered mandatory in the care of all hospitalized patients. Remember that many of the practices are designed to protect the staff as well as patients.

THE HIV-INFECTED PATIENT

Most patients with HIV infection who are admitted to the ICU have severe pneumonia with acute respiratory failure. Fewer are admitted

TABLE 34.2. THE AIDS EXPERIENCE IN THE UNITED STATES		
Year	New AIDS Cases	AIDS Deaths
1985	8,160	6,961
1990	41,761	31,339
1991	43,771	36,246
1992	45,961	40,072
1993	103,463	42,572
1994	77,767	46,810
1981–1994	461,383	332,644

Source: *Health United States, 1995.* National Center for Health Statistics, U.S. Department of Health and Human Services.

with severe cases of cryptococcal meningitis or toxoplasmic encephalitis. The description that follows is restricted to these problems. For information on the many other disorders associated with HIV infection, see Sande and Volberding (1995).

INCIDENCE OF HIV INFECTION

HIV infection is a worldwide epidemic. The diseases directly related to HIV infection (known collectively as acquired immunodeficiency syndrome, or AIDS) have become more prevalent each year in the United States, as indicated in Table 34.2. (The large increase in the number of reported cases of AIDS in 1993 is caused by the expanded number of AIDS-defining diseases proposed in that year.) Close to three-quarters of the reported cases of AIDS in the United States have had a fatal outcome.

Cell-Mediated Immunity

HIV has a propensity for invading lymphocytes and macrophages. Infection with HIV is followed by a long latency period that averages 10 to 11 years (3). During this time, the virus multiplies in lymphoid tissues, which eventually results in depression of cell-mediated immunity. When this occurs, there is an increased risk of infection, particularly with encapsulated microorganisms. These encapsulated microbes include bacteria (*Streptococcus pneumoniae, Hemophilus influenza*), fungi (*Cryptococcus neoformans*), and protozoans (*Pneumocystis carinii, Toxoplasma gondii*).

The depression of cell-mediated immunity in HIV infection is accompanied by a decrease in the density of certain immunologically distinct lymphocytes in blood. One of these is the CD4 lymphocyte, which is decreased below the normal level of 800 to 1200 cells per microliter (or mm^3) of blood. The number of circulating CD4 lymphocytes is therefore used as a marker of the severity of immunodepression in HIV-infected patients (3).

PNEUMONIA

The most common cause of pneumonia in HIV-infected patients has been the protozoan organism *P. carinii*. However, recent evidence indicates that bacterial pneumonia may be more common than *Pneumocystis* pneumonia in this patient population (6,7). Encapsulated bacteria such as *S. pneumoniae* (pneumococcus) and *H. influenza* are common offenders, along with *Staphylococcus aureus* (7). Other notable causes of lung infection in HIV-infected patients are cytomegalovirus (CMV), *Mycobacterium tuberculosis*, and *Mycobacterium avium*. Lung infections caused by fungi (e.g., *Aspergillus*) are usually seen only in the advanced stages of HIV infection (i.e., when CD4 lymphocyte counts fall below $50/mm^3$) (3,6).

Clinical Features

The clinical presentation of pneumonia is nonspecific and does not allow identification of the responsible pathogen (6). In particular, **the pattern of infiltration on the chest radiograph is not pathogen-specific.** To illustrate this point, review the portable chest radiographs shown in Figures 34.1 and 34.2. Both radiographs are from HIV-infected patients who presented with fever, nonproductive cough, and dyspnea. Neither patient could produce a sputum sample for analysis, and the results of blood cultures were either unrevealing or pending. Can you identify the pathogen based on the available information?

The clinical presentation of the patients just described is a common scenario. In the absence of sputum or pleural fluid to examine, bronchoscopy is usually required to identify the responsible pathogen.

Bronchoscopy

Bronchoscopy provides the diagnosis in 85% of lung infections caused by *P. carinii* (the organisms are apparent on microscopy using specialized stains), and in 95% of infections caused by *Mycobacterium tuberculosis* (6,8–10) Bronchoscopy can also have a high yield in the bacterial pneumonias, as described in Chapter 32. Bacterial cultures are performed quantitatively on specimens obtained by specialized protected-brush devices or bronchoalveolar lavage. However, the threshold for identifying infection on quantitative cultures may be higher in HIV-infected patients. The usual threshold of 10^3 colony-forming units per milliliter (CFU/mL) does not always indicate parenchymal infection in patients with HIV infection, and a higher threshold of 10^4 CFU/mL has been recommended for the diagnosis of pneumonia in HIV-infected patients (9).

In the patient with the radiograph shown in Figure 34.1, bronchoscopy revealed numerous *P. carinii* organisms in bronchoalveolar lavage fluid. In the other patient with the radiograph shown in Figure 34.2, bronchoscopy was unrevealing.

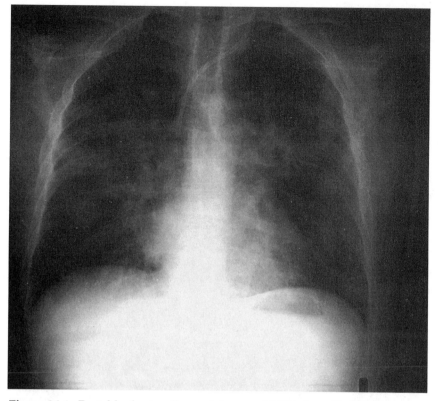

Figure 34.1. Portable chest radiograph from an HIV-infected patient who presented with fever, nonproductive cough, and dyspnea. Note the patchy infiltrates in both lungs. (Chest film courtesy of Dr. Richard Katz, M.D.)

Open-Lung Biopsy

When one or more bronchoscopies do not provide the diagnosis for suspected pneumonia, open-lung biopsy is a consideration. However, although open-lung biopsy can provide additional information, this information often does not lead to improved outcomes (8). In addition, severely ill patients with HIV infection may do poorly after open-lung biopsy (10). For these reasons, open-lung biopsy is not a popular procedure in the evaluation of pneumonia in HIV-infected (or otherwise immunocompromised) patients.

In the patient with the radiograph shown in Figure 34.2 who had an unrevealing bronchoscopy, open-lung biopsy was not performed. Therefore, the responsible pathogen was never identified. (The patient improved on empiric antibiotic therapy.) This case is included to emphasize that **in most cases of pneumonia in HIV-infected patients, the responsible pathogen is never identified.** In one study of apparent pneumonia in HIV infection, a pathogen was isolated in only 40% of the patients (7).

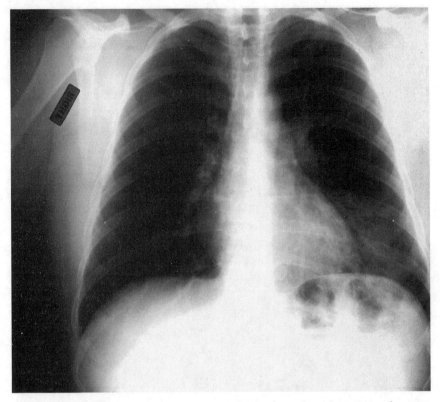

Figure 34.2. Portable chest radiograph of an HIV-infected patient who presented with fever, nonproductive cough, and dyspnea. Note infiltrate in left lower lung field. (Chest film courtesy of Dr. Richard Katz, M.D.)

P. CARINII PNEUMONIA

P. carinii pneumonia (PCP) is the most common cause for admission of HIV-infected patients to the ICU (11). In patients with PCP who are admitted to the ICU, the chest radiograph often looks like the one shown in Figure 34.3 (compare this film to the one in Fig. 34.1, which shows PCP in a less advanced stage). The radiographic changes in advanced stages of PCP are similar to the ones seen in the acute respiratory distress syndrome (ARDS). In fact, except for antimicrobial therapy, the management of patients with PCP and acute respiratory failure is the same as that of patients with ARDS. This management strategy is described in Chapter 23.

Trimethoprim–Sulfamethoxazole

As shown in Table 34.3, the initial antibiotic of choice for PCP is trimethoprim–sulfamethoxazole (TMP–SMX). The recommended dose is 20 mg/kg of TMP and 100 mg/kg of SMX daily, administered

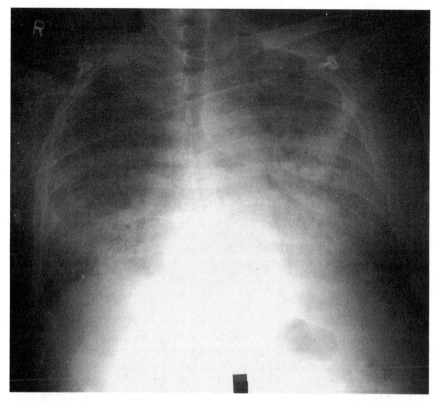

Figure 34.3. Portable chest radiograph of a patient with severe *P. carinii* pneumonia and acute respiratory failure. Note the similarity with the radiographic appearance of ARDS.

TABLE 34.3. RECOMMENDED TREATMENT FOR OPPORTUNISTIC INFECTIONS	
Infection	**Treatment**
Cytomegalovirus infections	(1) Ganciclovir: 5 mg/kg every 12 h
	(2) Foscarnet: 200 mg/kg/day
Invasive fungal infections	(1) Amphotericin: 0.5–1.0 mg/kg/day
	(2) Fluconazole: 200–400 mg/day
P. carinii pneumonia	(1) TMP–SMX: 20 mg/kg/day of TMP 100 mg/kg/day of SMX
	(2) Pentamidine: 4 mg/kg/day
Toxoplasma encephalitis	Pyrimethamine: 200 mg load, then 75 mg/day
	Folinic acid: 10 mg/day
	Clindamycin: 600 mg every 6 h
Numbers in parentheses indicate the order of preference for the antimicrobial agent.	

in three or four divided doses. Although TMP–SMX can be given orally, intravenous therapy is advised for patients with respiratory failure. A favorable response may not be apparent for 3 to 5 days, and there may be an initial period of deterioration. If a favorable response is not evident after 5 days of therapy, treatment is considered a failure. If evidence of improvement exists in the first few days of therapy, treatment is continued for a total of 3 weeks (11).

Adverse reactions to TMP–SMX develop in 30 to 50% of HIV-infected patients (11–14). These reactions usually appear during the second week of treatment, and they are often severe enough to warrant discontinuing the drug. The most common side effects are neutropenia (45 to 50%), fever (45 to 50%), skin rash (35 to 40%), elevated hepatic transaminase enzymes (30 to 35%), hyperkalemia (30%), and thrombocytopenia (10 to 15%). A case of fatal pancreatitis has also been linked to TMP–SMX (15). Only 35 to 45% of patients who receive TMP–SMX are able to complete the full course of therapy. The high incidence of adverse reactions to TMP–SMX is specific for HIV infection. In other groups of patients, adverse reactions to TMP–SMX develop in only 10% of the patients (11).

Pentamidine

When therapy with TMP–SMX fails or is not tolerated, the preferred second-line agent is pentamidine isethionate. The recommended dose is 4 mg/kg as a single daily dose. Pentamidine causes sterile abscesses when given by intramuscular injection, so intravenous therapy is preferred. The response time and duration of therapy are the same as for TMP–SMX. Treatment failures occur in one-third of patients (11).

Adverse reactions are also common with intravenous pentamidine (11,16–18). These side effects include neutropenia (5 to 30%), hyperglycemia and hypoglycemia (10 to 30%), prolonged Q–T interval (3 to 35%), torsade de pointes (up to 20%), renal insufficiency (3 to 5%), and pancreatitis (up to 1%). Of all patients who receive intravenous pentamidine, 40 to 50% are unable to complete therapy because of adverse reactions (11,16).

In patients who are unable to complete therapy with either TMP–SMX or pentamidine, a variety of other agents (e.g., dapsone and trimetrexate) are available. In this situation, you should consult an infectious disease expert pronto.

Steroids

Steroid therapy started at the time of antimicrobial therapy has been reported to improve outcomes in patients with PCP (19). Most trials have involved oral prednisone, but intravenous methylprednisolone (40 mg every 6 hours for at least 7 days) has also been recommended (11). Delay of treatment for 72 hours after the start of antimicrobial therapy negates any possible benefit from steroids (19). The response to steroids seems to vary in different clinical reports, and favorable responses can be short-lived (20).

CRYTOCOCCAL MENINGITIS

Cryptococcal meningitis is the most common life-threatening fungal infection in HIV-infected patients (21,22). It is expected in 10% of patients with HIV infection, and usually appears in the advanced stages of immunosuppression (i.e., when CD4 lymphocyte counts fall below 50/mm^3).

Clinical Features

The most common manifestations are fever and headache, each reported in approximately 85% of cases (21). Other findings include meningeal signs (35 to 40%), altered mental status (10 to 15%), and seizures (less than 10%) (21). Cryptococcal infections at other sites (e.g., pneumonia and skin rash) are seen in 20% of cases (22).

Diagnosis

Lumbar puncture is required for the diagnosis. Standard measurements in cerebrospinal fluid (CSF), such as glucose, protein, and leukocyte count, can be normal in up to 50% of cases (21). The organism can be demonstrated on india ink stains of CSF in 75% of cases (which is higher than the yield from india ink stains in non–HIV-infected patients) (21). CSF cultures and cryptococcal antigen titers are positive in over 90% of cases (21).

Treatment

The standard treatment of cryptococcal meningitis is intravenous **amphotericin** (Table 34.3). The administration of this antifungal agent is described in Chapter 35 (Table 35.3). Therapy with **fluconazole** (200 to 400 mg daily) has been reported to be as effective as amphotericin (23), but more experience is needed before fluconazole can be recommended as the preferred (i.e., less toxic) first-line agent for cryptococcal meningitis. (See Chapter 35 for more information on fluconazole.) Despite antifungal therapy, approximately one-third of HIV-infected patients with cryptococcal meningitis succumb to the infection (21).

TOXOPLASMIC ENCEPHALITIS

T. gondii encephalitis is the most common neurologic disorder in HIV-infected patients. Clinical evidence of toxoplasmic encephalitis is reported in 5 to 15% of HIV-infected patients, and autopsy evidence of the disease is present in up to 30% of patients (21).

Clinical Features

Toxoplasmic encephalitis is characterized by focal brain lesions. Hemiparesis and other focal neurologic deficits are seen in 60% of cases, and seizures are reported in 15 to 30% of patients (21). Other manifestations include fever (5 to 55%), confusion (60 to 65%), and choreiform movements (considered by some to be pathognomonic of toxoplasmic encephalitis) (21). Although extraneural disease is not common, disseminated toxoplasmosis with septic shock has been reported (24).

Diagnosis

Computerized tomography (CT) usually reveals solitary or multiple hypodense, contrast-enhancing mass lesions in the basal ganglia and frontoparietal regions of the cerebral hemispheres (21). Magnetic resonance imaging (MRI) is more sensitive and can reveal lesions when CT scans are negative (25). Lumbar puncture usually reveals abnormal findings, but these are nonspecific. Definitive diagnosis requires excisional brain biopsy (needle biopsy specimens are often unrevealing). The organism is demonstrated by immunoperoxidase staining.

Treatment

The treatment for toxoplasmic encephalitis is shown in Table 34.3. The preferred regimen is a combination of **pyrimethamine** (200 mg loading dose, then 75 mg daily) and **clindamycin** (600 mg every 6 hours). Because pyrimethamine is a folate antagonist, **folinic acid** (10 mg) is given with each dose of pyrimethamine to reduce the incidence of bone marrow suppression. All agents are given orally. Approximately 70% of cases show a favorable response to this regimen, and improvement is usually evident within the first week of therapy (26). The condition is considered uniformly fatal without appropriate therapy.

THE NEUTROPENIC PATIENT

Unlike the depression in cell-mediated immunity that occurs in HIV infections, isolated neutropenia (neutrophil count less than $500/mm^3$) results in a depression of humoral immunity. This results in an increased risk of infections with bacterial rather than opportunistic pathogens. The principal concern in the neutropenic patient is Gram-negative bacteremia, which can be accompanied by a rapid and fatal downhill course. Fortunately, bacteremia is uncommon in neutropenic patients unless the neutrophil count falls below $100/mm^3$ (27). In fact, most neutropenic patients with new-onset fever do not have a documented infection (28). Therefore, the rush to treatment in this situation is probably overkill in many instances.

EMPIRIC ANTIBIOTICS

A number of empiric antibiotic regimens have proven successful in febrile neutropenia, and these are shown in Table 34.4 (27–32). No one regimen has proven to be superior to the others.

TABLE 34.4. EMPIRIC ANTIBIOTIC THERAPY FOR FEBRILE NEUTROPENIA		
Antibiotics	Recommended Doses	Comment
Ceftazidime	2 g q 8 h	Is currently the popular choice, but doesn't cover Gram-positive pathogens.
Imipenem	500 mg q 6 h	Has a broader spectrum than ceftazidime, but risk for seizures (although low) limits its popularity.
Pipericillin + gentamicin	3 g q 4 h + 1.5 mg/kg q 8 h	Avoid aminoglycosides unless *Pseudomonas* is the suspected pathogen.
Vancomycin + any of the above	500 mg q 6 h + doses shown above	Add vancomycin if Gram-positive sepsis is a concern (that is, catheter sepsis).

Monotherapy with ceftazidime is a popular regimen and is currently the favored regimen at the National Cancer Institute (30). Monotherapy with imipenem is equally effective, but the popularity of this regimen has been hindered by the risk for seizures with imipenem (31), which is lower than perceived. The combination regimens are used when Gram-negative septicemia, particularly with *Pseudomonas* organisms, is suspected. The once popular aminoglycoside regimen is no longer favored because of the potential for toxicity with aminoglycosides. Finally, vancomycin can be added if a Gram-positive pathogen is suspected (e.g., catheter-related sepsis) or if methicillin-resistant staphylococci are prevalent at your hospital.

Pulmonary Infiltrates

If the fever is accompanied by pulmonary infiltrates (particularly diffuse infiltrates), the pathogens to consider are *Legionella pneumophila, Mycoplasma pneumoniae, Pneumocystis,* and CMV. In this setting, empiric therapy with erythromycin and TPM–SMX has been recommended, pending bronchoscopy (8). Because only a few doses of antibiotics can reduce the diagnostic yield from bronchoscopic cultures (see Chapter 32), the bronchoscopy should be performed as soon as possible after antibiotic therapy is started.

Persistent Fever

Continued fever after 1 week of empiric antibiotic therapy suggests possible invasive fungal disease (particularly disseminated candidiasis). In this situation, intravenous amphotericin (0.5 mg/kg daily) is recommended (8). As mentioned in the Chapter 33, blood cultures are negative in more than 50% of cases of disseminated candidiasis. The diagnosis of disseminated candidiasis is suggested by isolating *Can-*

dida at three separate sites (e.g., urine, sputum, and vascular catheter tips), and the diagnosis is confirmed by evidence of *Candida* ophthalmitis (see Reference 36 in Chapter 33).

THE TRANSPLANT RECIPIENT

A number of organ transplants can be encountered in the ICU, including of kidney, heart, liver, and bone marrow transplants. Infections in the first few weeks following organ transplantation are usually caused by bacterial pathogens (e.g., *S. aureus*), but infections that appear later (1 to 3 months) are often caused by opportunistic pathogens such as CMV, *Candida*, or other fungi (8,33,34). The change in microbial spectrum is explained by the chemotherapy used to prevent organ rejection.

CYTOMEGALOVIRUS

CMV is a herpesvirus that can cause a number of different infections in immunocompromised patients, including pneumonia, retinitis, hepatitis, pancreatitis, and esophageal ulcers. The virus is most pathogenic in transplant recipients and HIV-infected patients. Transplant recipients who have no CMV antibodies before surgery are most likely to develop CMV infections after transplantation.

Diagnosis

The diagnosis of CMV infection requires histologic evidence of cell invasion by the virus. Cultures of CMV in blood and urine are considered unreliable (35). The cytopathic action of CMV produces a characteristic cell with intranuclear inclusion bodies (36). The presence of this cell in tissue samples or bronchoscopy specimens is considered pathognomonic of CMV infection. Cytopathic changes in airway epithelial cells (from bronchoscopy) indicates CMV infection in the airways (tracheobronchitis). The diagnosis of CMV pneumonia requires cytopathic changes in alveolar macrophages or lung biopsies.

CMV pneumonia is accompanied by diffuse infiltrates in both lungs and can be confused with severe *Pneumocystis* pneumonia (as shown in Fig. 34.3). In fact, aprroximately 50% of HIV-infected patients with *P. carinii* pneumonia also have evidence of CMV infection (37). However, this is believed to represent colonization rather than infection in most cases. The situation is different in transplant recipients, in whom CMV is considered to be a common cause of pneumonia (38).

Treatment

The preferred agent for treating CMV infections is intravenous **ganciclovir** (Table 34.3). The recommended dose is 5 mg/kg every 8 to 12 hours (36). Lower doses (5 mg/kg/day) are used to prevent CMV infection in transplant recipients (39). Adverse reactions to ganciclovir, including neutropenia, thrombocytopenia, and skin rash, develop in 10% of patients.

In CMV infections that are refractory to ganciclovir, the antiviral agent **foscarnet** can be effective (40). The recommended dose is 200 mg/kg/day by continuous intravenous infusion. Adverse reactions to foscarnet develop in 20% of patients and include hypomagnesemia, hypocalcemia, hypophosphatemia, anemia, and renal insufficiency (36,40). Because of the greater incidence of adverse reactions, foscarnet is considered a second-line agent for the treatment of CMV infections.

REFERENCES

SUGGESTED READING

Greenbaum DM, ed. Management of the AIDS patient in the ICU. Critical care clinics. Vol. 9. Philadelphia: WB Saunders, 1993.

Sande MA, Volberding PA, eds. The medical management of AIDS. 4th ed. Philadelphia: WB Saunders, 1995.

INFECTION CONTROL

1. American College of Physicians and Infectious Disease Society of America. Human immunodeficiency virus (HIV) infection. Ann Intern Med 1994;120: 310–319.
2. Geberding JL. Limiting the risks of health care workers. In: Sande MA, Volberding PA, eds. The medical management of AIDS. 4th ed. Philadelphia: WB Saunders, 1995;89–101.
3. Levy JA. The transmission of HIV and factors influencing progression to AIDS. Am J Med 1993;95:86–100.
4. Berry AJ, Greene ES. The risk of needlestick injuries and needlestick-transmitted diseases in the practice of anesthesiology. Anesthesiology 1992;77: 1007–10021.
5. Garner JS. Universal precautions and isolation systems. In: Bennett JV, Brachman PS, eds. Hospital infections. 3rd ed. Boston: Little, Brown, 1992;231–244.

THE HIV-INFECTED PATIENT

6. Rosen MJ. Pneumonia in patients with HIV infection. Med Clin North Am 1994;78:1067–1079.
7. Hirschtick RE, Glassroth J, Jordan MC, et al. Bacterial pneumonia in persons infected with the human immunodeficiency virus. N Engl J Med 1995;333: 845–851.
8. Shelhammer JH, Toews GB, Masur H, et al. Respiratory disease in the immunosuppressed patient. Ann Intern Med 1992;117:415–431.
9. Ferrer M, Torres A, Xaubet A, et al. Diagnostic value of telescoping plugged catheters in HIV-infected patients with pulmonary infiltrates. Chest 1992;102: 76–83.
10. Trachiotis GD, Hafner GH, Hix WR, Aaron BL. Role of open lung biopsy

in diagnosing pulmonary complications of AIDS. Ann Thorac Surg 1992;54: 898–902.

PNEUMOCYSTIS CARINII PNEUMONIA

11. Brooks KR, Ong R, Spector RS, Greenbaum DM. Acute respiratory failure due to *Pneumocystis carinii* pneumonia. Crit Care Clin 1993;9:31–48.
12. Johnson MP, Goodwin D, Shands JW. Trimethoprim-sulfamethoxazole anaphylactoid reactions in patients with AIDS: case reports and literature review. Pharmacotherapy 1990;10:423–426.
13. van der Ven AJAM, Koopmans PP, Vree TB, van der Meer JWM. Adverse reactions to co-trimoxazole in HIV infection. Lancet 1991;338:431–433.
14. Greenberg S, Reiser IW, Chou S-Y, Porush JG. Trimethoprim-sulfamethoxazole induces reversible hyperkalemia. Ann Intern Med 1993;119:291–295.
15. Jost R, Stey C, Salomon F. Fatal drug-induced pancreatitis in HIV. Lancet 1993; 341:1412.
16. Dohn MN, Weinberg WG, Torres RA, et al. Oral atovaquone compared with intravenous pentamidine for *Pneumocystis carinii* pneumonia in patients with AIDS. Ann Intern Med 1994;121:174–180.
17. Eisenhauer MD, Eliasson AH, Taylor AJ, et al. Incidence of cardiac arrhythmias during intravenous pentamidine therapy in HIV-infected patients. Chest 1994;105:389–394.
18. Foisey MM, Slayter KL, Morse GD. Pancreatitis during intravenous pentamidine therapy in an AIDS patient with prior exposure to didanosine. Ann Pharmacother 1994;28:1025–1028.
19. National Institutes of Health—University of California Expert Panel for Corticosteroids as Adjunctive Therapy for *Pneumocystis* Pneumonia. Consensus statement on the use of corticosteroids as adjunctive therapy for *Pneumocystis* pneumonia in the acquired immunodeficiency syndrome. N Engl J Med 1990; 323:1500–1504.
20. Schiff MJ, Farber BF, Kaplan MH. Steroids for *Pneumocystis carinii* pneumonia and respiratory failure in the acquired immunodeficiency syndrome. Arch Intern Med 1990;150:1819–1821.

CRYPTOCOCCAL MENINGITIS

21. Levy RM, Berger JR. Neurologic critical care in patients with human immunodeficiency virus 1 infection. Clin Crit Care 1993;9:49–72.
22. Ennis DM, Saag MS. Cryptococcal meningitis in AIDS. Hosp Pract 1993;28: 99–112.
23. Saag MS, Powderly WG, Cloud GA, et al. Comparison of amphotericin B with fluconazole in the treatment of acute AIDS-associated cryptococcal meningitis. N Engl J Med 1992;326:83–89.

TOXOPLASMIC ENCEPHALITIS

24. Lucet J-C, Bailley M-P, Bedos J-P, et al. Septic shock due to toxoplasmosis in patients infected with the human immunodeficiency virus. Chest 1993;104: 1054–1058.
25. Knobel H, Graus F, Miro JM, et al. Toxoplasmic encephalitis with normal CT scan and pathologic MRI. Am J Med 1995;99:220–221.

26. Luft BJ, Hafner R, Korzun AH, et al. Toxoplasmic encephalitis in patients with the acquired immunodeficiency syndrome. N Engl J Med 1993;329:995–1000.

THE NEUROPENIC PATIENT

27. Shenep JL. Empiric antimicrobial treatment in febrile neutropenic cancer patients. Infect Med 1992;April:39–47.
28. Ranphal R, Gucalp R, Rotstein C, et al. Clinical experience with single agent and combination regimens in the management of infection in the febrile neutropenic patient. Am J Med 1996;100:83S–89S.
29. Hughes WT, Armstrong D, Bodey GP, et al. Guidelines for the use of antimicrobial agents in neutropenic patients with unexplained fever. J Infect Dis 1990;161:381–396.
30. Pizzo PA. Choosing empiric therapy for febrile neutropenic patients. J Crit Illness 1995;10:165–168.
31. Winston DJ, Ho WG, Bruckner DA, Champlin RE. Beta-lactam antibiotic therapy in febrile granulocytopenic patients. Ann Intern Med 1991;115:849–859.
32. De Pauw BE, Deresinski SC, Feld R, et al. for the Intercontinental Antimicrobial Study Group. Ceftazidime compared with piperacillin and tobramycin for the empiric treatment of fever in neutropenic patients with cancer. A multicenter randomized trial. Ann Intern Med 1994;120:833–844.

THE TRANSPLANT RECIPIENT

33. Kobasigawa JA, Stevenson LW. Managing complications in heart transplant recipients. J Crit Illness 1993;8:678–689.
34. Howard RJ. Infections in the immunocompromised patient. Surg Clin North Am 1994;74:609–620.

CYTOMEGALOVIRUS INFECTIONS

35. Zurlo JJ, O'Neill D, Polis M, et al. Lack of clinical utility of cytomegalovirus blood and urine cultures in patients with HIV infection. Ann Intern Med 1993; 118:12–17.
36. Goodgame RW. Gastrointestinal cytomegalovirus disease. Ann Intern Med 1993;119:924–935.
37. Jacobson MA, Mills J, Rush J, et al. Morbidity and mortality of patients with AIDS and first-episode *Pneumocystis carinii* pneumonia unaffected by concomitant pulmonary cytomegalovirus infection. Am Rev Respir Dis 1991;144:6–9.
38. Sommer SE, Emanuel D, Groeger J, et al. Successful management of CMV pneumonia in a mechanically ventilated patient. Chest 1991;100:856–858.
39. Goodrich JM, Bowden RA, Fisher L, et al. Ganciclovir prophylaxis to prevent cytomegalovirus disease after allogenic marrow transplant. Ann Intern Med 1993;118:173–178.
40. Lietman PS. Clinical pharmacology: foscarnet. Am J Med 1992;92(Suppl): 8S–11S.

chapter

35

ANTIMICROBIAL THERAPY

The danger with germ-killing drugs is that they may kill the patient as well as the germ.

JBS Haldane

Antimicrobial therapy is part of everyday life in the ICU. The agents listed here cover most of the infections encountered in the ICU, and each is presented briefly in the order listed. At the end of the chapter is a table listing the estimated daily cost of therapy with these agents (see Table 35.8).

Aminoglycosides
Antifungal agents (amphotericin, fluconazole)
Aztreonam
Cephalosporins
Imipenem
Penicillins
Quinolones
Vancomycin

A list of preferred antibiotics for specific pathogens is shown in Table 35.1.

AMINOGLYCOSIDES

The aminoglycosides (gentamicin, tobramycin, and amikacin) are the traditional agents used for serious Gram-negative infections (1). However because of the risk of nephrotoxicity, there has been a marked decline in aminoglycoside use in recent years. At one large teaching hospital, the use of gentamicin decreased 70% in the late 1980s (1).

ANTIBACTERIAL SPECTRUM

The aminoglycosides are active against all *Enterobacteriaceae,* including *Pseudomonas aeruginosa.* There is no emerging resistance to the ami-

562

TABLE 35.1. PARENTERAL ANTIBIOTIC SELECTIONS

Microorganisms	Preferred Agents	Alternatives
Aerobic Gram-positive cocci:		
Staphylococcus aureus	Nafcillin or oxacillin	Cefazolin* or vancomycin
Methicillin-resistant	Vancomycin ± gentamicin ± rifampin	Trimethoprim–sulfamethoxazole or ciprofloxacin
Staphylococcus epidermidis	Vancomycin	Rifampin
Streptococcus pneumoniae or	Penicillin G	Cefazolin*, erythromycin, or
Streptococcus pyogenes		vancomycin
Aerobic Gram-negative bacilli:		
Enterobacteriaceae:	Ceftazidime or ceftriaxone	Aminoglycosides, aztreonam, or
Escherichia coli		imipenem
Klebsiella pneumoniae		
Proteus, indole-positive		
Hemophilus influenza	Cefotaxime or ceftriaxone	Cefuroxime
Legionella species	Erthromycin + rifampin	Trimethoprim–sulfamethoxazole or ciprofloxacin
Pseudomonas aeruginosa (serious infections)	Antipseudomonal penicillin + aminoglycoside	Aztreonam, ceftazidime, or imipenem
Salmonella species	Ceftriaxone or ciprofloxacin	Ampicillin or trimethoprim–sulfamethoxazole
Anaerobic organisms:		
Bacteroides species		
Oropharyngeal strains	Penicillin G	Metronidazole
B. fragilis	Metronidazole	Clindamycin or imipenem
Clostridium difficile	Metronidazole	Vancomycin
Clostridium tetani	Penicillin G	Tetracycline
Enterococcus faecalis (serious infections)	Ampicillin + gentamicin	Vancomycin + gentamicin

* In patients with prior anaphylactic reactions to penicillin, cephalosporins should be avoided.
Adapted from The Medical Letter 1994;36:53–60.

noglycosides, which is one of the reasons for their continued popularity.

DOSING

Aminoglycoside dosing in critically ill patients is summarized in Table 35.2 (2). Drug doses are determined according to **ideal body**

TABLE 35.2. AMINOGLYCOSIDE THERAPY IN THE ICU

Agent	Dose in mg/kg*		Target Serum Levels‡ (mg/L)	
	Initial	Daily†	Peak	Trough
Gentamicin	3	3	>6	1–2
Tobramycin	3	3	>6	1–2
Amikacin	9	15	>30	5–10

* Use ideal body weight unless patient is morbidly obese (see text).
† Can be given once daily or in three divided doses. Doses shown are for normal renal function.
‡ Peak levels are obtained 30 minutes after the dose. Trough levels are drawn at the end of the dosing interval.
From Walting SM, Dasta JF. Aminoglycoside dosing considerations in intensive care unit patients. Ann Pharmacother 1993;27:351–357.

weight, except in patients who are morbidly obese; then the appropriate dosing weight is the ideal body weight plus half the difference between the ideal and actual body weight (3). The initial loading doses shown in Table 35.2 are larger than those recommended normally because of the larger volume of distribution for aminoglycosides in critically ill patients (4). The daily maintenance dose is traditionally given in three divided doses, but can also be given once daily. Because aminoglycosides are eliminated by the kidneys, dose adjustments are required when renal function is impaired. There are two methods for adjusting the dose when renal function is impaired:

The dose interval can be adjusted by multiplying the normal dose interval by the serum creatinine (in mg/dL).
The daily dose can be adjusted by dividing the normal daily dose by the serum creatinine (in mg/dL).

Once-Daily Dosing

The bactericidal effect of the aminoglycosides is concentration-dependent, so higher drug concentrations in the blood and tissues produce more bacterial killing (5). This has led to the recommendation that aminoglycosides be given in one daily dose, which produces higher drug concentrations in the tissues than the divided-dose regimen. The once-daily regimen has proven equivalent in efficacy and toxicity to the divided-dose regimen (2,6), while being less costly (because it eliminates the cost of extra intravenous infusion sets and reduces the need for monitoring serum drug levels). However, despite the potential advantages, once-daily dosing has been adopted in only 15 to 20% of hospitals in the United States (6).

Monitoring

Routine monitoring of serum aminoglycoside levels is recommended for three reasons (1,2). First, peak serum levels are directly related to clinical efficacy. Second, aminoglycoside toxicity shows a correlation with the minimal (trough) serum levels at the end of the dosing interval. Third, equivalent doses of aminoglycosides result in variable serum drug levels in individual patients. The recommended serum drug levels are shown in Table 35.2. The peak levels in this table have been shown to result in improved outcomes (2), whereas the trough levels are associated with reduced clinical toxicity. There is one report of spurious elevations in serum aminoglycoside levels when blood samples were drawn through central venous Silastic catheters (mechanism unknown).

TOXICITY

Nephrotoxicity

Approximately 20% of patients who receive aminoglycosides develop some degree of renal impairment, regardless of the agent used

(7). The onset is usually 3 to 7 days after the onset of therapy, and early signs include cylindrical casts in the urine, proteinuria, and inability to concentrate urine. This is followed by a rising serum creatinine concentration that culminates in acute renal failure. Nephrotoxicity is enhanced by hypovolemia, advanced age, preexisting renal impairment, hypokalemia, and hypomagnesemia (7). The acute renal failure is usually nonoliguric and reversible.

Ototoxicity

Aminoglycosides produce a dose-related and irreversible hearing loss for high-frequency sounds. Because the hearing loss occurs above the frequency range of normal human conversation, audiometry is required to document the ototoxicity (1).

Neuromuscular Blockade

In high doses, the aminoglycosides block acetylcholine release at presynaptic nerve terminals and reduce postsynaptic responsiveness to acetylcholine. These agents can aggravate the neuromuscular blockade associated with myasthenia gravis and nondepolarizing muscle relaxants (1,8,9). However, little evidence exists of this effect when the drugs are given in therapeutic doses (10).

COMMENT

The risk of aminoglycoside nephrotoxicity is reason to **avoid these agents whenever possible.** A number of less toxic agents are now available for treating Gram-negative infections, including the third-generation cephalosporins, aztreonam, and imipenem. Pharmaceutical companies apparently realize the bleak future for aminoglycosides because no new aminoglycoside agents have been introduced in over a decade.

ANTIFUNGAL AGENTS

AMPHOTERICIN

Amphotericin is the most effective antifungal agent in clinical use (11). However, therapy with this agent carries a considerable risk of toxicity, and several precautions are necessary.

Infusion-Related Side Effects

Amphotericin infusions are accompanied by fever, chills, nausea, vomiting, and rigors in approximately 70% of cases (12). Premedication with acetaminophen and diphenhydramine, given 30 minutes before the infusions, can reduce the incidence of infusion-related side

TABLE 35.3. GUIDELINES FOR AMPHOTERICIN ADMINISTRATION	
Premedication:	To avoid infusion-related side effects, give acetaminophen (650 mg PO) and diphenhydramine (25 mg PO or IV) 30 minutes before drug administration. For infusion-related rigors, premedicate with meperidine (25 mg IV).
Preparation:	
Diluent:	5% dextrose in water. DO NOT use NaCL solutions.
Concentration:	0.1 mg/mL.
Additives:	Add hydrocortisone (0.1 mg/mL) if fever persists despite the premedications.
Test dose:	1 mg over 30 min (not always necessary).
Daily dosing:	Start with initial dose of 0.25 mg/kg infused over 4 hr, then • For mild infections, double the dose on day 2 and continue a daily maintenance dose of 0.5 mg/kg. • For severe infections, increase each dose 0.25 mg/kg to a final daily dose of 0.75–1.0 mg/kg.
Adjustments:	• After 5 days, reduce infusion time to 1 hr unless there is renal impairment or drug-related hyperkalemia. • If serum creatinine rises above 3 mg/dL during therapy Stop drug Rx for 3 doses and infuse volume if possible. Restart Rx at ½ the prior maintenance dose, and advance the dose as recommended above
See Bult J, Franklin CM (12).	

effects (Table 35.3). Infusion-related rigors can be treated by premedication with meperidine (Demerol). An infusion-related phlebitis can appear days after amphotericin therapy is started, and it is particularly prominent when the drug is given through a peripheral vein. Heparin is often added to the infusate (1 U/mL) to prevent this complication, but no evidence exists that this is effective (11).

Dosing

Some recommendations for amphotericin administration are shown in Table 35.3 (12). A test dose is commonly given at the start of therapy, but this is unnecessary if premedications are given routinely. If fever persists despite premedications, hydrocortisone can be added to the infusate. The drug is given once daily, starting at a dose of 0.25 mg/kg and increasing to a final daily dose of 0.5 to 1.0 mg/kg (higher daily doses are used for more severe infections). The initial duration of drug infusion is 4 hours, and this can be reduced to a 1-hour infusion after 5 days of therapy if renal impairment or hyperkalemia does not occur. Daily infusions are continued until the cumulative dose reaches a specified level. The total amphotericin dose is dictated by the severity of the infection and can be as little as 500 mg (for catheter-related candidemia) or as much as 4 g (for life-threatening fungal infections).

Nephrotoxicity

The major complication of amphotericin therapy is impaired renal function. Nephrotoxic effects include renal vasoconstriction and a renal tubular acidosis (distal type) with increased urinary excretion of potassium and magnesium (13). The latter complication leads to **potassium and magnesium depletion.** The incidence of nephrotoxicity is unclear because amphotericin is often used in conditions that themselves cause renal impairment.

Preventive management of amphotericin nephrotoxicity includes routine monitoring of serum creatinine, potassium, and magnesium. If the serum creatinine rises above 3.0 mg/dL, the amphotericin infusion should be temporarily discontinued (Table 35.3) Daily magnesium supplements (300 to 600 mg elemental magnesium daily) should be given to counterbalance urinary losses. Serum magnesium is *not* a sensitive marker of magnesium depletion (see Chapter 42), so daily magnesium supplementation is important. **Sodium loading** (i.e., infusion of 1 L of isotonic saline) has been recommended before amphotericin infusions to maintain renal blood flow (13). However, sodium loading does not prevent amphotericin-induced renal failure, and it aggravates the renal tubular defect and promotes urinary potassium wasting (13). Thus, sodium loading should be viewed with caution. What may be more important is to avoid hypovolemia during amphotericin therapy.

FLUCONAZOLE

Fluconazole (Diflucan) is a member of the imidazole class of antifungal agents (the other members are itraconazole and ketoconazole) and was introduced for clinical use in 1990. The beneficial features of fluconazole include a broad spectrum of antifungal activity and fewer toxic side effects than amphotericin. Because of these favorable features, fluconazole could become a safer alternative to amphotericin for the treatment of severe fungal infections (14).

Indications

Fluconazole has proven effective in treating infections caused by *Candida* and *Cryptococcus* organisms in patients who are immunocompromised or have an intact immune system (15,16). It has also proven successful for preventing fungal infections in immunocompromised patients (17). In the ICU, the major use of fluconazole is in patients with documented or suspected disseminated candidiasis. In patients who are not immunocompromised, fluconazole (400 mg daily) can be used as an alternative to amphotericin (16). In those who are immunocompromised, combination therapy with fluconazole and amphotericin might be the wiser choice.

Dosing

Fluconazole is given once daily. The dose for serious infections is 400 mg/day. In patients with renal failure, the daily dose should be reduced by 50% (14). Serum drug levels can be used to guide drug dosing in renal failure. Trough levels should be maintained between 6 and 20 μg/mL (14).

Drug Interactions

Fluconazole can interfere with the metabolism of phenytoin and warfarin and potentiate the actions of both drugs. These interactions can be clinically significant, so it is important to monitor serum phenytoin levels and prothrombin times when fluconazole is given in concert with these drugs (18,19).

Hepatotoxicity

Severe and even fatal hepatic injury associated with fluconazole therapy has been reported (20). Most cases have been in patients with liver disease or human immunodeficiency virus (HIV) infection. Although this seems to be a rare event, liver enzymes probably should be monitored periodically during fluconazole therapy in patients who are HIV-positive or have liver disease (20).

AZTREONAM

Aztreonam (Azactam) is a synthetic antimicrobial agent that has a similar antibacterial spectrum to the aminoglycosides, but is devoid of nephrotoxicity (21).

DOSING

The usual intravenous dose of aztreonam in adults is **1 g every 8 hours** (21). Doubling the dose has been recommended for seriously ill patients, but no evidence exists that this improves efficacy. A dose reduction of 50 to 75% is recommended in patients with renal failure (22).

TOXICITY

Aztreonam is a relatively safe drug. In a survey of 2700 patients receiving aztreonam, adverse reactions were noted in 7% of patients. Most of these reactions were mild and nonspecific (e.g., nausea and diarrhea) (21).

COMMENT

Aztreonam provides a safe and effective alternative to the aminoglycosides for the management of serious Gram-negative infections.

		Gram⁺	Gram⁻			

TABLE 35.4. THE GENERATIONS OF PARENTERAL CEPHALOSPORINS

Agent	Generation	Gram⁺ Cocci*	Gram⁻ Bacilli	P. aeruginosa	B. fragilis	H. influenza
Cefazolin (Ancef)	1	+ + + +	+ +	—	—	+ +
Cefoxitin (Mefoxin)	2	+ +	+ + + +	—	+ +	+ +
Ceftriaxone (Rocephin)	3	+ +	+ + + +	—	—	+ + + +
Ceftazidime (Fortaz)	3	—	+ + + +	+ + + +	—	+ + + +
Cefepime (Maxipime)	4	+ +	+ + + +	+ + + +	—	+ + + +

* Does not include coagulase-negative or methicillin-resistant staphylococci, or enterococci.
Relative antibacterial activity is indicated by number of plus signs.
Adapted from information in References 23 and 24.

CEPHALOSPORINS

A small army of cephalosporins is available for clinical use. These agents are divided into *generations* based on the historical sequence of their introduction into clinical practice. Some of the parenteral agents in each generation are shown in Table 35.4 (23).

THE FAMILY OF CEPHALOSPORINS

The **first-generation** cephalosporins are primarily active against aerobic Gram-positive cocci, but are not active against *Staphylococcus epidermidis* or methicillin-resistant strains of *S. aureus*. The popular intravenous agent in this group is cefazolin (Ancef).

The **second-generation** cephalosporins exhibit stronger antibacterial activity against Gram-negative aerobic and anaerobic bacilli of enteric origin. The popular parenteral agents in this group are cefoxitin (Mefoxin) and cefamandole (Mandol).

The **third-generation** cephalosporins have greater antibacterial activity against Gram-negative aerobic bacilli, including *P. aeruginosa* and *Hemophilus influenza*, but are less active against aerobic Gram-positive cocci than the first-generation agents. The popular parenteral agents in this group are cefotaxime (Claforan), ceftriaxone (Rocephin), and ceftazidime (Fortaz). The latter agent is notable for its activity against *P. aeruginosa*.

The **fourth-generation** cephalosporins are just beginning to emerge. One of the agents in this group is cefepime (Maxipime), which has the Gram-negative antibacterial spectrum of ceftazidime (i.e., it covers *P. aeruginosa*), but is also active against aerobic Gram-positive cocci (eg. streptococci and methicillin-sensitive staphylococci) (24).

DOSING

The doses for some parenteral cephalosporins are shown in Table 35.5. Most agents are given in doses of 1 to 2 g every 6 to 8 hours.

TABLE 35.5. PARENTERAL CEPHALOSPORIN DOSING		
Agent	Dose for Serious Infections	Dose in Renal Failure*
Cefazolin	1 g q 6 h	1 g q 24 h
Cefotaxime	2 g q 8 h	2 g q 24 h
Ceftazidime	2 g q 8 h	2 g q 48 h
Ceftriaxone	2 g q 12 h	2 g q 12 h
* From Reference 22.		

Ceftriaxone is the exception, and can be given every 12 to 24 hours. The dose adjustments in renal failure are also included in Table 33.5 (22). Note that the dose is adjusted by extending the dosing interval rather than decreasing the amount of drug given with each dose. This is done to preserve concentration-dependent bacterial killing. Ceftriaxone requires no dose adjustment in renal failure.

TOXICITY

Adverse reactions to cephalosporins are uncommon and nonspecific (e.g., nausea, rash, and diarrhea). There is a 5 to 15% incidence of cross-antigenicity with penicillin (23), and cephalosporins should be avoided in patients with a prior anaphylactic reaction to penicillin.

COMMENT

The cephalosporins that see most action in the ICU setting are the third-generation agents (cefotaxime, ceftriaxone, and ceftazidime), which are used to treat infections caused by Gram-negative pathogens (Table 35.1). Ceftazidime is particularly popular because of its activity against *P. aeruginosa*. At the National Cancer Institute, monotherapy with ceftazidime is one of the preferred regimens for the empiric therapy of febrile neutropenia (25). The fourth-generation agent cefepime has also been used in febrile neutropenia (24), and this agent may replace ceftazidime because of its extended activity against Gram-positive pathogens.

IMIPENEM

Imipenem has the broadest spectrum of antibacterial activity of any antibiotic currently available (26). Because of its wide spectrum of activity, imipenem is useful for treating polymicrobial infections (e.g., bowel sepsis) and for empiric therapy of febrile neutropenic patients.

TABLE 35.6. THE ANTIBACTERIAL ACTIVITY OF IMIPENEM	
Covers	**Does Not Cover**
Aerobic streptococci	S. aureus (methicillin-resistant)
S. aureus (methicillin-sensitive)	Pseudomonas cepacia
S. epidermidis	
Anaerobic organisms	
Enterococcus faecalis	
Enterobacteriaceae	
Enterobacter	
Escherichia coli	
Klebsiella spp.	
Proteus spp.	
P. aeruginosa	

ANTIBACTERIAL SPECTRUM

As is evident in Table 35.6, the antibacterial spectrum of imipenem includes most of the pathogens involved in nosocomial infections. The most notable exception is methicillin-resistant staphylococci. In addition to its activity against the Enterobacteriaceae, imipenem covers all anaerobic pathogens, including B. fragilis and Enterococcus faecalis. Some strains of Pseudomonas (e.g., P. cepacia) are resistant to imipenem, and acquired resistance in P. aeruginosa is reported (26).

DOSING

Imipenem is inactivated by enzymes in the renal tubules, so it is impossible to achieve high levels of the drug in urine. To overcome this problem, the commercial preparation of imipenem contains an enzyme inhibitor, cilastatin. The combination imipenem–cilastatin preparation is available as Primaxin. The dose recommendations for imipenem–cilastatin represent the dose of imipenem. The usual intravenous dose in adults is **500 mg every 6 hours.** In suspected Pseudomonas infections, the dose is doubled to 1 g every 6 hours. In renal failure, the dose should be reduced by 50 to 75% (22).

TOXICITY

The major effect of toxicity associated with imipenem is **generalized seizures,** which occur in 1 to 3% of patients receiving the drug (26). Most patients have a history of a seizure disorder, an intracranial mass, or renal failure. Although this is an uncommon occurrence, a maximum daily dose of 2 g or 25 mg/kg has been recommended (26).

COMMENT

The ultimate antibiotic would be effective against all pathogens and produce no adverse reactions. Imipenem comes closer to this ideal

TABLE 35.7. USES FOR PARENTERAL PENICILLINS IN THE ICU		
Agents	Usual Dose	Uses
Penicillin G	6–24 million U/day	Infections caused by aerobic streptococci (such as pneumococcus).
Nafcillin Oxacillin	1–2 g q 6–8 h	Infections caused by methicillin-sensitive strains of S. aureus
Ticarcillin Pipericillin Mezlocillin	2–4 g q 4–6 h	Serious infections caused by P. aeruginosa

than any antibiotic currently available. Monotherapy with imipenem is a useful regimen for the empiric therapy of suspected sepsis, and it is one of the preferred regimens for the empiric therapy of febrile neutropenia (25,27). However, because of emerging resistance in *P. aeruginosa*, monotherapy with imipenem is not recommended for suspected *Pseudomonas* infections.

THE PENICILLINS

Almost 30 penicillins are available for clinical use. The few that are useful in the ICU are listed in Table 35.7.

NATURAL PENICILLINS

The penicillin discovered by Alexander Fleming in 1929 is benzyl-penicillin, or penicillin G. This substance is active against aerobic streptococci (*S. pneumoniae, S. pyogenes*) and anaerobic mouth flora. Penicillin G was active against staphylococci when first discovered, but these organisms have acquired a resistance to penicillin by virtue of an enzyme (called β-lactamase or penicillinase) that disrupts the penicillin molecule. The limited spectrum of penicillin G limits its use in the ICU. The major use for this agent is the occasional patient with pneumococcal pneumonia or disseminated pneumococcal sepsis.

PENICILLINASE-RESISTANT PENICILLINS

To regain the original activity against staphylococci, the penicillin G molecule was modified to make it resistant to the penicillinase enzyme. This resulted in the introduction of **methicillin, oxacillin,** and **nafcillin** to treat staphylococcal infections. However, staphylococci have demonstrated an increasing resistance to these agents over the last 15 to 20 years. These resistant organisms, known as *methicillin-resistant* staphylococci, have become prominent pathogens in hospitalized patients. The treatment of choice for these organisms is vancomycin.

EXTENDED-SPECTRUM PENICILLINS

The penicillins in this category have an extended antibacterial spectrum that covers Gram-negative aerobic bacilli. This category includes the aminopenicillins (**ampicillin and amoxicillin**), the carboxypenicillins (**carbenicillin and ticarcillin**), and the ureidopenicillins (**azlocillin, mezlocillin,** and **piperacillin**). All groups are active against Gram-negative enteric pathogens, but the latter two groups are active against *P. aeruginosa.* These agents are also known as antipseudomonal penicillins. In addition to treating serious infections caused by *Pseudomonas* organisms, these agents are also used for the empiric therapy of fever in neutropenic patients (25).

Dosing

The recommended doses for parenteral penicillins are shown in Table 35.7. Penicillin G has a short half-life (30 minutes) and is given by continuous intravenous infusion. The modified penicillins are usually given in a dose of 1 to 2 g every 4 to 6 hours. The penicillins are excreted by the kidneys, and dose reduction is advised in renal insufficiency. In renal failure, the dose interval should be extended to 8 to 12 hours (22).

Toxicity

The most common adverse reactions to the penicillins are allergic-type reactions. A rash develops in up to 4% of patients, but anaphylaxis occurs in only 0.05% of patients (28). A hypersensitivity nephritis has been linked to methicillin, but not to the other penicillins. A reversible neurotoxic syndrome with delirium and seizures has been linked to high-dose therapy with penicillin G, often in patients with renal insufficiency (28).

THE QUINOLONES

The quinolone antibiotics were introduced in the mid-1980s for the treatment of complicated urinary tract infections in outpatients. Two parenteral agents are currently available for clinical use: ciprofloxacin and ofloxacin.

ANTIBACTERIAL SPECTRUM

The quinolones are active against (methicillin-sensitive) staphylococci and most of the *Enterobacteriaceae,* including *P. aeruginosa.* They are less active against streptococci, and have no activity against anaerobic organisms. Emerging resistance in *Pseudomonas* isolates is a concern (29).

DOSING

The dose of intravenous ciprofloxacin is **400 mg every 12 hours** for serious infections (30). The drug is irritating to veins and should be either given via a central vein or infused slowly over 1 hour. In renal failure, the daily dose should be reduced by 25 to 50% (22).

TOXICITY

The quinolones are safe in most patients. There are rare reports of a hypersensitivity interstitial nephritis from ciprofloxacin (31), and one case of exacerbation of myasthenia gravis (32). The quinolones also **interfere with the hepatic metabolism of theophylline and warfarin** and can potentiate the actions of both of these drugs (29,33). Ciprofloxacin causes a 25% increase in serum theophylline levels, and combined therapy has resulted in symptomatic theophylline toxicity (34). Although no dose adjustments are necessary, serum theophylline levels and prothrombin times should be monitored carefully when ciprofloxacin is given in combination with these two agents.

COMMENT

Despite their popularity as oral agents, the quinolones have not found a niche in the treatment of infections in the ICU. Because of the rapid emergence of resistance in *Pseudomonas* organisms, the use of quinolones should be limited (29,34). They can be used to treat the occasional urinary tract infection caused by organisms that are not susceptible to other conventional agents.

VANCOMYCIN

Vancomycin may be the single most popular antibiotic in critical care. However, it is overused, which is creating problems with acquired resistance.

ANTIBACTERIAL SPECTRUM

Vancomycin is active against all Gram-positive cocci, including anaerobic streptococci (*E. faecalis*), coagulase-negative staphylococci (*S. epidermidis*), and methicillin-resistant strains of *S. aureus* (35). It is also one of the most active agents against *Clostridium difficile,* the pathogen responsible for antibiotic-associated pseudomembranous colitis. In recent years, nosocomial strains of *Enterococcus* have demonstrated an emerging resistance to vancomycin, and in a survey of U.S. hospitals conducted in 1993, 8% of all enterococcal isolates were vancomycin-resistant (36).

DOSING

The usual intravenous dose of vancomycin is **500 mg every 6 hours.** The drug must be infused slowly (**no faster than 10 mg/minute**) to minimize the risk of infusion-related reactions. Dose reduction is necessary in renal insufficiency. In patients with renal failure, the drug is given once every 4 days, and no supplemental doses are given after hemodialysis (22).

Serum drug levels are often monitored to limit toxicity and maintain efficacy. **Peak levels should be below 40 mg/L** to reduce the risk of ototoxicity, and **trough levels should be above 5 mg/L** to maintain antibacterial activity (37).

TOXICITY

Infusion-related Toxicity

Rapid administration of vancomycin is associated with vasodilation, flushing, and hypotension (38,39). The mechanism is vancomycin-induced histamine release from mast cells (38). Slow infusions (less than 10 mg/minute) reduce the risk of this reaction.

Ototoxicity

Vancomycin can cause reversible hearing loss for high-frequency sounds when serum drug levels exceed 40 mg/L (37). Irreversible deafness has been reported when serum levels exceed 80 mg/L (37). Both complications are uncommon, possibly because serum drug levels are monitored frequently.

Nephrotoxicity

Reversible renal insufficiency is reported in 5% of patients receiving vancomycin (37). There is no relationship to vancomycin dose, but the incidence is higher during combined therapy with aminoglycosides. Many of the patients are seriously ill and have other reasons for renal impairment, so the nephrotoxic potential of vancomycin may be overstated.

COMMENT

Vancomycin is a valuable drug in the ICU because of its activity for methicillin-resistant and coagulase-negative staphylococci. However, it is clearly overused, and the emergence of vancomycin-resistant en-

TABLE 35.8. COST OF ANTIMICROBIAL THERAPY		
Agents	**Daily Dose**	**Daily Cost**
Aminoglucosides		
Gentamicin	240 mg	$6.75
Tobramycin	240 mg	$15.75
Amikacin	1200 mg	$153.00
Antifungal Agents		
Amphotericin	35 mg	$17.50
Fluconazole	400 mg	$162.50
Cephalosporins		
Cefazolin	4 g	$14.25
Ceftazidime	6 g	$86.50
Ceftriaxone	6 g	$72.70
Penicillins		
Pencillin G	10 million U	$6.40
Nafcillin	8 g	$48.80
Ticarcillin–clavulenate	12 g	$53.40
Others		
Aztreonam	3 g	$46.85
Ciprofloxacin	800 mg	$60.00
Imipenem–cilastatin	2 g	$116.95
Vancomycin	2 g	$28.00

Daily cost of drugs estimated from the average wholesale prices listed in the 1996 Redbook. Montvale, NJ: Medical Economics, 1996.

terococci should prompt clinicians to curtail the use of this agent in hospitalized patients.

REFERENCES

AMINOGLYCOSIDES

1. Edson RS, Terrell CL. The aminoglycosides. Mayo Clin Proc 1991;66: 1158–1164.
2. Walting DM, Dasta JF. Aminoglycoside dosing considerations in intensive care unit patients. Ann Pharmacother 1993;27:351–357.
3. Pancoast SJ. Aminoglycoside antibiotics in clinical use. Med Clin North Am 1988;72:581–612.
4. Triginer C, Izquierdo I, Fernandez R, et al. Gentamicin volume of distribution in critically ill septic patients. Intensive Care Med 1990;16:303–306.
5. Rotschafer JC, Zabinski RA, Walker KJ. Pharmacodynamic factors in antibiotic efficacy. Pharmacotherapy 1992;12:64S–70S.
6. Schumock GT, Raber SR, Crawford SY, et al. National survey of once-daily dosing of aminoglycoside antibiotics. Pharmacotherapy 1995;15:201–209.
7. Wilson SE. Aminoglycosides: assessing the potential for nephrotoxicity. Surg Gynecol Obstet 1986;171(Suppl):24–30.
8. Isenstein DA, Venner DS, Duggan J. Neuromuscular blockade in the intensive care unit. Chest 1992;102:1258–1266.
9. Drachman DB. Myasthenia gravis. N Engl J Med 1994;330:179–1810.

10. Lippmann M, Yang E, Au E, Lee C. Neuromuscular blocking effects of tobramycin, gentamicin, and cefazolin. Anesth Analg 1982;61:767–770.

ANTIFUNGAL AGENTS

11. Gallis HA, Drew RH, Pickard WW. Amphotericin B: 30 years of clinical experience. Rev Infect Dis 1990;12:308–329.
12. Bult J, Franklin CM. Using amphotericin B in the critically ill: a new look at an old drug. J Crit Illness 1996;11:577–585.
13. Carlson MA, Condon RE. Nephrotoxicity of amphotericin B. J Am Coll Surg 1994;179:361–381.
14. Terrell CL, Hughes CE. Antifungal agents used in deep-seated mycotic infections. Mayo Clin Proc 1992;67:69–91.
15. Anaissie E, Bodey GP, Kantarjian H, et al. Fluconazole therapy for chronic disseminated candidiasis in patients with leukemia and prior amphotericin therapy. Am J Med 1991;91:142–150.
16. Rex JH, Bennett JE, Sugar AM, et al. A randomized trial comparing fluconazole with amphotericin B for the treatment of candidemia in patients without neutropenia. N Engl J Med 1994;331:1325–1330.
17. Goodman JL, Winston DJ, Greenfield RA, et al. A controlled trial of fluconazole to prevent fungal infections in patients undergoing bone marrow transplantation. N Engl J Med 1992;326:845–851.
18. Crussel-Porter LL, Rindone JP, Ford MA, Jaskar DW. Low-dose fluconazole therapy potentiates the hypoprothrombinemic effect of warfarin sodium. Arch Intern Med 1993;153:102–104.
19. Cadle RM, Zenon GJ, Rodriguez-Barradas MC, Hamill RJ. Fluconazole-induced symptomatic phenytoin toxicity. Ann Pharmacother 1994;28:191–194.
20. Gearhart MO. Worsening of liver function with fluconazole and a review of azole antifungal hepatotoxicity. Ann Pharmacother 1994;28:1177–1181.

AZTREONAM

21. Brewer NS, Hellinger WC. The monobactams. Mayo Clin Proc 1991;66:1152–1157.
22. Bennett WM, Aronoff GR, Golper TA, et al., eds. Drug prescribing in renal failure. 3rd ed. Philadelphia: American College of Physicians, 1994.

CEPHALOSPORINS

23. Gustafferro CA, Steckelberg JM. Cephalosporin antimicrobial agents and related compounds. Mayo Clin Proc 1991;66:1064–1073.
24. Ramphal R, Gucalp R, Rotstein C, et al. Clinical experience with single agent and combination regimens in the management of infection in the febrile neutropenic patient. Am J Med 1996;100(Suppl 6A):83S–89S.
25. Pizzo PA. Choosing empiric therapy for febrile neutropenic patients. J Crit Illness 1995;10:165–168.

IMIPENEM

26. Hellinger WC, Brewer NS. Imipenem. Mayo Clin Proc 1991;66:1074–1081.
27. Freifield A, Walsh T, Marshall D, et al. Monotherapy for fever and neutropenia

in cancer patients: a randomized comparison of ceftazidime versus imipenem. J Clin Oncol 1995;13:165–176.

PENICILLINS

28. McEvoy GK, ed. AHFS drug information monographs. Bethesda, MD: American Society of Hospital Pharmacists, 1995;225–338.

QUINOLONES

29. Walker RC, Wright AJ. The fluoroquinolones. Mayo Clin Proc 1991;66: 1249–1259.
30. Kljucar S, Heimesaat M, von Pritzbuer E, et al. A comparison of intravenous ciprofloxacin dosage regimens in severe nosocomial infections. Infect Med 1992;9(Suppl B):58–72.
31. Allon M, Lopez EJ, Min K-W. Acute renal failure due to ciprofloxacin. Arch Intern Med 1990;150:2187–2189.
32. Moore B, Safani M, Keesey J. Possible exacerbation of myasthenia gravis by ciprofloxacin. Lancet 1988;1:882.
33. Robson RA. The effects of quinolones on xanthine pharmacokinetics. Am J Med 1992;92(Suppl 4A):22S–26S.
34. Maddix DS. Do we need an intravenous fluoroquinolone? West J Med 1992; 157:55–59.

VANCOMYCIN

35. Wilhelm HP. Vancomycin. Mayo Clin Proc 1991;66:1170–1191.
36. Gin AS, Zhanel GG. Vancomycin-resistant enterococci. Ann Pharmacother 1996;30:615–623.
37. Saunders NJ. Why monitor peak vancomycin concentrations? Lancet 1994; 344:1748–1750.
38. Levy JH, Kettlekamp N, Goertz P, et al. Histamine release by vancomycin: the mechanism for hypotension in man. Anesthesiology 1987;67:122–125.
39. Romanelli VA, Howie MB, Myerowitz D, et al. Intraoperative and postoperative effects of vancomycin administration in cardiac surgery patients: a prospective, double-blind, randomized trial. Crit Care Med 1993;21:1124–1131.

GENERAL WORKS

Mayo Clinic Proceedings Symposium on Antimicrobial Agents. Rochester, MN: Mayo Clinic Proceedings, 1992.

section IX

ACID-BASE DISORDERS

*Life is a struggle, not against sin, not against
Money Power, . . . but against hydrogen ions.*
                                    H.L. Mencken

c h a p t e r

ACID-BASE INTERPRETATIONS

A little learning is a dangerous thing.
Drink deep, or taste not the Pyrean spring.
Alexander Pope

In a survey conducted at a university teaching hospital (1), 70% of the participating physicians claimed that they were well versed in the diagnosis of acid-base disorders and that they needed no assistance in the interpretation of arterial blood gases (ABGs). These same physicians were then given a series of ABG measurements to interpret, and they correctly interpreted only 40% of the test samples. A survey at another teaching hospital revealed that incorrect acid-base interpretations led to errors in patient management in one-third of the ABG samples analyzed (2). These surveys reveal serious deficiencies in an area that tends to be ignored. This can cause trouble in the ICU, where 9 of every 10 patients may have an acid-base disorder (3).

This chapter presents a structured approach to acid-base interpretations based on a set of well-defined rules that are applied to ABG analysis (4–8). This approach is taken from a computer program that interprets ABGs (8), so it should work.

BASIC CONCEPTS

The hydrogen ion concentration $[H^+]$ in extracellular fluid is determined by the balance between the partial pressure of carbon dioxide (P_{CO_2}) and the concentration of bicarbonate $[HCO_3]$ in the fluid. This relationship is expressed as follows (3):

$$[H^+] \text{ in nEq/L} = 24 \times (P_{CO_2}/[HCO_3]) \qquad (36.1)$$

Using a normal arterial P_{CO_2} of 40 mm Hg and a normal serum HCO_3 concentration of 24 mEq/L, the normal $[H^+]$ in arterial blood is $24 \times (40/24) = 40$ nEq/L.

[H$^+$] AND PH

Note that the [H$^+$] in extracellular fluid is expressed in *nano*equivalents (nEq) per liter. A nanoequivalent is *one-millionth* of a milliequivalent, so there are millions more sodium, chloride, and other ions measured in mEq than there are hydrogen ions. Because nanoequivalents is a cumbersome term, the [H$^+$] is routinely expressed in pH units, which are derived by taking the negative logarithm (base 10) of the [H$^+$] in nEq/L. The relationship between pH and [H$^+$] is shown in Figure 36.1. A normal [H$^+$] of 40 nEq/L corresponds to a pH of 7.40. Because the pH is a negative logarithm of the [H$^+$], changes in pH are inversely related to changes in [H$^+$] (e.g., a decrease in pH is associated with an increase in [H$^+$]). Note that as the pH decreases from its highest value (7.60), the slope of the curve progressively increases. Thus, as the pH decreases, a progressively larger change occurs in [H$^+$] associated with a given change in pH. The numbers above the curve indicate the change in [H$^+$] associated with each change of 0.1 pH units. Over the normal pH range from 7.36 to 7.44 (indicated by the shaded area in Figure 36.1), the change in [H$^+$] is less than 10 nEq/L (this shows how tightly the [H$^+$] is controlled). At the acidotic end of the curve, the change in [H$^+$] is more than threefold higher than at the alkalotic end of the curve (20 nEq/L versus 6 nEq/L per 0.1 pH unit, respectively). Therefore, the acid-base conse-

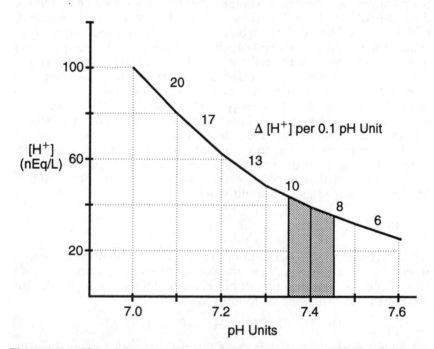

Figure 36.1. The relationship between hydrogen ion concentration [H$^+$] and pH. The numbers above the curve indicate the change in [H$^+$] associated with a change of 0.1 pH unit. The shaded area shows the normal pH range in extracellular fluid.

TABLE 36.1. PRIMARY AND SECONDARY ACID-BASE DERANGEMENTS

End-Point: A constant $\dfrac{P_{CO_2}}{HCO_3}$ ratio

Acid-Base Disorder	Primary Change	Compensatory Change
Respiratory acidosis	↑ P_{CO_2}	↑ HCO_3
Respiratory alkalosis	↓ P_{CO_2}	↓ HCO_3
Metabolic acidosis	↓ HCO_3	↓ P_{CO_2}
Metabolic alkalosis	↑ HCO_3	↑ P_{CO_2}

quences of a given change in pH depends on the underlying acid-base status of the patient.

COMPENSATORY CHANGES

According to the determinants of $[H^+]$ shown earlier, the stability of the extracellular pH is determined by the stability of the P_{CO_2}/HCO_3 ratio. Maintaining a constant P_{CO_2}/HCO_3 ratio will maintain a constant extracellular pH. This is the basis for the primary and compensatory acid-base changes shown in Table 36.1. When a primary acid-base disturbance alters one component of the P_{CO_2}/HCO_3 ratio, the compensatory response alters the other component in the same direction to keep the P_{CO_2}/HCO_3 ratio constant. Thus, when the primary disorder is metabolic (i.e., a change in HCO_3), the compensatory response is respiratory (i.e., a change in P_{CO_2}), and vice-versa. It is important to emphasize that compensatory responses limit rather than prevent changes in pH (i.e., compensation is not synonymous with correction).

Respiratory Compensation

The ventilatory control system provides the compensation for metabolic acid-base disturbances, and the response is prompt. The changes in ventilation are mediated by H^+-sensitive chemoreceptors located in the carotid body (at the carotid bifurcation in the neck) and in the lower brainstem. A metabolic acidosis excites the chemoreceptors and initiates a prompt increase in ventilation and a decrease in arterial P_{CO_2}. A metabolic alkalosis silences the chemoreceptors and produces a prompt decrease in ventilation and increase in arterial P_{CO_2}. When these ventilatory responses are fully functional, the compensatory, or expected, arterial P_{CO_2} can be defined according to the equations shown in Table 36.2. The compensatory response to metabolic alkalosis has varied in different reports; however, the equation shown in Table 36.2 has proven reliable, at least up to a HCO_3 level of 40 mEq/L (9).

Metabolic Compensation

The kidneys provide the compensation for respiratory acid-base disorders by adjusting HCO_3 reabsorption in the proximal tubules. Respiratory acidosis stimulates HCO_3 reabsorption, which increases the serum HCO_3 concentration, whereas respiratory alkalosis inhibits HCO_3 reabsorption, which decreases the serum HCO_3 concentration.

TABLE 36.2. EXPECTED CHANGES IN ACID-BASE DISORDERS	
Primary Disorder	**Expected Changes**
Metabolic acidosis	$P_{CO_2} = 1.5 \times HCO_3 + (8 \pm 2)$
Metabolic alkalosis	$P_{CO_2} = 0.7 \times HCO_3 + (21 \pm 2)$
Acute respiratory acidosis	$\Delta pH = 0.008 \times (P_{CO_2} - 40)$
Chronic respiratory acidosis	$\Delta pH = 0.003 \times (P_{CO_2} - 40)$
Acute respiratory alkalosis	$\Delta pH = 0.008 \times (40 - P_{CO_2})$
Chronic respiratory alkalosis	$\Delta pH = 0.017 \times (40 - P_{CO_2})$

However, the compensatory response in the kidneys is not immediate. It begins to appear in 6 to 12 hours and slowly increases to a steady-state response over the next few days. Because of this delay in renal compensation, respiratory acid-base disorders are classified as acute (before renal compensation begins) and chronic (after renal compensation is fully developed). The changes in pH that accompany the acute and chronic respiratory disorders can be defined using the equations shown in Table 36.2.

THE RULES OF ACID-BASE INTERPRETATION

The approach that follows is based on three acid-base variables: pH, P_{CO_2}, and HCO_3. The reference ranges for each of these variables is shown below (3). Any measurement that falls outside of these ranges is considered to be abnormal.

$$pH = 7.36 \text{ to } 7.44$$
$$P_{CO_2} = 36 \text{ to } 44 \text{ mm Hg}$$
$$HCO_3 = 22 \text{ to } 26 \text{ mEq/L} \tag{36.2}$$

PRIMARY METABOLIC DISORDERS

Rule 1. A primary metabolic acid-base disorder is present if the pH is abnormal and the pH and P_{CO_2} change in the same direction.

Thus, a primary *metabolic acidosis* is present if the arterial pH is below 7.36 and the arterial P_{CO_2} (Pa_{CO_2}) is decreased, whereas a primary *metabolic alkalosis* is present if the pH is above 7.44 and the Pa_{CO_2} is increased. If a primary metabolic acid-base disorder is identified, proceed to Rule 2.

Rule 2. A superimposed respiratory acid-base disorder is present if any of the following conditions are satisfied.

The measured P_{CO_2} is normal.
The measured P_{CO_2} is higher than the expected P_{CO_2} (this indicates a superimposed respiratory *acidosis*).
The measured P_{CO_2} is less than the expected P_{CO_2} (this indicates a superimposed respiratory *alkalosis*).

Thus, once a primary metabolic disorder has been identified, the appropriate equation in Table 36.2 should be used to define the P_{CO_2} that is expected with full respiratory compensation. If the measured

P_{CO_2} is above or below the expected P_{CO_2}, a *combined* (metabolic and respiratory) acid-base disorder is present.

PRIMARY RESPIRATORY DISORDERS

Rule 3. A primary respiratory acid-base disorder is present if the Pa_{CO_2} is abnormal and the Pa_{CO_2} and pH change in opposite directions.

Thus, a primary *respiratory acidosis* is present if the Pa_{CO_2} is above 44 mm Hg and the arterial pH is decreased, whereas a *respiratory alkalosis* is present if the Pa_{CO_2} is below 36 mm Hg and the arterial pH is increased. If a primary respiratory acid-base disorder is identified, proceed to Rule 4.

Rule 4. The expected change in pH (determined by using the equations in Table 36.2) is used to determine whether the respiratory disorder is acute or chronic and whether a superimposed metabolic acid-base disorder is present.

> If the change in pH is 0.008 times the change in Pa_{CO_2}, the respiratory disorder is *acute* (uncompensated).
> If the change in pH is 0.003 to 0.008 times the change in Pa_{CO_2}, the respiratory disorder is *partially compensated*.
> If the change in pH is 0.003 times the change in Pa_{CO_2}, the respiratory disorder is *chronic* (fully compensated).
> If the change in pH is more than 0.008 times the change in Pa_{CO_2}, a superimposed metabolic acid-base disorder is present.

For example, if the P_{CO_2} has increased to 50 mm Hg, then an acute respiratory acidosis would have a decrease in pH of (0.008 × 10 mm Hg) 0.08 pH units, a chronic respiratory acidosis would have a change in pH of (0.003 × 10 mm Hg) 0.03 pH units, and a partially compensated respiratory acidosis would have a change in pH between 0.03 and 0.08 pH units. If the decrease in pH is greater than 0.08 pH units, then a superimposed metabolic acidosis is present.

MIXED DISORDERS

Rule 5. A mixed (acidosis and alkalosis) acid-base disorder is present if the Pa_{CO_2} is abnormal and the pH is unchanged or normal, or if the pH is abnormal and the Pa_{CO_2} is unchanged or normal.

This rule is based on the fact that compensatory responses to primary acid-base disorder do not completely correct the primary abnormality. Therefore, if the Pa_{CO_2} is 50 mm Hg and the pH is 7.40, the compensatory change in pH is more than expected, indicating that there is a metabolic alkalosis in addition to the compensated respiratory acidosis.

RULE-ORIENTED ACID-BASE INTERPRETATIONS

This section illustrates how the 5 rules just described can be applied to the interpretation of ABGs. Each of the interpretation begins with the arterial pH.

ACIDEMIA

If the pH is below 7.36, check the P_{CO_2} and proceed as follows:

A low or normal Pa_{CO_2} indicates a primary metabolic acidosis (Rule 1).

The difference between the measured and expected Pa_{CO_2} is then used to identify a superimposed respiratory disorder (Rule 2).

A high P_{CO_2} indicates a primary respiratory acidosis (Rule 3).

The change in pH is then used to determine whether the disorder is acute or chronic, or whether a superimposed metabolic acid-base disorder is present (Rule 4).

ALKALEMIA

If the pH is above 7.44, check the P_{CO_2} and proceed as follows:

A normal or high Pa_{CO_2} indicates a primary metabolic alkalosis (Rule 1).

A comparison of the measured and expected Pa_{CO_2} is then used to identify an associated respiratory disorder (Rule 2).

A low Pa_{CO_2} indicates a primary respiratory alkalosis (Rule 3).

The change in pH is then used to determine whether the disorder is acute or chronic, or whether a superimposed metabolic disorder is present (Rule 4).

NORMAL PH

If the arterial pH is unchanged or normal, the P_{CO_2} should be checked:

A high P_{CO_2} indicates a mixed respiratory acidosis-metabolic alkalosis (Rule 5).

A low P_{CO_2} indicates a mixed respiratory alkalosis-metabolic acidosis (Rule 5).

A normal pH combined with a normal Pa_{CO_2} is not absolute evidence against an acid-base disorder because a metabolic acidosis coexisting with a metabolic alkalosis can be accompanied by a normal pH and Pa_{CO_2}.

THE ANION GAP

The anion gap (AG) is an acid-base parameter that is used to evaluate patients with a metabolic acidosis to determine whether the problem is an accumulation of hydrogen ions (e.g., lactic acidosis) or a loss of bicarbonate (e.g., diarrhea). Although it does not perform well in certain situations, the AG can still provide valuable information when it is used judiciously (10).

THE CONCEPT

To achieve electrochemical balance the ionic elements in the extracellular fluid must have a net charge of zero. Thus, the concentration of negatively-charged anions and positively-charged cations must balance. All ions participate in this balance, both those that are routinely measured, such as sodium (Na), chloride (Cl), and bicarbonate (HCO_3), and those that are not measured. The unmeasured cations (UC) and unmeasured anions (UA) have the following relationships to the commonly measured electrolytes:

$$Na + UC = (Cl + HCO_3) + UA \qquad (36.3)$$

or when the terms are rearranged:

$$Na - (CL + HCO_3) = UA - UC \qquad (36.4)$$

The relationship (UA − UC) is a measurement of the relative abundance of unmeasured anions and is called the AG.

Determinants

The anions and cations that contribute to the AG are shown in Table 36.3. The plasma proteins are the major source of unmeasured anions, whereas potassium and calcium make up the bulk of the unmeasured cations (describing these electrolytes as unmeasured is hardly appropriate). The charge difference between the two groups reveals an anion excess (anion gap) of 12 mEq/L. Much of this difference is due to the plasma proteins. For example, **a 50% reduction in plasma proteins can result in a 75% reduction in the AG** (from 12 to 4 mEq/L), as indicated at the bottom of Table 36.3. Most of the charge donated by plasma proteins is from albumin, so hypoalbuminemia can have a significant influence in reducing the AG (3).

Reference Range

The normal range for the AG was originally defined as 8 to 16 mEq/L (11,12). However this range was defined using automated systems for electrolyte measurements (the SMA-6 and SMA-12) that are no longer used in most clinical laboratories. Using the newer automated systems (e.g., the ASTRA), the normal range for the AG is 3 to 11 mEq/L (12), which is lower than the original reference range. The significance of this lower reference range is unclear, and it adds more confusion to the interpretation of the AG.

METABOLIC ACIDOSIS

As mentioned previously, the AG has been used to identify certain types of metabolic acidosis. Specifically, it is used to differentiate be-

TABLE 36.3. DETERMINANTS OF THE ANION GAP	
Unmeasured Anions	Unmeasured Cations
Proteins (15 mEq/L)	Calcium (5 mEq/L)
Organic acids (5 mEq/L)	Potassium (4.5 mEq/L)
Phosphates (2 mEq/L)	Magnesium (1.5 mEq/L)
Sulfates (1 mEq/L)	
UA: 23 mEq/L	UC: 11 mEq/L
Anion Gap = UA − UC = 12 mEq/L	
If plasma proteins are reduced by 50%, Anion gap = 4 mEq/L	

tween metabolic acidoses caused by an accumulation of hydrogen ions and metabolic acidoses caused by a loss of bicarbonate ions.

High Anion Gap

When a metabolic acidosis is due to the accumulation of hydrogen ions in the extracellular fluid (e.g., lactic acidosis), the hydrogen ions combine with bicarbonate to form carbonic acid. This decreases the bicarbonate concentration in the extracellular fluid, which in turn increases the AG (as predicted by the relationship $AG = Na - [CL + HCO_3]$). Therefore, **a metabolic acidosis with a high AG is most likely caused by** organic acid accumulation (i.e., **lactic acid or ketoacids**) or **renal failure** with impaired hydrogen ion excretion.

Although a high AG can be helpful in the setting of a metabolic acidosis, it should not be used as evidence of a metabolic acidosis unless it exceeds 30 mEq/L (13). In fact, an elevated AG can be a sign of an underlying metabolic *alkalosis*. That is, alkalosis can elevate the AG, presumably by increasing the strength of the negative charge on albumin molecules (10,11).

Normal Anion Gap

When a metabolic acidosis is caused by the loss of bicarbonate ions from the extracellular fluid (e.g., diarrhea), the bicarbonate loss is counterbalanced by a gain of chloride ions to maintain electrical charge neutrality. Because the increase in chloride concentration is proportional to the decrease in bicarbonate concentration, the AG remains unchanged. Therefore, **a metabolic acidosis with a normal AG** is taken as a sign of a bicarbonate-wasting process, such as **diarrhea** or increased bicarbonate losses in the urine in **early renal failure.**

Reliability

The AG has not been proven to be a sensitive marker of organic acid accumulation (i.e., lactic acidosis). Although lactic acid accumulation should be accompanied by a high AG, **numerous reports of lactic acidosis with a normal anion gap** exist (14,15). In a recent case report, the AG was only 11 mEq/L, despite a markedly elevated serum lactate of 13 mEq/L (15). Some of these cases can be explained by the presence of conditions that could prevent the AG from increasing in response to acid accumulation (e.g., hypoalbuminemia) (16). However, this does not add to the poor performance of the AG as a screen for lactic acidosis.

MIXED METABOLIC DISTURBANCES

Mixed metabolic disturbances (e.g., high AG from ketoacidosis plus normal AG from diarrhea) can be identified using the relationship between the increase in AG and the decrease in serum HCO_3. This relationship is expressed as the AG excess/HCO_3 deficit ratio, which is sometimes called the *gap-gap*.

$$\text{AG excess/HCO}_3 \text{ deficit} = (AG - 12/24 - HCO_3) \quad (36.5)$$

MIXED METABOLIC ACIDOSES

When hydrogen ions accumulate in blood, the decrease in serum HCO_3 is equivalent to the increase in AG and the AG excess/HCO_3 deficit ratio is unity. When a hyperchloremic acidosis is present, the ratio approaches zero. When a mixed acidosis (high AG + normal AG) is present, the AG excess/HCO_3 deficit ratio indicates the relative contribution of each type to the acidosis. For example, a ratio of 0.5 indicates an equivalent contribution from high AG and normal AG acidoses.

Diabetic Ketoacidosis

Diabetic ketoacidosis is expected to present as a high AG metabolic acidosis. However, **after therapy** with fluids and insulin **begins, the high AG acidosis changes to a normal AG acidosis** (17). This is partly due to the chloride load in the intravenous fluids. In this situation, the serum bicarbonate remains low (dilutional effect) but the AG excess/HCO_3 deficit ratio shows a steady decline. In this situation, the persistent decrease in serum HCO_3 will create a false impression that the ketoacids are not being cleared. This illustrates the value of the AG excess/HCO_3 deficit ratio for the management of patients with ketoacidosis.

MIXED ACIDOSIS–ALKALOSIS

When alkali is added in the presence of a high AG acidosis, the decrease in serum bicarbonate is less than the decrease in AG and the AG excess/HCO_3 deficit ratio is greater than unity. Metabolic alkalosis is common in the ICU because of the popularity of nasogastric suction and diuretics. Therefore, mixed metabolic acidosis and alkalosis may be more common than suspected.

VENOUS BLOOD GASES

ABG analysis continues to thrive, despite the fact that the acid-base status in arterial blood is not likely to reflect the acid-base status in the peripheral tissues. The discrepancy between arterial and venous blood gases is shown in Figure 36.2. (18). These data are taken from a study of 16 patients in the ICU with indwelling pulmonary artery catheters who had experienced a cardiac arrest. The measurements were obtained during cardiopulmonary resuscitation. Note that the arterial blood appears reasonably normal (pH is 7.41 and Pco_2 is 32 mm Hg) and that the venous blood reveals severe acidemia (pH of 1.5) and hypercapnia (Pco_2 of 74 mm Hg). Thus, even in the most extreme conditions, the arterial blood is not a sensitive marker of the acid-base conditions at the tissue level. Remember this when performing cardiopulmonary resuscitation.

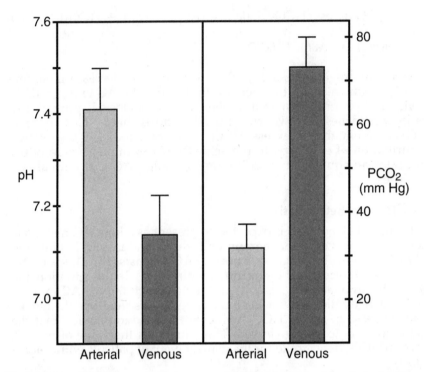

Figure 36.2. Acid-base parameters in arterial and venous blood during cardiopulmonary resuscitation. Height of the vertical columns indicates the mean; cross-bars indicate standard deviation. Study group: 16 adult patients. (From Weil MH, Rackow EC, Trevino R, et al. Difference in acid-base state between venous and arterial blood during cardiopulmonary resuscitation. N Engl J Med 1986;315:153–156.)

REFERENCES

SUGGESTED READINGS

Arieff AI, DeFronzo RA, eds. Fluid electrolyte and acid-base disorders. New York: Churchill Livingstone, 1985.
Rose BD. Clinical physiology of acid-base and electrolyte disorders. 4th ed. New York: McGraw-Hill, 1994.

INTRODUCTION

1. Hingston DM. A computerized interpretation of arterial pH and blood gas data: do physicians need it? Respir Care 1982;27:809–815.
2. Broughton JO, Kennedy TC. Interpretation of arterial blood gases by computer. Chest 1984;85:148–149.
3. Gilfix BM, Bique M, Magder S. A physical chemical approach to the analysis of acid-base balance in the clinical setting. J Crit Care 1993;8:187–197.

COMPREHENSIVE REVIEWS

4. Narins RG, Emmett M. Simple and mixed acid-base disorders: a practical approach. Medicine 1980;59:161–187 (89 references).
5. Laski ME, Kurtzman NA. Acid-base disorders in medicine. Dis Mon 1996; XLII:57–128 (200 references).

MINIREVIEWS

6. Morganroth M. An analytical approach to diagnosing acid-base disorders. J Crit Illness 1990;5:138–150 (5 references).
7. Haber RJ. A practical approach to acid-base disorders. West J Med 1991;155: 146–151 (22 references).

SOFTWARE

8. Krasner J, Marino PL. Respiratory expert. Philadelphia: WB Saunders, 1987.

SELECTED REFERENCES

9. Javaheri S, Kazemi H. Metabolic alkalosis and hypoventilation in humans. Am Rev Respir Dis 1987;136:1011–1016.
10. Emmet M, Narins RG. Clinical use of the anion gap. Medicine 1977;56:38–54.
11. Oster JR, Perez GO, Materson BJ. Use of the anion gap in clinical medicine. South Med J 1988;81:229–237.
12. Winter SD, Pearson JR, Gabow PA, et al. The fall of the serum anion gap. Arch Intern Med 1990;150:311–313.
13. Gabow PA, Kaehny WD, Fennessey PV. Diagnostic importance of an increased anion gap. N Engl J Med 1980;303:854–858.
14. Iberti TS, Liebowitz AB, Papadakos PJ, et al. Low sensitivity of the anion gap as a screen to detect hyperlactatemia in critically ill patients. Crit Care Med 1990;18:275–277.
15. Schwartz-Goldstein B, Malik AR, Sarwar A, Brandtsetter RD. Lactic acidosis associated with a normal anion gap. Heart Lung 1996;25:79–80.
16. Ernest D, Herkes RG, Raper RF. Alterations in the anion gap following cardiopulmonary bypass. Crit Care Med 1992;20:52–56.
17. Paulson WD. Anion gap-bicarbonate relationship in diabetic ketoacidosis. Am J Med 1986;81:995–1000.
18. Weil MH, Rackow EC, Trevino R. Difference in acid-base state between venous and arterial blood during cardiopulmonary resuscitation. N Engl J Med 1986; 315:153–156.

37

THE ORGANIC ACIDOSES

This chapter focuses on the clinical disorders produced by the accumulation of organic acids (i.e., lactic acid and ketoacids) in the extracellular fluid. The important dictum to emphasize in these conditions is that the acid-base disturbance is not the primary illness, but it is a clinical marker of an underlying pathologic disorder. Therefore, the focus should be on identifying and correcting the pathologic disorder rather than treating the acid-base disturbance.

LACTIC ACIDOSIS

LACTATE METABOLISM

Lactate is the end-product of anaerobic glycolysis and is normally produced at a rate of 1 mmol/kg/hour (or 1920 mmol/day for a 175-lb adult) (1–4). The overall reaction for anaerobic glycolysis is as follows:

$$\text{Glucose} + 2\ \text{ATP} + 2\ H_2PO_4 \rightarrow 2\ \text{Lactate} + 2\ \text{ADP} + 2\ H_2O$$

$$(37.1)$$

Note that the reaction produces lactate, a negatively-charged ion, *not* lactic acid. The hydrogen ions needed to convert lactate to lactic acid must be generated by the hydrolysis of ATP (5). Therefore, lactate production is not synonymous with lactic acid production. Most of the lactate production occurs in skeletal muscle, bowel, brain, and circulating erythrocytes. The lactate generated in these tissues can be taken up by the liver and converted to glucose (via gluconeogenesis) or can be used as a primary oxidative fuel.

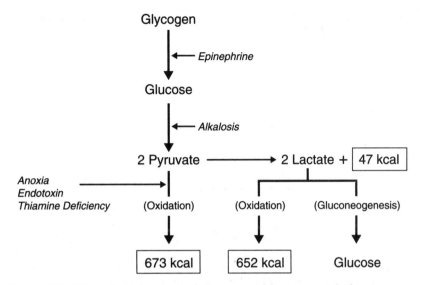

Figure 37.1. The salient features of glucose and lactate metabolism.

Energetics

The energy yield from glucose metabolism is outlined in Figure 37.1 (see also Table 13.5). The anaerobic metabolism of glucose generates 47 kilocalories (kcal) of energy per mole of glucose, whereas the aerobic metabolism of glucose generates 673 kcal per mole of glucose (6). Therefore, the energy yield from anaerobic glycolysis is only 7% of the energy yield from aerobic glucose metabolism. However, **lactate can serve as an oxidative fuel,** and the oxidative use of lactate can correct the energy deficit associated with anaerobic glycolysis. The oxidation of lactate generates 326 kcal per mole of lactate (6), and because 1 mole of glucose generates 2 moles of lactate, the energy yield from anaerobic glycolysis will be increased by 652 (2 × 326) kcal per mole of glucose if the lactate that is generated is completely oxidized. This role of lactate as an oxidative fuel (called the lactate shuttle) has been described in exercise (7), and it may also be operative in the developing stages of clinical shock. For example, when the skeletal muscles become anaerobic in the early stages of clinical shock, the lactate that is generated could be used as a source of energy by other vital organs that are not yet anaerobic, such as the heart and central nervous system.

Hyperlactatemia

The normal concentration of lactate in blood is less than 2 mmol/L while at rest, and up to 5 mmol/L during exercise (2–4). Therefore, a resting blood lactate level above 2 mmol/L is considered abnormal. However, mild elevations in blood lactate (2 to 4 mmol/L) may not be accompanied by an acidosis. Therefore, **hyperlactatemia is not synonymous with lactic acidosis.**

ETIOLOGIES

The principal causes of hyperlactatemia and lactic acidosis are indicated in italicized print in Figure 37.1.

Oxygen Deprivation

The single most important cause of lactic acidosis is deficient cell oxygenation in shock (e.g., hypovolemic, cardiogenic, and septic shock). **Hypoxemia and anemia,** which are presumed to cause impaired cellular oxygenation, **are rarely accompanied by lactic acidosis.** The lack of association between severe hypoxemia and hyperlactatemia is shown in Table 24.1. The inability of severe anemia to produce hyperlactatemia is described in Chapter 44.

In patients with clinical shock, the severity of the hyperlactatemia has prognostic value (2–4,8–10). This is demonstrated in Figure 37.2. Note that when the blood lactate level rises to 10 mmol/L, the chances of survival are negligible. The prognostic value of blood lactate levels pertains only to patients with clinical shock.

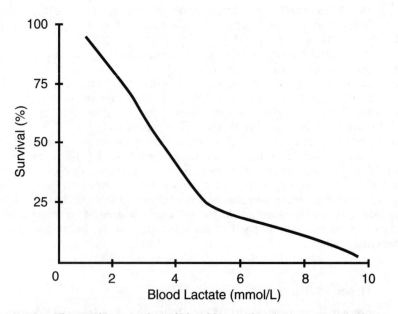

Figure 37.2. The predictive value of blood lactate levels in patients with circulatory shock. (From Weil MH, Afifi AA. Experimental and clinical studies on lactate and pyruvate as indicators of the severity of acute circulatory failure [shock]. Circulation 1970;16:989–1001.)

Endotoxemia

As described in Chapter 13, endotoxemia can elevate blood lactate levels without producing cellular oxygen deprivation (see Figure 13.5). This effect is due to endotoxin-mediated inhibition of pyruvate dehydrogenase, the enzyme that initiates pyruvate oxidation in the mitochondria (11). This effect implies that **sepsis** with endotoxin-producing gram-negative organisms **can be a source of hyperlactatemia in the absence of septic shock.** This may explain the reported association between lactic acidosis and the acquired immunodeficiency syndrome (12).

Thiamine Deficiency

Thiamine serves as a co-factor for the pyruvate dehydrogenase enzyme that initiates pyruvate oxidation in the mitochondria. Therefore, thiamine deficiency can be accompanied by hyperlactatemia (13). As with endotoxemia, the hyperlactatemia in thiamine deficiency may not be accompanied by evidence of clinical shock. Because thiamine deficiency may be common in critically ill patients (see Chapter 46), this diagnosis should be considered in all cases of unexplained hyperlactatemia in the ICU.

Alkalosis

Severe alkalosis (respiratory or metabolic) can raise blood lactate levels (14) because the increased activity in pH-dependent enzymes in the glycolytic pathway promotes lactate production. When liver function is normal, the liver clears the extra lactate generated during alkalosis and hyperlactatemia becomes evident only when the pH of the blood is 7.6 or higher. However, in patients with impaired liver function, hyperlactatemia can be seen with less severe alkalemia. Alkalosis-enhanced lactate formation is an undesirable consequence of alkali therapy for lactic acidosis.

Others

Other possible causes of hyperlactatemia in patients in the ICU are **seizures** (from increased lactate production), **hepatic insufficiency** (from reduced lactate clearance), **epinephrine infusions** (from enhanced glycogenolysis with increased lactate production), **nitroprusside toxicity** (from cyanide accumulation), and **acute asthma** (possibly from enhanced lactate production by the respiratory muscles) (15–17). Hyperlactatemia associated with epinephrine infusions and hepatic insufficiency is often mild and not accompanied by lactic acidosis (15). Hyperlactatemia that accompanies generalized seizures can be severe but is transient (16). Hyperlactatemia during nitroprusside infusions is a manifestation of cyanide intoxication and is an ominous sign (see Chapter 53).

DIAGNOSIS

Hyperlactatemia is a possible cause of any metabolic acidosis in a critically ill patient, regardless of the anion gap.

The Anion Gap

As described in Chapter 36, the anion gap should be elevated in lactic acidosis, but there are numerous reports of a normal anion gap in patients with lactic acidosis (16,18). Therefore, **the anion gap should not be used as a screening test for possible lactic acidosis.** For more information on the anion gap, see Chapter 36.

Blood Lactate

Lactate concentrations can be measured in plasma or whole blood. A lactate-specific electrode that requires a blood sample of only 0.13 mL is available and can complete the lactate measurement in less than 2 minutes (10). This electrode is combined with other substrate-specific electrodes in a portable chemistry analyzer (NOVA SP7, NOVA Biomedical, Waltham, Massachusetts) that can be used at the bedside. If immediate measurements are unavailable, the blood sample should be placed on ice to retard lactate production by red blood cells in the sample.

A lactate level above 2 mmol/L (in plasma or whole blood) is abnormal, and in patients with circulatory shock, a blood lactate level above 4 mmol/L is evidence of significant tissue oxygen deficits (see Table 13.1). The prognostic value of the 2 mmol/L versus 4 mmol/L threshold in patients with suspected shock is shown in Table 13.4.

D-LACTIC ACIDOSIS

The lactate produced by mammalian tissues is a levo-isomer (bends light to the left), whereas a dextro-isomer of lactate (bends light to the right) is produced by certain strains of bacteria that can populate the bowel (19). D-lactate generated by bacterial fermentation in the bowel can gain access to the systemic circulation and produce a metabolic acidosis, often combined with a metabolic encephalopathy (20). Most cases of D-lactic acidosis have been reported after extensive small bowel resection or after jejunoileal bypass for morbid obesity (19–21).

Diagnosis

D-lactic acidosis can produce an elevated anion gap. However, the standard laboratory assays for blood lactate measure only L-lactate and will miss D-lactic acidosis. Most clinical laboratories will perform a specific assay for D-lactate on request.

ALKALI THERAPY FOR LACTIC ACIDOSIS

The primary goal of therapy in lactic acidosis is to correct the under-lying metabolic abnormality. Alkali therapy aimed at preventing se-vere acidemia (i.e., serum pH below 7.2) has also been popular (22) but is of questionable value. The alkali therapy's lack of value is evident in the most recent recommendations of the American Heart Association to avoid bicarbonate therapy during cardiac arrest (see Table 17.5). The following issues are relevant to the use of alkali therapy in lactic acidosis.

RATIONALE

The principal fear in acidosis is the risk of impaired myocardial contractility (23). However, in the intact organism, acidemia is often accompanied by an increase in cardiac output (24). This is explained by the ability of acidosis to stimulate catecholamine release from the adrenals and to produce vasodilation. Therefore, impaired contractil-ity from acidosis is less of a concern in the intact organism. Further-more, acidosis may have a protective role in the setting of clinical shock. For example, extracellular acidosis has been shown to protect energy-depleted cells from cell death (25).

PROTOCOL

Alkali therapy is carried out with sodium bicarbonate solutions such as the ones shown in Table 37.1. Bicarbonate administration is guided by the estimated deficit in the bicarbonate (HCO_3) buffer pool:

$$HCO_3 \text{ deficit (mEq)} = 0.6 \times wt\,(kg)$$

(37.2)

$$\times (\text{desired } HCO_3 - \text{measured } HCO_3)$$

The body weight in this equation is *lean body weight*. The factor 0.6 represents the apparent bicarbonate space (a reflection of total body buffering capacity), which is 60% of the body weight in mild to moder-ate acidosis (26). In severe acidosis (serum HCO_3 less than 10 mEq/L), the apparent bicarbonate space is increased to 70% of the body

TABLE 37.1. BICARBONATE-CONTAINING BUFFER SOLUTIONS		
	7.5% NaHCO$_3$	Carbicarb
Sodium	0.9 mEq/mL	0.9 mEq/mL
Bicarbonate	0.9 mEq/mL	0.3 mEq/mL
Dicarbonate	—	0.3 mEq/mL
Pco$_2$	>200 mm Hg	3 mm Hg
Osmolality	1461 mOsm/kg	1667 mOsm/Kg
pH (25°C)	8.0	9.6

weight, so 0.7 can be used in Equation 37.2 when the measured serum HCO_3 is below 10 mEq/L (26).

In the absence of a superimposed respiratory acid-base disorder, a serum HCO_3 of 15 mEq/L should be sufficient to keep the serum pH in a safe range. Therefore, a desired HCO_3 of 15 mEq/L can be used to calculate the bicarbonate deficit. One-half of the bicarbonate deficit is replaced immediately, and the remaining deficit is infused over the next 4 to 6 hours.

EFFICACY

The administration of sodium bicarbonate has limited success in raising the serum pH in patients with lactic acidosis (27). This has been attributed to the tendency of bicarbonate to generate CO_2, a volatile acid. However, a simpler explanation is provided by examining the titration curve for the carbonic acid-bicarbonate buffer system, which is shown in Figure 37.3. The HCO_3 buffer pool is generated by the dissociation of carbonic acid (H_2CO_3):

$$CO_2 + H_2O \leftrightarrow H_2CO_3 \leftrightarrow H^+ + HCO_3^- \qquad (37.3)$$

The dissociation constant (pK) for carbonic acid (i.e., the pH at which the acid is 50% dissociated) is 6.1, as indicated on the titration curve. Buffers are most effective within 1 pH unit on either side of the pK

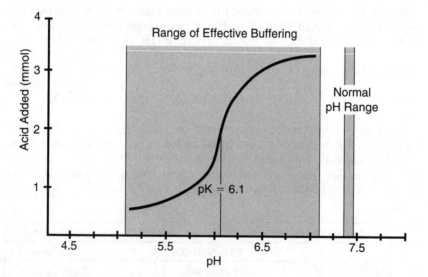

Figure 37.3. The titration curve for the carbonic acid-bicarbonate buffer system. The large, shaded area indicates the effective pH range for the bicarbonate buffer system, which does not coincide with the normal pH range for extracellular fluid. (Adapted from Comroe JH. Physiology of respiration. Chicago: Yearbook Medical Publishers, 1974;203.)

(28), so the effective range of the bicarbonate buffer system should be an extracellular pH between 5.1 and 7.1 pH units (indicated by the shaded area on the titration curve). Therefore, **bicarbonate is not expected to be an effective buffer in the usual pH range of extracellular fluid.** The limited buffer capacity for bicarbonate in the physiologic pH range, as predicted by its titration curve, deserves more emphasis in discussions of bicarbonate therapy for the organic acidoses. In fact, bicarbonate is best described as a transport form for carbon dioxide in blood (see Figure 2.3), and not as a buffer.

Hemodynamics

Bicarbonate therapy has also shown a limited ability to correct the hemodynamic alterations in shock-associated lactic acidosis (29). In fact, whatever hemodynamic improvements are produced by bicarbonate administration may be the result of the sodium load (Table 37.1) and not the alkali therapy (30).

ADVERSE EFFECTS

A number of undesirable effects are associated with sodium bicarbonate therapy. One of the principal disadvantages is the ability of sodium bicarbonate to **generate CO_2** and raise the P_{CO_2} in both intracellular and extracellular fluids (24,29–31). Considering the P_{CO_2} of the sodium bicarbonate solution in Table 37.1, this effect is not surprising. The increase in P_{CO_2} is undesirable because it creates a (volatile) acid load that must be excreted by the lungs and reduces the buffering capacity of sodium bicarbonate. Infusions of sodium bicarbonate can also increase blood lactate levels (29). This effect is attributed to alkalosis-induced augmentation of lactate production, and it hardly seems desirable in the setting of hyperlactatemia. Finally, bicarbonate can bind calcium and lower the concentration of ionized calcium in the blood. This can impair myocardial contractility and promote hypotension (27).

OTHER BUFFER SOLUTIONS

Carbicarb

Carbicarb is a commercially available buffer solution that is a 1:1 mixture of sodium bicarbonate and disodium carbonate. As shown in Table 37.1, Carbicarb has less bicarbonate and a much lower P_{CO_2} than the standard 7.5% sodium bicarbonate solution. As a result, Carbicarb does not produce the increase in P_{CO_2} seen with sodium bicarbonate infusions. Because of this, Carbicarb is a more effective buffer than sodium bicarbonate (29,30).

Tromethamine

The amine buffer tromethamine (TRIS or THAM) provides intracellular and extracellular buffering without generating CO_2 (31). The buffer reaction for THAM has a pK of 7.8 at body temperatures, so THAM provides effective buffering over the pH range of 6.8 to 8.8 (a more appropriate pH range than seen with bicarbonate). THAM is available as a 0.3 M solution (0.3 mEq/mL) and is given according to the base deficit: THAM (mEq/L) = 0.3 × body weight (kg) × base deficit. THAM is excreted in the urine and should be avoided in patients with renal failure. This buffer may prove beneficial in protecting the brain from local tissue acidosis during and after cardiac arrest (31). However, the clinical experience with THAM is limited at present.

SUMMARY

Alkali therapy has a limited role in the management of patients with lactic acidosis. First, it is unclear if acidosis is detrimental. Furthermore, therapy with sodium bicarbonate has limited efficacy in raising the pH, and it produces an undesirable increase in the Pco_2 of the body fluids. Buffers that do not generate CO_2 are available, but their clinical value is unproven.

Recommendation

If severe lactic acidosis develops (pH below 7.1) and the patient is deteriorating, a trial infusion of bicarbonate can be attempted by administering one-half of the estimated bicarbonate deficit. If cardiovascular improvement occurs, bicarbonate therapy can be continued. If no improvement or further deterioration occurs, further bicarbonate administration is not warranted.

KETOSIS

In conditions of reduced nutrient intake, adipose tissue releases free fatty acids, which are then taken up in the liver and metabolized to form the ketones acetoacetate and β-hydroxybutyrate. These ketones are released from the liver and can be used as oxidative fuels by vital organs such as the heart and central nervous system. The oxidative metabolism of ketones yields 4 kcal/g, which is a greater energy yield than the 3.4 kcal/g produced by carbohydrate metabolism (see Chapter 46).

The normal concentration of ketones in the blood is negligible (less than 0.1 mmol/L), but after 3 days of starvation, blood ketone levels increase tenfold. Ketones are strong acids, and thus progressive ketosis eventually produces a metabolic acidosis. The prevalence of acetoacetate (AcAc) and β-hydroxybutyrate (BOHB) in blood is determined by the following redox reaction:

$$AcAc + NADH \leftrightarrow BOHB + NAD \qquad (37.4)$$

The balance of this reaction favors the formation of β-hydroxybuty-

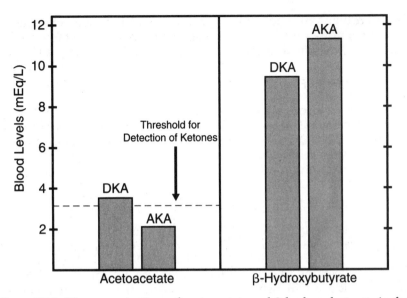

Figure 37.4. The concentrations of acetoacetate and β-hydroxybutyrate in the blood in diabetic ketoacidosis (DKA) and alcoholic ketoacidosis (AKA). The horizontal hatched line represents the minimum concentration of acetoacetate required to produce a positive nitroprusside reaction.

rate. In conditions of enhanced ketone production, the BOHB:AcAc ratio ranges from 3:1 (in diabetic ketoacidosis) to as high as 8:1 (in alcoholic ketoacidosis). The concentration of ketones in the blood in diabetic and alcoholic ketoacidosis is shown in Figure 37.4. Note the preponderance of β-hydroxybutyrate in both conditions. Because of this preponderance, ketoacidosis is more accurately called β-hydroxybutyric acidosis.

NITROPRUSSIDE REACTION

The nitroprusside reaction is a colorimetric method for detecting acetoacetate and acetone in blood and urine. The test can be performed with tablets (Acetest) or reagent strips (Ketostix, Labstix, Multistix). A detectable reaction requires a minimum acetoacetate concentration of 3 mEq/L. Because this reaction **does not detect the predominant ketoacid β-hydroxybutyrate** (32), it is an insensitive method for monitoring the severity of ketoacidosis. This is illustrated in Figure 37.4. In alcoholic ketoacidosis, the total concentration of ketoacids in blood is 13 mEq/L, which represents more than a hundredfold increase over the normal concentration of blood ketones, yet the nitroprusside reaction will be negative because the acetoacetate concentration is below 3 mEq/L.

While discussing the nitroprusside reaction, it may be worth mentioning that acetylcysteine can produce a falsely-negative nitroprusside reaction (33). The clinical significance of this interaction seems marginal; however, the antioxidant properties of acetylcysteine (see Chapter 3) may lead to more common use of this agent in the ICU.

DIABETIC KETOACIDOSIS

Diabetic ketoacidosis (DKA) is usually seen in insulin-dependent diabetic patients, but in 20% of cases, there is no previous history of diabetes mellitus (34). DKA is most often the result of inappropriate insulin dosing, but 50% of patients can have a concurrent illness, most commonly an infection (34).

CLINICAL FEATURES

The hallmark of DKA is the combination of hyperglycemia and a serum bicarbonate level below 20 mEq/L. The blood glucose is usually above 250 mg/dL, but may not be above 350 mg/dL. No correlation exists between the severity of the hyperglycemia and the severity of the ketoacidosis (35). Semiquantitative methods for detecting ketones (acetoacetate) in blood and urine will be positive; however, as mentioned earlier, these methods underestimate the degree of ketonemia.

Anion Gap

The increase in ketoacids should produce an elevated anion gap; however, this is variable, and the anion gap can be normal in DKA (36). The renal excretion of ketones is accompanied by an increase in chloride reabsorption in the renal tubules, and the resulting hyperchloremia limits the increase in the anion gap.

MANAGEMENT

The management of DKA is summarized in Table 37.2. The following are some of the details.

TABLE 37.2. MANAGEMENT OF DIABETIC KETOACIDOSIS		
Insulin:	0.1 U/kg IV push, then 0.1 U/kg/hr by continuous infusion. Decrease dose rate 50% when serum HCO_3 rises above 16 mEq/L.	
Fluids:	Start with 0.9% saline, 1 L/hr for the first 2 hours. Follow with 0.45% saline at 250–500 mL/hr. Total fluid deficit is usually 50–100 mL/kg.	
Potassium:	If serum K = _____ mEq/L, give _____ mEq over next hour	
	<3	40
	3–4	30
	4–5	20
	5–6	10
	>6	0
Phosphate:	If serum PO_4 is below 1.0 mg/dL, give 7.7 mg/kg over 4 hours.	

Insulin

Insulin therapy is given intravenously, starting with a bolus dose of 0.1 units per kilogram body weight (37). Because intravenous insulin has a half-life of only 5 minutes, it must be given by continuous infusion. The initial dose rate is 0.1 U/kg/hour. The blood glucose should fall 10% in the first hour of therapy. If it does not, the insulin dose rate should be doubled. The blood glucose levels should be measured every 1 to 2 hours during intravenous insulin therapy. Fingerstick glucose determinations can be performed if the blood glucose is below 500 mg/dL (34).

Fluids

Volume deficits average 50 to 100 mL/kg (or 4 to 8 L for a 175-lb adult). If no evidence of hypovolemic shock exists, crystalloid fluids are appropriate for volume replacement. Fluid therapy begins with 0.9% (isotonic) saline infused at a rate of approximately 1 L/hour for the first 2 hours. This is followed by infusion of 0.45% (half-normal) saline at 250 to 500 mL/hour. When the blood glucose falls to 250 mg/dL, dextrose can be used in the intravenous fluids and the infusion rate is dropped to 100 to 250 mL/hour.

If evidence of hypovolemia shock (e.g., hypotension, reduced urine output) does exist, fluid replacement should begin with colloid fluids (5% albumin or 6% hetastarch). Colloid resuscitation is given at one-third the volume recommended for crystalloid fluid replacement.

Potassium

Potassium depletion is almost universal in DKA, and the average deficit is 3 to 5 mEq/kg. However, the serum potassium is often normal (74% of patients) or elevated (22% of patients) at presentation. The serum potassium falls during insulin therapy (transcellular shift), and this fall can be dramatic. Therefore, potassium replacement should be started as soon as possible (Table 37.2), and the serum potassium should be monitored hourly for the first 4 to 6 hours of therapy.

Phosphate

Phosphorous depletion is also common in DKA and averages 1 to 1.5 mmol/kg. However, phosphorous replacement seems to have little impact on the outcome in DKA, and therefore phosphate replacement is not recommended routinely (34). The serum phosphate level should be measured 4 hours after the start of therapy. If the level is severely depressed (less than 1 mg/dL), phosphate replacement is advised (see Table 37.1 for the recommended replacement dose).

Alkali Therapy

Bicarbonate therapy does not improve the outcome in DKA, and because of the disadvantages of alkali therapy described earlier, bicarbonate therapy is not recommended in DKA, regardless of the severity of the acidemia (34).

MONITORING

The serum bicarbonate level may not be a reliable parameter for following the course of the ketoacidosis. Fluid replacement therapy often produces a hyperchloremic acidosis by promoting ketoacid excretion in the urine, which increases chloride reabsorption in the renal tubules. This can keep the bicarbonate from rising despite a resolving ketoacidosis. In this situation, the *pattern* of the acidosis is changing (i.e., changing from a high anion gap to a low anion gap acidosis). Therefore, monitoring the pattern of the acidosis as therapy proceeds can be more informative. This is accomplished by monitoring the **anion gap excess : bicarbonate deficit ratio,** as described in Chapter 36. This ratio is 1.0 in pure ketoacidosis, and decreases toward zero as the ketoacidosis resolves and is replaced by the hyperchloremic acidosis. When the ketones have been cleared from the bloodstream, the ratio approaches zero.

ALCOHOLIC KETOACIDOSIS

Alcoholic ketoacidosis (AKA) is a complex acid-base disorder that occurs in chronic alcoholics and usually appears 1 to 3 days after a period of heavy binge drinking (38). Several mechanisms seem to be involved in the ketosis, including reduced nutrient intake (which initiates enhanced ketone production), hepatic oxidation of ethanol (which generates NADH and enhances β-hydroxybutyrate formation), and dehydration (which impairs ketone excretion in the urine).

CLINICAL FEATURES

Patients with AKA tend to be chronically ill and have several concurrent disorders (e.g., pancreatitis, upper gastrointestinal bleeding, hepatitis, ethanol withdrawal, seizures). The presentation usually includes nausea, vomiting, and abdominal pain (38). Electrolyte abnormalities are common, particularly the *hypos* (e.g., hyponatremia, hypokalemia, hypophosphatemia, hypomagnesemia, hypoglycemia). Mixed acid-base disorders are also common in AKA. More than half the patients can have lactic acidosis (caused by other concurrent conditions), and a hyperchloremic acidosis is common (possibly caused by ketone excretion in the urine). A metabolic alkalosis is also seen in patients with protracted vomiting.

DIAGNOSIS

The diagnosis of AKA is suggested by the clinical setting (i.e., after a period of binge drinking), an elevated anion gap, and the presence of ketones in the blood or urine. However, the nitroprusside reaction for detecting ketones can be negative in AKA. The oxidation of ethanol in the liver generates NADH, and this favors the conversion of acetoacetate to β-hydroxybutyrate. As a result, the acetoacetate in blood and urine are low and may be below the threshold for ketone detection by the nitroprusside reaction, as shown in Figure 37.4. However most cases of AKA have a positive nitroprusside reaction for ketones (38).

MANAGEMENT

The management of AKA is notable for its simplicity. Infusion of dextrose-containing saline solutions is all that is required. The glucose helps retard hepatic ketone production, while the infused volume promotes the renal clearance of ketones. The ketoacidosis usually resolves within 24 hours. Other electrolyte deficiencies are corrected as needed. Bicarbonate therapy is unnecessary (38).

REFERENCES

SUGGESTED READINGS

Cohn RM, Roth KS. Biochemistry and disease. Baltimore: Williams & Wilkins, 1996.
Rose BD. Clinical physiology of acid-base and electrolyte disorders. 4th ed. New York: McGraw-Hill, 1994.

GENERAL REVIEWS

1. Laski ME, Kurtzman NA. Acid-base disorders in medicine. Dis Mon 1996; XLII:57–128 (200 references).

LACTIC ACIDOSIS: REVIEWS

2. Mizock BA. Lactic acidosis. Dis Mon 1989;XXXV:235–300 (322 references).
3. Mizock BA, Falk JL. Lactic acidosis in critical illness. Crit Care Med 1992;20: 80–93 (144 references).
4. Stacpoole PW. Lactic acidosis. Endocrinol Metab Clin North Am 1993;22: 221–245.

LACTIC ACIDOSIS: SELECTED REFERENCES

5. Aberti KGMM, Cuthbert C. The hydrogen ion in normal metabolism: a review. CIBA Foundation Symposium 87. Metabolic acidosis. London: Pitman Books, 1982;1–15.
6. Lehninger AL. Bioenergetics. New York: WA Benjamin, 1965;16.

7. Brooks GA. Lactate production under fully aerobic conditions: the lactate shuttle during rest and exercise. Fed Proc 1986;45:2924–2929.

8. Weil MH, Afifi AA. Experimental and clinical studies on lactate and pyruvate as indicators of the severity of acute circulatory failure (shock). Circulation 1970;16:989–1001.

9. Stacpoole PW, Wright EC, Baumgartner TG, et al. Natural history of acquired lactic acidosis in adults. Am J Med 1994;97:47–54.

10. Aduen J, Bernstein WK, Khastgir T, et al. The use and clinical importance of a substrate-specific electrode for rapid determinations of blood lactate concentrations. JAMA 1994;272:1678–1684.

11. Curtis SE, Cain SM. Regional and systemic oxygen delivery/uptake relations and lactate flux in hyperdynamic, endotoxin-treated dogs. Am Rev Respir Dis 1992;145:348–354.

12. Chattha G, Arieff AI, Cummings C, Tierney LM. Lactic acidosis complicating the acquired immunodeficiency syndrome. Ann Intern Med 1993;118:37–39.

13. Campbell CH. The severe lactic acidosis of thiamine deficiency: acute, pernicious or fulminating beriberi. Lancet 1984;1:446–449.

14. Bersin RM, Arieff AI. Primary lactic alkalosis. Am J Med 1988;85:867–871.

15. Kruse JA, Zaidi SAJ, Carlson RW. Significance of blood lactate levels in critically ill patients with liver disease. Am J Med 1987;83:77–82.

16. Brivet F, Bernadin M, Cherin P, et al. Hyperchloremic acidosis during grand mal seizure acidosis. Intensive Care Med 1994;20:27–31.

17. Mountain RD, Heffner JE, Brackett NC, Sahn SA. Acid-base disturbances in acute asthma. Chest 1990;98:651–655.

18. Iberti TS, Liebowitz AB, Papadakos PJ, et al. Low sensitivity of the anion gap as a screen to detect hyperlactatemia in critically ill patients. Crit Care Med 1990;18:275–277.

LACTIC ACIDOSIS

19. Anonymous. The colon, the rumen, and d-lactic acidosis. Lancet 1990;336: 599–600 (editorial).

20. Thurn JR, Pierpoint GL, Ludvigsen CW, Eckfeldt JH. D-lactate encephalopathy. Am J Med 1985;79:717–720.

21. Bustos D, Ponse S, Pernas JC et al. Fecal lactate and the short bowel syndrome. Dig Dis Sci 1994;39:2315–2319.

ALKALI THERAPY

22. Biebuyck JF. Sodium bicarbonate in the treatment of subtypes of acute lactic acidosis: physiologic considerations. Anesthesiology 1990;72:1064–1076.

23. Sonnett J, Pagani FD, Baker LS, et al. Correction of intramyocardial hypercarbic acidosis with sodium bicarbonate. Circ Shock 1994;42:163–173.

24. Mehta PM, Kloner RA. Effects of acid-base disturbance, septic shock, and calcium and phosphorous abnormalities on cardiovascular function. Crit Care Clin 1987;3:747–758.

25. Gores GJ, Nieminen AL, Fleischman KE, et al. Extracellular acidosis delays onset of cell death in ATP-depleted hepatocytes. Am J Physiol 1988;255: C315–C322.

26. Rose BD. Clinical physiology of acid-base and electrolyte disorders. 4th ed. New York: McGraw-Hill, 1994;590.

27. Graf H, Arieff AI. The use of sodium bicarbonate in the therapy of organic acidoses. Intensive Care Med 1986;12:286–288.

28. Comroe JH. Physiology of respiration. Chicago: Yearbook Medical Publishers, 1974;203.
29. Rhee KY, Toro LO, McDonald GG, et al. Carbicarb, sodium bicarbonate, and sodium chloride in hypoxic lactic acidosis. Chest 1993;104:913–918.
30. Benjamin E, Oropello JM, Abalos A, et al. Effects of acid-base correction on hemodynamics, oxygen dynamics, and resuscitability in severe canine hemorrhagic shock. Crit Care Med 1994;22:1616–16723.
31. Rosenberg JM, Martin GB, Paradis NA, et al. The effect of CO_2 and non–CO_2-generating buffers on cerebral acidosis after cardiac arrest: a ^{31}P NMR study. Ann Emerg Med 1989;18:341–347.

DIABETIC KETOACIDOSIS

32. Umpierrez GE, Kitabachi AE. A rational approach to diagnosing diabetic ketoacidosis. J Crit Illness 1996;11:428–432.
33. Holcombe BJ, Messick CR. Drug:lab interactions: implications for nutrition support. Nutr Clin Pract 1994;9:196–198.
34. Fish LH. Diabetic ketoacidosis. Postgrad Med 1994;96:75–96.
35. Brandt KR, Miles JM. Relationship between severity of hyperglycemia and metabolic acidosis in diabetic ketoacidosis. Mayo Clin Proc 1988;63:1071–1074.
36. Gamblin GT, Ashburn RW, Kemp DG, Beuttel SC. Diabetic ketoacidosis presenting with a normal anion gap. Am J Med 1986;80:758–760.
37. Umpierrez GE, Kitabachi AE. Management strategies for diabetic ketoacidosis. J Crit Illness 1996;11:437–443.

ALCOHOLIC KETOACIDOSIS

38. Wrenn KD, Slovis CM, Minion GE, Rutkowsli R. The syndrome of alcoholic ketoacidosis. Am J Med 1991;91:119–128.

38

METABOLIC ALKALOSIS

Metabolic alkalosis does not have the notoriety of metabolic acidosis, yet it is the most common acid-base disorder in hospitalized patients (1). One of the features of metabolic alkalosis that makes it so prevalent is its self-sustaining ability after the inciting condition resolves. This is attributed to chloride depletion, which enhances bicarbonate reabsorption in the renal tubules (to maintain electrical neutrality in the extracellular fluids). In fact, chloride depletion and repletion are the *yin* and *yang* of metabolic alkalosis in hospitalized patients.

COMMON ETIOLOGIES

The following is a brief description of the common causes of metabolic alkalosis (1,2).

NASOGASTRIC SUCTION

Each milliequivalent of hydrogen ion (H^+) that is secreted by the gastric mucosa generates 1 mEq of bicarbonate (HCO_3). The gastric juice has a H^+ concentration of 50 to 100 mEq/L, so a considerable quantity of HCO_3 is generated by gastric acid secretion. However, this is not normally accompanied by an increase in plasma HCO_3 because the acidic gastric juice also stimulates pancreatic secretion of HCO_3, which counterbalances the HCO_3 generated by gastric acid secretion. The loss of HCO_3 in pancreatic secretions is eliminated when gastric acid is removed by vomiting or nasogastric suction, and this allows the plasma HCO_3 to rise. Additional factors that promote metabolic alkalosis during nasogastric suction are loss of potassium and hypovolemia.

DIURETICS

Diuretics promote alkalosis by increasing the urinary loss of electrolytes and free water. The following electrolytes are involved:

1. **Chloride** excretion is enhanced by diuretics because chloride follows the sodium that is lost in the urine. To maintain electrical neutrality in the extracellular fluid, the urinary chloride loss is counterbalanced by an increase in HCO_3 reabsorption across the renal tubules. This results in an increase in extracellular (plasma) HCO_3 concentration.
2. **Potassium** loss in the urine is enhanced by diuretics because sodium delivery to the distal tubules is increased, and this promotes potassium secretion via the sodium–potassium exchange pump in the distal tubule. The resultant potassium depletion can then produce an extracellular alkalosis by promoting the intracellular accumulation of H^+ (transcellular H^+–K^+ exchange) and by promoting the secretion of H^+ in the distal renal tubules.
3. **Magnesium** is also lost in the urine during diuresis, and this promotes potassium depletion through unclear mechanisms. Magnesium depletion is an important factor in diuretic-induced potassium depletion, as discussed in Chapter 42.

VOLUME DEPLETION

Volume depletion can promote metabolic alkalosis in two ways. First, loss of free water concentrates the existing HCO_3 stores and raises the HCO_3 concentration in extracellular fluids. Second, a decrease in circulating blood volume stimulates the renin–angiotensin–aldosterone axis, and the aldosterone release promotes the loss of potassium and hydrogen ions in the distal tubule. The importance of volume depletion as a cause of metabolic alkalosis is unclear because fluid losses are almost always accompanied by electrolyte losses and the latter condition could promote the alkalosis, as described previously. In fact, volume depletion can be accompanied by a decrease in the glomerular filtration rate (GFR), and this should promote a metabolic *acidosis* (as occurs in renal failure).

ORGANIC ANIONS

The administration of organic anions such as lactate (in lactated Ringer's solution), acetate (in parenteral nutrition solutions), and citrate (in banked blood) could produce a metabolic alkalosis. Of these, only citrate administration in blood transfusions seems to be capable of causing a metabolic alkalosis (3). However, at least 8 units of blood must be transfused before the plasma HCO_3 begins to rise (2).

POSTHYPERCAPNIA

The compensatory response to CO_2 retention is a decrease in renal bicarbonate excretion, which produces a compensatory metabolic alkalosis. If chronic hypercapnia is corrected acutely (e.g., by overventilation during mechanical ventilation), the compensatory metabolic alkalosis will become a primary acid-base disorder. However, this should be a transient condition because the decrease in arterial P_{CO_2} promotes renal bicarbonate excretion.

ADVERSE EFFECTS

Metabolic alkalosis has several potential adverse effects. The following ones deserve mention, although their clinical significance is unclear.

NEUROLOGIC MANIFESTATIONS

The neurologic manifestations attributed to alkalosis include depressed consciousness, generalized seizures, and carpopedal spasms. However, these manifestations are almost always associated with respiratory alkalosis, not metabolic alkalosis. This is explained by the greater tendency for respiratory alkalosis to influence the acid-base status of the central nervous system.

HYPOVENTILATION

Metabolic alkalosis can depress ventilation, and this has been mentioned as a contributing factor in failed weaning from mechanical ven-

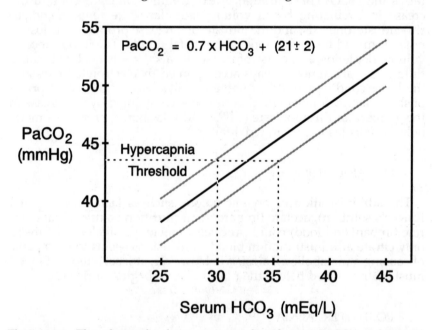

Figure 38.1. The relationship between serum bicarbonate (HCO_3) and arterial P_{CO_2} (Pa_{CO_2}) as predicted by the equation shown at the top of the graph. Note that the serum HCO_3 must rise above 30 to 35 mEq/L to produce hypercapnia (i.e., Pa_{CO_2} above 44 mm Hg).

tilation (1). However, as mentioned in Chapter 36, the ventilatory depression in metabolic alkalosis is a variable and often minor effect. The lack of hypoventilation in metabolic alkalosis is easily demonstrated in patients who receive chronic diuretic therapy (i.e., most of these patients have a metabolic alkalosis, but few have CO_2 retention). The expected arterial P_{CO_2} at any given serum HCO_3 concentration is described by the equation shown in Table 36.2 (4). This equation is used to plot the relationship between serum HCO_3 and arterial P_{CO_2} shown in Figure 38.1. As shown in the graph, hypercapnia is not expected until the serum HCO_3 rises above 30 to 35 mEq/L.

The relative lack of ventilatory depression in metabolic alkalosis may be a reflection of the baseline activity in the peripheral chemoreceptors, where metabolic acid-base disorders exert most of their influence on ventilation. That is, the peripheral chemoreceptors show minimal activity under normal conditions (5), so there is little baseline activity for alkalosis to inhibit.

TISSUE OXYGENATION

Metabolic alkalosis has several effects that could impair tissue oxygenation. These are demonstrated in Figure 38.2. Alkalosis can decrease tissue oxygen delivery in two ways. First, alkalosis increases the fraction of serum calcium that is bound to albumin, and the resultant decrease in ionized (free) calcium can impair myocardial contractility

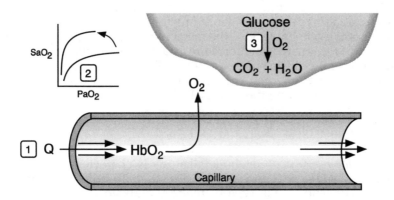

EFFECTS OF METABOLIC ALKALOSIS

1. Decreases Cardiac Output
2. Shifts HBO_2 Curve to the Left
3. Increases Tissue O_2 Consumption

Figure 38.2. Effects of metabolic alkalosis on the determinants of tissue oxygenation.

TABLE 38.1. CLASSIFICATION OF METABOLIC ALKALOSIS	
Chloride-Responsive	Chloride-Resistant
Urinary chloride <15 mEq/L:	Urinary chloride >25 mEq/L:
1. Loss of gastric acid	1. Mineralocorticoid excess
2. Diuretics	2. Potassium depletion
3. Volume depletion	
4. Posthypercapnia	

and reduce cardiac output. Second, alkalosis shifts the oxyhemoglobin dissociation curve to the left (Bohr effect), which decreases the tendency for hemoglobin to release oxygen in the tissue capillaries. In addition, intracellular alkalosis stimulates glycolysis, which can increase tissue oxygen requirements (6). Therefore, metabolic alkalosis can decrease tissue oxygen availability while increasing tissue oxygen demands. Although the effects of metabolic alkalosis on tissue oxygenation are unknown (because it is impossible to directly monitor tissue oxygenation), the potential for impaired tissue oxygenation is an important consideration in patients with shock (in whom tissue oxygenation is already impaired).

EVALUATION

The cause of a metabolic alkalosis is often readily apparent (e.g., nasogastric suction, diuretics). However, the **urinary chloride concentration** can also be useful in identifying the source of a metabolic alkalosis. As shown in Table 38.1, the metabolic alkaloses can be classified as chloride-responsive or chloride-resistant based on the urinary chloride concentration. The only exception to this rule is in the early stages of diuretic therapy, when the urinary chloride concentration is elevated but the resulting metabolic alkalosis is chloride-responsive.

CHLORIDE-RESPONSIVE ALKALOSIS

A *chloride-responsive* metabolic alkalosis is characterized by a low urinary chloride concentration (i.e., less than 15 mEq/L), indicating chloride depletion. This type of metabolic alkalosis is the result of gastric acid loss, diuretic therapy, volume depletion, or renal compensation for hypercapnia. As indicated by the inciting conditions, volume depletion is common in chloride-responsive metabolic alkalosis. The majority of cases of metabolic alkalosis in hospitalized patients are the chloride-responsive variety.

CHLORIDE-RESISTANT ALKALOSIS

A *chloride-resistant* metabolic alkalosis is characterized by an elevated urinary chloride concentration (i.e., above 25 mEq/L). Most cases of chloride-resistant alkalosis are caused by mineralocorticoid excess (e.g., hyperadrenal conditions) or potassium depletion (these two conditions often co-exist). This type of metabolic alkalosis is characterized by volume expansion rather than volume depletion. The disorders associated with chloride-resistant alkalosis are not commonly seen in patients in the ICU, with the possible exception of aggressive corticosteroid therapy.

SPOT URINE CHLORIDE

When the cause of a metabolic alkalosis is unclear, the concentration of chloride in a random (spot) urine sample can help identify the possible sources of the problem. One source of error occurs in the early stages of diuretic therapy, when the urinary chloride concentration is elevated in a chloride-responsive metabolic alkalosis. Another benefit of measuring the spot urinary chloride concentration is in selecting the appropriate therapy to correct the alkalosis. These are described below.

MANAGEMENT

Because most metabolic alkaloses that occur in hospitalized patients are chloride-responsive, chloride replacement is the mainstay of therapy for metabolic alkalosis in most patients. The chloride can be replaced as sodium chloride, potassium chloride, or hydrochloric acid (HCl).

SALINE INFUSION

Because volume depletion is common in chloride-responsive metabolic alkalosis, infusion of isotonic saline (0.9% sodium chloride) is the most common method of chloride replacement in this condition.

Method

The volume of isotonic saline needed can be determined by estimating the chloride deficit, as shown in Table 38.2. For example, if a patient weighs 80 kg (175 lb) and the serum chloride concentration is 80 mEq/L, the chloride deficit will be $0.3 \times 80 \times 20 = 480$ mEq. The chloride

TABLE 38.2. SALINE INFUSION FOR METABOLIC ALKALOSIS
Chloride deficit (mEq) $= 0.3 \times$ wt (kg) $\times$ (100 $-$ Plasma [CL^-])
Volume of isotonic saline (L) $= \dfrac{\text{Chloride deficit}}{154}$

concentration in isotonic saline is 154 mEq/L, so the volume of saline needed to replace the chloride deficit will be 480/154 = 3.1 L.

POTASSIUM CHLORIDE

The administration of potassium chloride is not an effective method of chloride repletion because the maximum rate of potassium infusion that is safe is 40 mEq/hour (see Chapter 41). Therefore, potassium chloride administration is indicated only for patients who are hypokalemic. However, because hypokalemia can promote metabolic alkalosis, correcting hypokalemia is an important measure for correcting a metabolic alkalosis.

It is important to emphasize that the administration of **potassium chloride will not replenish potassium stores if there is concurrent magnesium depletion** (7). Therefore, it is important to identify and correct magnesium depletion before attempting to replace potassium deficits (see Chapter 42 for information on identifying and correcting magnesium deficiency).

HYDROCHLORIC ACID

Infusion of dilute solutions of HCl produces the most rapid correction of metabolic alkalosis (1). This method can be used when rapid correction of severe alkalemia (pH greater than 7.5) is desirable, particularly when the cause of the alkalosis is loss of gastric acid.

Method

The amount of HCl required to correct a metabolic alkalosis can be determined by estimating the hydrogen ion (H^+) deficit, as shown in Table 38.3. A plasma HCO_3 concentration of 35 mEq/L can be used as the desired plasma HCO_3 level because immediate correction of the plasma HCO_3 to normal is rarely necessary. Once the H^+ deficit is calculated, the corresponding volume and infusion rate of the HCl solution can be determined. A popular solution is 0.1N HCl, which contains 100 mEq of H^+ per liter (equivalent to the H^+ concentration in gastric secretions, which is 50 to 100 mEq/L). Because HCl solutions are corrosive, they must be infused through a large, central vein (8).

**TABLE 38.3. HYDROCHLORIC ACID INFUSION
FOR METABOLIC ALKALOSIS**

A. H^+ deficit (mEq) = 0.3 × wt (kg) × (Measured [HCO_3] − Desired [HCO_3])
B. Rate of H^+ replacement = 0.2 mEq/kg/hr
C. For a 0.1N HCl solution (H^+ = 100 mEq/L):
   1. Volume (L) = H^+ deficit/100
   2. Infusion rate (L/hr) = 0.2 × wt (kg)/100

To illustrate the use of the equations in Table 38.3, consider a patient who weighs 80 kg and has a plasma HCO_3 of 50 mEq/L. Using a desired plasma HCO_3 of 35 mEq/L, one can calculate the H^+ deficit as follows: $0.3 \times 80 \times (50 \text{ ms } 35) = 360$ mEq. The corresponding volume of 0.1N is $360/100 = 3.6$ L. The infusion rate of the 0.1N HCl solution is $(0.2 \times 80)/100 = 0.16$ L/hour, or 2.6 ml/minute.

Adverse Effects

The major concern with HCl infusions is the corrosive effects of the HCl solutions. Extravasation of HCl solutions can produce severe tissue necrosis, even when the solution is infused through a central vein (9). Solutions more concentrated than 0.1N HCl can also promote corrosion of intravascular catheters (10). To limit the risk for corrosion, HCl solutions that are more concentrated than the 0.1N solution should be avoided.

OTHER CHLORIDE SOLUTIONS

Ammonium chloride can be converted to ammonia and HCl in the liver, and this can correct a metabolic alkalosis indirectly. However, ammonium chloride infusions are discouraged because the ammonia that is generated can produce an encephalopathy (with obtundation and coma), particularly in patients with hepatic or renal insufficiency (1,2).

Arginine hydrochloride is also broken down to arginine and HCl in the liver. However, the movement of arginine (a cation) into cells is coupled with the movement of potassium out of cells, and this can lead to severe and life-threatening hyperkalemia (1,2).

HISTAMINE H_2 BLOCKERS

Inhibition of gastric acid secretion with histamine H_2 receptor antagonists has been used to prevent metabolic alkalosis during prolonged periods of nasogastric suctioning (1,2). However, considering the consequences of gastric acid suppression on colonization of the upper gastrointestinal tract (described in Chapter 6 and Chapter 33), this approach should be discouraged.

CHLORIDE-RESISTANT ALKALOSIS

The management of chloride-resistant metabolic alkalosis is aimed at treating the underlying cause of the mineralocorticoid excess (e.g., hyperadrenalism, renal artery stenosis) and correcting potassium deficits. Because this type of metabolic alkalosis usually is accompanied by extracellular volume expansion (not volume contraction), the diuretic corrective measures described below can also be used.

Acetazolamide

Acetazolamide (Diamox) is a carbonic anhydrase inhibitor that blocks HCO_3 reabsorption in the proximal renal tubules and promotes urinary HCO_3 excretion. Acetazolamide has diuretic effects, and because chloride-resistant metabolic alkalosis usually is accompanied by a high extravascular volume, acetazolamide is well-suited for correcting chloride-resistant metabolic alkaloses. The recommended dose is 5 to 10 mg/kg IV (or PO), and the maximum effect is seen after an average of 15 hours (11). Acetazolamide promotes potassium depletion as well as volume depletion, and thus it should not be used in chloride-resistant metabolic alkalosis that is accompanied by hypokalemia.

REFERENCES

SUGGESTED READING

Rose BD. Clinical physiology of acid-base and electrolyte disorders. 4th ed. New York: McGraw-Hill, 1994.

REVIEWS

1. Friedman BS, Lumb PD. Prevention and management of metabolic alkalosis. J Intensive Care Med 1990;5(Suppl):S22–S27.
2. Rose BD. Metabolic alkalosis. In: Clinical physiology of acid-base and electrolyte disorders. 4th ed. New York: McGraw-Hill, 1994;515–539.

SELECTED REFERENCES

3. Driscoll DF, Bistrian BR, Jenkins RL. Development of metabolic alkalosis after massive transfusion during orthotopic liver transplantation. Crit Care Med 1987;15:905–908.
4. Javaheri S, Kazemi H. Metabolic alkalosis and hypoventilation in humans. Am Rev Respir Dis 1987;136:1011–1016.
5. Marino PL. Brainstem chemoreception. Ann Arbor: University of Michigan Press, 1974.
6. Rastegar HR, Woods M, Harken AH. Respiratory alkalosis increases tissue oxygen demand. J Surg Res 1979;26:687–692.
7. Whang R, Flink EB, Dyckner T, et al. Mg depletion as a cause of refractory potassium depletion. Arch Intern Med 1985;145:1686–1689.
8. Brimioulle S, Vincent JL, Dufaye P, et al. Hydrochloric acid infusion for treatment of metabolic alkalosis: effects on acid-base balance and oxygenation. Crit Care Med 1985;13:738–742.
9. Jankauskas SJ, Gursel E, Antonenko DR. Chest wall necrosis secondary to hydrochloric acid use in the treatment of metabolic alkalosis. Crit Care Med 1989;17:963–964.
10. Kopel R, Durbin CG. Pulmonary artery catheter deterioration during hydrochloric infusion for the treatment of metabolic alkalosis. Crit Care Med 1989;17:688–689.
11. Marik PE, Kussman BD, Lipman J, Kraus P. Acetazolamide in the treatment of metabolic alkalosis in critically ill patients. Heart Lung 1991;20:455–458.

section X
FLUID AND ELECTROLYTE DISORDERS

Man is a bundle of relations.
Ralph Waldo Emerson

chapter

39

ACUTE OLIGURIA

Lack of urine output in the acutely hypovolemic patient is renal success, not renal failure.

Ronald V. Maier, MD

An acute decrease in urine output can represent a functional adaptation, as Dr. Maier points out, but more often it represents trouble. The trouble is acute renal failure, which can have a mortality of 80% in critically ill patients (1,2). Furthermore, *the introduction of acute hemodialysis has not reduced the mortality in acute renal failure* (1,2), which has serious implications. Let's hope this information does not fall into the hands of the "outcomes analysts," who believe that an intervention is not justified if it does not improve the outcome.

OVERVIEW

Oliguria (urine output less than 400 mL/day) may not be associated with abnormal renal function (4). This condition (which can be caused by antidiuretic hormone [ADH] excess) differs from the oliguria described in this chapter, which should be accompanied by any of the following:

1. An increase in serum creatinine of at least 0.5 mg/dL above baseline
2. An increase in serum creatinine of at least 50% over baseline
3. A reduction in calculated creatinine clearance of at least 50%
4. Severe renal dysfunction requiring some form of renal replacement therapy

---

TABLE 39.1. QUANTITATIVE ASSESSMENT OF RENAL FUNCTION

Creatinine Clearance (Men):

$$CL_{Cr} \text{ (mL/min)} = \frac{(140 - \text{age}) \times \text{weight (kg)}}{72 \times \text{Serum creatinine (mg/dL)}}$$

Creatinine Clearance (Women):

$$CL_{Cr} \text{ (mL/min)} = 0.85 \times CL_{Cr} \text{ for men}$$

Fractional Excretion of Sodium:

$$FE_{Na} = \frac{\text{Urine [Na]/Plasma [Na]}}{\text{Urine [Cr]/Plasma [Cr]}} \times 100$$

The creatinine clearance can be estimated using the formulas shown in Table 39.1 (5). This helps not only to determine the degree of renal functional impairment, but also to determine appropriate drug dosages.

The four criteria listed above identify the condition known as acute oliguric renal failure (AORF). The causes of AORF are traditionally separated into three categories, as shown in Figure 39.1 (1,6). Each category is named according to the anatomic location of the problem responsible for the oliguria.

PRERENAL DISORDERS

The prerenal sources of AORF are located proximal to the kidneys and are characterized by a decrease in renovascular flow. The disorders in this category include hypovolemia, severe cardiac dysfunction, loss of vascular tone, drugs that promote renal vasoconstriction (e.g., nonsteroidal antiinflammatory agents), and drugs that reduce glomerular filtration pressure (e.g., angiotensin-converting enzyme inhibitors). Prerenal disorders are responsible for roughly half of the cases of AORF (1–3).

INTRINSIC RENAL DISORDERS

The intrinsic renal disorders involve the renal parenchyma and are characterized by impaired glomerular filtration, renal tubular dysfunction, or both. These disorders are traditionally described as three entities: acute glomerulonephritis, acute tubular necrosis (ATN), and acute interstitial nephritis (AIN). ATN is the most common intrinsic renal disorder in AORF. It is most often caused by sepsis, circulatory shock, and nephrotoxins (6). The toxins include drugs (e.g., aminoglycosides), radiocontrast dye, and pigments (e.g., myoglobin).

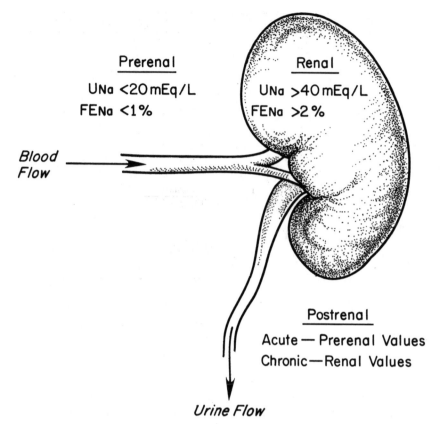

Figure 39.1. Causes of acute oliguria based on anatomic location of the problem.

Acute Tubular Necrosis

Acute renal failure is characterized by ineffective filtration across the glomeruli. However, in ATN (an unfortunate term because there may be no tubular necrosis), the pathologic defect does not involve the glomerulus, but rather involves the renal tubules and adjacent parenchyma (i.e., tubulointerstitial injury). If the glomerulus is not involved, what shuts off the glomerular filtration rate (GFR)? This is explained in the photomicrograph in Figure 39.2. The center of this picture is a proximal tubule that is filled with tubular epithelial cells that have sloughed into the lumen of the tubule. This mass of cells creates an obstruction, and this produces a back pressure that is exerted on the proximal to the obstruction. This back pressure then serves to reduce the net filtration pressure across the glomerular capillaries. This tubulo-glomerular feedback pressure reduces the GFR.

The damage to the renal tubules in ATN is believed to be the result of ischemia as well as inflammatory cell injury (7). The latter process can be widespread, and it can be accompanied by dysfunction in multi-

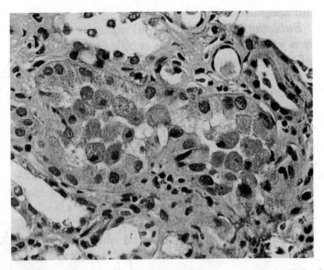

Figure 39.2. Photomicrograph of acute tubular necrosis (ATN) showing a proximal tubule filled with exfoliated epithelial cells (magnification × 400). (From Racusen LC. Histopathology of acute renal failure. New Horiz 1995; 3:662–668.)

ple organs (the multiorgan dysfunction syndrome, described in Chapter 31). In this situation, the intrinsic renal failure is part of a more widespread systemic illness and is not an isolated organ injury. This is an important consideration because it means that the therapy for acute intrinsic renal failure should not be directed solely at the kidneys (as it usually is).

POSTRENAL DISORDERS

The postrenal causes of AORF occur distal to the renal parenchyma and are characterized by obstruction of urinary flow. The disorder in this category can involve obstruction in the collecting system (papillary necrosis), the ureters (retroperitoneal tumors), or the bladder outlet (strictures, prostatism). Postrenal obstruction is an uncommon cause of oliguria unless a solitary functional kidney is present.

URINARY PARAMETERS

The initial evaluation of the oliguric patient should include a microscopic and, if necessary, chemical analysis of the urine. The methods described below will help distinguish prerenal from intrinsic renal disorders. The urinary evaluation is less valuable for identifying postrenal obstruction (except in papillary necrosis, where sloughed papilla can be evident on urine microscopy).

URINE MICROSCOPY

Microscopic examination of the urine sediment is the easiest and least expensive diagnostic procedure. The presence of abundant tubular epithelial cells with epithelial cell casts is virtually pathognomonic of ATN. In addition, the presence of white cell casts identifies an interstitial nephritis, and the presence of pigmented casts identifies myoglobinuria. Urine microscopy is not a valuable procedure for identifying prerenal causes of oliguria. If the urine microscopy is unrevealing, the urinary sodium determination can be useful.

URINE SODIUM

When renal perfusion is diminished, sodium reabsorption increases and urinary sodium excretion decreases. On the other hand, intrinsic renal failure is associated with impaired sodium reabsorption and an increase in urinary sodium excretion. Therefore, in the setting of oliguria, **a urine sodium below 20 mEq/L usually indicates a prerenal disorder.** However, a urine sodium above 40 mEq/L does not necessarily rule out a prerenal disorder. An elevated urine sodium can occur when a prerenal disorder is superimposed on intrinsic renal dysfunction (with obligatory sodium loss) or when there is ongoing diuretic therapy. Elderly patients often have obligatory sodium loss in the urine, and they can have a high urine sodium in the face of prerenal disorders. Therefore, a urine sodium above 40 mEq/L is not absolute evidence in favor of renal over prerenal disorders.

FRACTIONAL EXCRETION OF SODIUM

The fractional excretion of sodium (FE_{Na}) is the fraction of sodium filtered at the glomerulus that is excreted in the urine. This is equivalent to the sodium clearance divided by the creatinine clearance, as shown in Table 39.1 (8). The FE_{Na} is normally less than 1%; i.e., less than 1% of the filtered sodium is excreted in the urine. In the setting of oliguria, the FE_{Na} provides the following information:

$$FE_{Na} < 1\% = \text{Prerenal disorder}$$

$$(39.1)$$

$$FE_{Na} > 2\% = \text{Intrinsic renal disorder}$$

Although exceptions to these criteria exist (i.e., the FE_{Na} can be less than 1% in an occasional case of intrinsic renal failure), the FE_{Na} is one of the most reliable urinary parameters for distinguishing prerenal from renal causes of AORF. However, it is a cumbersome determination to perform, which limits its popularity.

BEDSIDE MANAGEMENT

The principal task in the early management of the oliguric patient is to identify and correct any prerenal disorders that might be responsible for the oliguria. This is a simple task when invasive hemodynamic monitoring is available.

OPTIMIZE CENTRAL HEMODYNAMICS

The approach to optimizing central hemodynamics is very similar to the initial part of the flow diagram shown in Figure 13.3. The first step is to determine the adequacy of cardiac filling.

Cardiac Filling Pressures

The cardiac filling pressures (central venous pressure [CVP] and wedge pressures) should be normal or unchanged (a decrease in the filling pressures in excess of 4 mm Hg is considered a significant change). If the filling pressures are low (CVP less than 4 mm Hg, wedge pressure less than 8 mm Hg), then volume should be infused until the CVP increases to 6 to 8 mm Hg and the wedge pressure reaches 12 to 15 mm Hg. Once the filling pressures are in these ranges, the cardiac output should be measured.

Cardiac Output

If the cardiac output is low, more volume should be infused until the CVP reaches 10 to 12 mm Hg and the wedge pressure is close to 20 mm Hg. If the cardiac output is still low despite filling pressures in the high-normal range, then the appropriate cardiac support drug is selected using the blood pressure. If the blood pressure is normal, dobutamine is given (start at 5 µg/kg/min) for inotropic support. If the blood pressure is low, dopamine is given (start at 5 µg/kg/min) for pressure and flow support. The goal should be a cardiac index above 3 L/min/m^2.

GLOMERULOTUBULAR FLOW

If the oliguria persists despite adequate systemic pressure and flow, the likely source of the problem is intrinsic renal failure. In this situation, little else can be done. The following two maneuvers are popular but ineffective.

LOW-DOSE DOPAMINE

Despite thirty years of use as a renal vasodilator, low-dose dopamine (2 µg/kg/min) has shown no evidence of benefit when used in patients with acute oliguric renal failure (9–12). A summary of the

TABLE 39.2. LOW-DOSE DOPAMINE IN AORF		
	Yes	No
Increases renal blood flow ?	■	□
Increases urine output ?	■	□
Improves renal function ?	□	■
Decreases need for dialysis ?	□	■
Improves outcome ?	□	■
From References 9–12.		

experience with dopamine in this setting is shown in Table 39.2. Although dopamine can augment renal blood flow and promote a diuresis, these effects are not accompanied by improved renal function or better outcomes. The diuretic effect of dopamine is unrelated to its vascular effects, so the increase in urine output is not a reflection of an increase in GFR.

In addition to being ineffective, low-dose dopamine has also been identified as a potential risk because of the actions of dopamine as a splanchnic vasoconstrictor (which could predispose to bowel ischemia) (12). Therefore, as a result of its unproven value and potential for harm, **low-dose dopamine is no longer recommended for the management of acute oliguric renal failure** (1,11).

FUROSEMIDE

The goal of diuretic administration in acute tubular injury is to promote tubular flow and reduce the back pressure that impedes glomerular filtration. However, furosemide has shown little value in promoting a diuresis in this setting. Considering that less than 10% of a furosemide dose reaches the lumen of the renal tubules in renal failure (13), the lack of diuretic effect in renal failure is not surprising. When furosemide is given by continuous intravenous infusion, the diuretic effects are much greater than seen with bolus drug administration (the diuretic effect of furosemide is a function of the drug delivery time) (14). Therefore, this may be the preferred method of attempted diuresis in acute renal failure. The optimal dose is unknown, but the dose rate in clinical reports averages 1 to 9 mg/hour, although dose rates up to 0.75 mg/kg/hour have been reported (14). There is no evidence that a loading dose is required before the infusion.

SPECIFIC RENAL DISORDERS

DYE-INDUCED RENAL FAILURE

Standard iodinated radiocontrast agents can produce a hyperosmotic endothelial injury in the small vessels of the renal medulla, which leads to ischemic injury and an ATN-like picture. The renal

TABLE 39.3. DRUGS THAT CAN CAUSE INTERSTITIAL NEPHRITIS		
Allopurinol	Ciprofloxacin	Phenytoin
Captopril	Furosemide	Rifampin
Cephalothin	NSAIDs	Thiazides
Cimetidine	Penicillins	TMP–SMX

injury usually becomes apparent as a rising serum creatinine within 48 hours of the procedure. Oliguria is uncommon (10% of cases), and most cases resolve within 2 weeks (15,16).

This type of injury is common in diabetic patients with renal insufficiency, and dehydration is considered a risk factor. Saline infusions (150 to 200 mL/hour) before, during, and after the procedure are effective in reducing the incidence of dye-induced ATN. Despite the introduction of more isotonic dyes, the problem persists.

INTERSTITIAL NEPHRITIS

AIN is caused by infections (usually viral or atypical pathogens) and hypersensitivity drug reactions. Virtually any drug can produce AIN, but the most notorious offenders are listed in Table 39.3 (3). Many of these drugs are common in the ICU, so you should be aware of their nephrotoxic potential.

AIN can be difficult to distinguish from ATN. The characteristic signs of a hypersensitivity reaction (e.g., fever, rash, eosinophilia) may not be present. Ongoing therapy with a high-risk drug can raise suspicion for AIN, but the renal injury can occur months and even years after the onset of drug therapy (17). This can direct attention away from the possibility of a drug-induced nephropathy. One of the aids to the diagnosis of AIN is the presence of white cell casts on urine microscopy.

No specific treatment exists for AIN other than removing the offending drug. Therefore, in cases where the cause of acute renal failure is uncertain, it is wise to stop use of as many medications as possible.

MYOGLOBINURIC ATN

Widespread muscle breakdown (rhabdomyolysis) leads to the release of myoglobin into the bloodstream, and when the myoglobin is filtered in the kidneys, it damages the renal tubules and produces an ATN-like illness. However, this is usually a milder form of renal failure and is nonoliguric in most cases. Most cases of rhabdomyolysis are toxin-induced or traumatic. The number of potential toxins is staggering; one review lists over 150 candidates (18).

Diagnosis

A positive urinary dipstick test for occult blood, combined with the absence of erythrocytes on urine microscopy, is diagnostic of myoglo-

TABLE 39.4 CONSEQUENCES OF RENAL SHUTDOWN	
Variable	Daily Change
Blood urea nitrogen	20–30 mg/dL
Creatinine	1–2 mg/dL
Potassium	0.3–0.5 mEq/L
Bicarbonate	1–2 mEq/L

binuria (except in the rare case of severe intravascular hemolysis with hemoglobinuria). Rhabdomyolysis may be suspected when serum creatinine rises at a rate that is greater than expected. As shown in Table 39.4, the serum creatinine will rise 1 to 2 mg/dL daily in the absence of renal function. However, in the presence of widespread muscle breakdown, the serum creatinine will rise by more than 2 mg/dL each day. The diagnosis of rhabdomyolysis is secured by measuring any one of several muscle enzymes in blood (e.g., creatine phosphokinase, lactate dehydrogenase). I prefer the aldolase enzyme, because it is specific for skeletal muscle.

Management

The management of myoglobinuric ATN includes volume infusion and careful monitoring of potassium and phosphate levels in blood (these electrolytes are released from muscle, and their serum concentration can rise quickly to dangerous levels). Volume infusion is very important because the damaging effects of myoglobin in the kidneys is markedly enhanced by volume depletion. Alkalinization of the urine is often recommended in myoglobinuria, but is rarely necessary.

HEMOFILTRATION

Although hemodialysis is the standard method of blood purification in renal failure, a number of alternative methods have surfaced in recent years (19). One of these is *hemofiltration*, which is described below.

BASIC FEATURES

Whereas hemodialysis removes solutes by diffusion, hemofiltration uses convection (solvent drag) to remove solutes. This is a less efficient method of solute removal. However, the membranes used for hemofiltration are porous, and they allow large molecules (molecular weights up to 25,000 daltons) to pass through the membranes. This facilitates both solute and fluid removal.

CONTINUOUS HEMOFILTRATION

Although hemofiltration removes solutes at a slower rate than hemodialysis, this allows hemofiltration to be used for longer periods

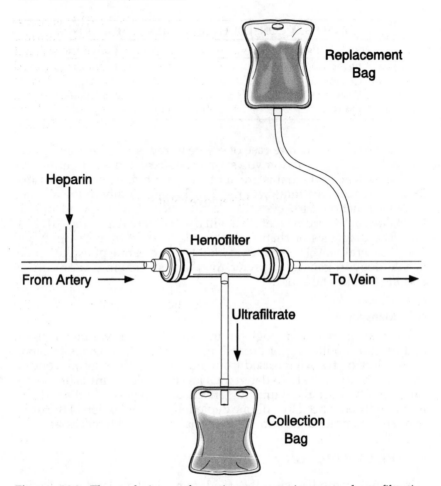

Figure 39.3. The technique of continuous arteriovenous hemofiltration (CAVH).

(days). The technique of continuous hemofiltration is shown in Figure 39.3. In this case, the filter is placed between an artery and a vein. This is called continuous arteriovenous hemofiltration (CAVH). The hemofilter can also be placed between two veins. This method is called continuous venovenous hemofiltration (CVVH).

Continuous Arteriovenous Hemofiltration

No pumps are involved in CAVH. The arteriovenous pressure difference is the pressure gradient for flow through the filter. The pressure gradient for filtration is the vertical distance between the filter and the ultrafiltrate collection bag. The filtration pressure can thus be adjusted by adjusting the position of the collection bag relative to the filter.

Also note the replacement fluid in the CAVH circuit. This is necessary because the concentration of solutes in the ultrafiltrate is the same as in the blood. Therefore, the concentration of solutes in blood will not decrease during hemofiltration unless a replacement fluid is infused (dilutional effect). The use of a replacement fluid allows CAVH to reduce the concentration of toxins that accumulate in renal failure (i.e., it allows CAVH to function as a method of dialysis). Over a 24-hour period, CAVH can remove 10 L of fluid (which is replaced) and 12 g of urea (20).

Uses

Hemofiltration can be used to remove solutes or fluids (e.g., in renal failure or heart failure). Because the removal rate of fluid is slower than with hemodialysis, hemofiltration is better tolerated in patients who are hemodynamically compromised. The ability to remove large molecules also has several potential applications. One of these is in severe sepsis, in which hemofiltration has been used to remove potentially harmful inflammatory mediators (21). This type of *radiator flush* is likely to become a very popular practice in the near future (if it works).

REFERENCES

SUGGESTED READINGS

Bellomo R, ed. Acute renal failure. New horizons. Vol. 3, No. 4. Baltimore: Williams & Wilkins, 1995.

REVIEWS

1. Thadani R, Pascual M, Bonventre JV. Acute renal failure. N Engl J Med 1996; 334:1448–1460 (153 references).

OVERVIEW

2. Anderson RA. Prevention and management of acute renal failure. Hosp Pract 1993;28:61–75.
3. Garella S. Drug-induced renal disease. Hosp Pract 1993;28:129–140.
4. Zaloga GP, Hughes SS. Oliguria in patients with normal renal function. Anesthesiology 1990;72:598–602.
5. Cockroft DW, Gault MN. Prediction of creatinine clearance from serum creatinine. Nephron 1976;16:31–41.
6. Brivet FG, Kleinknecht DJ, Loirat P, et al. Acute renal failure in intensive care units: causes, outcome, and prognostic factors of hospital mortality: a prospective multicenter study. Crit Care Med 1996;24:192–198.
7. Johnson JP, Rockaw MD. Sepsis or ischemia in experimental acute renal failure: what have we learned? New Horiz 1995;3:608–614.

URINARY PARAMETERS

8. Steiner RW. Interpreting the fractional excretion of sodium. Am J Med 1984; 77:699–702.

LOW-DOSE DOPAMINE

9. Bersten AD, Holt AW. Vasoactive drugs and the importance of renal perfusion pressure. New Horiz 1995;3:650–661.
10. Marik PE. Low-dose dopamine in critically ill oliguric patients. Heart Lung 1993;22:171–175.
11. Chertow GM, Sayegh MH, Allgren RL, Lazarus JM. Is the administration of dopamine associated with adverse or favorable outcomes in acute renal failure? Am J Med 1996;1:49–53.
12. Thompson BT, Cockrill BA. Renal-dose dopamine: a Siren song? Lancet 1994; 344:7–8.

FUROSEMIDE

13. Brater DC, Anderson SA, Brown-Cartwright D. Response to furosemide in chronic renal insufficiency: rationale for limited doses. Clin Pharmacol Ther 1986;40:134–139.
14. Martin SJ, Danzinger LH. Continuous infusion of loop diuretics in the critically ill: a review of the literature. Crit Care Med 1994;22:1323–1329.

RENAL DISORDERS

15. Wish JB, Moritz CE. Preventing radiocontrast-induced acute renal failure. J Crit Illness 1990;5:16–31.
16. Hock R, Anderson RJ. Prevention of drug-induced nephrotoxicity in the intensive care unit. J Crit Care 1995;10:33–43.
17. Ten RM, Torres VE, Millner DS, et al. Acute interstitial nephritis. Mayo Clin Proc 1988;3:921–930.
18. Curry SC, Chang D, Connor D. Drug and toxin-induced rhabdomyolysis. Ann Emerg Med 1989;18:1068–1084.

HEMOFILTRATION

19. Ronco C, Barbacini S, Digito A, Zoccali G. Achievements and new directions in continuous renal replacement therapy. New Horiz 1995;3:708–716.
20. Merrill RH. Techniques of continuous arteriovenous hemofiltration and hemodialysis. J Crit Illness 1991;6:381–387.
21. Vincent J-L, Tielemans C. Continuous hemofiltration in severe sepsis: is it beneficial? J Crit Care 1995;10:27–32.

40

HYPERTONIC AND HYPOTONIC SYNDROMES

This chapter describes the clinical disorders that are characterized by an abnormal distribution of total body water (TBW) in the intracellular and extracellular fluid compartments. These disorders are characterized by a change in the effective osmolarity of the extracellular fluid, and many are associated with an abnormal plasma sodium concentration.

BASIC CONCEPTS

The following is a description of the forces that determine the movement of water between the intracellular and extracellular fluid compartments (1–4).

OSMOTIC ACTIVITY

The activity (concentration) of solute particles in a solution is inversely related to the activity (concentration) of water molecules in the solution. The solute activity in a solution is also called the *osmotic activity* and is expressed in osmoles (osm). The total osmotic activity in a solution is the sum of the individual osmotic activities of all the solute particles in the solution. For monovalent ions, the osmotic activity in milliosmoles (mOsm) per unit volume is equivalent to the concentration of the ions in milliequivalents (mEq) per unit volume. Thus, the osmotic activity in isotonic saline (0.9% sodium chloride) is as follows:

$$0.9\% \text{ NaCl} = 154 \text{ mEq Na/L} + 154 \text{ mEq Cl/L}$$

$$= 154 \text{ mOsm Na/L} + 154 \text{ mOsm Cl/L} \quad (40.1)$$

$$= 308 \text{ mOsm/L}$$

Osmolarity is the osmotic activity per volume of solution (solutes plus water) and is expressed as mOsm/L. **Osmolality** is the osmotic activity per volume of water and is expressed as mOsm/kg H_2O. The osmotic activity of body fluids usually is expressed in relation to the volume of water (i.e., osmolality). However, the volume of water in body fluids is far greater than the volume of solutes, so there is little difference between the osmolality and osmolarity of body fluids. Thus, the terms osmolality and osmolarity can be used interchangeably to describe the osmotic activity in body fluids.

TONICITY

When two solutions are separated by a membrane that allows the passage of water but not solutes, the water passes from the solution with the lower osmotic activity to the solution with the higher osmotic activity. The relative osmotic activity in the two solutions is called the effective osmolality, or *tonicity*. The solution with the higher osmolality is described as hypertonic, and the solution with the lower osmolality is described as hypotonic. Thus, the tendency for water to move into and out of cells is determined by the relative tonicity of the intracellular and extracellular fluids.

When the membrane separating two fluids is permeable to both solutes and water and a solute is added to one of the fluids, the solute equilibrates fully across the membrane. In this situation, the solute increases the osmolality of both fluids but does not change the relative tonicity of either fluid. Therefore, the water will not move from one fluid compartment to the other. An example of a solute that behaves in this manner is urea. Urea is freely permeable across cell membranes, so an increase in the urea concentration in extracellular fluid (i.e., an increase in the plasma blood urea nitrogen [BUN]) increases the osmolality of the extracellular fluids but does not increase the tonicity of the extracellular fluids or cause a net movement of water out of cells. Thus, azotemia (an increase in BUN) is a hyperosmotic condition, but not a hypertonic condition.

PLASMA OSMOLALITY

The osmolality of the extracellular fluids can be measured in the clinical laboratory using the freezing point of plasma (a solution containing 1 osm/L will freeze at $-1.86°$ C). This is the *freezing point depression* method for measuring osmolality.

The osmolality of the extracellular fluids can also be calculated using the concentrations of sodium, chloride, glucose, and urea in plasma (these are the major solutes in extracellular fluid). The calculation below uses a plasma [Na] of 140 mEq/L, a plasma [glucose] of 90 mg/dL, and a plasma [BUN] of 14 mg/dL.

$$\text{Plasma Osmolality} = (2 \times [\text{Na}]) + \frac{[\text{Glucose}]}{18} + \frac{[\text{BUN}]}{2.8}$$

$$= (2 \times 140) + \frac{90}{18} + \frac{14}{2.8} \qquad (40.2)$$

$$= 290 \text{ mOsm/kg H}_2\text{O}$$

The sodium concentration is doubled to include the osmotic contribution of chloride. The serum glucose and urea are measured in milligrams per deciliter, and the factors 18 and 2.8 (the atomic weights divided by 10) are used to convert mg/dL to mOsm/kg H_2O.

OSMOLAL GAP

Because solutes other than sodium, chloride, glucose, and urea are present in the extracellular fluid, the measured plasma osmolality will be greater than the calculated plasma osmolality. This osmolar gap (i.e., the difference between the measured and calculated plasma osmolality) is normally as much as 10 mOsm/kg H_2O (4,5). An increase in the osmolar gap occurs when certain toxins (e.g., ethanol, methanol, ethylene glycol, or the unidentified toxins that accumulate in renal failure) are in the extracellular fluid. Therefore, the osmolar gap has been proposed as a screening test for identifying the presence of toxins in the extracellular fluid. In the case of renal failure, the osmolar gap has been recommended as a reliable test for distinguishing acute from chronic renal failure: the osmolar gap is expected to be normal in acute renal failure and elevated in chronic renal failure (4). In reality, the osmolar gap is used infrequently.

PLASMA TONICITY

Because urea passes freely across cell membranes, the effective osmolality or tonicity of the extracellular fluid can be calculated by eliminating urea (BUN) from the plasma osmolality equation.

$$\text{Plasma tonicity} = (2 \times [\text{Na}]) + \frac{[\text{Glucose}]}{18}$$

$$= (2 \times 140) + \frac{90}{18} \qquad (40.3)$$

$$= 285 \text{ mOsm/kg H}_2\text{O}$$

Because the concentration of urea contributes little to the total solute concentration in extracellular fluids, there is little difference between the osmolality and tonicity of the extracellular fluid. This equation

TABLE 40.1. CHANGES IN TOTAL BODY SODIUM AND WATER IN HYPERNATREMIA AND HYPONATREMIA

Condition	Extracellular Volume	Total Body Sodium	Total Body Free Water
Hypernatremia	Decreased	↓	↓↓
	Normal	→	↓
	Increased	↑↑	↑
Hyponatremia	Decreased	↓↓	↓
	Normal	→	↑
	Increased	↑	↑↑

establishes the plasma sodium concentration as the principal determinant of the effective osmolality of extracellular fluid. Because the effective osmolality determines the tendency for water to move into and out of cells, **the plasma sodium concentration is the principal determinant of the relative volumes of the intracellular and extracellular fluids.**

HYPERNATREMIA

The normal plasma (serum) sodium concentration is 135 to 145 mEq/L. Therefore, hypernatremia (i.e., a serum sodium concentration above 145 mEq/L) can be the result of loss of fluid that has a sodium concentration below 135 mEq/L (hypotonic fluid loss) or gain of fluid that has a sodium concentration above 145 mEq/L (hypertonic fluid gain). Each of these conditions can be identified by assessing the state of the extracellular volume, as shown in Table 40.1.

EXTRACELLULAR VOLUME

If invasive hemodynamic monitoring is available, the intravascular volume (IVV) can be evaluated by noting the cardiac filling pressures and the cardiac output (as described in Chapters 10, 11, 14, and 16). In the absence of hypoproteinemia (which shifts fluids from the intravascular to extravascular space), the state of the IVV can be used as a reflection of the state of the extracellular volume (ECV).

If invasive hemodynamic monitoring is unavailable, the state of the ECV can be inferred from a few clinical variables. The first is the sudden loss of weight (i.e., in a nonedematous person, a sudden loss of weight over a few days is an indication of a decreased ECV). The second is the presence of peripheral edema (i.e., in the absence of hypoproteinemia, the presence of peripheral edema is an indication of an increased ECV). The third is the concentration of sodium in a random (spot) urine sample (i.e., a urine sodium concentration less than 10 mEq/L is an indication of a decreased ECV). Finally, the clini-

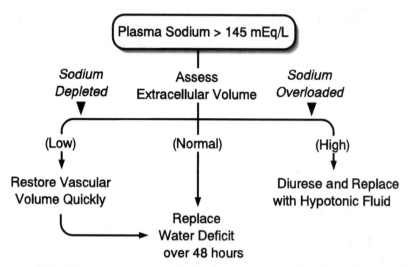

Figure 40.1. Management strategies for hypernatremia based on the extracellular volume. (From Marino PL, Krasner J, O'Moore P. Fluid and electrolyte expert. Philadelphia: WB Saunders, 1987.)

cal manifestations shown in Table 14.2 can be used as evidence for a decreased ECV.

Once the state of the ECV is determined, the strategies shown in Figure 40.1 can be applied.

Low ECV indicates loss of hypotonic fluids. Common causes are excessive diuresis, vomiting, and diarrhea. The management strategy is to replace the sodium deficit quickly (to maintain IVV) and to replace the free water deficit slowly (to prevent intracellular overhydration).

Normal ECV indicates a net loss of free water. This can be seen in diabetes insipidus, or when loss of hypotonic fluids (e.g., diuresis) is treated by replacement with isotonic saline in a 1:1 volume-to-volume ratio. The management strategy is to replace the free water deficit slowly (to prevent intracellular overhydration).

High ECV indicates a gain of hypertonic fluids. This is seen with aggressive use of hypertonic saline or sodium bicarbonate solutions. The management strategy is to induce sodium loss in the urine with diuresis and to replace the urine volume loss with fluids that are hypotonic to the urine.

Each of these conditions is described in more detail in the following sections.

HYPOVOLEMIC HYPERNATREMIA

The most common cause of hypernatremia is loss of hypotonic body fluids. The concentration of sodium in the body fluids that are com-

TABLE 40.2. SODIUM CONCENTRATION IN BODY FLUIDS	
Fluids Commonly Lost	**Sodium Concentration (mEq/L)**
Urine*	<10
Diarrhea	40
Gastric secretions	55
Sweat	80
Furosemide diuresis	75
Pancreatic secretions	145
Small bowel secretions	145
* Urinary sodium concentration varies according to daily sodium intake.	

monly lost is shown in Table 40.2. With the exception of small bowel secretions and pancreatic secretions, loss of any of these body fluids will result in hypernatremia.

CONSEQUENCES

All of the body fluids listed in Table 40.2 contain sodium, so the loss of these fluids will be accompanied by deficits in total body sodium as well as TBW. The sodium deficits predispose to hypovolemia, whereas the free water deficits predispose to hypertonicity in the extracellular fluids. Therefore, the two consequences of hypotonic fluid loss are hypovolemia and hypertonicity.

Hypovolemia

The most immediate threat with hypotonic fluid loss is hypovolemia, which predisposes to hypoperfusion of the vital organs. Fortunately, hypovolemia is not as prominent when hypotonic fluids are lost as when whole blood is lost. This is because the resultant hypertonicity draws water out of cells, and this helps maintain the volume of the extracellular (intravascular) fluid compartment.

Hypertonicity

The hypertonicity of the extracellular fluids predisposes to cellular dehydration. The most serious consequence of hypertonic hypernatremia is a metabolic encephalopathy (6). Clinical findings include depressed consciousness that can progress to frank coma, generalized seizures, and focal neurologic deficits. Hypernatremic encephalopathy has an associated mortality of up to 50% (6), but management should proceed slowly.

VOLUME REPLACEMENT

The most immediate concern in hypovolemic hypernatremia is to replace volume deficits and to maintain the cardiac output. Volume replacement can be guided by the cardiac filling pressures and the cardiac output, or by the clinical variables shown in Table 14.2. When solute losses are severe and hemodynamic compromise is present, colloid fluid replacement with 5% albumin or 6% hetastarch can rapidly restore the IVV, as described in Chapter 15. When crystalloid fluids are given for volume replacement, isotonic saline should always be used and less concentrated fluids (e.g., half-normal saline), which predispose to cellular overhydration, should be avoided.

FREE WATER REPLACEMENT

When hypovolemia has been corrected, the next step is to calculate and replace the free water deficit. The calculation of free water deficit is based on the assumption that the product of TBW and plasma sodium concentration (P_{Na}) is always constant.

$$\text{Current TBW} \times \text{Current } P_{Na} = \text{Normal TBW} \times \text{Normal } P_{Na} \quad (40.4)$$

Using a normal plasma sodium concentration of 140 mEq/L and rearranging terms yields the following relationship:

$$\text{Current TBW} = \text{Normal TBW} \times (140/\text{Current } P_{Na}) \quad (40.5)$$

The normal TBW (in liters) usually is 60% of lean body weight (in kg) in men and 50% of lean body weight in women. However, in hypernatremia associated with free water deficits, the normal TBW should be approximately 10% less than usual (3). Thus in men, the normal TBW is 0.5 × body weight (kg), and in women, the normal TBW is 0.4 × body weight (in kg). Once the current TBW is calculated, the water deficit is taken as the difference between the normal TBW and the current TBW.

$$\text{TBW deficit (L)} = \text{Normal TBW} - \text{Current TBW} \quad (40.6)$$

Example Calculation

Assume that an adult man with a lean body weight of 70 kg has a plasma sodium of 160 mEq/L. The normal TBW will be 0.5 × 70 = 35 L. The current TBW will be 35 × 140/160 = 30.5 L. The TBW deficit will be 35 − 30.5 = 4.5 L.

Replacement Volume

The volume of the replacement fluid needed to correct the water deficit is determined by the concentration of sodium in the replacement fluid. The replacement volume can be determined as follows (1):

$$\text{Replacement volume (L)} = \text{TBW deficit} \times (1/1 - X) \quad (40.7)$$

where X is the ratio of the sodium concentration in the replacement fluid to the sodium concentration in isotonic saline (X = replacement fluid Na/154). If the water deficit is 4.5 L and the replacement fluid is half-normal saline (Na = 75 mEq/L), the replacement volume will be 4.5 × (1/0.5) = 9 L.

Cerebral Edema

The brain cells initially shrink in response to a hypertonic extracellular fluid, but cell volume is restored within hours. This restoration of cell volume is attributed to the generation of osmotically active substances called idiogenetic osmoles (6). Once the brain cell volume is restored to normal, the aggressive replacement of free water can predispose to cerebral edema. To limit the risk of cerebral edema, **free water deficits should be replaced slowly, over 48 to 72 hours** (6).

DIABETES INSIPIDUS

The most noted cause for hypernatremia without apparent volume deficits is diabetes insipidus (DI), which is a condition of impaired renal water conservation (7). This condition results in excessive loss of urine that is almost pure water (devoid of solute). The underlying problem in DI is related to antidiuretic hormone (ADH), a hormone secreted by the posterior pituitary gland that promotes water reabsorption in the distal tubule. Two defects related to ADH can occur in DI:

Central DI is caused by inhibition of ADH release from the posterior pituitary. Common causes of central DI in critically ill patients include closed head injury, anoxic encephalopathy, and meningitis (5,7). The onset is heralded by polyuria that usually is evident within 24 hours of the inciting event.

Nephrogenic DI is caused by defective end-organ responsiveness to ADH. Possible causes of nephrogenic DI in critically ill patients includes hypokalemia, aminoglycosides, amphotericin, radiocontrast dyes, and the polyuric phase of ATN. The defect in urine concentrating ability in nephrogenic DI is not as severe as it is in central DI.

DIAGNOSIS

The hallmark of DI is a dilute urine in the face of plasma hypertonicity. In central DI, the urine osmolarity is often below 200 mOsm/L, whereas in nephrogenic DI, the urine osmolarity is usually between 200 and 500 mOsm/L (5). The diagnosis of DI is confirmed by noting the urinary response to fluid restriction. Failure of the urine osmolarity to increase more than 30 mOsm/L in the first hours of complete fluid restriction is diagnostic of DI. The fluid losses can be excessive during fluid restriction in DI (particularly central DI), and thus fluid restriction must be monitored carefully. Once the diagnosis of DI is confirmed, the response to vasopressin (5 units intravenously) will differentiate central from nephrogenic DI. In central DI, the urine osmolality increases by at least 50% almost immediately after vasopressin administration, whereas the urine osmolality remains unchanged after vasopressin in nephrogenic DI.

MANAGEMENT

The fluid loss in DI is almost pure water, so the replacement strategy is aimed at replacing free water deficits only. The water deficit is calculated as described previously, and the free water deficit is corrected slowly (over 2 to 3 days) to limit the risk of cerebral edema. In central DI, vasopressin administration is also required to prevent ongoing free water losses. The usual dose is 5 to 10 units of aqueous vasopressin subcutaneously every 6 to 8 hours (5,7). The serum sodium must be monitored carefully during vasopressin therapy because water intoxication and hyponatremia can occur if the central DI begins to resolve.

HYPERVOLEMIC HYPERNATREMIA

Hypernatremia from hypertonic fluid gain is uncommon. Possible causes are hypertonic saline resuscitation, sodium bicarbonate infusions for metabolic acidosis (see Table 37.1), and ingestion of excessive amounts of table salt (8).

MANAGEMENT

In patients with normal renal function, excess sodium and water are excreted rapidly. When renal sodium excretion is impaired, it might be necessary to increase renal sodium excretion with a diuretic (e.g., furosemide). Because the sodium concentration in urine during furosemide diuresis is approximately 75 mEq/L, excessive urine output will aggravate the hypernatremia (because the urine is hypotonic to plasma). Therefore, urine volume losses must be partially replaced with a fluid that is hypotonic to the urine.

HYPERGLYCEMIA

The formula for plasma tonicity presented earlier predicts that hyperglycemia will be accompanied by a hypertonic extracellular fluid. When progressive hyperglycemia does not result in ketosis, the major clinical consequence is a hypertonic encephalopathy similar to the one described for hypernatremia (6). The syndrome of **nonketotic hyperglycemia** (NKH) usually is seen in patients who have enough endogenous insulin to prevent ketosis. The condition usually is precipitated by a physiological stress (e.g., infection, trauma), and the patients may or may not have a prior history of diabetes mellitus (9). The plasma glucose is often 1000 mg/dL or higher (9) (whereas in ketoacidosis, the plasma glucose is usually below 800 mg/dL). The persistent loss of glucose in the urine produces an osmotic diuresis that can lead to profound volume losses.

CLINICAL MANIFESTATIONS

Patients with NKH usually have an altered mental status and may show signs of hypovolemia. The altered mental status can progress to frank coma when the plasma tonicity rises above 330 mOsm/kg H_2O (9). Advanced cases of encephalopathy can be accompanied by generalized seizures and focal neurologic deficits, as described for hypernatremic encephalopathy.

MANAGEMENT

The fluid management of NKH is similar to that described for hypovolemic hypernatremia. Volume deficits tend to be more profound in NKH than in simple hypovolemic hypernatremia because of the osmotic diuresis that accompanies the glycosuria. Therefore, rapid correction of the IVV (i.e., with 5% albumin or isotonic saline) may be necessary.

Free Water Deficit

Once the IVV is restored, free water deficits are estimated and replaced slowly. However when calculating the free water deficit that accompanies hyperglycemia, it is necessary to correct the plasma sodium for the increase in plasma glucose. This is because the hyperglycemia draws water from the intracellular space, and this creates a dilutional effect on the plasma sodium concentration. The decrease in plasma sodium in hypernatremia can vary according to the state of the ECV. In general, **for every 100 mg/dL increment in the plasma glucose, the plasma sodium should fall by 1.6 to 2 mEq/L** (10). Therefore, for a patient with a plasma glucose of 1000 mg/dL and a measured plasma sodium of 145 mEq/L, the actual or corrected plasma sodium will average 145 + (900/100 × 1.8) = 161 mEq/L (the factor 1.8 is taken as the average value between 1.6 and 2 mEq/L).

The restoration of brain cell volume can occur rapidly in hypertonic states due to hyperglycemia (9). Therefore, the free water replacement should be particularly judicious in NKH.

Insulin Therapy

Because insulin drives both glucose and water into cells, insulin therapy can aggravate hypovolemia. Therefore, in patients who are hypovolemic, insulin should be withheld until the IVV is restored. Once this is accomplished, insulin therapy can be given as advised for diabetic ketoacidosis (see Table 37.2). The insulin requirement will diminish as the hypertonic condition is corrected, so plasma glucose concentrations should be monitored hourly during intravenous insulin therapy in NKH.

HYPONATREMIA

Hyponatremia (serum sodium less than 135 mEq/L) is found in up to 4.5% of hospitalized elderly patients (11) and in 1% of postoperative patients (12). It is particularly prevalent in patients with the acquired immunodeficiency syndrome (AIDS) and can be seen in up to 40% of hospitalized patients with AIDS (13). The mortality in hyponatremic patients is as much as double the mortality in patients with a normal plasma sodium concentration (11,13). This increase in mortality can be a reflection of the treatment as well as the consequences of hyponatremia.

PSEUDOHYPONATREMIA

Extreme elevations in plasma lipids or proteins increase the plasma volume and can reduce the measured plasma sodium concentration. The increase in plasma volume in these situations is in the nonaqueous phase of plasma, and because the sodium is contained in the aqueous phase of plasma, the hyponatremia in this situation does not represent a decrease in extracellular sodium relative to extracellular water (i.e., true or hypotonic hyponatremia). This condition is therefore called *pseudohyponatremia*. Because the nonaqueous phase of plasma represents only 7% of the total plasma volume, large increases in plasma lipids and plasma proteins are needed to produce significant decreases in the measured plasma sodium concentration. The correction factors for hyperlipidemia and hyperproteinemia are as follows (1):

1. Plasma triglycerides (g/L) $\times$ 0.002 = mEq/L decrease in plasma Na.
2. Plasma protein level minus 8 (g/dL) $\times$ 0.025 = mEq/L decrease in plasma Na.

Ion-Specific Electrodes

The conventional method for measuring plasma sodium (flame emission spectrophotometry) includes both the aqueous and nonaqueous phases of plasma. However, the newer ion-specific sodium electrodes measure the sodium concentration only in the aqueous phase of plasma. Therefore, pseudohyponatremia will not occur when ion-specific electrodes are used to measure the plasma sodium concentration (14).

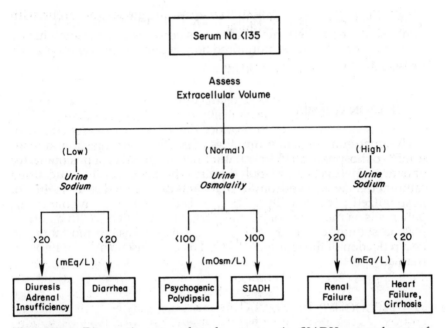

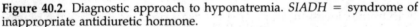

Figure 40.2. Diagnostic approach to hyponatremia. *SIADH* = syndrome of inappropriate antidiuretic hormone.

HYPOTONIC HYPONATREMIA

True or hypotonic hyponatremia represents an increase in free water relative to sodium in the extracellular fluids. It does *not* necessarily represent an increase in the volume of extracellular fluids. As shown in Table 40.1, the ECV can be low, normal, or high in patients with hyponatremia. The diagnostic approach to hyponatremia can begin with an assessment of the ECV, as shown in Figure 40.2 (14,15). (The assessment of ECV is described earlier, for the assessment of hyperna-tremia.)

HYPOVOLEMIC HYPONATREMIA

This condition is characterized by fluid losses combined with vol-ume replacement using a fluid that is hypotonic to the lost fluid (e.g., diuresis replaced by drinking tap water). The result is a net loss of sodium relative to free water, which decreases both the ECV and the extracellular sodium concentration. The concentration of sodium in a random (spot) urine sample can sometimes help determine if the so-dium loss is renal or extrarenal in origin.

Site of Sodium Loss	Urine Sodium
Renal	>20 mEq/L
Extrarenal	<10 mEq/L

Renal sodium losses would be seen in diuretic overuse and in adrenal insufficiency, whereas extrarenal sodium losses can occur with diarrhea and persistent vomiting.

ISOVOLEMIC HYPONATREMIA

Isovolemic hyponatremia is characterized by a small gain in free water, but not enough to be clinically detected (approximately 5 L of excess water is necessary to produce detectable peripheral edema in the average-size adult). In this situation, the major disorders to consider are inappropriate (nonosmotic) release of ADH and acute water intoxication (psychogenic polydipsia). The urine sodium and urine osmolality will help distinguish between these two disorders.

Clinical Disorder	Urine Sodium	Urine Osmolality
Inappropriate ADH	>20 mEq/L	>100 mOsm/kg H_2O
Water intoxication	<10 mEq/L	<100 mOsm/kg H_2O

The inappropriate (nonosmotic) release of ADH is characterized by an inappropriately concentrated urine (urine osmolality above 100 mOsm/kg H_2O) in the face of a hypotonic plasma (plasma tonicity below 290 mOsm/kg H_2O). This condition can be seen in certain groups of "stressed" patients, such as patients who have undergone recent surgery. It can also be produced by a variety of tumors and infections. This latter condition is known as the *syndrome of inappropriate ADH* (SIADH), and it can be accompanied by severe hyponatremia (plasma sodium below 120 mEq/L).

HYPERVOLEMIC HYPONATREMIA

Hypervolemic hyponatremia represents an excess of sodium and water, with the water gain exceeding the sodium gain. In this situation, the urine sodium can sometimes help identify the source of the problem.

Common Causes	Urine Sodium
Heart failure	<20 mEq/L
Renal failure	>20 mEq/L
Hepatic failure	<20 mEq/L

The urine sodium can be misleading if the patient is also receiving diuretics (which are commonly used in these conditions). The clinical picture is usually helpful, although these conditions can co-exist in critically ill patients.

SYMPTOMATIC HYPONATREMIA

The major complication of hyponatremia is a metabolic encephalopathy, which can be both irreversible and fatal (12,16,17). This condition is due to cerebral edema and increased intracranial pressure (17). In addition to having the same manifestations as the encephalopathy associated with the hypertonic syndromes (i.e., depressed level of consciousness, seizures, and focal neurologic findings), this encephalopathy can be accompanied by the acute respiratory distress syndrome (18).

In addition to hyponatremic encephalopathy another distinct encephalopathy is associated with the therapy of hyponatremia, particularly when the hyponatremia is corrected too rapidly (17). This encephalopathy is characterized by diffuse demyelinating lesions and can be accompanied by pituitary damage and oculomotor nerve palsies. A specific type of demyelinating disorder known as central pontine myelinolysis has also been attributed to rapid correction of hyponatremia (19). As described in the following section, the risk of this second encephalopathy has led to specific recommendations for limiting the maximum rate and end-point of corrective therapy.

MANAGEMENT STRATEGIES

The management of hyponatremia is determined by the state of the ECV (i.e., low, normal, or high) and by the presence or absence of neurologic symptoms. Symptomatic hyponatremia requires more aggressive corrective therapy than asymptomatic hyponatremia. However, to limit the risk of a demyelinating encephalopathy, **the rate of rise in plasma sodium should not exceed 0.5 mEq/L/hour and the final plasma sodium concentration should not exceed 130 mEq/L** (17). The general management strategies based on the ECV are as follows:

Low ECV: Infuse hypertonic saline (3% NaCl) in symptomatic patients, and isotonic saline in asymptomatic patients.

Normal ECV: Combine furosemide diuresis with infusion of hypertonic saline in symptomatic patients, or isotonic saline in asymptomatic patients.

High ECV: Use furosemide-induced diuresis in asymptomatic patients. In symptomatic patients, combine furosemide diuresis with judicious use of hypertonic saline.

SODIUM REPLACEMENT

When corrective therapy requires the infusion of isotonic saline or hypertonic saline, the replacement therapy can be guided by the calculated sodium deficit. This is determined as follows (using a plasma sodium of 130 mEq/L as the desired end-point of replacement therapy):

$$\text{Sodium deficit (mEq)} = \text{Normal TBW} \times (130 - \text{Current } P_{Na})$$

$$(40.8)$$

The normal TBW (in liters) is 60% of the lean body weight (in kg) in men, and 50% of the lean body weight in women. Thus, for a 60 kg woman with a plasma sodium of 120 mEq/L, the sodium deficit will be $0.5 \times 60 \times (130 - 120) = 300$ mEq.

Because 3% sodium chloride contains 513 mEq of sodium per liter, the volume of hypertonic saline needed to correct a sodium deficit of 300 mEq will be $300/513 = 585$ mL. Using a maximum rate of rise of 0.5 mEq/L/hour for the plasma sodium (to limit the risk of a demyelinating encephalopathy), the sodium concentration deficit of 10 mEq/L in the previous example should be corrected over at least 20 hours. Thus, the maximum rate of hypertonic fluid administration will be $585/20 = 29$ mL/hour. If isotonic saline is used for sodium replacement, the replacement volume will be 3.3 times the replacement volume of the hypertonic 3% saline solution.

REFERENCES

SUGGESTED READING

Rose BD. Clinical physiology of acid-base and electrolyte disorders. 4th ed. New York: McGraw-Hill, 1994.

REVIEWS

1. Marino PL, Krasner J, O'Moore P. Fluid and electrolyte expert. Philadelphia: WB Saunders, 1987 (software).
2. Oh MS, Carroll HJ. Disorders of sodium metabolism: hypernatremia and hyponatremia. Crit Care Med 1992;20:94–103 (34 references).

BASIC CONCEPTS

3. Rose BD. The total body water and the plasma sodium concentration. In: Clinical physiology of acid-base and electrolyte disorders. 4th ed. New York: McGraw-Hill, 1994;219–234.
4. Sklar AK, Linas SL. The osmolal gap in renal failure. Ann Intern Med 1983; 98:481–482.

HYPERNATREMIA

5. Geheb M. Clinical approach to the hyperosmolar patient. Crit Care Clin 1987; 5:797–815.
6. Arieff AI, Ayus JC. Strategies for diagnosing and managing hypernatremic encephalopathy. J Crit Illness 1996;11:720–727.
7. Blevins LS, Wand GS. Diabetes insipidus. Crit Care Med 1992;20:69–79.
8. Moder KG, Hurley DL. Fatal hypernatremia from exogenous salt intake: report of a case and review of the literature. Mayo Clin Proc 1990;65:1587–1594.

HYPERGLYCEMIA

9. Rose BD. Hyperosmolal states: hyperglycemia. In Clinical physiology of acid-base and electrolyte disorders. 4th ed. New York: McGraw-Hill, 1994;737–762.
10. Moran SM, Jamison RL. The variable hyponatremic response to hyperglycemia. West J Med 1985;142:49–53.

HYPONATREMIA

11. Terzian C, Frye EB, Piotrowski ZH. Admission hyponatremia in the elderly. J Gen Intern Med 1994;9:89–91.
12. Ayus JC, Wheeler JM, Arieff AI. Postoperative hyponatremic encephalopathy in menstruant women. Ann Intern Med 1992;117:891–897.
13. Tang WW, Kaptien EM, Feinstein EI, Massry SG. Hyponatremia in hospitalized patients with the acquired immunodeficiency syndrome (AIDS) and the AIDS-related complex. Am J Med 1993;94:169–174.
14. Weisberg LS. Pseudohyponatremia: a reappraisal. Am J Med 1988;86:315–318.
15. Schrier RW, Briner VA. The differential diagnosis of hyponatremia. Hosp Pract 1990;25:29–37.
16. Ayus JC, Arieff AI. Symptomatic hyponatremia: making the diagnosis rapidly. J Crit Illness 1990;5:846–856.
17. Arieff AI, Ayus JC. Pathogenesis of hyponatremic encephalopathy. Chest 1993;103:607–610.
18. Ayus JC, Arieff AI. Pulmonary complications of hyponatremic encephalopathy: noncardiogenic pulmonary edema and hypercapnic respiratory failure. Chest 1995;107:517–521.
19. Bruner JE, Redmond JM, Haggar AM, et al. Central pontine myelinolysis and pontine lesions after rapid correction of hyponatremia: a prospective magnetic resonance imaging study. Ann Neurol 1990;27:61–66.

41

POTASSIUM

Early sea-living organisms exhibited a preference for intracellular potassium and a disdain for intracellular sodium, which eventually changed the composition of the oceans from a potassium salt solution to a sodium salt solution. This behavior is also found in mammalian organisms, in whom potassium is the major intracellular cation and sodium is the major extracellular cation. This pattern is the result of the sodium–potassium exchange pump on cell membranes, which sequesters potassium and extrudes sodium. In humans, only 2% of the total body potassium stores are found outside cells. This lack of extracellular representation limits the value of the plasma (extracellular) potassium concentration as an index of total body potassium stores.

POTASSIUM DISTRIBUTION

The marked discrepancy between the intracellular and extracellular content of potassium is illustrated in Figure 41.1. The total body potassium content in healthy adults is approximately 50 mEq/kg (1), so a 70-kg adult will have 3500 mEq of total body potassium. However, only 70 mEq (2% of the total amount) is found in the extracellular fluids. Because the plasma accounts for approximately 20% of the extracellular fluid volume, the potassium content of plasma will be about 15 mEq, which is 0.004% of the total amount of potassium in the body. This suggests that the plasma potassium will be an insensitive marker of changes in total body potassium stores.

SERUM POTASSIUM

The relationship between changes in total body potassium and changes in serum potassium is curvilinear, as shown in Figure 41.2 (2,3). The slope of the curve decreases on the "deficit" side of the graph, indicating that the change in serum potassium is much smaller

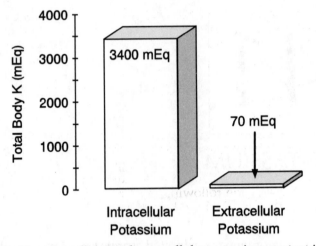

Figure 41.1. The intracellular and extracellular potassium content in a 70-kg adult with a total body potassium of 50 mEq/L.

when potassium is depleted than when potassium accumulates. In an averaged-size adult with a normal serum potassium concentration (i.e., 3.5 to 5.5 mEq/L), a total body potassium deficit of 200 to 400 mEq is required to produce a 1 mEq/L decrease in serum potassium, whereas a total body potassium excess of 100 to 200 mEq is required to produce a 1 mEq/L rise in serum potassium (3). In other words, potassium depletion must be twice as great as potassium accumulation

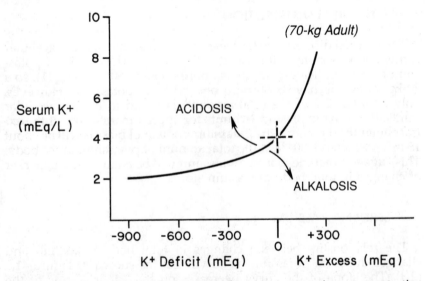

Figure 41.2. The relationship between the serum potassium concentration and changes in total body potassium content. (Redrawn from Brown RS. Extrarenal potassium homeostasis. Kidney Int 1986;30:116–127.)

to produce a significant (1 mEq/L) change in the serum potassium concentration. This difference is due to the large pool of intracellular potassium, which can replenish extracellular stores when potassium is lost.

HYPOKALEMIA

Hypokalemia is a serum potassium concentration below 3.5 mEq/L. The causes of hypokalemia can be classified according to whether an intracellular shift of potassium (transcellular shift) occurred or whether a decrease in total body potassium content (potassium depletion) occurred (4). The following are some of the possible causes of hypokalemia that are likely to be encountered in the ICU.

TRANSCELLULAR SHIFT

Potassium movement into cells is facilitated by stimulation of β_2-adrenergic receptors on muscle cell membranes. Inhaled **β-agonist bronchodilators** (e.g., albuterol) are well known for their ability to reduce the serum potassium concentration, but this effect is mild (0.5 mEq/L or less) in the usual therapeutic doses (5). A more significant effect is seen when inhaled β-agonists are given in combination with diuretics (6). Other factors that promote the transcellular shift of potassium into cells include **alkalosis** (respiratory or metabolic), **hypothermia** (accidental or induced), and **insulin.** Alkalosis has a variable and unpredictable effect on the serum potassium (7). Hypothermia causes a transient drop in serum potassium that resolves during rewarming. Lethal cases of hypothermia can be accompanied by *hyper*kalemia because of widespread cell death (8).

POTASSIUM DEPLETION

Potassium depletion can be the result of either renal or extrarenal potassium losses. The site of potassium loss can often be identified by using a combination of urinary potassium and chloride concentrations, as shown in Figure 41.3.

Renal Potassium Loss

The leading cause of renal potassium wasting is **diuretic therapy.** Other causes likely to be seen in the ICU include nasogastric drainage, alkalosis, and magnesium depletion. The urinary chloride is low (less than 15 mEq/L) when nasogastric drainage or alkalosis is involved, and it is high (greater than 25 mEq/L) when magnesium depletion or diuretics are responsible. **Magnesium depletion** impairs potassium reabsorption across the renal tubules and may play a very important

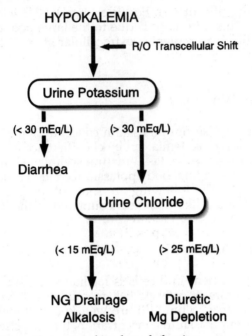

HYPOKALEMIA

R/O Transcellular Shift

Urine Potassium

(< 30 mEq/L)   (> 30 mEq/L)

Diarrhea

Urine Chloride

(< 15 mEq/L)   (> 25 mEq/L)

NG Drainage   Diuretic
Alkalosis   Mg Depletion

Figure 41.3. Diagnostic approach to hypokalemia.

role in promoting and sustaining potassium depletion in critically ill patients, particularly those receiving diuretics (9).

Extrarenal Potassium Loss

The major cause of extrarenal potassium loss is **diarrhea.** The potassium concentration in stool is 75 mEq/L, but because the stool volume is normally 200 mL or less each day, little potassium is lost. In diarrheal states, the daily volume of stool can be as high as 10 L, and thus severe or prolonged diarrhea can result in significant potassium depletion.

CLINICAL MANIFESTATIONS

Severe hypokalemia (serum K^+ below 2.5 mEq/L) can be accompanied by diffuse muscle weakness and mental status changes. Milder degrees of hypokalemia (serum K^+ 2.5 to 3.5 mEq/L) are often asymptomatic. Abnormalities in the ECG, including prominent U waves (more than 1 mm in height), flattening and inversion of T waves, and prolongation of the QT interval, can be present in more than half of the cases (10). None of these changes are specific for hypokalemia. The T wave changes and U waves can be seen with digitalis or left ventricular hypertrophy, and QT prolongation can be seen with hypocalcemia and hypomagnesemia.

TABLE 41.1. POTASSIUM DEFICITS IN HYPOKALEMIA*		
Serum Potassium (mEq/L)	Potassium Deficit	
	mEq	% Total Body K
3.0	175	5
2.5	350	10
2.0	470	15
1.5	700	20
1.0	875	25

* Estimated deficits for a 70 kg adult with a total body potassium content of 50 mEq/kg.

Arrhythmias

There is a misconception about the ability of hypokalemia to promote cardiac arrhythmias. **Hypokalemia alone does not produce serious cardiac arrhythmias** (10). Hypokalemia is often combined with other conditions that can promote arrhythmias (e.g., magnesium depletion, digitalis), and the hypokalemia may enhance the proarrhythmic effects of these other conditions. Hypokalemia is well known for its ability to promote digitalis-induced arrhythmias (see Chapter 53).

MANAGEMENT OF HYPOKALEMIA

The first concern in hypokalemia is to eliminate or treat any condition that promotes transcellular potassium shifts (e.g., alkalosis). If the hypokalemia is due to potassium depletion, proceed as described in the following section.

POTASSIUM DEFICIT

If the hypokalemia is due to potassium depletion, a potassium deficit of 10% of the total body potassium stores is expected for every 1 mEq/L decrease in the serum potassium (11). The correlation between potassium deficits and the severity of hypokalemia is shown in Table 41.1. These estimates do not consider any contribution from transcellular potassium shifts, and thus they are meant only as rough guidelines for gauging the severity of potassium depletion.

POTASSIUM REPLACEMENT

Solutions

The usual replacement fluid is potassium chloride, which is available as a concentrated solution (1.5 and 2 mEq/mL) in ampules containing 10, 20, 30, and 40 mEq of potassium. These solutions are extremely hyperosmotic (the 2 mEq/L solution has an osmolality of 4000 mOsm/kg H_2O) and must be diluted (12). A potassium phosphate solution is also available (contains 4.5 mEq potassium and 3 mM phosphate per mL) and is preferred by some for potassium replacement in diabetic ketoacidosis (because of the phosphate depletion that accompanies ketoacidosis).

Infusion Rate

The standard method of intravenous potassium replacement is to add 20 mEq of potassium to 100 mL of isotonic saline and infuse this mixture over 1 hour (13). The maximum rate of intravenous potassium replacement is usually set at 20 mEq/hour (13), but dose rates up to 40 mEq/hour occasionally may be necessary (e.g., with serum K^+ below 1.5 mEq/L or serious arrhythmias), and dose rates as high as 80 mEq/hour have been used safely (4). A large central vein should be used for infusion because of the irritating properties of the hyperosmotic potassium solutions. However, if the desired replacement rate is greater than 20 mEq/hour, the infusion should not be given through a central venous catheter because of the theoretical risk of transient hyperkalemia in the right heart chambers, which can predispose to cardiac standstill. In this situation, the potassium dose can be split and administered via two peripheral veins.

Response

The serum potassium may be slow to rise at first, because of the position on the flat part of the curve in Figure 41.2. Full replacement usually takes a few days, particularly if potassium losses are ongoing. If the hypokalemia seems refractory to replacement therapy, the serum magnesium level should be checked. **Magnesium depletion** promotes urinary potassium losses and **can cause refractory hypokalemia** (14). The management of hypomagnesemia is presented in Chapter 42.

HYPERKALEMIA

While hypokalemia is often well tolerated, hyperkalemia (serum K^+ greater than 5.5 mEq/L) can be a serious and life-threatening condition (15).

PSEUDOHYPERKALEMIA

Potassium release from traumatic hemolysis during the venipuncture can produce a spurious elevation in serum potassium. This is more common than suspected, and has been reported in 20% of blood samples with an elevated serum potassium (16). Potassium release from muscles distal to a tourniquet can also be a source of spuriously high serum potassium levels (17). Because of the risk of spurious hyperkalemia, an unexpected finding of hyperkalemia in an asymptomatic patient should always prompt a repeat measurement before any diagnostic or therapeutic measures are initiated.

Potassium release from cells during clot formation in the specimen tube can also produce pseudohyperkalemia when severe leukocytosis (white blood cell count greater than $50,000/mm^3$) or thrombocytosis (platelet count greater than 1 million/mm^3) is present. When this condition is suspected, the serum potassium should be measured in an unclotted blood sample.

URINE POTASSIUM

Hyperkalemia can be caused by potassium release from cells (transcellular shift) or by impaired renal potassium excretion. If the source of the hyperkalemia is unclear, the urinary potassium concentration can be helpful. A high urine potassium (greater than 30 mEq/L) suggests a transcellular shift, and a low urine potassium (less than 30 mEq/L) indicates impaired renal excretion.

TRANSCELLULAR SHIFT

Acidosis traditionally has been listed as a cause of hyperkalemia because of the tendency for acidosis to both enhance potassium release from cells and reduce renal potassium excretion. However, hyperkalemia does not always accompany respiratory acidosis (18), and **no clear evidence exists that organic acidoses** (i.e., lactic acidosis and ketoacidosis) **can produce hyperkalemia** (7,18,19). Although hyperkalemia can accompany acidoses associated with renal failure and renal tubular acidosis, hyperkalemia in these instances may be caused by impaired renal potassium excretion.

Myonecrosis can release large amounts of potassium into the extracellular fluid, but if renal function is normal, the extra potassium is promptly cleared by the kidneys. For example, severe exercise can raise the serum potassium to 8 mEq/L, but the hyperkalemia resolves with a half-time of 25 seconds (20).

Drugs that can promote hyperkalemia via transcellular potassium shifts include β-receptor antagonists and digitalis (Table 41.2). Serious

TABLE 41.2. DRUGS THAT CAN CAUSE HYPERKALEMIA	
ACE Inhibitors	NSAIDs
β-Blockers	Pentamidine
Cyclosporine	Potassium penicillin
Digitalis	THAM
Diuretics (K-sparing)	TMP–SMX
Heparin	Succinylcholine

ACE = Angiotensin-converting enzyme, *NSAIDs* = nonsteroidal antiinflammatory drugs, *TMP–SMX* = trimethoprim–sulfamethoxadole.

hyperkalemia (i.e., serum potassium above 7 mEq/L) is possible only with digitalis toxicity.

IMPAIRED RENAL EXCRETION

Renal insufficiency can produce hyperkalemia when the glomerular filtration rate falls below 10 mL/minute or the urine output falls below 1 L/day (21). Exceptions are interstitial nephritis and hyporeninemic hypoaldosteronism (21). The latter condition is seen in elderly diabetic patients who have defective renin release in response to reduced renal blood flow.

Adrenal insufficiency is a well known cause of hyperkalemia from impaired renal potassium excretion, but is not a common cause of hyperkalemia in the ICU.

Drugs that impair renal potassium excretion are considered one of the leading causes of hyperkalemia. A list of common offenders is shown in Table 41.2. The drugs most commonly implicated are angiotensin-converting enzyme inhibitors, potassium sparing diuretics, and nonsteroidal antiinflammatory drugs (15,16). Other potential offenders in the ICU are heparin, trimethoprim–sulfamethoxazole, and pentamidine (22–24). All of these agents promote hyperkalemia by inhibiting or blocking the renin–angiotensin–aldosterone system, and all promote hyperkalemia particularly when given with potassium supplements.

BLOOD TRANSFUSIONS

Massive blood transfusions (i.e., when the transfusion volume exceeds the estimated blood volume) can promote hyperkalemia when given to patients with circulatory shock. Potassium leakage from erythrocytes results in a steady rise in plasma potassium levels in stored blood. In whole blood, the plasma potassium rises an average of 1 mEq/L/day. However, because one unit of whole blood contains 250 mL of plasma, this represents an increase of only 0.25 mEq/day in the plasma potassium content per unit of whole blood. After 14 days of storage, the plasma potassium load is 4.4 mEq per unit of whole blood and 3.1 mEq per unit of packed red cells (25).

The potassium load in blood transfusions normally is cleared by the kidneys, and thus no sustained rise in plasma potassium occurs. However, in patients with circulatory shock, the extra potassium from blood transfusions can accumulate and produce hyperkalemia. Furthermore, when the volume of distribution for potassium is curtailed by widespread hypoperfusion, the potassium accumulation can be rapid and life-threatening.

CLINICAL MANIFESTATIONS

The most serious consequence of hyperkalemia is the slowing of electrical conduction in the heart. The ECG can begin to change when the serum potassium reaches 6.0 mEq/L, and it is always abnormal when the serum potassium reaches 8.0 mEq/L (21). Figure 41.4 illustrates the ECG changes associated with progressive hyperkalemia.

The earliest change in the ECG is a tall, tapering (tented) T wave that is most evident in precordial leads V_2 and V_3. Similar "peaked T" waves have been observed in metabolic acidosis (26). As the hyperkalemia progresses, the P wave amplitude decreases and the PR interval lengthens. The P waves eventually disappear and the QRS duration becomes prolonged. The final event is ventricular asystole.

MANAGEMENT OF HYPERKALEMIA

The acute management of hyperkalemia is guided by the serum potassium level and the ECG. The therapeutic maneuvers are outlined in Table 41.3.

MEMBRANE ANTAGONISM

Calcium directly antagonizes the membrane actions of potassium. When hyperkalemia is severe (i.e., above 7 mEq/L) or accompanied by advanced ECG changes (i.e., loss of P waves and prolonged QRS duration), **calcium gluconate** is administered in the dose shown in Table 41.3. If there is no response to calcium within a few minutes, a second dose can be given. A third dose will not be effective if there was no response to the second dose of calcium. The response to calcium lasts only 20 or 30 minutes, so other therapies should be initiated to enhance potassium clearance.

Calcium must be given cautiously to patients on digitalis because hypercalcemia can potentiate digitalis cardiotoxicity. For patients receiving digitalis, the calcium gluconate should be added to 100 mL of isotonic saline and infused over 20 to 30 minutes. If the hyperkalemia is a manifestation of digitalis toxicity, calcium is contraindicated.

When hyperkalemia is accompanied by evidence of circulatory compromise, **calcium chloride** is preferred to calcium gluconate. One ampule (10 mL) of 10% calcium chloride contains three times more elemental calcium than one ampule of 10% calcium gluconate (see Table 43.3), and the extra calcium in calcium chloride may prove beneficial in promoting cardiac contraction and maintaining peripheral vascular tone.

TRANSCELLULAR SHIFT

Insulin–Dextrose

Combined therapy with insulin and dextrose will drive potassium into muscle cells and decrease the serum potassium by an average of 1 mEq/L. However, this is a temporary effect, and other maneuvers aimed at enhancing potassium clearance are also required.

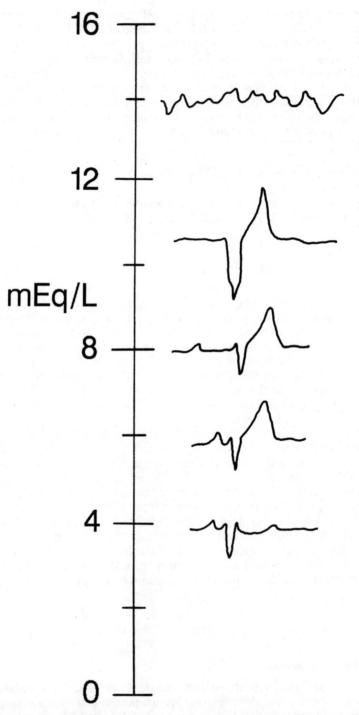

Figure 41.4. The ECG manifestations of progressive hyperkalemia. (Adapted from Burch GE, Winsor T. A primer of electrocardiography. Philadelphia: Lea & Febiger, 1966;143.)

TABLE 41.3. ACUTE MANAGEMENT OF HYPERKALEMIA		
Condition	**Treatment**	**Comment**
ECG changes or serum K >7 mEq/L	Calcium gluconate (10%): 10 mL IV over 3 minutes; can repeat in 5 minutes	Response lasts only 20 to 30 minutes. *Do not* give bicarbonate after calcium.
ECG changes and circulatory compromise	Calcium chloride (10%): 10 mL IV over 3 minutes	Calcium chloride contains 3 times more calcium than calcium gluconate.
AV block refractory to calcium treatment	1. 10 U regular insulin in 500 mL of 20% dextrose: infuse over 1 hour 2. Transvenous pacemaker	Insulin–dextrose treatment should drop the serum K by 1 mEq/L for 1 to 2 hours.
Digitalis cardiotoxicity	1. Magnesium sulfate: 2 g as IV bolus 2. Digitalis-specific antibodies if necessary	*Do not* use calcium for the hyperkalemia of digitalis toxicity. See Chapter 53 for more on the treatment of digitalis toxicity.
After acute phase or when no ECG changes	Kayexalate: oral dose of 30 g in 50 mL of 20% sorbitol, or rectal dose of 50 g in 200 mL 20% sorbitol as a retention enema	Oral dosing is preferred. Enemas poorly tolerated by patients and nurses.

Sodium Bicarbonate

The administration of sodium bicarbonate (44 to 88 mEq) can also shift potassium into cells. However, the most common acidotic condition associated with hyperkalemia is renal failure, and in this condition, insulin–dextrose is much more effective in lowering the serum potassium than bicarbonate (27). Furthermore, bicarbonate binds calcium and should not be given after calcium is administered. For these reasons, there is little value in using bicarbonate to treat hyperkalemia.

ENHANCED CLEARANCE

Measures aimed at enhancing the removal of potassium from the body can be used alone in mild cases of hyperkalemia (i.e., serum K less than 7 mEq/L) without advanced ECG changes or can serve as a follow-up to calcium and insulin–dextrose therapy.

Exchange Resin

Polystyrene sulfonate (Kayexalate) is a cation exchange resin that can enhance potassium clearance across the gastrointestinal mucosa (gastrointestinal dialysis). This resin can be given orally or by retention enema, and it is mixed with 20% sorbitol to prevent concretion. For each mEq of potassium removed, 2 to 3 mEq of sodium are added. If there is concern about the added sodium, one or two doses of furosemide can be used to enhance natriuresis.

Loop Diuretics

The loop diuretics furosemide and ethacrynic acid enhance urinary potassium excretion. These agents can be used as a follow-up measure to calcium and insulin–dextrose. This approach is ineffective in renal failure.

Hemodialysis

Hemodialysis is the most effective method of lowering the serum potassium in patients with renal failure (27).

REFERENCES

SUGGESTED READING

Androgue HJ, Wesson DE. Potassium. Boston: Blackwell Scientific, 1994.

POTASSIUM DISTRIBUTION

1. Rose BD. Potassium homeostasis. In: Clinical physiology of acid-base and electrolyte disorders. 4th ed. New York: McGraw-Hill, 1994;346–376.
2. Brown RS. Extrarenal potassium homeostasis. Kidney Int 1986; 30:116-127.
3. Sterns RH, Cox M, Feig PU, Singer I. Internal potassium balance and the control of the plasma potassium balance. Medicine 1981;60:339–351.

HYPOKALEMIA

4. Freedman BI, Burkhart JM. Hypokalemia. Crit Care Clin 1991;7:143–153.
5. Bodenhammer J, Bergstrom R, Brown D, et al. Frequently nebulized beta-agonists for asthma: effects on serum electrolytes. Ann Emerg Med 1992;21: 1337–1342.
6. Lipworth BJ, McDevitt DG, Struthers AD. Prior treatment with diuretic augments the hypokalemic and electrocardiographic effects of inhaled albuterol. Am J Med 1989;86:653–657.
7. Androgue HJ, Madias NE. Changes in plasma potassium concentration during acute acid-base changes. Am J Med 1981;71:456–467.
8. Schaller MD, Fischer AP, Perret CH. Hyperkalemia: a prognostic factor during acute, severe hypothermia. JAMA 1990;264:1842–1845.
9. Salem M, Munoz R, Chernow B. Hypomagnesemia in critical illness. Crit Care Clin 1991;7:225–252.
10. Flakeb G, Villarread D, Chapman D. Is hypokalemia a cause of ventricular arrhythmias? J Crit Illness 1986;1:66–74.
11. Stanaszek WF, Romankiewicz JA. Current approaches to management of potassium deficiency. Drug Intell Clin Pharmacol 1985;19:176–184.

12. Trissel LA. Handbook on injectable drugs. 8th ed. Bethesda, MD: American Society for Hospital Pharmacists, 1994;886–902.
13. Kruse JA, Carlson RW. Rapid correction of hypokalemia using concentrated intravenous potassium chloride infusions. Arch Intern Med 1990;150:613–617.
14. Whang R, Flink EB, Dyckner T, et al. Mg depletion as a cause of refractory potassium depletion. Arch Intern Med 1985;145:1686–1689.

HYPERKALEMIA

15. Williams ME. Hyperkalemia. Crit Care Clin 1991;7:155–174.
16. Rimmer JM, Horn JF, Gennari FJ. Hyperkalemia as a complication of drug therapy. Arch Intern Med 1987;147:867–869.
17. Don BR, Sebastian A, Cheitlin M, et al. Pseudohyperkalemia caused by fist clenching during phlebotomy. N Engl J Med 1990;322:1290–1293.
18. Burger GA, Howard R. Acidosis and [K^+]. Anesth Analg 1993;76:680.
19. Orringer CE, Eustace JC, Wunsch CD, Gardner LB. Natural history of lactic acidosis after grand-mal seizure. N Engl J Med 1977;297:796–799.
20. Medbo JL, Sejersted OM. Plasma potassium changes with high intensity exercise. J Physiol 1990;42:105–122.
21. Williams ME, Rosa RM. Hyperkalemia: disorders of internal and external potassium balance. J Intensive Care Med 1988;3:52–64.
22. Oster JR, Singer I, Fishman LM. Heparin-induced aldosterone suppression and hyperkalemia. Am J Med 1995;98:575–586.
23. Greenberg S, Reiser IW, Chou SY, Porush JG. Trimethoprim–sulfamethoxazole induces reversible hyperkalemia. Ann Intern Med 1993;119:291–295.
24. Peltz S, Hashmi S. Pentamidine-induced severe hyperkalemia. Am J Med 1989;87:698–699.
25. Michael JM, Dorner I, Burns D, et al. Potassium load in CPD-preserved whole blood and two types of packed red cells. Transfusion 1975;15:144–149.
26. Dreyfuss D, Jondeau G, Couturier R, et al. Tall T waves during metabolic acidosis without hyperkalemia: a prospective study. Crit Care Med 1989;17:404–408.
27. Blumberg A, Weidmann P, Gnadinger M. Effect of various therapeutic approaches on plasma potassium and major regulating factors in terminal renal failure. Am J Med 1988;85:507–512.

42

MAGNESIUM

Magnesium is the second most abundant intracellular cation in the human body (potassium being the first), where it serves as a cofactor for more than 3000 enzyme reactions that involve adenosine triphosphate (1). One of the magnesium-dependent enzyme systems is the membrane pump that generates the electrical gradient across cell membranes. As a result, magnesium plays an important role in the activity of electrically excitable tissues (1–4). Magnesium also regulates the movement of calcium into smooth muscle cells, which gives it a pivotal role in the maintenance of cardiac contractile strength and peripheral vascular tone (2).

MAGNESIUM BALANCE

The content and distribution of magnesium in the human body is shown in Table 42.1 (1). The average-size adult contains approximately 24 g (1 mole, or 2000 mEq) of magnesium; a little over half is located in bone, whereas less than 1% is located in plasma. This lack of representation in the plasma limits the value of the plasma magnesium concentration as an index of total body magnesium stores. This is particularly true in patients with magnesium deficiency, in whom **serum magnesium levels can be normal in the face of total body magnesium depletion** (5,6).

SERUM MAGNESIUM

Serum is favored over plasma for magnesium assays because the anticoagulant used for plasma samples can be contaminated with citrate or other anions that bind magnesium (6). The normal range for serum magnesium depends on the daily magnesium intake, which

TABLE 42.1. MAGNESIUM DISTRIBUTION IN ADULTS			
Tissue	Wet Weight (kg)	Magnesium Content (mmol)	Total Body Magnesium (%)
Bone	12	530	53
Muscle	30	270	27
Soft Tissue	23	193	19
RBC	2	5	0.7
Plasma	3	3	0.3←
Total	70 kg	1001 mmol	100%

From Elin RJ. Magnesium metabolism in health and disease. Dis Mon 1988; 34:161–219.

varies according to geographic region. The normal range for healthy adults residing in the United States is shown in Table 42.2 (7).

Ionized Magnesium

Only 55% of the magnesium in plasma is in the ionized (active) form, and the remaining 45% is either bound to plasma proteins (33% of the total) or chelated with divalent anions such as phosphate and sulfate (12% of the total) (1,3,4). The standard assay for magnesium (i.e., spectrophotometry) measures all three fractions of magnesium. Therefore, when the serum magnesium is abnormally low, it is impossible to determine whether the problem is a decrease in the ionized (active) fraction or a decrease in the bound fractions (e.g., hypoproteinemia) (8). The level of ionized magnesium can be measured with an ion-specific electrode (9) or by ultrafiltration of plasma (10), but these techniques are not routinely available for clinical use. However, because the total amount of magnesium in plasma is small, the difference between the ionized and bound magnesium *content* may not be large enough to be clinically relevant.

URINARY MAGNESIUM

The normal range for urinary magnesium excretion is shown in Table 42.2. Under normal circumstances, only small quantities of mag-

TABLE 42.2. REFERENCE RANGES FOR MAGNESIUM*		
Fluid	Traditional Units	SI Units
Serum magnesium:		
Total	1.4–2.0 mEq/L	0.7–1.0 mmol/L
Ionized	0.8–1.1 mEq/L	0.4–0.6 mmol/L
Urinary magnesium	5–15 mEq/24 hr	2.5–7.5 mmol/24 hr

* Pertains to healthy adults residing in the United States (see Reference 7).

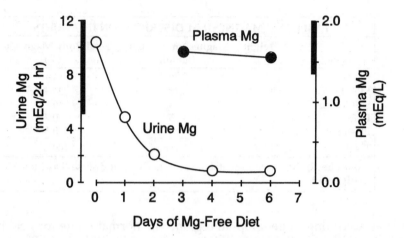

Figure 42.1. Urinary and plasma magnesium levels in a healthy volunteer placed on a magnesium-free diet. Solid bars on the vertical axes indicate the normal range for urine and plasma magnesium. (Adapted from Shils ME. Experimental human magnesium deficiency. Medicine 1969;48:61–82.)

nesium are excreted in the urine. When magnesium intake is deficient, the kidneys conserve magnesium and urinary magnesium excretion falls to negligible levels. This is shown in Figure 42.1 (11). After the start of a magnesium deficient diet, the urinary magnesium excretion promptly falls to negligible levels and the serum magnesium remains in the normal range. This illustrates the relative value of urinary magnesium over serum magnesium levels in the detection of magnesium deficiency. This is discussed again later in this chapter.

MAGNESIUM DEFICIENCY

Magnesium deficiency is common in hospitalized patients (12–20). Hypomagnesemia is reported in 10 to 20% of patients on general medical wards (15–17) and in 60 to 65% of patients in ICUs (18,19). Because magnesium depletion may not be accompanied by hypomagnesemia, the incidence of magnesium depletion is even higher than indicated by the surveys of hypomagnesemia. In fact, magnesium depletion has been described as "the most underdiagnosed electrolyte abnormality in current medical practice" (20).

PREDISPOSING CONDITIONS

Because serum magnesium levels have a limited ability to detect magnesium depletion, recognizing the conditions that predispose to magnesium depletion may be the only clue of an underlying electro-

TABLE 42.3. MARKERS OF POSSIBLE MAGNESIUM DEPLETION	
Predisposing Conditions	**Clinical Findings**
Drug therapy*:	Electrolyte abnormalities*:
Furosemide (50%)	Hypokalemia (40%)
Aminoglycosides (30%)	Hypophosphatemia (30%)
Amphotericin, pentamidine	Hyponatremia (27%)
Digitalis (20%)	Hypocalcemia (22%)
Cisplatin, cyclosporine	Cardiac manifestations:
Diarrhea (secretory)	Ischemia
Alcohol abuse (chronic)	Arrhythmias (refractory)
Diabetes mellitus	Digitalis toxicity
Acute MI	Hyperactive CNS Syndrome
* Numbers in parentheses indicate incidence of associated hypomagnesemia.	

lyte imbalance. The common predisposing conditions for magnesium depletion are listed in Table 42.3.

Diuretic Therapy

Diuretics are the leading cause of magnesium deficiency. Drug-induced inhibition of sodium reabsorption also interferes with magnesium reabsorption, and the resultant urinary magnesium losses can parallel urinary sodium losses. Urinary magnesium excretion is most pronounced with the loop diuretics (furosemide and ethacrynic acid). Magnesium deficiency has been reported in 50% of patients receiving chronic therapy with furosemide (21). The thiazide diuretics show a similar tendency for magnesium depletion, but only in elderly patients (22). Magnesium depletion is not a complication of therapy with "potassium-sparing" diuretics such as triamterene (23).

Antibiotic Therapy

The antibiotics that promote magnesium depletion are the aminoglycosides, amphotericin and pentamidine (24,25). The aminoglycosides block magnesium reabsorption in the ascending loop of Henle, and hypomagnesemia has been reported in 30% of patients receiving aminoglycoside therapy (25). The other risk associated with antibiotic use occurs with antibiotic-associated diarrhea, which can be accompanied by significant magnesium losses in the stool.

Other Drugs

A variety of other drugs have been associated with magnesium depletion, including digitalis (26), adrenergic agents (27), and the chemotherapeutic agents cisplatin (28) and cyclosporine (29). The first two agents shift magnesium into cells, whereas the latter two promote renal magnesium excretion.

Alcohol-Related Illness

Hypomagnesemia is reported in 30% of hospital admissions for alcohol abuse, and in 85% of admissions for delirium tremens (30,31). The magnesium depletion in these conditions is due to a number of factors, including generalized malnutrition and chronic diarrhea. In addition, there is an association between magnesium deficiency and thiamine deficiency (32). Magnesium is required for the transformation of thiamine into thiamine pyrophosphate, so magnesium deficiency can promote thiamine deficiency in the face of adequate thiamine intake. For this reason, the magnesium status should be monitored periodically in patients receiving daily thiamine supplements.

Secretory Diarrhea

A high concentration of magnesium (10 to 14 mEq/L) is present in secretions from the lower gastrointestinal tract (33), and thus secretory diarrhea can be accompanied by profound magnesium depletion (31). Upper tract secretions are not rich in magnesium (1 to 2 mEq/L), so vomiting does not pose a risk for magnesium depletion.

Diabetes Mellitus

Magnesium depletion is common in insulin-dependent diabetic patients, probably as a result of urinary magnesium losses that accompany glycosuria (34). Hypomagnesemia is reported in only 7% of admissions for diabetic ketoacidosis, but the incidence increases to 50% over the first 12 hours after admission (35), probably as a result of insulin-induced movement of magnesium into cells.

Acute Myocardial Infarction

As many as 80% of patients with acute myocardial infarction (MI) can have hypomagnesemia in the first 48 hours after the event (36). The mechanism is unclear but may be due to an intracellular shift of magnesium caused by endogenous catecholamines excess. The importance of magnesium in patients with acute MI is discussed in Chapter 19.

CLINICAL MANIFESTATIONS

Although no clinical manifestations are specific for magnesium deficiency, the following clinical findings are suggestive of an underlying magnesium deficiency (Table 42.3).

Associated Electrolyte Abnormalities

Magnesium depletion is often accompanied by depletion of other electrolytes, such as potassium, phosphate, calcium, and phosphate (See Table 42.3) (37). As mentioned in Chapter 41, the **hypokalemia** that accompanies magnesium depletion can be refractory to potassium replacement therapy (see Reference 14 in Chapter 41), and magnesium repletion is often necessary before potassium repletion is possible.

The **hypocalcemia** that accompanies magnesium depletion is due to impaired parathormone release (38) combined with an impaired end-organ response to parathormone (39). In addition, magnesium deficiency may act on bone directly to reduce calcium release, independent of parathyroid hormone (40). As with the hypokalemia, the hypocalcemia from magnesium depletion is difficult to correct unless magnesium deficits are corrected.

Hypophosphatemia is a cause rather than effect of magnesium depletion. The mechanism is enhanced renal magnesium excretion (41). Therefore, when hypophosphatemia accompanies hypomagnesemia, the phosphate stores should be replenished to ensure adequate repletion of magnesium stores.

Arrhythmias

Because magnesium is required for proper function of the membrane pump on cardiac cell membranes, magnesium depletion will depolarize cardiac cells and promote tachyarrhythmias. Because both digitalis and magnesium deficiency act to inhibit the membrane pump, magnesium deficiency will magnify the digitalis effect and promote **digitalis cardiotoxicity.** Intravenous magnesium is effective in suppressing digitalis-toxic arrhythmias, even when serum magnesium levels are normal (42,43). Intravenous magnesium can also be effective in abolishing **refractory arrhythmias** (i.e., unresponsive to traditional antiarrhythmic agents) in the absence of hypomagnesemia (44). This effect may be due to a membrane-stabilizing effect of magnesium that is unrelated to magnesium repletion.

One of the most serious arrhythmias associated with magnesium depletion is **torsades de pointes** (polymorphous ventricular tachycardia). The role of magnesium in this arrhythmia is discussed in Chapter 20.

Neurologic Findings

The neurologic manifestations of magnesium deficiency include altered mentation, generalized seizures, tremors, and hyperreflexia. All are uncommon, nonspecific, and have little diagnostic value.

A neurologic syndrome described recently that can abate with magnesium therapy deserves mention. The clinical presentation is characterized by ataxia, slurred speech, metabolic acidosis, excessive salivation, diffuse muscle spasms, generalized seizures, and progressive obtundation (45). The clinical features are often brought out by loud noises or bodily contact, and thus the term **reactive central nervous system magnesium deficiency** has been used to describe this disorder. This syndrome is associated with reduced magnesium levels in cerebrospinal fluid, and it resolves with magnesium infusion. The prevalence of this disorder is unknown at present.

DIAGNOSIS

As mentioned several times, the serum magnesium level is an insensitive marker of magnesium depletion. When magnesium depletion is due to nonrenal factors (e.g., diarrhea), the urinary magnesium excretion is a more sensitive test for magnesium depletion (46). However, because most cases of magnesium depletion are due to enhanced renal magnesium excretion, the diagnostic value of urinary magnesium excretion may be limited.

Magnesium Retention Test

In the absence of renal magnesium wasting, the urinary excretion of magnesium in response to a magnesium load may be the most sensitive index of total body magnesium stores (47,48). This method is outlined in Table 42.4. The normal rate of magnesium reabsorption is close to the maximum tubular reabsorption rate (T_{max}), so most of the infused magnesium will be excreted in the urine when magnesium stores are normal. However, when magnesium stores are deficient, the magnesium reabsorption rate is much lower than the T_{max}, so more of the infused magnesium will be reabsorbed and less will be excreted in the urine. When less than 50% of the infused magnesium is recovered in the urine, magnesium deficiency is likely, and when more than 80% of the infused magnesium is excreted in the urine, magnesium deficiency is *un*likely. This test can be particularly valuable in determining the end-point of magnesium replacement therapy (i.e., magnesium replacement is continued until urinary magnesium excretion is at least 80% of the infused magnesium load). It is important to

---

TABLE 42.4. RENAL MAGNESIUM RETENTION TEST

Indications:
1. For suspected magnesium deficiency when the serum magnesium concentration is normal.
2. Can be useful for determining the end-point of magnesium replacement therapy.
3. Is *not* reliable in the setting of renal magnesium wasting or when renal function is impaired.

Contraindications:
1. Cardiovascular instability or renal failure.

Methodology*:
1. Add 24 mmol of magnesium (6 g of $MgSO_4$) to 250 mL of isotonic saline and infuse over 1 hour.
2. Collect urine for 24 hours, beginning at the onset of the magnesium infusion.
3. A urinary magnesium excretion of less than 12 mmol (24 mEq) in 24 hours (i.e., less than 50% of the infused magnesium) is evidence of total body magnesium depletion.

*Magnesium infusion protocol from Reference 48.

emphasize that this test will be unreliable in patients with impaired renal function or when there is ongoing renal magnesium wasting.

MAGNESIUM REPLACEMENT THERAPY

PREPARATIONS

The magnesium preparations available for oral and parenteral use are listed in Table 42.5 (49,50). The oral preparations can be used for daily maintenance therapy (5 mg/kg in normal subjects) and for correcting mild, asymptomatic magnesium deficiency. However, because intestinal absorption of oral magnesium is erratic, parenteral magnesium is preferred for treating symptomatic or severe magnesium deficiency.

Magnesium Sulfate

The standard intravenous preparation is magnesium sulfate ($MgSO_4$). **Each gram of magnesium sulfate has 8 mEq (4 mmol) of elemental magnesium** (3). A 50% magnesium sulfate solution (500 mg/mL) has an osmolarity of 4000 mOsm/L (50), so it must be diluted to a 10% (100 mg/mL) or 20% (200 mg/mL) solution for intravenous use. Saline solutions should be used as the diluent for magnesium sulfate. Ringer's solutions should not be used because the calcium in Ringer's solutions will counteract the actions of the infused magnesium.

REPLACEMENT PROTOCOLS

The following magnesium replacement protocols are recommended for patients with normal renal function (51).

Mild, Asymptomatic Hypomagnesemia

The following guidelines can be used for patients with mild hypomagnesemia and no apparent complications (51):

TABLE 42.5. ORAL AND PARENTERAL MAGNESIUM PREPARATIONS	
Preparation	**Elemental Magnesium**
Oral preparations:	
Magnesium chloride enteric coated tablets	64 mg (5.3 mEq)
Magnesium oxide tablets (400 mg)	241 mg (19.8 mEq)
Magnesium oxide tablets (140 mg)	85 mg (6.9 mEq)
Magnesium gluconate tablets (500 mg)	27 mg (2.3 mEq)
Parenteral solutions:	
Magnesium sulfate (50%)*	500 mg/mL (4 mEq/mL)
Magnesium sulfate (20%)	200 mg/mL (1.6 mEq/mL)
*Should be diluted to a 20% solution for intravenous injection.	

1. Assume a total magnesium deficit of 1 to 2 mEq/kg.
2. Because 50% of the infused magnesium can be lost in the urine, assume that the total magnesium requirement is twice the magnesium deficit.
3. Replace 1 mEq/kg for the first 24 hours, and 0.5 mEq/kg daily for the next 3 to 5 days.
4. If the serum magnesium is greater than 1 mEq/L, oral magnesium can be used for replacement therapy.

Moderate Hypomagnesemia

The following therapy is intended for patients with a serum magnesium level less than 1 mEq/L or when hypomagnesemia is accompanied by other electrolyte abnormalities:

1. Add 6 g $MgSO_4$ (48 mEq Mg) to 250 or 500 mL isotonic saline and infuse over 3 hours.
2. Follow with 5 g $MgSO_4$ (40 mEq Mg) in 250 or 500 mL isotonic saline infused over the next 6 hours.
3. Continue with 5 g $MgSO_4$ every 12 hours (by continuous infusion) for the next 5 days.

Life-Threatening Hypomagnesemia

When hypomagnesemia is associated with serious cardiac arrhythmias or generalized seizures, do the following:
1. Infuse 2 g $MgSO_4$ (16 mEq Mg) intravenously over 2 minutes.
2. Follow with 5 g $MgSO_4$ (40 mEq Mg) in 250 or 500 mL isotonic saline infused over the next 6 hours.
3. Continue with 5 g $MgSO_4$ every 12 hours (by continuous infusion) for the next 5 days.

Serum magnesium levels will rise after the initial magnesium bolus but will begin to fall after 15 minutes. Therefore, it is important to follow the bolus dose with a continuous magnesium infusion. Serum magnesium levels may normalize after 1 to 2 days, but it will take several days to replenish the total body magnesium stores.

Hypomagnesemia and Renal Insufficiency

Hypomagnesemia is not common in renal insufficiency but can occur when severe or chronic diarrhea is present and the creatinine clearance is greater than 30 mL/minute. When magnesium is replaced in the setting of renal insufficiency, no more than 50% of the magnesium in the standard replacement protocols should be administered, (51) and the serum magnesium should be monitored carefully.

MAGNESIUM ACCUMULATION

Magnesium accumulation occurs almost exclusively in patients with impaired renal function. In one survey of hospitalized patients, hypermagnesemia (i.e., a serum magnesium greater than 2 mEq/L) was reported in 5% of patients (15).

PREDISPOSING CONDITIONS

Hemolysis

The magnesium concentration in erythrocytes is approximately three times greater than that in serum (1), so hemolysis can increase the plasma magnesium. This can occur either in vivo from a hemolytic anemia or in vitro from traumatic disruption of erythrocytes during phlebotomy. In hemolytic anemia, the serum magnesium is expected to rise by 0.1 mEq/L for every 250 mL of erythrocytes that lyse completely (1), so hypermagnesemia is expected only with massive hemolysis.

Renal Insufficiency

The renal excretion of magnesium becomes impaired when the creatinine clearance falls below 30 mL/minute (52). However, hypermagnesemia is not a prominent feature of renal insufficiency unless magnesium intake is increased.

Others

Other conditions that can predispose to mild hypermagnesemia are diabetic ketoacidosis (transient), adrenal insufficiency, hyperparathyroidism, and lithium intoxication (52).

CLINICAL FEATURES

The clinical consequences of progressive hypermagnesemia are listed below (52).

Serum Magnesium	Clinical Finding
4.0 mEq/L	Hyporeflexia
>5.0 mEq/L	Prolonged atrioventricular conduction
>10 mEq/L	Complete heart block
>13 mEq/L	Cardiac arrest

Magnesium has been described as nature's physiologic calcium blocker (53), and most of the serious consequences of hypermagnesemia are due to calcium antagonism in the cardiovascular system. Most of the cardiovascular depression is the result of cardiac conduction delays. Depressed contractility and vasodilation are not prominent.

MANAGEMENT

Hemodialysis is the treatment of choice for severe hypermagnesemia. Intravenous calcium gluconate (1 g IV over 2 to 3 minutes) can be used to antagonize the cardiovascular effects of hypermagnesemia *temporarily*, until dialysis is started (52). If fluids are permissible and some renal function is preserved, aggressive volume infusion combined with furosemide may be effective in reducing the serum magnesium levels in less advanced cases of hypermagnesemia.

REFERENCES

GENERAL REVIEWS

1. Elin RJ. Magnesium metabolism in health and disease. Dis Mon 1988;34: 161–219 (238 references).
2. White RE, Hartzell HO. Magnesium ions in cardiac function. Biochem Pharmacol 1989;38:859–867 (109 references).
3. McLean RM. Magnesium and its therapeutic uses: a review. Am J Med 1994; 96:63–76 (130 references).
4. Marino PL. Calcium and magnesium in critical illness: a practical approach. In: Sivak ED, Higgins TL, Seiver A, eds. The high risk patient: management of the critically ill. Baltimore: Williams & Wilkins, 1995;1183–1195 (87 references).

MAGNESIUM BALANCE

5. Reinhart RA. Magnesium metabolism: a review with special reference to the relationship between intracellular content and serum levels. Arch Intern Med 1988;148:2415–2420.
6. Elin RJ. Assessment of magnesium status. Clin Chem 1987;33:1965–1970.
7. Lowenstein FW, Stanton MF. Serum magnesium levels in the United States 1971–1974. J Am Coll Nutr 1986;5:399–414.
8. Kroll MH, Elin RJ. Relationship between magnesium and protein concentrations in serum. Clin Chem 1985;31:244–246.
9. Alvarez-Lefmans FJ, Giraldez F, Gamino SM. Intracellular free magnesium in excitable cells: its measurement and its biologic significance. Can J Physiol Pharmacol 1987;65:915–925.
10. Munoz R, Khilnani P, Salem M, et al. Ionized hypomagnesemia: a frequent problem in critically ill neonates. Crit Care Med 1991;19:S48.
11. Shils ME. Experimental human magnesium depletion. Medicine 1969;48: 61–82.

MAGNESIUM DEPLETION
Reviews

12. Salem M, Munoz R, Chernow B. Hypomagnesemia in critical illness. Crit Care Clin 1991;7:225–252 (154 references.
13. Reinhart RA. Magnesium deficiency: recognition and treatment in the emergency medicine setting. Am J Emerg Med 1992;10:78–83.
14. Whang RW, Hampton EM, Whang DD. Magnesium homeostasis and clinical disorders of magnesium deficiency. Ann Pharmacother 1994;28:220–225 (66 references).

Prevalence

15. Whang R, Ryder KW. Frequency of hypomagnesemia and hypermagnesemia: requested vs routine. JAMA 1990;263:3063–3064.
16. Martin BJ, Black J, McLelland AS. Hypomagnesemia in elderly hospital admissions: a study of clinical significance. Q J Med 1991;78:177–184.
17. Rubeiz GJ, Thill-Baharozian M, Hardie D, Carlson RW. Association of hypomagnesemia with mortality in acutely ill medical patients. Crit Care Med 1993; 21:203–209.
18. Ryzen E, Wagers PW, Singer FR, Rude RK. Magnesium deficiency in a medical ICU population. Crit Care Med 1985;13:19–21.
19. Chernow B, Bamberger S, Stoiko M, et al. Hypomagnesemia in patients in postoperative intensive care. Chest 1989;95:391–397.
20. Whang R. Magnesium deficiency: pathogenesis, prevalence, and clinical implications. Am J Med 1987;82(3A):24–29.

Predisposing Factors

21. Dykner T, Wester PO. Potassium/magnesium depletion in patients with cardiovascular disease. Am J Med 1987;82(Suppl 3A):11–17.
22. Hollifield JW. Thiazide treatment of systemic hypertension: effects on serum magnesium and ventricular ectopic activity. Am J Med 1989;63:22G–25G.
23. Ryan MP: Diuretics and potassium/magnesium depletion. Am J Med 1987; 82(Suppl 3A):38–47.
24. Shah GM, Kirschenbaum MA. Renal magnesium wasting associated with therapeutic agents. Miner Electrolyte Metab 1991;17:58–64.
25. Zaloga G, Chernow B, Pock A, et al. Hypomagnesemia is a common complication of aminoglycoside therapy. Surg Gynecol Obstet 1984;158:561–564.
26. Whang R, Oci TO, Watawabe A. Frequency of hypomagnesemia in hospitalized patients receiving digitalis. Arch Int Med 1985;145:655–656.
27. Whyte K, Addis GJ, Whitesmith R, Reid JL. Adrenergic control of plasma magnesium in man. Clin Sci 1987;72:135–138.
28. Ashraf M, Scotchel PL, Krall JM, et al. Cis-platinum-induced hypomagnesemia and peripheral neuropathy. Gynecol Oncol 1983;16:309–318.
29. Thompson CB, June CH, Sullied KM, Themes ED. Association between cyclosporin neurotoxicity and hypomagnesemia. Lancet 1984;ii:1116–1120.
30. Balesteri FJ. Magnesium metabolism in the critically ill. Crit Care Clin 1985; 5:217–226.
31. Martin HE. Clinical magnesium deficiency. Ann N Y Acad Sci 1969;162: 891–903.
32. Dyckner T, Ek B, Nyhlin H, Wester PO. Aggravation of thiamine deficiency by magnesium depletion. Acta Med Scand 1985;218:129–131.
33. Kassirer JP, Hrick DE, Cohen JJ. Repairing body fluids: principles and practice. Philadelphia: WB Saunders, 1989;118–129.
34. Sjogren A, Floren CH, Nilsson A. Magnesium deficiency in IDDM related to level of glycosylated hemoglobin. Diabetes 1986;35:459–463.
35. Lau K. Magnesium metabolism: normal and abnormal. In: Arieff AI, DeFronzo RA, eds. Fluids, electrolytes, and acid-base disorders. New York: Churchill Livingstone, 1985;575–623.
36. Abraham AS, Rosenmann D, Kramer M, et al. Magnesium in the prevention of lethal arrhythmias in acute myocardial infarction. Arch Intern Med 1987; 147:753–755.

Clinical Findings

37. Whang R, Oei TO, Aikawa JK, et al. Predictors of clinical hypomagnesemia. Arch Intern Med 1984;144:1794–1796.
38. Anast CS, Winnacker JL, Forte LR. Impaired release of parathyroid hormone in magnesium deficiency. J Clin Endocrinol Metab 1976;42:707–717.
39. Rude RK, Oldham SB, Singer FR. Functional hypoparathyroidism and parathyroid hormone end-organ resistance in human magnesium deficiency. Clin Endocrinol 1976;5:209–224.
40. Graber ML, Schulman G. Hypomagnesemic hypocalcemia independent of parathyroid hormone. Ann Intern Med 1986;104:804–805.
41. Dominiquez JH, Gray RW, Lemann J Jr. Dietary phosphate deprivation in women and men: effects on mineral and acid balances, parathyroid hormone and metabolism of 25-OH-vitamin D. J Clin Endocrinol Metab 1976;43: 1056–1068.
42. Cohen L, Kitzes R. Magnesium sulfate and digitalis-toxic arrhythmias. JAMA 1983;249:2808–2810.
43. French JH, Thomas RG, Siskind AP, et al. Magnesium therapy in massive digoxin intoxication. Ann Emerg Med 1984;13:562–566.
44. Tsivoni DT, Keren A. Suppression of ventricular arrhythmias by magnesium. Am J Cardiol 1990;65:1397–1399.
45. Langley WF, Mann D. Central nervous system magnesium deficiency. Arch Intern Med 1991;151:593–596.

Diagnosis

46. Fleming CR, George L, Stoner GL, et al. The importance of urinary magnesium levels in patients with gut failure. Mayo Clin Proc 1996;71:21–24.
47. Rasmussen HS, McNair P, Goransson L, et al. Magnesium deficiency in patients with ischemic heart disease with and without acute myocardial infarction uncovered by an intravenous loading test. Arch Intern Med 1988;148: 329–332.
48. Clague JE, Edwards RHT, Jackson MJ. Intravenous magnesium loading in chronic fatigue syndrome. Lancet 1992;340:124–125.

Magnesium Replacement Therapy

49. Dipalma JR. Magnesium replacement therapy. Am Fam Physician 1990;42: 173–176.
50. Trissel LA. Handbook on injectable drugs. 8th ed. Bethesda, MD: American Society of Hospital Pharmacists, 1994;633–639.
51. Oster JR, Epstein M. Management of magnesium depletion. Am J Nephrol 1988;8:349–354.

Magnesium Acculmulation

52. Van Hook JW. Hypermagnesemia. Crit Care Clin 1991;7:215–223.
53. Iseri LT, French JH. Magnesium: nature's physiologic calcium blocker. Am Heart J 1984;108:188–193.

43

CALCIUM AND PHOSPHORUS

Calcium and phosphorus are responsible for much of the structural integrity of the bony skeleton. Although neither is found in abundance in the soft tissues, both play an important role in vital cell functions. Phosphorus participates in aerobic energy production, whereas calcium participates in several diverse processes, such as blood coagulation, neuromuscular transmission, and smooth muscle contraction. Considering the important functions of these electrolytes, it is surprising that abnormalities in calcium and phosphorus balance are so well tolerated.

CALCIUM

Calcium is the most abundant electrolyte in the human body (the average adult has more than half a kilogram of calcium), but 99% is in bone (1). In the soft tissues, calcium is 10,000 times more concentrated in the extracellular fluids (2). This preference for the extracellular fluid seems odd because calcium seems most involved with smooth muscle contraction (3), which is an intracellular process.

PLASMA CALCIUM

The calcium in plasma is present in three forms, as depicted in Figure 43.1. Approximately 50% of the calcium is bound to plasma proteins, and albumin is responsible for 80% of the protein binding. An additional 5 to 10% is chelated to plasma anions such as sulfates and phosphates. The remainder is present as free or unattached calcium ions. This ionized fraction is the physiologically active fraction of calcium in plasma. The concentration of total and ionized calcium in plasma

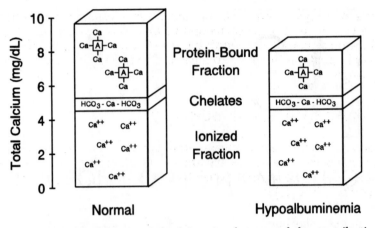

Figure 43.1. The three fractions of calcium in plasma and the contribution of each to the total plasma calcium concentration. The column on the right shows how a decrease in plasma albumin can reduce the total plasma calcium without affecting the ionized calcium.

is shown in Table 43.1. These values may vary slightly in different clinical laboratories.

Total versus Ionized Calcium

The calcium assay used by most clinical laboratories measures all three fractions of calcium, which can be misleading. The column on the right in Figure 43.1 demonstrates the effects of a decrease in the concentration of albumin in plasma. Because albumin is responsible for 80% of the protein-bound calcium in plasma, a decrease in albumin decreases the amount of calcium in the protein-bound fraction. The total calcium in plasma decreases by the same amount, but the ionized calcium remains unchanged. Because the ionized calcium is the physiologically active fraction, the hypocalcemia caused by hypoalbuminemia is not physiologically significant. The hypocalcemia that is physiologically significant is *ionized* hypocalcemia.

Various correction factors have been proposed for determining the

TABLE 43.1. NORMAL RANGES FOR CALCIUM AND PHOSPHOROUS IN BLOOD			
Serum Electrolyte	Traditional Units (mg/dL)	Conversion Factor*	SI Units (mmol/L)
Total calcium	8.0–10.2	0.25	2.2–2.5
Ionized calcium	4.0–4.6	0.25	1.0–1.5
Phosphorous	2.5–5.0	0.32	0.8–1.6
* Multiply traditional units by conversion factor to derive SI Units or divide SI units by conversion factor to derive tranditional units.			

effects of hypoalbuminemia on the plasma calcium concentration. However, none of these correction factors have proven reliable (4,5), and the only method of identifying true (ionized) hypocalcemia in the face of hypoalbuminemia is to measure the ionized fraction of calcium in plasma.

IONIZED CALCIUM MEASUREMENT

Ionized calcium can be measured in whole blood, plasma, or serum with ion-specific electrodes that are now available in most clinical laboratories (4–6). The normal concentration of ionized calcium in plasma is shown in Table 43.1.

Blood Collection

Several conditions can alter the level of ionized calcium in blood samples (5). Acidosis decreases the binding of calcium to albumin and increases the ionized calcium, whereas alkalosis has the opposite effect. Loss of carbon dioxide from a blood sample could falsely lower the ionized calcium, so it is important to avoid gas bubbles in the blood sample. Anticoagulants (e.g., heparin, citrate, and EDTA) can bind calcium, so blood samples should not be placed in collection tubes that contain these anticoagulants. Tubes with red stoppers ("red top" tubes) contain silicone and are adequate for measuring ionized calcium in serum samples. Heparinized syringes can be used for measuring ionized calcium in whole blood. Although heparin also binds calcium, the effect is minimal if the heparin level is less than 15 U/ mL of blood (5).

IONIZED HYPOCALCEMIA

Ionized hypocalcemia has been reported in 50 to 65% of admissions to the ICU (6,7). The common disorders associated with ionized hypocalcemia in patients in the ICU are listed in Table 43.2. Hypoparathyroidism is a leading cause of hypocalcemia in outpatients, but it is not

TABLE 43.2. CAUSES OF IONIZED HYPOCALCEMIA IN THE ICU	
Alkalosis	Fat embolism
Blood transfusions (15%)	Magnesium depletion (70%)
Cardiopulmonary bypass	Pancreatitis
Drugs:	Renal insufficiency (50%)
Aminoglycosides (40%)	Sepsis (30%)
Cimetidine (30%)	
Heparin (10%)	
Theophylline (30%)	
Numbers in parentheses show the frequency of ionized hypocalcemia reported in each condition.	

a consideration in the ICU unless neck surgery has been performed recently.

PREDISPOSING CONDITIONS

Magnesium Depletion

Magnesium depletion promotes hypocalcemia by inhibiting parathormone secretion and reducing end-organ responsiveness to parathormone (see Chapter 42). Hypocalcemia from magnesium depletion is refractory to calcium replacement therapy, and magnesium repletion often corrects the hypocalcemia without calcium replacement.

Sepsis

Sepsis is a common cause of hypocalcemia in the ICU (6–9). The mechanism is unclear, but it may involve an increase in calcium binding to albumin caused by elevated levels of circulating free fatty acids. Hypocalcemia is independent of the vasodilation that accompanies sepsis (9), and thus the clinical significance of the hypocalcemia in sepsis is questioned.

Alkalosis

As mentioned earlier, alkalosis promotes the binding of calcium to albumin and can reduce the fraction of ionized calcium in blood. Symptomatic hypocalcemia is more common with respiratory alkalosis than with metabolic alkalosis. Infusions of sodium bicarbonate can also be accompanied by ionized hypocalcemia because calcium directly binds to the infused bicarbonate.

Blood Transfusions

Ionized hypocalcemia has been reported in 15% of patients receiving blood transfusions (6). The mechanism is calcium binding by the citrate preservative in banked blood. Hypocalcemia from blood transfusions usually is transient, and resolves when the infused citrate is metabolized by the liver and kidneys (1). In patients with renal or hepatic failure, a more prolonged hypocalcemia can result. Although hypocalcemia from blood transfusions could impede blood coagulation, this is not considered to be a significant effect and calcium infusions are no longer recommended in massive blood transfusions.

Drugs

A number of drugs can bind calcium and promote ionized hypocalcemia (1,6,7). The ones most often used in the ICU are aminoglycosides, cimetidine, heparin, and theophylline.

Renal Failure

Ionized hypocalcemia can accompany renal failure as a result of phosphate retention and impaired conversion of vitamin D to its active form in the kidneys. The treatment in this setting is aimed at lowering the phosphate levels in blood with antacids that block phosphorus absorption in the small bowel. However, the value of this practice is unproven. The acidosis in renal failure can decrease the binding of calcium to albumin, so hypocalcemia in renal failure does not imply ionized hypocalcemia.

Pancreatitis

Severe pancreatitis can produce ionized hypocalcemia through several mechanisms. The prognosis is adversely affected by the appearance of hypocalcemia (10), although a causal relationship has not been proven.

CLINICAL MANIFESTATIONS

The clinical manifestations of hypocalcemia are related to enhanced cardiac and neuromuscular excitability and reduced contractile force in cardiac muscle and vascular smooth muscle.

Neuromuscular Excitability

Hypocalcemia can be accompanied by hyperreflexia, generalized seizures, and tetany. Chvostek's and Trousseau's signs are often listed as manifestations of hypocalcemia. However, **Chvostek's sign is nonspecific** (it is present in 25% of normal adults), and **Trousseau's sign is insensitive** (it can be absent in 30% of patients with hypocalcemia) (1).

Cardiovascular Effects

The cardiovascular complications of hypocalcemia include hypotension, decreased cardiac output, and ventricular ectopic activity. These complications are rarely seen in mild cases of ionized hypocalcemia (i.e., ionized calcium 0.8 to 1.0 mmol/L). However, advanced stages of ionized hypocalcemia (i.e., ionized calcium less than 0.65 mmol/L) can be associated with ventricular tachycardia and refractory hypotension (1).

CALCIUM REPLACEMENT THERAPY

The treatment of ionized hypocalcemia should be directed at the underlying cause of the problem. However, symptomatic hypocalcemia is considered a medical emergency (1), and the treatment of choice is intravenous calcium. The calcium solutions and dosage rec-

TABLE 43.3. INTRAVENOUS CALCIUM REPLACEMENT THERAPY			
Solution	Elemental Calcium	Unit Volume	Osmolarity
10% Calcium chloride	27 mg (1.36 mEq)/mL	10-mL ampules	2000 mOsm/L
10% Calcium gluconate	9 mg (0.46 mEq)/mL	10-mL ampules	680 mOsm/L

For symptomatic hypocalcemia:
1. Infuse calcium into a large central vein if possible. If a peripheral vein is used, calcium gluconate should be less irritating.
2. Give a bolus dose of 200 mg elemental calcium (8 mL of 10% calcium chloride or 22 mL of 10% calcium gluconate) in 100 mL isotonic saline over 10 minutes.
3. Follow with a continuous infusion of 1–2 mg elemental calcium per kg per hour for 6–12 hours.

ommendations for intravenous calcium replacement are shown in Table 43.3.

Calcium Salt Solutions

The two most popular calcium solutions for intravenous use are 10% calcium chloride and 10% calcium gluconate. Both solutions have the same concentration of calcium salt (i.e., 100 mg/mL), but **calcium chloride contains three times more elemental calcium than calcium gluconate.** One 10-mL ampule of 10% calcium chloride contains 272 mg (13.6 mEq) of elemental calcium, whereas one 10-mL ampule of 10% calcium gluconate contains only 90 mg (4.6 mEq) of elemental calcium (11).

Dosage Recommendations

The intravenous calcium solutions are hyperosmolar and should be given through a large central vein if possible. If a peripheral vein is used, calcium gluconate is the preferred solution because of its lower osmolarity (Table 43.3). A bolus dose of 200 mg elemental calcium (diluted in 100 mL isotonic saline and given over 10 minutes) should raise the total serum calcium by 1 mg/dL (1), but levels will begin to fall after 30 minutes. Therefore, the bolus dose of calcium should be followed by a continuous infusion at a dose rate of 1 to 2 mg (elemental calcium) per kilogram of body weight per hour. This should be continued for at least 6 hours. Subsequent doses of calcium should be guided by the level of ionized calcium in blood.

Maintenance Therapy

The daily maintenance dose of calcium is 2 to 4 g in adults. This can be administered orally using calcium carbonate (e.g., Oscal) or calcium gluconate tablets (500 mg calcium per tablet).

Caution

Intravenous calcium replacement can be risky in select patient populations. Calcium infusions can promote vasoconstriction and ischemia in any of the vital organs (12). The risk of calcium-induced ischemia should be particularly high in patients with low cardiac output who are already vasoconstricted. In addition, aggressive calcium replacement can promote intracellular calcium overload, which can produce a lethal cell injury (13), particularly in patients with circulatory shock. Because of these risks, calcium infusions should be used judiciously. **Intravenous calcium is indicated only for patients with symptomatic hypocalcemia or an ionized calcium level below 0.65 mmol/L (1).**

HYPERCALCEMIA

Hypercalcemia is not nearly as common as hypocalcemia: it is reported in less than 1% of hospitalized patients (14). In 90% of cases, the underlying cause is hyperparathyroidism or malignancy (15). Less common causes include prolonged immobilization, thyrotoxicosis, and drugs (lithium, thiazide diuretics). Malignancy is the most common cause of severe hypercalcemia (i.e., total serum calcium above 14 mg/dL or ionized calcium above 3.5 mmol/L) (16).

CLINICAL MANIFESTATIONS

The manifestations of hypercalcemia usually are nonspecific and can be categorized as follows:

1. **Gastrointestinal (GI):** nausea, vomiting, constipation, ileus, and pancreatitis
2. **Cardiovascular:** hypovolemia, hypotension, and shortened QT interval
3. **Renal:** polyuria and nephrocalcinosis
4. **Neurologic:** confusion and depressed consciousness, including coma

These manifestations can become evident when the total serum calcium rises above 12 mg/dL (or the ionized calcium rises above 3.0 mmol/L), and they are almost always present when the serum calcium is greater than 14 mg/dL (or the ionized calcium is above 3.5 mmol/L) (16).

MANAGEMENT

Treatment is indicated when the hypercalcemia is associated with adverse effects, or when the serum calcium is greater than 14 mg/dL (ionized calcium above 3.5 mmol/L). The management of hypercalcemia is summarized in Table 43.4 (15,16).

Saline Infusion

Hypercalcemia usually is accompanied by hypercalciuria, which produces an osmotic diuresis. This eventually leads to hypovolemia,

TABLE 43.4. MANAGEMENT OF SEVERE HYPERCALCEMIA		
Agent	Dose	Comment
Isotonic saline	Variable	Initial treatment of choice. Goal is rapid correction of hypovolemia.
Furosemide	40–80 mg IV every 2 hours	Add to isotonic saline to maintain a urine output of 100–200 mL/hr.
Calcitonin	4 U/kg IM or SC every 12 hours	Response is evident within a few hours. Maximum drop in serum calcium is only 0.5 mmol/L.
Hydrocortisone	200 mg IV daily in 2–3 divided doses	Used as an adjunct to calcitonin.
Pamidronate	90 mg by continuous IV infusion over 24 hours	Delayed response (maximum effect in 4–5 days) but much more potent than calcitonin.
Plicamycin	25 μg/kg IV over 4 hours; can repeat every 24 hours	More rapid effect than pamidronate, but potential for toxic side effects limits the use of this agent.

which reduces calcium excretion in the urine and precipitates a rapid rise in the serum calcium. Therefore, volume infusion to correct hypovolemia and promote renal calcium excretion is the first goal of management for hypercalcemia. Isotonic saline is recommended for the volume infusion because natriuresis itself promotes renal calcium excretion.

Furosemide

Saline infusion will not return the calcium to normal levels. To do this requires the addition of furosemide (40 to 80 mg IV every 2 hours) to further promote urinary calcium excretion. The goal is an hourly urine output of 100 to 200 mL/minute. The hourly urine output *must* be replaced with isotonic saline. Failure to replace urinary volume losses will favor a return to hypovolemia, which is counterproductive.

Calcitonin

Although saline and furosemide will correct the hypercalcemia acutely, this approach does not treat the underlying cause of the problem, which (in malignancy) is enhanced bone resorption. Calcitonin is a naturally occurring hormone that inhibits bone resorption. It is available as salmon calcitonin, which is given subcutaneously or intramuscularly in a dose of 4 U/kg every 12 hours. The response is rapid (onset within a few hours), but the effect is mild (the maximum drop in serum calcium is 0.5 mmol/L).

Hydrocortisone

Corticosteroids can reduce the serum calcium by impeding the growth of lymphoid neoplastic tissue and enhancing the actions of vitamin D. Steroids are usually combined with calcitonin and can be particularly useful in the hypercalcemia associated with multiple myeloma or renal failure (15,16). The standard regimen uses hydrocortisone, 200 mg IV daily in 2 or 3 divided doses.

Pamidronate

Calcitonin can be used for rapid reduction of serum calcium, but the mild response will not keep the calcium in the normal range. A group of compounds known as *biphosphonates* (pyrophosphate derivatives) are more potent inhibitors of bone resorption and maintain a normal serum calcium. However, their onset of action is delayed, and thus they are not useful when rapid control of serum calcium is desired.

Pamidronate is currently the *biphosphonates* of choice for the management of severe hypercalcemia (15). The dose is 90 mg, which is given by continuous intravenous infusion over 24 hours. The peak effect is seen in 4 to 5 days, and the dose can be repeated at that time if necessary.

Plicamycin

Plicamycin (formerly mithramycin) is an antineoplastic agent that inhibits bone resorption. It is similar to pamidronate in that it is more potent than calcitonin but has a delayed onset of action. The dose is 25 µg/kg (intravenously over 4 hours), which can be repeated in 24 to 48 hours if necessary. Because of the potential for serious side effects (e.g., bone marrow suppression), plicamycin has largely been replaced by pamidronate.

Dialysis

Dialysis is effective in removing calcium in patients with renal failure. Either hemodialysis or peritoneal dialysis can be used (15).

PHOSPHORUS

The average adult has 500 to 800 g of phosphorus (17). Most phosphorus is contained in organic molecules such as phospholipids and phosphoproteins, and 85% is located in the bony skeleton. The remaining 15% in soft tissues is present as free, inorganic phosphorus. Unlike calcium, inorganic phosphorus is predominantly intracellular in location, where it participates in glycolysis and high energy phosphate production. The normal concentration of inorganic phosphorus in plasma is shown in Table 43.1. This reference range pertains only to adults; the normal range in children is higher (17).

HYPOPHOSPHATEMIA

Hypophosphatemia (serum PO_4 less than 2.5 mg/dL or 0.8 mmol/L) can be the result of an intracellular shift of phosphorus, an increase in the renal excretion of phosphorus, or a decrease in phosphorus absorption from the GI tract. Most cases of hypophosphatemia are due to movement of PO_4 into cells.

PREDISPOSING CONDITIONS

Glucose Loading

The movement of glucose into cells is accompanied by a similar movement of PO_4 into cells, and if the extracellular content of PO_4 is marginal, this intracellular PO_4 shift can result in hypophosphatemia. Glucose loading is the most common cause of hypophosphatemia in hospitalized patients (18,19), usually seen during refeeding in alcoholic, malnourished, or debilitated patients. It can occur with oral feedings, enteral tube feedings, or with total parenteral nutrition. The influence of parenteral nutrition on serum PO_4 levels is shown in Figure 43.2. Note the gradual decline in the serum PO_4 and the severe degree of hypophosphatemia (serum PO_4 below 1 mg/dL) seen after 7 days of intravenous nutrition. This trend in serum PO_4 is one of the reasons why parenteral nutrition regimens are advanced gradually for the first few days after being started.

As mentioned, oral and enteral feedings create a similar risk of hypophosphatemia, particularly in debilitated or malnourished patients. In fact, hypophosphatemia may be responsible for the progressive weakness and inanition that characterizes the refeeding syndrome in malnourished patients (20).

Respiratory Alkalosis

Respiratory alkalosis can increase intracellular pH, and this accelerates glycolysis. The increase in glucose use then increases glucose and

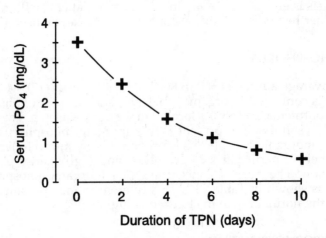

Figure 43.2. The cumulative effect of total parenteral nutrition (*TPN*) on the serum phosphate level. (Data from Knochel JP. The pathophysiology and clinical characteristics of severe hypophosphatemia. Arch Intern Med 1977; 137:203–220.)

phosphorus movement into cells. This may be an important source of hypophosphatemia in ventilator-dependent patients because overventilation and respiratory alkalosis is common in these patients.

β-Receptor Agonists

Stimulation of β-adrenergic receptors can move PO_4 into cells and promote hypophosphatemia. This effect is evident in patients treated with β-agonist bronchodilators. In one study of patients with acute asthma who were treated aggressively with nebulized albuterol (2.5 mg every 30 minutes), the serum PO_4 decreased by 1.25 mg/dL (0.4 mmol/L) 3 hours after the onset of therapy [21]. However, the significance of this effect is unclear.

Sepsis

There is a common association between septicemia and hypophosphatemia in some studies [19]. A causal relationship is unproven, but sepsis could promote a transcellular shift of PO_4 as a result of elevated levels of endogenous catecholamines.

Phosphorus-Binding Agents

Aluminum can form insoluble complexes with inorganic phosphorus. As a result, aluminum-containing compounds, such as sucralfate (Carafate), or antacids that contain aluminum hydroxide (e.g., Amphojel) can impede the absorption of phosphate in the upper GI tract and promote phosphate depletion [18]. The major concern is sucralfate, which is being used with increasing frequency for the prophylaxis of stress ulcer bleeding in critically ill patients (see Chapter 6). Sucralfate administration is associated with an increased incidence of hypophosphatemia in patients in the ICU [21]. However a direct cause-and-effect relationship between sucralfate and phosphate depletion remains to be established.

Diabetic Ketoacidosis

The osmotic diuresis from glycosuria promotes the urinary loss of PO_4, and patients with prolonged or severe hyperglycemia are often phosphate depleted. As mentioned in Chapter 37, phosphate depletion is almost universal in patients who have diabetic ketoacidosis, but it does not become evident until insulin therapy drives PO_4 into cells. Because phosphate supplementation does not alter the outcome in diabetic ketoacidosis (see Chapter 37), the significance of the phosphate depletion in this disorder is unclear.

CLINICAL MANIFESTATIONS

Hypophosphatemia is often clinically silent, even when the serum PO_4 falls to extremely low levels. In one study of patients with severe hypophosphatemia (i.e., serum PO_4 less than 1.0 mg/dL), none of the

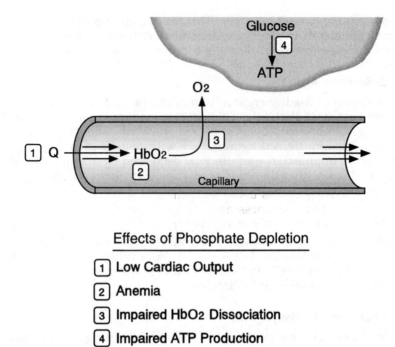

Effects of Phosphate Depletion

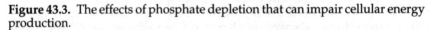

1 Low Cardiac Output

2 Anemia

3 Impaired HbO2 Dissociation

4 Impaired ATP Production

Figure 43.3. The effects of phosphate depletion that can impair cellular energy production.

patients showed evidence of harmful effects (23). Despite the apparent lack of harm, phosphate depletion creates a risk for impaired energy production in all aerobic cells.

Aerobic Energy Production

Phosphate depletion has several effects that could impair cellular energy production. These are summarized in Figure 43.3. To begin with, each of the following determinants of systemic oxygen delivery can be adversely affected by phosphate depletion.

1. **Cardiac output:** Phosphate depletion can impair myocardial contractility and reduce cardiac output. Hypophosphatemic patients with heart failure have shown improved cardiac performance after phosphate supplementation (24).
2. **Hemoglobin:** Reduction of high energy phosphate production from glycolysis in erythrocytes can reduce the deformability of red cells. This may explain why severe hypophosphatemia can be accompanied by a hemolytic anemia (18).
3. **Oxyhemoglobin dissociation:** Phosphate depletion is accompanied by depletion of 2,3-diphosphoglycerate, and this shifts the oxyhemoglobin dissociation curve to the left. When this occurs, hemoglobin is less likely to release oxygen to the tissues.

In addition to the adverse effects on tissue oxygen availability, phosphate depletion can directly impede cellular energy production by reducing the availability of inorganic phosphorus for high-energy phosphate production and decreasing the activity of the glycolytic pathway.

Muscle Weakness

One of the possible consequences of impaired energy production from phosphate depletion is skeletal muscle weakness. Biochemical evidence of skeletal muscle disruption (e.g., elevated creatine kinase levels in blood) is common in patients with hypophosphatemia, but overt muscle weakness is usually absent (25). There is one report of respiratory muscle weakness and failure to wean from mechanical ventilation in patients with severe hypophosphatemia (26). However, other studies show that respiratory muscle weakness is common in hyposphaphatemia but is not clinically significant in most patients (27). At present, the evidence linking phosphate depletion with clinically significant skeletal muscle weakness is scant.

PHOSPHORUS REPLACEMENT THERAPY

Intravenous phosphorus replacement is recommended for all patients with severe hypophosphatemia (i.e., serum PO_4 below 1.0 mg/dL or 0.3 mmol/L) and for patients with hypophosphatemia of any degree who also have cardiac dysfunction, respiratory failure, muscle weakness, or impaired tissue oxygenation. The phosphate solutions and dosage recommendations are shown in Table 43.5 (21,22).

Once the serum PO_4 rises above 2 mg/dL, phosphate replacement can be continued using oral phosphate preparations like Neutra-Phos or K-Phos. The oral replacement dosage is 1200 to 1500 mg phosphorus daily. Remember that sucralfate and phosphate-binding antacids need to be discontinued when oral phosphate preparations are used. The

TABLE 43.5. INTRAVENOUS PHOSPHATE REPLACEMENT THERAPY		
Solution	**Phosphorous Content**	**Other Content**
Sodium phosphate	93 mg (3 mmol)/mL	Na^+: 4.0 mEq/mL
Potassium phosphate	93 mg (3 mmol)/mL	K^+: 4.3 mEq/mL

Dosage Recommendations*
For severe hypophosphatemia (PO_4 <1 mg/dL) without adverse effects: IV dose is 0.6 mg (0.02 mmol) per kg body weight per hour
For hypophosphatemia (PO_4 <2 mg/dL) with adverse effects: IV dose is 0.9 mg (0.03 mmol) per kg body weight per hour
Monitor serum PO_4 level every 6 hours.

* From Reference 1. In patients with renal dysfunction, slower dose rates are advised.

TABLE 43.6. THE PHOSPHORUS CONTENT OF ENTERAL TUBE FEEDINGS			
Formula	Phosphorous (mg/L)	Formula	Phosphorous (mg/L)
Altra Q	733	Nutrivent	1200
Attain	800	Osmolite/HN	530/758
Compleat Regular	1200	Peptamen	700
Criticare HN	530	Perative	866
Ensure/HN	530/758	Pulmocare	1056
Ensure Plus/HN	704/1056	Reabilan/HN	499/499
Entrition 0.5/1.0	250/500	Replete	1000
Entrition 1.5/HN	1000/770	Resource/Plus	530/620
Glucerna	704	Sustacal/Plus	930/850
Impact	800	Traumacal	750
Isocal/HN	530/850	Travasorb STD/HN	501/501
Isosource/HN	670/670	Twocal HN	1052
Jevity	759	Ultracal	850
Magnacal	1000	Vitaneed	667
Nutren 1.0/2.0	700/1040	Vivonex TEN	500

tendency for oral phosphate preparations to promote diarrhea limits the use of high-dosage oral PO_4 replacement therapy.

Maintenance Therapy

The normal daily maintenance dosage of phosphate is 1200 mg if given orally (1). As shown in Table 43.6, the content of enteral feeding formulas varies widely, and thus thus enteral nutrition may not provide the daily phosphorus requirements without additional phosphate supplementation.

In patients who cannot tolerate enteral nutrition, daily phosphate requirements are provided intravenously. The IV maintenance dosage of PO_4 is approximately 800 mg/day (this dosage is lower than the oral maintenance dosage because only 70% of orally administered phosphate is absorbed from the GI tract).

HYPERPHOSPHATEMIA

Most cases of hyperphosphatemia in the ICU are the result of impaired PO_4 excretion from **renal insufficiency** or PO_4 release from cells because of **widespread cell necrosis** (e.g., rhabdomyolysis or tumor lysis). Hyperphosphatemia can also be seen in diabetic ketoacidosis, but as described earlier, this disorder is almost always accompanied by phosphate depletion, which becomes evident after the onset of insulin therapy.

CLINICAL MANIFESTATIONS

The clinical manifestations of hyperphosphatemia are not well documented. The most noted concern is the formation of insoluble calcium–phosphate complexes that are deposited in soft tissues and promote tissue damage. However, little information exists on this subject.

MANAGEMENT

There are two approaches to hyperphosphatemia. The first is to promote PO_4 binding in the upper GI tract, which can lower the serum PO_4 even in the absence of any oral intake of phosphate (i.e., GI dialysis). Sucralfate or aluminum-containing antacids can be used for this purpose. In patients with significant hypocalcemia, calcium acetate tablets (PhosLo, Braintree Labs) can help raise the serum calcium while lowering the serum PO_4. Each calcium acetate tablet (667 mg) contains 8.45 mEq elemental calcium. The recommended dosage is 2 tablets three times a day.

The other approach to hyperphosphatemia is to enhance PO_4 clearance with hemodialysis. This is reserved for patients with renal failure, and is rarely necessary.

REFERENCES

GENERAL REFERENCES

1. Zaloga GP, Chernow B. Divalent cations: calcium, magnesium and phosphorus. In: Chernow B, ed. The pharmacologic approach to the critically ill patient. 3rd ed. Baltimore: Williams & Wilkins, 1994;777–804 (190 references).

CALCIUM REVIEWS

2. Marino PL. Calcium and magnesium in serious illness: a practical approach. In: Sivak ED, Higgins TL, Seiver A, eds. The high risk patient: management of the critically ill. Baltimore: Williams & Wilkins, 1995;1183–1195 (87 references).
3. Smith JB. Calcium homeostasis in smooth muscle. New Horiz 1996;4:2–18 (137 references).

PLASMA CALCIUM

4. Weaver CA. Assessing calcium status and metabolism. J Nutr 1990;120(Suppl 11):1470–1473.
5. Foreman DT, Lorenzo L. Ionized calcium: it's significance and clinical usefulness. Ann Clin Lab Sci 1991;21:297–304.
6. Cagir B, Walsh CB, Mahoney WD, Herz BL. Hypocalcemia in surgical critical care patients: measurements of ionized calcium. Contemp Surg 1994;45:71–78.

HYPOCALCEMIA

7. Zaloga GP. Hypocalcemia in critically ill patients. Crit Care Med 1992;20:251–262.
8. Desai TK, Carlson RW, Geheb MA. Prevalence and clinical implications of hypocalcemia in acutely ill patients in a medical intensive care setting. Am J Med 1988;84:209–214.

9. Burchard KW, Simms H, Robinson A, et al. Hypocalcemia during sepsis. Arch Surg 1992;127:265–272.
10. Steinberg W, Tenner S. Acute pancreatitis. N Engl J Med 1994;330:1198–1210.
11. Trissel LA. Handbook of injectable drugs. 8th ed. Bethesda, MD: American Society of Hospital Pharmacists, 1994;134–148.
12. Shapiro MJ, Mistry M. Calcium regulation and nonprotective properties of calcium in surgical ischemia. New Horiz 1995;4:134–138.
13. Trump BF, Berezesky IK. Calcium-mediated cell injury and cell death. New Horiz 1995;4:139–150.

HYPERCALCEMIA

14. Shek CC, Natkunam A, Tsang V, et al. Incidence, causes and mechanism of hypercalcemia in a hospital population in Hong Kong. Q J Med 1990;77:1277–1285.
15. Mundy GR. Evaluation and treatment of hypercalcemia. Hosp Pract 1994;29:79–86.
16. Bilezikian JP. Management of acute hypercalcemia. N Engl J Med 1992;326:1196–1203.

PHOSPHORUS REVIEWS

17. Peppers M, Geheb M, Desai T. Hypophosphatemia and hyperphosphatemia. Crit Care Clin 1991;7:201–214 (64 references).

HYPOPHOSPHATEMIA

18. Brown GR, Greenwood JK. Drug- and nutrition-induced hypophosphatemia: mechanisms and relevance in the critically ill. Ann Pharmacother 1994;28:626–632.
19. Halevy J, Bulvik S. Severe hypophosphatemia in hospitalized patients. Arch Intern Med 1988;148:153–155.
20. Solomon SM, Kirby DF. The refeeding syndrome: a review. J Parenter Enteral Nutr 1990;14:90–97.
21. Bodenhamer J, Berstrom R, Brown D, et al. Frequently nebulized beta-agonists for asthma: effects on serum electrolytes. Ann Emerg Med 1992;21:1337–1342.
22. Miller SJ, Simpson J. Medication-nutrient interactions: hypophosphatemia associated with sucralfate in the intensive care unit. Nutr Clin Pract 1991;6:199–201.
23. King AL, Sica DA, Miller G, Pierpaoli S. Severe hypophosphatemia in a general hospital population. South Med J 1987;80:831–835.
24. Davis SV, Olichwier KK, Chakko SC. Reversible depression of myocardial performance in hypophosphatemia. Am J Med Sci 1988;295:183–187.
25. Singhal PC, Kumar A, Desroches L, et al. Prevalence and predictors of rhabdomyolysis in patients with hypophosphatemia. Am J Med 1992;92:458–464.
26. Agusti AG, Torres A, Estopa R, Agusti-Vidal A. Hypophosphatemia as a cause of failed weaning: the importance of metabolic factors. Crit Care Med 1984;12:142–143.
27. Gravelyn TR, Brophy N, Siegert C, Peters-Golden M. Hypophosphatemia-associated respiratory muscle weakness in a general inpatient population. Am J Med 1988;84:870–875.

section XI
BLOOD COMPONENT THERAPY

The maintenance of blood volume is such an important factor in determining the symptoms resulting from loss of blood.

> William Castle and George Minot. Pathologic physiology and clinical description of the anemias, 1936.

c h a p t e r

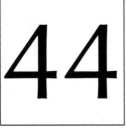

ERYTHROCYTE TRANSFUSIONS

*One of the important discoveries, I believe . . . is the realization that anemia is well
tolerated . . . providing blood volume is maintained.*
Daniel J. Ullyott. J Thoracic Cardiovasc Surg 1992;103:1007.

The transfusion of erythrocyte products to correct anemia is one of
the least scientific practices to be encountered in the ICU. One of the
problems, as highlighted in Figure 44.1, is an apparent confusion about
the relative merits of blood *cells* versus blood *volume* in maintaining
tissue viability. As indicated in the introductory quote, the human
organism suffers little from deficits of red blood cells (anemia), as long
as deficits of blood volume are prevented. The relative importance of
blood volume over blood cells is shown by the fact that hypovolemia
is a well-known cause of shock (impaired tissue oxygenation), whereas
anemic shock is a nonentity.

This chapter begins by examining some of the basic assumptions
for the use of erythrocyte transfusions to correct anemia. Following
this is a more practical discussion of the indications, methods, and
complications of erythrocyte transfusions (1–5).

ASSUMPTIONS

The transfusion of erythrocyte products to correct anemia is rooted
in the following three assumptions.

1. It is possible to accurately monitor anemia.
2. It is possible to identify when an anemia impairs tissue oxygenation.
3. Erythrocyte transfusions improve tissue oxygenation.

This section briefly evaluates the validity of these assumptions.

MONITORING ANEMIA

Anemia is a condition that is characterized by **a decrease in the
oxygen carrying capacity of blood** (5). Because the oxygen carrying

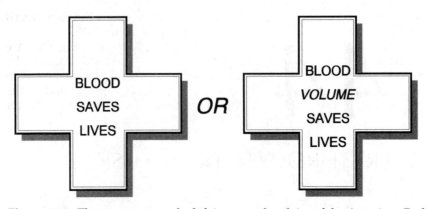

Figure 44.1. The statement on the left is a popular claim of the American Red Cross. However, the statement on the right is more accurate and would help foster a more judicious use of erythrocyte transfusions.

capacity of blood is determined by the mass of circulating red blood cells, anemia can be defined as a decrease in the red cell mass. The red cell mass is measured as a volume using chromium-tagged autologous erythrocytes; the normal values in adults are shown in Table 44.1.

Because red cell volume is not easily measured in the clinical setting, the clinical definition of anemia is based on the hematocrit and hemoglobin concentration in whole blood. Anemia is defined as any hematocrit or hemoglobin concentration that falls below the normal ranges shown in Table 44.1.

Reliability

The problem with the clinical definition of anemia is the influence of the plasma volume on the hematocrit and hemoglobin concentration. For example, an increase in the plasma volume (e.g., from hydration) will decrease the hematocrit and hemoglobin concentration and give the impression of a developing or worsening anemia, even though the oxygen carrying capacity of the blood (i.e., the red cell volume) remains unchanged. Therefore, changes in the hemoglobin and hematocrit can be misleading because they may not reflect a change in the oxygen carrying capacity of the blood. This is revealed in clinical stud-

TABLE 44.1. NORMAL VALUES FOR RED CELL PARAMETERS IN ADULTS			
	Red Cell Volume	Hematocrit	Hemoglobin
Males	26 mL/kg	40–54%	13.5–18.0 g/dL
Females	24 mL/kg	38–47%	12.0–16.0 g/dL
From the American Association of Blood Banks Technical Manual. 10th ed. Arlington, VA: AABB, 1990;649–650.			

ies that show a poor correlation between changes in the hematocrit and hemoglobin and changes in the red cell volume (6,7).

Thus the clinical markers of anemia are unreliable because they are relative measurements (i.e., relative to plasma volume), whereas the true marker of anemia is an absolute measurement (i.e., a deficit in red cell volume). This means that the first assumption stated at the beginning of the section (i.e., that it is possible to accurately monitor an anemia and determine its severity) is invalid.

CONSEQUENCES OF ANEMIA

Cardiac Output

A decrease in the number of circulating erythrocytes will decrease the viscosity of blood (see Table 1.2), and according to the Hagen–Poiseuille equation shown in Equation 44.1 (where μ is the symbol for viscosity), this will favor an increase in the rate of blood flow. (See Chapter 1 for a description of the Hagen–Poiseuille equation.)

$$\text{Flow Rate} = \Delta P \left(\frac{\pi r^4}{8\ \mu L} \right) \tag{44.1}$$

Anemia will therefore be accompanied by an increase in cardiac output, and this helps maintain the rate of oxygen delivery to the peripheral tissues.

The severity of anemia required to elicit an increase in cardiac output varies in different reports. Early observations showed that cardiac output begins to rise when the hemoglobin falls below 7 g/dL (8). However, subsequent studies have shown that hemoglobin levels as low as 4.5 g/dL (both acute and chronic) may not be accompanied by an increase in cardiac output (9,10).

Systemic Oxygenation

Another compensatory response to anemia that helps maintain tissue oxygenation is an increase in oxygen extraction from the systemic capillaries. This is demonstrated in Figure 44.2. As the hematocrit decreases below normal, there is a decrease in systemic oxygen delivery (DO_2), but the oxygen extraction ratio (O_2ER) increases, which helps maintain a constant oxygen uptake (VO_2) into the tissues. However, when the hematocrit falls below 10%, the increase in oxygen extraction is no longer sufficient to maintain a constant VO_2 and tissue oxygenation begins to fall. Further decreases in hematocrit beyond this point result in impaired tissue oxygenation, as shown by the increase in blood lactate levels (lower graph).

Figure 44.2 shows a threshold hematocrit of 10% (which corresponds to a hemoglobin of 3 g/dL) for impaired tissue oxygenation. These results are taken from a study of anesthetized primates breathing 100%

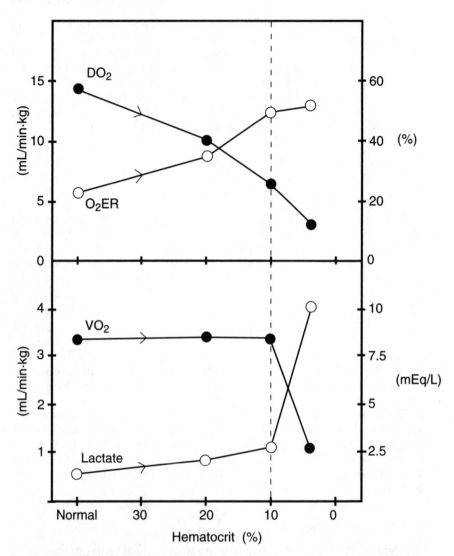

Figure 44.2. The effects of progressive isovolemic anemia on oxygen delivery (DO_2), oxygen extraction ratio (O_{2ER}), oxygen uptake (VO_2), and blood lactate levels in anesthetized primates breathing 100% oxygen. (From Wilkerson DK et al. Oxygen extraction ratio: a valid indicator of myocardial metabolism in anemia. J Surg Res 1987;42:629–634.)

oxygen (14). Similar results have been reported in anesthetized humans (both children and adults) breathing 100% oxygen (11,12) and in nonanesthetized primates breathing room air (13). However, impaired tissue oxygenation is expected at higher levels of hematocrit and hemoglobin in awake patients who are breathing less than 100% oxygen and who have either cardiac dysfunction or hypermetabolism. Because these latter conditions are common in patients in the ICU, the level of anemia that compromises tissue oxygenation is expected to vary in individual patients.

TRANSFUSION TRIGGER

As just indicated, a single hematocrit or hemoglobin level cannot be used as the transfusion trigger for all patients in the ICU. This is stated in the *Clinical Practice Guideline on Elective Red Blood Cell Transfusion* from the American College of Physicians, which cautions to avoid an empiric, automatic transfusion threshold, such as a hemoglobin less than 10 g/dL (2).

Physiologic Parameters

The physiologic markers of impaired tissue oxygenation (see Table 13.1) should be superior to the hemoglobin and hematocrit as transfusion triggers in individual patients in the ICU (1,13–16). The oxygen extraction ratio has been specifically recommended for this purpose (14,15). As demonstrated in Figure 44.2, the point at which the compensatory increase in oxygen extraction begins to fail corresponds to an O_2ER of 0.5 (50%). Therefore, **an O_2ER of 0.5 can be used as a transfusion trigger** (14,15). Oxygen extraction can be monitored continuously in the ICU by using pulse oximetry (for arterial O_2 saturation) combined with mixed venous oximetry (for venous O_2 saturation), as described in Chapter 22.

Therefore, the second assumption stated at the beginning of the section (i.e., that it is possible to identify when an anemia impairs tissue oxygenation) is not valid if the hemoglobin and hematocrit are monitored, but can be valid if the physiologic parameters of tissue oxygenation are monitored.

EFFICACY OF RED CELL TRANSFUSIONS

Cardiac Output

Just as anemia can increase the cardiac output by reducing blood viscosity, correcting anemia can reduce the cardiac output by increasing blood viscosity (16). This tendency to reduce cardiac output limits the ability of erythrocyte transfusions to improve systemic oxygen transport.

Systemic Oxygenation

Erythrocyte transfusions have a variable effect on systemic oxygenation in individual patients (17–19). This is demonstrated in Figure 44.3. Each line in this graph shows the effects of erythrocyte transfusions on the hemoglobin concentration and systemic oxygen uptake (Vo_2) in individual postoperative patients with isovolemic anemia. The

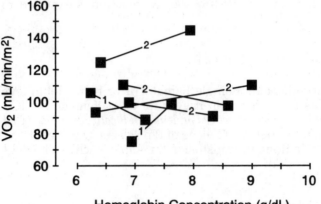

Figure 44.3. The effects of erythrocyte transfusions on hemoglobin concentration and systemic oxygen uptake (Vo_2) in individual postoperative patients with isovolemic anemia. Each line on the graph represents the changes recorded in an individual patient. The number of packed cells transfused in each case is indicated by the numbers that transect each line. (Data from personal observations.)

number of units of packed cells transfused in each patient is indicated by the numbers intersecting each line in the graph. Of the six patients who were transfused, three patients showed an increase in Vo_2 and three patients showed a decrease in Vo_2. Note that the direction of change in the Vo_2 after the erythrocyte transfusions is unrelated to either the baseline level of anemia (the baseline hemoglobin is less than 7 g/dL in all patients) or the magnitude of increase in the serum hemoglobin concentration. This graph demonstrates that an increase in hemoglobin concentration after erythrocyte transfusions does not necessarily indicate that tissue oxygenation has also improved.

Therefore, the third assumption stated at the beginning of this section (i.e., that erythrocyte transfusions improve tissue oxygenation) is valid for some but not all patients. Furthermore, some parameter of systemic oxygenation, and not just the hematocrit and hemoglobin concentration, should be monitored to identify which patients benefit from blood transfusions.

INDICATIONS FOR ERYTHROCYTE TRANSFUSIONS

The following statements are relevant regarding the need for erythrocyte concentrates (packed red cells) in individual patients with normovolemic anemia. These statements represent a summary of the recommendations in References 1–5.

1. Erythrocyte transfusions are **not indicated** for the following:
   a. Enhancing a sense of well-being

b. Promoting wound healing
c. Expanding the intravascular volume
d. Correcting a hemoglobin below 10 g/dL in a patient who has no evidence of ongoing tissue ischemia (e.g., angina, ischemic stroke, hyperlactatemia)
e. Correcting anemia of any degree in patients who do not have cardiac dysfunction, coronary artery disease, or cerebrovascular disease

2. Erythrocyte transfusions **are indicated** for the following:
a. Evidence of impaired tissue oxygenation (e.g., Vo_2 less than 100 mL/min/m^2 or hyperlactatemia) or ongoing coronary or cerebrovascular ischemia in patients with an adequate blood volume
b. An O_2ER above 0.5 in patients with an adequate cardiac output
c. Correction of hemoglobin below 7 g/dL in patients with a history of active coronary artery disease, cerebrovascular insufficiency, or significant cardiac dysfunction

When erythrocyte products are given to improve systemic oxygen transport in asymptomatic patients, 1 or 2 units of packed cells should be transfused and the effects on oxygen transport variables should be measured approximately 15 to 30 minutes after the transfusion is completed. If a significant rise in hemoglobin occurs but no improvement in systemic oxygen transport is seen, no further transfusions should be given at that time.

ERYTHROCYTE PRODUCTS

All blood products containing erythrocytes are stored at 4° C using a liquid anticoagulant preservative that contains citrate, phosphate, and dextrose (CPD). The citrate binds ionized calcium and acts as an anticoagulant. The phosphate helps retard the breakdown of 2,3-diphosphoglycerate, and the dextrose serves as a fuel source for the erythrocytes. Erythrocytes stored in CPD at 4° C are viable for at least 21 days (20).

WHOLE BLOOD

A unit of whole blood contains an average of 510 mL (blood plus CPD solution) (21). Most blood banks will store whole blood only on request. Otherwise, the blood is fractionated into erythrocyte and plasma fractions within a few hours of collection. The separation of whole blood into its component fractions allows more efficient use of blood products to achieve specific transfusion goals.

PACKED RED CELLS

Erythrocyte concentrates, or *packed red cells,* are prepared by centrifuging whole blood and removing 250 mL of the plasma supernatant

(20). Each unit of packed cells contains approximately 200 mL of cells (mostly erythrocytes) and 50 to 100 mL of plasma and CPD solution. The hematocrit is usually between 60 and 80%, and the hemoglobin concentration is between 23 and 27 g/dL (20).

LEUKOCYTE-POOR RED CELLS

Removal of the leukocytes in packed red cells is recommended when transfusing patients with a history of febrile, nonhemolytic transfusion reactions (which are caused by antibodies to leukocytes in donor blood) (21). The leukocytes can be separated by centrifugation or filters, but separation is never complete and up to 30% of the leukocytes remain in the sample.

WASHED RED CELLS

Packed cells can be washed with isotonic saline to remove leukocytes and residual plasma. The removal of plasma helps prevent allergic reactions caused by prior sensitization to plasma proteins in donor blood. Washed red cells are therefore used for transfusing patients with a history of hypersensitivity transfusion reactions.

INFUSING ERYTHROCYTE PRODUCTS

A standard infusion system for transfusing erythrocyte products is shown in Figure 44.4. Each of the numbered components in the system is described briefly in the following paragraphs.

PRESSURIZED INFUSIONS

The gravity-driven flow of whole blood and packed cells is shown in Table 44.2 (22). Because these flow rates do not approach the 250 mL/min or greater flow rates needed for the resuscitation of trauma victims, pressure-generating devices are used to speed infusion rates. The most common device used for this purpose is a standard blood pressure cuff that is wrapped around the collapsible plastic blood containers. When the cuff is inflated to a pressure of 200 mm Hg, the infusion rate of whole blood and packed cells increases approximately threefold, as shown in Table 44.2. Manual hand pumps are also available for increasing infusion rates. These hand pumps are not as effective as the blood pressure cuff (at 200 mm Hg) for infusing whole blood but are equivalent to the pressure cuffs for infusing packed cells (Table 44.2).

SALINE DILUTION

As described in Chapter 14 (see Figure 14.4), the infusion rate of blood products is inversely related to the density of erythrocytes in

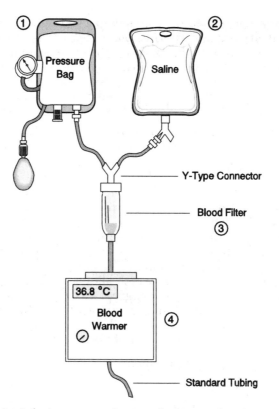

Figure 44.4. An infusion system for transfusing erythrocyte products. Each of the numbered components is described in the text.

		Infusion Rate (mL/min)*		
Fluid	Catheter Size	Gravity Flow	Hand Pump	Pressure Cuff (200 mm Hg)
Tap water	16-gauge 2″ length	100	180	285
Whole blood	↓	65	125	185
Packed cells		20	80	70

TABLE 44.2. PRESSURIZED INFUSION OF ERYTHROCYTE PRODUCTS

*Infusion rates for fluids at room temperature. Refrigerated blood products infuse at 30 to 50% slower rates.

Data from Dula DJ et al. Flow rate variance of commonly used IV infusion techniques. J Trauma 1981;21:480–482.

the fluid (a viscosity effect). As a result, packed cells infuse at approximately one-third the rate of whole blood. Special Y-configured tubing in blood infusion sets allows packed cells to be diluted with an equal volume of isotonic saline. When this is done, the infusion rate of packed cells is comparable to that of whole blood. Only isotonic saline should be used as a diluent for packed red cells. Ringer's solutions are not advised for diluting erythrocyte products because the calcium in Ringer's solutions can promote clotting in the blood sample (23).

BLOOD FILTERS

Erythrocyte products are infused through filters that trap small clots and other cellular debris (e.g., decomposed platelets and fibrin-coated leukocytes). These filters can become an impediment to flow as they collect trapped debris, and thus they should be replaced periodically (e.g., after every 4 units of blood). The standard filters have a pore size of 170 to 260 microns (23), which allows small fibrin microaggregates to pass freely. These microaggregates can become lodged in the pulmonary capillaries and create abnormalities in gas exchange. Smaller microaggregate filters are available, but their value in preventing pulmonary complications has not been proven (24).

BLOOD WARMERS

Warming reduces the viscosity of refrigerated blood and can increase infusion rates by 30 to 50% (see footnote in Table 44.2). However, the major value of warming blood is considered to be the prevention of hypothermia from rapid transfusions (when 1 unit of blood is transfused every 5 to 10 minutes) (25). The recommended temperature for infused blood is 33° to 35° C (25). Temperatures of 37° C or higher can promote hemolysis.

A simple method for warming blood is to immerse the blood storage bags in hot water before transfusion. However, this rewarming method can take up to 30 minutes, and can produce hemolysis from overheating. Controlled warming devices that can warm blood to the desired infusion temperatures at flow rates slightly in excess of 100 mL/minute are available (26). However, at the infusion rates often used to resuscitate trauma victims (i.e., greater than 250 mL/minute), blood warming devices are often unable to warm blood to the desired temperature (26).

ADVERSE REACTIONS

The complications of homologous blood transfusion (i.e., blood donor from the same species) that are most noted are listed in Table

TABLE 44.3. RISKS OF HOMOLOGOUS BLOOD TRANSFUSION	
Complication	Frequency (per units transfused)
Immune:	
Fever, chills, urticaria	1 in 100
Hemolysis	1 in 6,000
Fatal hemolysis	1 in 100,000
Anaphylaxis	1 in 500,000
Infectious:	
Bacterial contamination	1 in 25,000
Viral hepatitis*	1 in 80,000
Human immunodeficiency virus infection*	1 in 500,000

* Risks for blood transfusions in 1996.
Data from References 27–33.

44.3 (27–33). The acute transfusion reactions are described briefly in the following paragraphs.

ACUTE HEMOLYTIC REACTIONS

Acute hemolytic transfusion reactions are uncommon and are rarely severe enough to be life-threatening (27–29). These reactions are produced by antibodies in the recipient that bind to ABO surface antigens on donor erythrocytes. These antibodies fix complement and can produce rapid lysis. One unit of packed red cells can be completely lysed in less than 1 hour (27). Lysis of red cells somehow provokes a severe systemic inflammatory response that can lead to hypotension and progressive multiorgan dysfunction. This type of transfusion reaction is usually the result of identification errors leading to transfusion of ABO mismatched blood (28).

Clinical Manifestations

Severe reactions require as little as 10 mL of donor blood (27) and are usually evident within a few minutes after the transfusion is started. Fever, dyspnea, chest pain, and low back pain are common (27–29). Hypotension can develop suddenly and may be the only sign in comatose patients. Severe reactions are accompanied by a consumptive coagulopathy and progressive multiorgan dysfunction. Acute renal failure is prominent in 5 to 10% of cases (29).

Bedside Strategy

The following approach is recommended for any patient who develops a fever soon after the onset of a homologous blood transfusion.

1. *Stop* the transfusion immediately. This is imperative because the

morbidity and mortality in hemolytic reactions is a function of the volume of incompatible blood transfused (27).

2. Check the blood pressure immediately. If the pressure is dropping, do the following:
   a. Infuse volume (colloids may be preferred because of their ability to rapidly expand the vascular volume).
   b. Start dopamine (at 5 μg/kg/minute). This agent has been preferred for its renal vasodilating effects because renal failure is a poor prognostic sign in hemolytic transfusion reactions (29). However, the relative benefits of dopamine over other pressor agents is unproven.

Once the patient is stabilized, do the following:

3. Obtain a blood sample and inspect the plasma for the pink-to-red hue of hemoglobin.
4. Obtain a freshly voided urine specimen and perform a dipstick test for blood.
5. Send a blood sample for a direct Coomb's test. A positive test confirms a hemolytic transfusion reaction. However, a negative test is possible if most of the donor erythrocytes have already lysed.

FEBRILE NONHEMOLYTIC REACTIONS

Fever that is not related to hemolysis is the most common acute transfusion reaction, appearing in approximately 1% of transfusions. This reaction is the result of antibodies in the recipient to leukocytes in donor blood. The antileukocyte antibodies are produced in response to prior transfusions or prior pregnancies, so this type of response is usually seen in multiparous women or in patients with a history of prior transfusions.

Clinical Manifestations

The fever usually appears 1 to 6 hours after starting the transfusion (later than the onset of fever associated with hemolytic transfusion reactions), and it is not usually accompanied by signs of systemic illness. However, severe reactions can occur, and patients can have a toxic appearance.

Bedside Strategy

The bedside approach is the same as outlined for hemolytic transfusion reactions. The diagnosis of a nonhemolytic febrile reaction is confirmed by excluding the presence of hemolysis with the tests described previously. Bacterial contamination of blood products is a potential cause of fever, but it is uncommon (32). However, some recommend routine culture of donor and recipient blood for any febrile transfusion reaction accompanied by other signs of systemic illness (e.g., rigors, dyspnea).

Future Transfusions

More than 50% of patients who develop a febrile nonhemolytic transfusion reaction will not experience a similar reaction during subsequent blood transfusions. Therefore, no special precautions are necessary for future transfusions. If a second febrile reaction develops, leukocyte-poor red cell preparations are advised for all further erythrocyte transfusions.

ALLERGIC REACTIONS

Hypersensitivity reactions (rash, anaphylaxis) are the result of sensitization to plasma proteins in prior transfusions. Patients with IgA deficiency are particularly prone to hypersensitivity reactions to blood transfusions, and can do so without prior exposure to plasma products (33).

Clinical Manifestations

The usual manifestation is mild urticaria that appears during the transfusion and may be accompanied by fever. Anaphylactic reactions are rare (Table 44.3).

Bedside Strategy

Mild urticaria without fever does not require interruption of the transfusion. However, the common practice is to stop the transfusion temporarily and administer antihistamines (diphenhydramine, 25 to 50 mg orally or intramuscularly every 6 hours). Antihistamines may help alleviate the pruritus associated with urticaria but otherwise are without benefit.

The rare instance of transfusion-associated anaphylaxis should be managed as described in Chapter 31 (see Table 31.4). Patients who develop anaphylaxis should be tested for an underlying IgA deficiency.

Future Transfusions

Future transfusions should be avoided if possible for all cases of transfusion-associated anaphylaxis. For less severe allergic reactions, washed red cell preparations (plasma removed) are advised for subsequent transfusions. Antihistamine premedication is a popular but unproven practice.

ACUTE LUNG INJURY

Acute respiratory failure is a much talked about but uncommon transfusion reaction, with an estimated incidence of 1 per 5000 transfusions (34). It has been observed after a single transfusion of either whole blood or packed red cells (15). The prevailing theory is that antileukocyte antibodies in donor blood bind to circulating granulocytes in the recipient and promote leukocyte sequestration in the pulmonary microcirculation. This then leads to granulocyte-mediated lung injury, which presents as acute respiratory distress syndrome (ARDS). However, unlike most cases of ARDS, this lung injury is rarely fatal.

Clinical Manifestations

Signs of respiratory compromise (dyspnea, hypoxemia) usually develop within a few hours after the transfusion begins. Fever is common, and hypotension has been reported (34). The chest x-ray film eventually shows diffuse pulmonary infiltrates. Although the acute syndrome can be severe, the process usually resolves within a week. As mentioned, fatalities are rare.

Bedside Strategy

The transfusion should be stopped (if still running) at the first signs of respiratory compromise. The remainder of the management is similar to that described for ARDS in Chapter 23.

Future Transfusions

There are no firm recommendations regarding future transfusions in patients who develop transfusion-associated ARDS. Some advocate the use of washed red cells (to remove any antibody-containing plasma in the donor sample), while others caution against any future transfusions unless absolutely necessary (34).

AUTOLOGOUS TRANSFUSION

Reinfusion of the patient's own blood (autologous transfusion) not only eliminates many of the risks associated with homologous transfusions, but also reduces the strain on the nation's blood supply. The following is a brief description of the different approaches to autologous blood transfusion (35).

PREOPERATIVE DEPOSIT

Patients undergoing elective surgical procedures with minimal blood losses (e.g., orthopedic procedures) can donate their own blood before the procedure. The patients must have a baseline hemoglobin of 11 g/dL or higher and be free of any conditions that pose a risk for phlebotomy (e.g., frequent angina, aortic stenosis). One unit of blood can be removed every 4 days (usually weekly) for 2 or 3 weeks before the procedure. Any blood transfusions required during or after surgery are then performed with the patient's own blood.

INTRAOPERATIVE SALVAGE

Reinfusion of lost blood is a popular practice for "bloody" surgical procedures such as open-heart surgery and liver transplantation. It is also allowed by some Jehovah's Witnesses (35). Blood is aspirated with a modified suction wand and fed to a specialized "cell-saver" instrument that centrifuges the blood to concentrate the erythrocytes and washes the specimen with saline. High-speed instruments that can process a unit of packed cells in less than 5 minutes are now available (35).

Complications

Surprisingly few risks are associated with intraoperative blood salvage. Dilutional coagulopathy is probably the most common complication, and it occurs with larger volume reinfusions. Consumptive coagulopathy and ARDS are the most serious complications (salvaged blood syndrome) and may be caused by reinfusion of activated leukocytes (36).

POSTOPERATIVE SALVAGE

The most common method of postoperative blood salvage is the reinfusion of shed mediastinal blood after median sternotomy procedures (37). Chest tube drainage from the mediastinum is directed to a rigid cannister that contains two collection bags. The first bag contains a 170-micron filter to trap large clots and cellular debris. Because the blood has undergone endogenous defibrination in the chest, no anticoagulants need to be added. The blood passes through the filter and drains into the second collection bag, which has an 800 mL capacity. When this bag is filled, it is detached and hung on an IV pole for reinfusion.

This method differs from intraoperative salvage in that there is no centrifugation or saline washing of the sample. Traumatic disruption of cells is common, and the hematocrit of the reinfused blood is only 15 to 25%. This low hematocrit may explain why reinfusion of shed mediastinal blood does not always reduce homologous transfusion needs (38). Complications are considered uncommon. However, the supernatant in shed mediastinal blood contains high concentrations of leukocyte elastase (39), and this could produce a clinical syndrome similar to the salvaged blood syndrome seen with intraoperative blood salvage.

REFERENCES

CONSENSUS STATEMENTS

1. Consensus Conference on Perioperative Red Blood Cell Transfusion. JAMA 1988;260:2700–2702.
2. Practice strategies for elective red blood cell transfusion. A Clinical Practice Guideline from the American College of Physicians. Ann Intern Med 1992; 116:403–406.

REVIEWS

3. Robertie PG, Gravlee GP. Safe limits of isovolemic hemodilution and recommendations for erythrocyte transfusions. Int Anesthesiol Clin 1990;28:197–204 (54 references).
4. Welch HG, Meehan KR, Goognough LT. Prudent strategies for elective red blood cell transfusion. Ann Intern Med 1992;116:393–402 (120 references).
5. Spence RK, Cernaianu AC, Carson J, DelRossi AJ. Transfusion and surgery. Curr Probl Surg 1993;30:1101–1192 (212 references).

MONITORING ANEMIA

6. Jones JG, Holland BM, Wardrop CAJ. Total circulating red cells versus hematocrit as a primary descriptor of oxygen transport by the blood. Br J Hematol 1990;76:228–232.
7. Cordts PR, LaMorte WW, Fisher JB, et al. Poor predictive value of hematocrit and hemodynamic parameters for erythrocyte deficits after extensive elective vascular operations. Surg Gynecol Obstet 1992;175:243–248.

CONSEQUENCES OF ANEMIA

8. Brannon ES, Merrill AJ, Warren JV, Stead EA Jr. Cardiac output in patients with chronic anemia as measured by the technique of right heart catheterization. J Clin Invest 1945;24:332–337.
9. Duke M, Abelmann WH. The hemodynamic response to chronic anemia. Circulation 1969;39:503–515.
10. Rosen AL, Gould S, Sehgal LR, et al. Cardiac output response to extreme hemodilution with hemoglobin solutions of various P_{50} values. Crit Care Med 1979;7:380–382.
11. Fontana JL, Welborn L, Mongan PD, et al. Oxygen consumption and cardiovascular function in children during profound intraoperative normovolemic hemodilution. Anesth Analg 1995;80:219–225.
12. Messmer K. Therapeutic threshold values for acute alterations in hemoglobin concentration. In: Zander R, Mertzlufft F, eds. The oxygen status of arterial blood. Basel, Switzerland: Karger Publishers, 1991;167–173.
13. Levine E, Rosen A, Sehgal L, et al. Physiologic effects of acute anemia: implications for a reduced transfusion trigger. Transfusion 1990;30:11–14.

TRANSFUSION TRIGGER

14. Wilkerson DK, Rosen AL, Gould SA, et al. Oxygen extraction ratio: a valid indicator of myocardial metabolism in anemia. J Surg Res 1987;42:629–634.
15. Levy PS, Chavez RP, Crystal GJ, et al. Oxygen extraction ratio: a valid indicator of transfusion need in limited coronary vascular reserve? J Trauma 1992;32: 769–774.

EFFICACY OF RED CELL TRANSFUSIONS

16. Shah DM, Gottlieb M, Rahm R, et al. Failure of red cell transfusions to increase oxygen transport or mixed venous Po_2 in injured patients. J Trauma 1982;22: 741–746.
17. Silverman H, Tuma P. Gastric tonometry in patients with sepsis: effects of dobutamine and packed red cell transfusions. Chest 1992;102:184–188.
18. Marik PE, Sibbald W. Effect of stored-blood transfusion on oxygen delivery in patients with sepsis. JAMA 1993;269:3024–3029.
19. Robbins JM, Keating K, Orlando R, Yeston N. Effects of blood transfusion on oxygen delivery and consumption in critically ill surgical patients. Contemp Surg 1993;43:281–285.

ERYTHROCYTE PRODUCTS

20. American Association of Blood Banks Technical Manual. 10th ed. Arlington, VA: American Association of Blood Banks, 1990;37–58, 635–637.
21. Davies SC. Transfusion of red cells. In: Contreras M, ed. ABC of transfusion. London: British Medical Journal, 1990;9–13.

INFUSING ERYTHROCYTE PRODUCTS

22. Dula DJ, Muller A, Donovan SW. Flow rate variance of commonly used IV infusion techniques. J Trauma 1981;21:480–482.
23. Blood Transfusion Practice. In: American Association of Blood Banks Technical Manual. 10th ed. Arlington, VA: American Association of Blood Banks, 1990;341–375.
24. Kruskall MS, Bergen JJ, Klein HG, et al. Transfusion therapy in emergency medicine. Ann Emerg Med 1988;17:327–335.
25. Iserson KV, Huestis DW. Blood warming: current applications and techniques. Transfusion 1991;31:558–571.
26. Uhl L, Pacini D, Kruskall MS. A comparative study of blood warmer performance. Anesthesiol 1992;77:1022–1028.

RISKS OF HOMOLOGOUS TRANSFUSION

27. Seyfried H, Walewska I. Immune hemolytic transfusion reactions. World J Surg 1987;11:25–29.
28. Gloe D. Common reactions to transfusions. Heart Lung 1991;20:506–512.
29. Nicholls MD. Transfusion: morbidity and mortality. Anesth Intensive Care 1993;21:15–19.

30. Schreiber GB, Busch MP, Akinman S, et al. The risk of transfusion-transmitted viral infections. N Engl J Med 1996;334:1685–1690.
31. Klein HG. New insights into the management of anemia in the surgical patient. Am J Med 1996;101(Suppl 2A):12S–15S.
32. Gottlieb T. Hazards of bacterial contamination of blood products. Anesth Intensive Care 1993;21:20–23.
33. Isbister JP. Adverse reactions to plasma and plasma components. Anesth Intensive Care 1993;21:31–38.
34. Gans ROB, Duurkens VAM, van Zundert AA, et al. Transfusion-related acute lung injury. Intensive Care Med 1988;14:654–657.

AUTOLOGOUS TRANSFUSIONS

35. Ereth MH, Oliver WC Jr, Santrach PJ. Perioperative interventions to decrease transfusion of allogenic blood products. Mayo Clin Proc 1994;69:575–586.
36. Bull BS, Bull MH. The salvaged blood syndrome: a sequel to mechanochemical activation of platelets and leukocytes? Blood Cells 1990;16:5–20.
37. Ward HB, Smith RR, Landis KP, et al. Prospective, randomized trial of autotransfusion after routine cardiac operations. Ann Thorac Surg 1993;56:137–141.
38. Roberts SR, Early G, Brown B, et al. Autotransfusion of unwashed mediastinal shed blood fails to decrease banked blood requirements in patients undergoing aortocoronary bypass surgery. Am J Surg 1991;162:477–480.
39. Harbison S, Chung S, Kucick B, Marino PL. Leukocyte disruption and elastase release in autotransfused blood. Crit Care Med 1989;17:S42.

SUGGESTED READINGS

Anderson KC, Ness P. Scientific basis of transfusion medicine: implications for clinical practice. Philadelphia: WB Saunders, 1994.
Blood: Bearer of life and death: New ways to fight diseases caused by faults in the bloodstream. A report from the Howard Hughes Medical Institute. Chevy Chase, MD: Howard Hughes Medical Institute, 1993.
Contreras M, ed. ABC of transfusion. London: British Medical Journal, 1990.
Gravlee GP, ed. Blood conservation. Int Anesthesiol Clin 1990;28:183–243.
Hillman RS, Finch CA. Red cell manual. 6th ed. Philadelphia: FA Davis, 1992.
Spence RK, ed. New insights into the management of anemia in the surgical patient. Am J Med 1996;101(Suppl 2A):1S–44S.

c h a p t e r

PLATELET DISORDERS
AND REPLACEMENT

Platelet disorders fall into two categories: those characterized by abnormal numbers of circulating platelets and those characterized by abnormal platelet function. This chapter introduces the common causes of both types of platelet disorders in the ICU population. This is followed by a brief description of the indications, methods, and complications of platelet transfusion therapy (1–4).

PLATELETS AND HEMOSTASIS

The normal adult has an average of 250 billion platelets per liter of blood. Assuming a normal blood volume of 5.5 L, the total number of platelets in the bloodstream will be slightly in excess of 1 trillion. To keep this platelet count constant, as many as 45 billion new platelets must be added to each liter of blood daily (5). For a blood volume of 5.5 L, this corresponds to a total production of 248 billion platelets each day. These numbers are astounding, and indicate the level of marrow activity needed to maintain normal platelet homeostasis.

THROMBOSIS

Platelets are not really cells because they contain no nucleus and cannot synthesize proteins. They are a portion of megakaryocyte cytoplasm that has been pinched off and completely surrounded by a cell membrane. This cytoplasm is composed of dense granules that are rich in calcium. When the vascular endothelium is denuded, platelets adhere to the exposed subendothelium (by virtue of membrane glycoproteins called *integrins* that act as adhesion receptors) and release the contents of their granules. The calcium that is released helps initiate the coagulation cascade that ends in the production of fibrin strands.

709

The strands of fibrin then form an interlacing meshwork with the platelets to produce a thrombus.

THROMBOCYTOPENIA

Thrombocytopenia is defined as a platelet count below $150,000/mm^3$ (or $150 \times 10^9/L$ in SI Units) (6). However, the ability to form a hemostatic plug is retained until the platelet count falls below $100,000/mm^3$. Therefore, clinically significant thrombocytopenia can be defined as a platelet count below $100,000/mm^3$. The bleeding tendency in thrombocytopenia is determined primarily by the presence or absence of a structural lesion that is prone to bleeding and is not a function of the platelet count. Although the traditional teaching has been that spontaneous hemorrhage in the absence of a structural lesion can occur when the platelet count falls below $20,000/mm^3$ (1), this is no longer considered valid (7). In the absence of risk factors for bleeding, platelet counts below $5000/mm^3$ can be tolerated without troublesome bleeding (8).

PLATELET ADHESION

When the ability of platelets to adhere to the subendothelium is diminished (e.g., as in uremia), the risk of hemorrhage can be increased despite platelet counts exceeding $100,000/mm^3$. Defects in platelet adhesion can be detected by a prolonged bleeding time. However, no correlation exists between the bleeding time and the tendency for bleeding (9), and thus the bleeding time is not useful for detecting clinically significant abnormalities in platelet adhesion. The recognition of platelet adhesion abnormalities in individual patients is accomplished by identifying the conditions that alter platelet adhesiveness.

THROMBOCYTOPENIA

The only survey of thrombocytopenia in patients in the ICU is from a medical ICU, where 23% of the patients had platelet counts below $100,000/mm^3$ at some time during their ICU stay (10). The causes of thrombocytopenia that are most likely to be encountered in the ICU are listed in Table 45.1.

| TABLE 45.1. CAUSES OF PLATELET DISORDERS IN THE ICU ||
Thrombocytopenia	Abnormal Platelet Function
Heparin (1–3%)	Renal insufficiency
Sepsis (>50%)	Cardiopulmonary bypass
AIDS (40–60%)	Aspirin
DIC	Dextran
TTP	
Incidence of platelet disorders is indicated in parentheses.	

HEPARIN

Heparin can combine with a heparin-binding protein (platelet factor 4) in platelets to form an antigenic complex that induces the formation of IgG. This immunoglobulin can then bind to platelets and promote platelet clumping. If severe enough, this process can result in a consumptive thrombocytopenia and clinically apparent thrombosis (11).

Clinical Features

Thrombocytopenia is reported in 1 to 3% of patients receiving heparin (12). It usually appears within 14 days after heparin is started and is independent of the heparin dose. Even the small doses of heparin used for **heparin flushes and** the small amounts on **heparin-coated pulmonary artery catheters can induce thrombocytopenia** (13). Thrombocytopenia is less common with low–molecular-weight heparin than with unfractionated heparin (14).

The **major complication** of heparin-induced thrombocytopenia **is thrombosis, not bleeding.** In a 14-year survey of patients with heparin-induced thrombocytopenia, venous thromboembolism was identified in 70% of the patients and arterial thrombosis was identified in 15% of the patients (12). In approximately half the patients surveyed, the disorder was first recognized after a thrombotic episode had occurred. In the other patients who had isolated thrombocytopenia, 50% developed a thrombosis within the next 30 days *despite the discontinuation of heparin therapy* (12).

Diagnosis

There are two criteria for the diagnosis of heparin-induced thrombocytopenia (14). The first is thrombocytopenia that develops more than 5 days after the initial exposure to heparin. The second is a positive assay for heparin-induced IgG antibodies. The antibody is detected by the release of ^{14}C-labeled serotonin from platelets that are added to a sample of the patient's serum. This assay is available in most clinical laboratories and is costly [$222 for the assay performed by the Smith Kline Clinical Laboratories (Philadelphia, PA) in 1996].

Management

In patients with isolated thrombocytopenia (without thrombosis), heparin administration should be discontinued. **Remember to discontinue heparin flushes and remove any heparin-coated intravascular catheters.** If anticoagulation is necessary, Coumadin can be started. Dextran (500 mL of Dextran-40 daily) can be used as a temporary antithrombotic measure until the Coumadin achieves therapeutic levels of anticoagulation.

The management of heparin-induced thrombosis is difficult. Coumadin is usually ineffective (15), and alternative anticoagulants (e.g., danaproid and hirudin) are currently not available in the United States. Thrombolytic therapy may prove useful here (16).

INFECTIONS

Thrombocytopenia is reported in more than 50% of patients with systemic sepsis (4), and in 50% of patients with acquired immunodeficiency syndrome (AIDS) (17). In both conditions platelet destruction is enhanced; but in AIDS it is immune-mediated, and in sepsis it is not. Bleeding is not common in either condition unless the thrombocytopenia is accompanied by other coagulation abnormalities.

DISSEMINATED INTRAVASCULAR COAGULATION

Widespread endothelial damage, as can occur with septicemia or multiple trauma, releases a protein known as *tissue factor* that activates the endogenous coagulation cascade and the fibrinolytic system. This can result in a severe coagulopathy characterized by widespread microvascular thrombosis accompanied by depletion of circulating platelets and procoagulant proteins (18). This condition is called *disseminated intravascular coagulation* (DIC).

Clinical Features

The microvascular thrombosis in DIC produces multiorgan dysfunction. The lungs are commonly involved, and the clinical picture is similar to the acute respiratory distress syndrome, which is described in Chapter 23. Advanced cases are accompanied by acute oliguric renal failure and progressive hepatocellular injury. Depletion of platelets and coagulation factors can be accompanied by bleeding from multiple sites, particularly the gastrointestinal tract.

Diagnosis

The diagnosis of DIC is based on the clinical setting (i.e., severe sepsis or multiple trauma) combined with laboratory evidence of widespread coagulation defects. Thrombocytopenia can be severe and is accompanied by prolongation of the prothrombin time and activated partial thromboplastin time (from depleted coagulant proteins) and elevated fibrin degradation products (from fibrinolysis). Fibrinogen levels can be misleading because fibrinogen is an acute phase reactant, and this can result in normal fibrinogen levels in the face of increased fibrinogen use (19).

Management

Acute, fulminant DIC often has a fatal outcome. Heparin usually is ineffective in retarding the microvascular thrombosis, probably because of depletion of antithrombin-III (20). Antithrombin-II concentrates can be given with heparin (the AT-III dosage is 90 to 120 Units-as a load, then 90 to 120 Units daily for 4 days), but the value of this practice remains unproven (21). Bleeding is particularly troublesome to manage because the administration of coagulation factors and platelets can aggravate the microvascular thrombosis.

THROMBOTIC THROMBOCYTOPENIA PURPURA

Thrombotic thrombocytopenia purpura (TTP) is a rare but life-threatening condition caused by immune-mediated platelet aggregation with widespread microvascular thrombosis (similar to DIC). It usually is seen in young adults, particularly women, and often follows a nonspecific illness.

Clinical Features

A combination of five clinical features (pentad) is characteristic of TTP: fever, neurologic changes, acute renal failure, thrombocytopenia, and microangiopathic hemolytic anemia.

Patients usually experience fever and depressed consciousness that can progress rapidly to coma and generalized seizures. Thrombocytopenia is not associated with other coagulation abnormalities, which distinguishes TTP from DIC. The diagnosis is confirmed by the presence of schistocytes in the blood smear (indicating a microangiopathic hemolytic anemia).

Management

The treatment of choice for TTP is plasma exchange (22,23). This can be performed with plasmapheresis equipment that removes blood and separates the plasma from the red cells. The plasma is discarded and the red cells are reinfused with fresh frozen plasma. This is continued until 1.5 times the plasma volume has been exchanged (the normal plasma volume is 40 mL/kg in adult men and 36 mL/kg in adult women). This is repeated daily for approximately 1 week.

If plasmapheresis equipment is unavailable, a "poor man's" plasma exchange can be performed by inserting an arterial catheter into the femoral artery and withdrawing 500 mL aliquots of blood (equivalent to 1 Unit of whole blood) into a blood collection bag. This is then sent to the blood bank for centrifugation to separate the plasma from the blood cells. The cells are then returned and reinfused with a unit of fresh frozen plasma. This is continued until at least one plasma volume has been exchanged.

Acute, fulminant TTP is almost always fatal if untreated. **With prompt use of plasma exchange, as many as 90% of patients can survive** the acute episode (22,23). Platelet transfusions can aggravate the underlying thrombosis in TTP, and thus are contraindicated.

BLOOD TRANSFUSIONS

The viability of platelets in whole blood and erythrocyte concentrates (packed cells) is almost completely lost after 24 hours of storage.

Therefore, large-volume transfusions can produce dilutional thrombocytopenia. This effect becomes prominent when the transfusion volume exceeds 1.5 times the blood volume (24).

A rare type of posttransfusion thrombocytopenia appears approximately 1 week after transfusion, usually in multiparous women, and is caused by antiplatelet antibodies. This condition is called *posttransfusion purpura*, and thrombocytopenia is often severe and prolonged (25). Platelet counts can fall to $10,000/mm^3$ or lower for as long as 40 days (18). If hemorrhage ensues, plasma exchange is the treatment of choice.

ABNORMAL PLATELET FUNCTION

The common causes of impaired platelet aggregation in patients in the ICU are listed in Table 45.1 (26).

RENAL INSUFFICIENCY

Impaired platelet adhesion is seen in both acute and chronic renal insufficiency. No correlation exists between the severity of the renal dysfunction and the severity of the platelet function abnormality. The problem is corrected by hemodialysis or peritoneal dialysis. It is unclear if this platelet function abnormality is clinically significant (26).

CARDIOPULMONARY BYPASS

Platelet adhesiveness is impaired by unknown mechanisms when blood passes through the oxygenator apparatus used during cardiopulmonary bypass. The severity of the platelet function defect is directly related to the duration of bypass (26). In most cases, the abnormality resolves within a few hours after bypass is completed. However, defects in platelet adhesion may contribute to troublesome mediastinal bleeding in the immediate postoperative period.

Aprotinin

Aprotinin (Trasylol) is a proteinase inhibitor that can prevent the platelet dysfunction associated with cardiopulmonary bypass (27). When administered intraoperatively at the dosage shown below, aprotinin can reduced the requirement for platelets and erythrocyte products (28).

Dose: 280 mg IV as a loading dose, followed by a continuous infusion of 70 mg/hour. Also add 280 mg to the oxygenator prime solution.

The drug is infused for the duration of the operative procedure. Although there is a concern that aprotinin might promote thrombosis in the bypass grafts, no evidence exists to support this concern (28).

ASPIRIN

Aspirin inhibits platelet aggregation by blocking prostaglandin-mediated platelet degranulation. The effect is irreversible and lasts for the entire life span of the platelets (10 days). One aspirin tablet (325 mg) is enough to produce the platelet defect.

Emergency Surgery

The effects of aspirin on platelet adhesion becomes an important consideration in patients taking aspirin daily (e.g., as a preventive measure for coronary thrombosis) who require emergency surgery. This is particularly true for cardiopulmonary bypass surgery because aspirin can add to the risk of bleeding from bypass-induced platelet dysfunction. Most studies of emergency bypass surgery show increased bleeding associated with recent aspirin use (26). This aspirin effect is less pronounced when aprotinin is given during the bypass procedure (29).

OTHER DRUGS

A variety of other drugs can impair platelet adhesion, including β-lactam antibiotics, nonsteroidal anti-inflammatory agents, and dextrans (26). However, the clinical significance of these drug-induced platelet effects is unclear.

INDICATIONS FOR PLATELET TRANSFUSIONS

The following guidelines for platelet transfusions are summarized from the first four references listed at the end of this chapter.

ACTIVE BLEEDING

The following statements apply to all instances of active bleeding other than ecchymotic and petechial hemorrhage.
Platelet transfusions are **indicated** in the following situations:
1. The platelet count is below 50,000/mm^3 and the thrombocytopenia is not the result of immune mechanisms.
2. The platelet count is above 50,000/mm^3 and a condition that significantly impairs platelet adhesion (e.g., cardiopulmonary bypass) is present.
Platelet transfusions are **not indicated** in the following situations:
1. The platelet count is above 50,0000/mm^3 and platelet function is normal.
2. Thrombocytopenia is caused by antiplatelet antibodies.

MASSIVE TRANSFUSION

The traditional practice of giving platelet transfusions after transfusion of 8 to 10 Units of whole blood or packed cells is no longer recommended. Platelet counts should be monitored and platelets transfused if the platelet count falls to below $50,000/mm^3$ and evidence of continued bleeding is present. As mentioned previously, significant dilutional thrombocytopenia is not expected until the transfused blood volume exceeds 1.5 times the blood volume.

PROPHYLAXIS

The following statements apply to patients with no evidence of active bleeding other than ecchymotic or petechial hemorrhage.

Platelet transfusions are **indicated** in the following situations:
1. The platelet count is below $5,000/mm^3$.
2. The platelet is below $20,000/mm^3$ and a high-risk condition for bleeding (e.g., peptic ulcer disease, prior hemorrhage from diverticulosis or arteriovenous malformations) is present.
3. The platelet count is below $50,000/mm^3$, and the following procedures are planned:
   Endoscopic biopsy
   Lumbar puncture
   Major surgery

Platelet transfusions are **not indicated** in the following situations:
1. The platelet count is 5000 to $20,000/mm^3$ but no risk factors for bleeding are present.
2. Thrombocytopenia is caused by antiplatelet antibodies.

PLATELET TRANSFUSIONS

Platelet concentrates are prepared by centrifuging fresh whole blood and suspending the platelet pellet in a small volume of plasma. Each platelet concentrate (from 1 Unit of whole blood) contains 50 to 100 billion platelets in 50 mL of plasma (30). Platelets can be stored for up to 7 days, but viability begins to decline after 3 days. Platelet transfusions are usually given as multiples of 6 to 10 individual platelet concentrates that are pooled together.

EFFICACY

In the average-size adult, each platelet concentrate should raise the circulating platelet count by 5000 to $10,000/mm^3$ (30) and the effect should last approximately 8 days. Smaller increments for a shorter duration are expected when the rate of platelet destruction increases, either in the platelet concentrate or in the patient.

COMPLICATIONS

Because one platelet transfusion involves platelet concentrates from 6 to 8 individual donors, the infectious risks associated with homologous blood transfusions (see Table 44.3) are increased sixfold to eightfold with platelet transfusions. Febrile nonhemolytic reactions are also more common with platelet transfusions, and fever has been reported in up to 30% of platelet transfusion recipients (31). Hypersensitivity reactions triggered by proteins in the plasma fraction of platelet concentrates can also occur.

Although platelet membranes have ABO antigens, transfusion reactions as a result of ABO incompatibility do not occur with platelet transfusions. However, recipients of multiple platelet transfusions can develop antiplatelet antibodies that limit the effectiveness of platelet transfusions. If this becomes a problem, platelets can be harvested by apheresis from single, HLA-matched donors.

REFERENCES

CLINICAL PRACTICE GUIDELINE

1. College of American Pathologists, Administration Practice Guidelines Development Task Force. Fresh frozen plasma, cryoprecipitate, and platelets. JAMA 1994;271:777–781.

REVIEWS

2. Rintels PB, Kenney RM, Cowley JP. Therapeutic support of the patient with thrombocytopenia. Hematol Oncol Clin North Am 1994;8:1131–1157.
3. Machin SJ, Kelsey H, Seghatchian MJ. Platelet transfusion. Thromb Haemost 1995;74:246–252.
4. Chang JC. Postoperative thrombocytopenia with etiologic, diagnostic, and therapeutic considerations. Am J Med Sci 1996;311:96–105.

PLATELETS AND HEMOSTASIS

5. Tomer A, Harker LA. Megakaryocytopoiesis and platelet kinetics. In: Rossi EC, Simon TL, Moss GS, eds. Principles of transfusion therapy. Baltimore: Williams & Wilkins, 1991;167–179.
6. American Association of Blood Banks Technical Manual. 10th ed. Arlington, VA: American Association of Blood Banks, 1990;649.
7. Beutler E. Platelet transfusions: the 20,000 per microliter trigger. Blood 1993; 81:1411–1413.
8. Beutler E. Commentary. Abstr Clin Care Guidelines 1994;6:4.
9. Rodgers RP, Levin J. A critical reappraisal of the bleeding time. Semin Thromb Hemost 1990;16:1–20.

THROMBOCYTOPENIA

10. Baughman RP, Lower EF, Flessa HC, Tollerud DJ. Thrombocytopenia in the intensive care unit. Chest 1993;104:1243–1247.

11. Aster RH. Heparin-induced thrombocytopenia and thrombosis. N Engl J Med 1995;332:1374–1376.
12. Warkentin TE, Kelton JG. A 14-year study of heparin-induced thrombocytopenia. Am J Med 1996;101:502–507.
13. Laster J, Silver D. Heparin-coated catheters and heparin-induced thrombocytopenia. J Vasc Surg 1988;7:667–672.
14. Warkentin TE, Levine MN, Hirsh J, et al. Heparin-induced thrombocytopenia in patients treated with low-molecular-weight heparin or unfractionated heparin. N Engl J Med 1995;332:1330–1335.
15. Warkentin TE, Hirsh J, Kelton JG. Heparin-induced thrombocytopenia. N Engl J Med 1995;333:1007.
16. Dieck JA, Rizo-Patron C, Unisa A, et al. A new manifestation and treatment alternative for heparin-induced thrombosis. Chest 1990;98:1524–1526.
17. Doweiko JP, Groopman JE. Hematologic consequences of HIV infection. In: Broder S, Merigan TC, Bolognesi D, eds. Textbook of AIDS medicine. Baltimore: Williams & Wilkins, 1994;617–628.
18. Bell WR. The pathophysiology of disseminated intravascular coagulation. Semin Hematol 1994;31(Suppl 1):19–24.
19. Bovill EG. Laboratory diagnosis of disseminated intravascular coagulation. Semin Hematol 1994;31(Suppl 1):35–39.
20. Clark J, Rubin RN. A practical approach to managing disseminated intravascular coagulation. J Crit Illness 1994;9:265–280.
21. Fourrier F, Chopin C, Huart J-J, et al. Double-blind, placebo-controlled trial of antithrombin II concentrates in septic shock with disseminated intravascular coagulation. Chest 1993;104:882–888.
22. Rock GA, Shumack KH, Buskard NA, et al. Comparison of plasma exchange with plasma infusion in the treatment of thrombotic thrombocytopenia purpura. N Engl J Med 1991;325:393–397.
23. Hayward CP, Sutton DMC, Carter WH Jr, et al. Treatment outcomes in patients with adult thrombotic thrombocytopenic purpura-hemolytic uremic syndrome. Arch Intern Med 1994;154:982–987.
24. Reiner A, Kickler TS, Bell W. How to administer massive transfusions effectively. J Crit Illness 1987;2:15–24.
25. Heffner JE. What caused post-op thrombocytopenia in this 82 year-old man? J Crit Illness 1996;11:666–671.

ABNORMAL PLATELET FUNCTION

26. George JN, Shattil SJ. The clinical importance of acquired abnormalities of platelet function. N Engl J Med 1991;324:27–39.
27. Mohr R, Goor DA, Lusky A, Lavee J. Aprotinin prevents cardiopulmonary bypass-induced platelet dysfunction. Circulation 1992;86(Suppl II):405–409.
28. Lemmer JH Jr, Stanford W, Bonney SL, et al. Aprotinin for coronary bypass operations: efficacy, safety, and influence on early saphenous vein graft patency. J Thorac Cardiovasc Surg 1994;107:543–553.
29. Murkin JM, Lux J, Shannon NA, et al. Aprotinin significantly decreases bleeding and transfusion requirements in patients receiving aspirin and undergoing cardiac operations. J Thorac Cardiovasc Surg 1994;107:554–561.

PLATELET TRANSFUSIONS

30. Simon TL. Platelet transfusion therapy. In: Rossi EC, Simon TL, Moss GS, eds. Principles of transfusion medicine. Baltimore: Williams & Wilkins, 1991; 219–222.
31. Heddle NM, Klama L, Singer J, et al. The role of the plasma from platelet concentrates in transfusion reactions. N Engl J Med 1994;331:625–628.

section XII
NUTRITION AND METABOLISM

What is food to one man may be fierce poison to others.
Lucretius

chapter

46

NUTRIENT AND ENERGY REQUIREMENTS

The fundamental goal of nutritional support is to provide individual patients with their daily nutritional requirements. This chapter explains how to determine the nutrient and energy needs of each patient in the ICU (1–3).

OXIDATIVE ENERGY CONVERSION

OXIDATIVE COMBUSTION

According to the Laws of Thermodynamics, energy can neither be produced nor destroyed. Therefore, the only way to obtain energy is to transfer it from an energy source in nature. Natural substances that are rich in stored energy are called *fuels,* and the device that performs the energy transfer is called an *engine.* The process of energy transfer by two types of engines is illustrated in Figure 46.1. The automobile has a mechanical engine that mixes oxygen with a fossil fuel (e.g., gasoline) at high temperatures, and this releases the energy from the fuel that is then used to power the automobile. Likewise, the human body has a biochemical engine (metabolism) that mixes oxygen with an organic fuel (e.g., carbohydrates) at high temperatures, and this releases energy from the fuel that is then used to power the human body. The process that allows the energy to be released from a fuel is called oxidation, or the chemical reaction between oxygen and a fuel (see Chapter 3). If the oxidation reaction is conducted at high temperatures, the energy release from the fuel is more rapid. Such high-temperature oxidation reactions are called *combustion* reactions. Thus, both the automobile engine and oxidative metabolism are internal combustion engines that capture the energy stored in natural fuels.

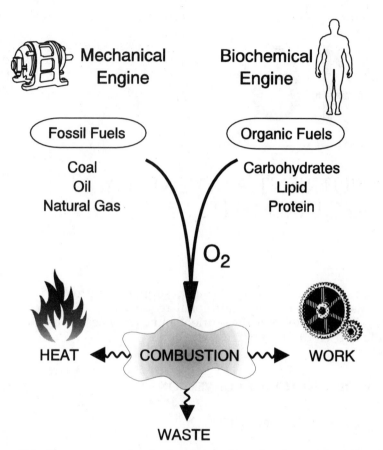

Figure 46.1. Energy conversion by two internal combustion engines. One engine is mechanical, and the other is biochemical.

ORGANIC FUELS

The three organic (carbon-based) fuels used by the human body are carbohydrates, proteins, and lipids. The energy yield from the combustion of these fuels is measured as heat production in kilocalories (kcal) per gram of substrate. The energy yield from the combustion of each of the organic fuels is shown in Table 46.1. The information in this table can be stated as follows:

Fuel	V_{O_2} (L/g)	V_{CO_2} (L/g)	RQ*	Energy Yield (kcal/g)
Lipid	2.00	1.40	0.70	9.1
Protein	0.96	0.78	0.80	4.0
Glucose	0.74	0.74	1.00	3.7

TABLE 46.1. THE OXIDATIVE METABOLISM OF ORGANIC FUELS

* Respiratory quotient: $RQ = V_{CO_2}/V_{O_2}$.

$$1 \text{ g Glucose} + 0.74 \text{ L of } O_2 \text{ yields } 0.74 \text{ L of } CO_2 + 3.75 \text{ kcal} \quad (46.1)$$

The summed metabolism of all three organic substrates determines the total-body O_2 consumption (V_{O_2}), CO_2 production (V_{CO_2}), and energy expenditure (EE) for any given period. The 24-hour EE then determines the daily calorie requirements that must be provided by nutrition support.

DAILY ENERGY EXPENDITURE

The daily energy expenditure of each individual patient can be estimated or measured.

PREDICTIVE EQUATIONS

In the early part of the twentieth century, the daily energy expenditure of a group of healthy adults (136 men and 103 women) was measured (4). The results of this study were expressed as regression equations for daily energy expenditure based on sex, body weight (in kilograms), and height (in inches). These equations are known as the Harris–Benedict equations (named after the principal investigators in the study), and they are shown in Table 46.2. The daily energy expenditure is expressed as the basal energy expenditure (BEE), which is the heat production of basal metabolism in the resting and fasted state. Because the body weight in the Harris–Benedict equations does not allow for changes in body weight caused by obesity or edema fluid, the ideal body weight should be used in these predictive equations.

Another more simplified predictive equation for the BEE is as follows:

$$\text{BEE (kcal/day)} = 25 \times \text{wt (in kg)} \quad (46.2)$$

TABLE 46.2. METHODS FOR DETERMINING DAILY ENERGY REQUIREMENTS

Predictive equations*:
  Men:
      BEE (kcal/24 hr) = 66 + (13.7 × wt) + (5.0 × ht) − (6.7 × Age)
  Women:
      BEE (kcal/24 hr) = 655 + (9.6 × wt) + (1.8 × ht) − (4.7 × Age)

  REE (kcal/24 hr) = BEE × 1.2
Indirect calorimetry†:
  REE (kcal/24 hr) = (3.9 × V_{O_2}) + (1.1 × V_{CO_2}) − 61

---

* BEE = Basal energy expenditure, Wt = ideal body weight in kg, Ht = height in inches, REE = resting energy expenditure (the BEE plus the thermal effect of food intake).
† V_{O_2} and V_{CO_2} are measured in mL/min but are extrapolated to L/24 hr. Equation taken from Reference 9.

This relationship has proven to be equivalent to the more complicated Harris–Benedict equations (5). Although it has not been tested rigorously, this simple relationship provides a "ballpark" estimate of BEE for determining nutritional needs.

Adjustments in BEE

To allow for the thermal effect of food intake, the BEE is multiplied by 1.2 to derive the resting energy expenditure (REE), which is the energy expenditure of basal metabolism in the resting but not fasted state. Other adjustments in the BEE that allow for enhanced energy expenditure in hypermetabolic conditions are shown below:

Fever: BEE × 1.1 (for each °C above the normal body temperature)
Mild stress: BEE × 1.2
Moderate stress: BEE × 1.4
Severe stress: BEE × 1.6

The actual adjustments for severe illness can vary widely in individual patients (6). Studies comparing predicted and actual energy expenditure in critically ill patients have shown that the predictive equations (with adjustments for degree of stress) overestimate daily energy needs by 20 to 60% (6–8). For this reason, measurements of energy expenditure are more accurate than predictive equations in patients in the ICU.

INDIRECT CALORIMETRY

Because it is impossible to measure metabolic heat production in clinical practice, the metabolic energy expenditure is measured indirectly by measuring the whole-body V_{O_2} and V_{CO_2}. This technique is called indirect calorimetry (2). The REE can be derived from the whole-body V_{O_2} and V_{CO_2} by using the equation shown in Table 46.2 (9). The original REE equation, which incorporated a measurement of the daily urinary nitrogen excretion, was proposed by the Scottish physiologist J. B. de V. Weir in 1949 (10). A number of adaptations of the original Weir equation have been proposed (11,12), but the REE equations used in the clinical setting do not include the urinary nitrogen excretion.

Method

Indirect calorimetry is performed with specialized instruments called metabolic carts that measure the exchange of O_2 and CO_2 across the lungs. These instruments can be placed at the bedside, and gas exchange measurements are obtained over 15 to 30 minutes. The V_{O_2} and V_{CO_2} are then extrapolated to a 24-hour period, and the 24-hour REE is calculated by using an equation similar to the one shown in Table 46.2.

Total Energy Expenditure

The REE obtained from indirect calorimetry is usually measured for 15 to 30 minutes, and then extrapolated to a 24-hour period. The total energy expenditure (TEE), measured over 24 hours, is equivalent to the extrapolated REE in patients who are not hypermetabolic (13), but the TEE can be as much as 40% higher than the extrapolated REE in hypermetabolic septic patients (13). Therefore, the REE measured over limited periods is not necessarily equivalent to the total daily energy expenditure in hypermetabolic patients in the ICU.

Limitations

Indirect calorimetry is the most accurate method for determining the daily energy requirements of individual patients in the ICU. However, several factors limit the popularity of indirect calorimetry in the clinical setting. First and foremost, the technique requires relatively expensive equipment and specially trained personnel, and it is not universally available. In addition, the oxygen sensor in most metabolic carts is not reliable at inspired oxygen levels above 50%, so indirect calorimetry can be unreliable in patients with respiratory failure who require inhaled oxygen concentrations above 50% (2). Because of all these limitations, daily caloric needs are often estimated using predictive formulas such as the Harris–Benedict equations, whereas indirect calorimetry (if available) is reserved for selected patients who require careful titration of daily energy intake (e.g., ventilator-dependent patients).

NONPROTEIN CALORIES

The daily energy requirement should be provided by calories derived from carbohydrates and lipids, and protein intake should be used to maintain the stores of essential enzymatic and structural proteins. The proportion of daily calories that is provided by lipids and carbohydrates is a matter of some debate, but no clear evidence shows one substrate to be superior to the other as a source of calories (2).

CARBOHYDRATES

Carbohydrates supply approximately 70% of the nonprotein calories in the average American diet. Because the human body has limited carbohydrate stores (Table 46.3), daily intake of carbohydrates is neces-

TABLE 46.3. ENDOGENOUS FUEL STORES IN HEALTHY ADULTS		
Fuel Source	**Amount (kg)**	**Energy Yield (kcal)**
Adipose tissue fat	15.0	141,000
Muscle protein	6.0	24,000
Total glycogen	0.09	900
		Total: 165,900
Data from Cahill GF Jr. N Engl J Med 1970;282:668–675.		

sary to ensure proper functioning of the central nervous system, which relies heavily on glucose as its principal fuel source. However, excessive intake of carbohydrates can prove detrimental for the following reasons.

1. Carbohydrates stimulate the release of insulin, and insulin inhibits the mobilization of free fatty acids from adipose tissue. Because adipose tissue fat is the major source of endogenous calories (Table 46.3), excessive carbohydrate intake impairs the ability of the body to rely on endogenous fat stores during periods of inadequate nutrition.
2. The oxidative metabolism of glucose produces an abundance of CO_2 relative to the oxygen consumed, as indicated by the respiratory quotients listed in Table 46.1. Furthermore, ingestion of excessive carbohydrates leads to de novo lipogenesis, which has a respiratory quotient of 8.0. Therefore, the ingestion of excessive carbohydrates can be accompanied by an exaggerated production of CO_2 (14), and this could promote hypercapnia in patients with compromised lung function. In fact, excessive calories from any nutrient source can be accompanied by excessive CO_2 production (15).

LIPIDS

Dietary lipids have the highest energy yield of the three organic fuels (Table 46.1), and lipid stores in adipose tissues represent the major endogenous fuel source in healthy adults (Table 46.3). Most nutritional regimens use exogenous lipids to provide approximately 30% of the daily energy needs.

Linoleic Acid

Dietary lipids are triglycerides, which are composed of a glycerol molecule linked to three fatty acids. The only dietary fatty acid that is considered essential (i.e., must be provided in the diet) is linoleic acid, a long chain, polyunsaturated fatty acid with 18 carbon atoms (16). A deficient intake of this essential fatty acid produces a clinical disorder characterized by a scaly dermopathy, cardiac dysfunction, and increased susceptibility to infections (16). This disorder is prevented by providing 0.5% of the dietary fatty acids as linoleic acid. Safflower oil is used as the source of linoleic acid in most nutritional support regimens.

PROTEIN REQUIREMENTS

The goal of protein intake is to match the rate of protein catabolism in the individual patient. Protein intake can be estimated by using the following generalized predictions for normal and hypercatabolic patients (17):

Condition	Daily Protein Intake
Normal metabolism	0.8 to 1.0 g/kg
Hypercatabolism	1.2 to 1.6 g/kg

The estimated protein intake in hypercatabolic patients is limited by the inability to determine the severity of protein catabolism. A more accurate assessment of daily protein requirements requires some measure of protein catabolism. This measure is the urinary excretion of nitrogen, as described below.

NITROGEN BALANCE

Two-thirds of the nitrogen derived from protein breakdown is excreted in the urine (17). Because protein is 16% nitrogen, each gram of urinary nitrogen (UN) represents 6.25 g of degraded protein. The total-body nitrogen (N) balance can therefore be determined as follows (18):

$$\text{N Balance (g)} = (\text{Protein intake (g)}/6.25) - (\text{UUN} + 4) \qquad (46.3)$$

where UUN is the urinary urea nitrogen excretion (in grams) in 24 hours, and the factor 4 represents the daily nitrogen loss (in grams) other than UUN. If the UUN is greater than 30 (g/24 hours), a factor of 6 is more appropriate for the daily nitrogen losses other than UUN (19). The goal of the nitrogen balance is to maintain a positive balance of 4 to 6 grams.

Total versus Urea Nitrogen

Under normal circumstances, approximately 85% of the nitrogen in the urine is contained in urea and the remainder is contained in ammonia and creatinine. However, in certain groups of patients in the ICU (e.g., postoperative patients), urea may contain less than 50% of the total nitrogen in the urine (20). Therefore, the UUN can underestimate urinary nitrogen losses in patients in the ICU. Measuring the urinary ammonia excretion in addition to the UUN will provide a more accurate assessment of the TUN in these patients (21). However, the clinical significance of this added measurement is unknown at present.

NITROGEN BALANCE AND CALORIC INTAKE

The first step in achieving a positive nitrogen balance is to **provide enough nonprotein calories to spare proteins from being degraded**

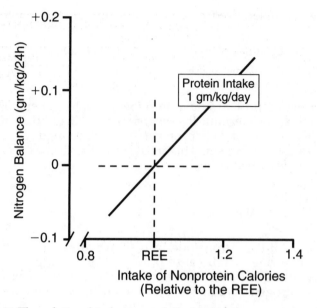

Figure 46.2. The relationship between daily intake of nonprotein calories (in relation to the resting energy expenditure) and the nitrogen balance at a constant protein intake. *REE* = Resting energy expenditure.

to provide energy. This is demonstrated in Figure 46.2, which shows the relationship between the intake of nonprotein calories and the nitrogen balance. When the daily protein intake is constant, the nitrogen balance becomes positive only when the intake of nonprotein calories is sufficient to meet the daily energy needs (i.e., the REE). If the nonprotein calorie intake is insufficient, some of the protein provided in the diet will be broken down to provide calories, which will produce a negative nitrogen balance. Therefore, when the daily intake of nonprotein calories is insufficient, increasing the protein intake becomes an inefficient method of achieving a positive nitrogen balance.

VITAMIN REQUIREMENTS

Twelve vitamins are considered an essential part of the daily diet. The recommended daily dose of individual vitamins in enteral and parenteral nutritional regimens is shown in Table 46.4 (2). It is important to emphasize that the daily vitamin requirements may be much higher than indicated in this table in seriously ill, hypermetabolic patients. In fact, deficiencies in several vitamins have been documented in hospitalized patients, despite the daily provision of vitamins in nutritional support regimens (22,23). The normal vitamin levels in blood are included in the section on Reference Ranges in the Appendix at the end of this text.

Although it is impossible to comment on the importance of each of

**TABLE 46.4. RECOMMENDED DAILY REQUIREMENTS
FOR VITAMINS**

Vitamin	Enteral Dose	Parenteral Dose
Vitamin A	1000 μg	3300 IU
Vitamin B_{12}	3 μg	5 μg
Vitamin C	60 mg	100 mg
Vitamin D	5 μg	200 IU
Vitamin E	10 mg	10 IU
Vitamin K*	100 μg	10 mg
Thiamine (B_1)*	2 mg	3 mg
Riboflavin (B_2)*	2 mg	4 mg
Pyridoxine (B_6)*	2 mg	4 mg
Pantothenic acid*	6 mg	15 mg
Biotin*	150 μg	60 μg
Folate	400 μg	400 μg

Adapted from Dark DS, Pingleton SK. Nutrition and nutritional support in critically ill patients. Intensive Care Med 1993;8:16–33. Doses for vitamins indicated by asterisks (*) are averaged or rounded off to the nearest whole number.

the vitamins in ICU patients, the following comments on thiamine and the antioxidant vitamins are deserved.

THIAMINE

Thiamine (vitamin B_1) is a component of thiamine pyrophosphate, an essential cofactor in carbohydrate metabolism. Thiamine deficiency is likely to be common in patients in the ICU for the following reasons. First, the normal body content of thiamine is only approximately 30 mg (24), so assuming a daily thiamine requirement of 3 mg in patients in the ICU (Table 46.4), lack of thiamine intake could result in depletion of endogenous thiamine stores after just 10 days. Second, the use of thiamine is increased beyond expected levels in hypercatabolic conditions (25) and may also be increased in patients receiving nutritional support with glucose-rich formulas. Third, urinary thiamine excretion is increased by furosemide (26), which is a commonly used diuretic in the ICU. Finally, magnesium is necessary for the conversion of thiamine into thiamine pyrophosphate, so magnesium depletion (which is common in patients in the ICU) causes a "functional" form of thiamine deficiency (27).

Clinical Features

Four clinical disorders are associated with thiamine deficiency (24,28–30): (*a*) cardiac dysfunction (beriberi heart disease), (*b*) a metabolic (Wernicke's) encephalopathy, (*c*) lactic acidosis (see Fig. 37.1), and (*d*) a peripheral neuropathy. Similar disorders, such as cardiac dysfunction and metabolic encephalopathy, are common in patients

TABLE 46.5. LABORATORY EVALUATION OF THIAMINE STATUS	
Plasma thiamine levels:	
Thiamine fraction	Normal range
Total	3.4–4.8 μg/dL
Free	0.8–1.1 μg/dL
Phosphorylated	2.6–3.7 μg/dL
Erythrocyte transketolase activity:	
Enzyme activity measured in response to the addition of thiamine pyrophosphate (TPP).	
Increased activity after TPP	Interpretation
Less than 20%	Normal
Greater than 25%	Thiamine deficiency

Plasma thiamine levels taken from Reference 29. Erythrocyte transketolase activities taken from Reference 31.

in the ICU, and thiamine deficiency should be considered in each case in which one of these disorders is unexplained.

Diagnosis

The laboratory evaluation of thiamine status is shown in Table 46.5. Although plasma levels of thiamine can be useful in detecting thiamine depletion, the most reliable assay of functional intracellular thiamine stores is the erythrocyte transketolase assay (31). This assay measures the activity of a thiamine pyrophosphate–dependent (transketolase) enzyme in the patient's red blood cells in response to the addition of thiamine pyrophosphate (TPP). An increase in enzyme activity of greater than 25% after the addition of TPP indicates a functional thiamine deficiency. I use the plasma thiamine levels to screen for thiamine depletion and reserve the transketolase assay for determining the endpoint of thiamine repletion in patients with documented thiamine deficiency.

ANTIOXIDANT VITAMINS

Two vitamins serve as important endogenous antioxidants: vitamin C and vitamin E. Both of these antioxidant vitamins are described in Chapter 3 (see Table 3.1), and they will not be described further here. Considering the important role that oxidation-induced cell injury may have in multiorgan damage in serious illnesses (see Table 3.2), it is wise to maintain adequate body stores of the antioxidant vitamins in critically ill patients. The increased rates of biological oxidation that are common in critical illness are likely to increase the daily requirements for vitamin C and vitamin E far above those listed in Table 46.4. Therefore, it is important to monitor vitamin C and vitamin E status carefully in seriously ill patients in the ICU (see the Appendix for the normal plasma levels of vitamins C and E).

ESSENTIAL TRACE ELEMENTS

A trace element is a substance that is present in the body in amounts less than 50 μg per gram of body tissue (32). Seven trace elements are considered essential in humans (i.e., associated with a deficiency syndrome), and these are listed in Table 46.6 along with their recommended daily maintenance doses (2). As with the vitamin requirements, the trace element requirements in Table 46.6 are for healthy adults; the requirements in hypermetabolic patients in the ICU may be far greater.

The following trace elements are mentioned because of their relevance to oxidation-induced cell injury.

IRON

One of the interesting features of iron in the human body is how little is allowed to remain as free, unbound iron. The normal adult has approximately 4.5 g of iron, yet there is virtually no free iron in plasma (33). Most of the iron is bound to hemoglobin, and the remainder is bound to ferritin in tissues and transferrin in plasma. Furthermore, the transferrin in plasma is only approximately 30% saturated with iron, so any increase in plasma iron will be quickly bound by transferrin, thus preventing any rise in plasma free iron.

Iron and Oxidation Injury

One reason why the body may be so concerned with binding iron is the ability of free iron to promote oxidation-induced cell injury (see References 27 and 28 in Chapter 3). As described in Chapter 3, iron in the reduced state (Fe-II) promotes the formation of hydroxyl radicals (see Figure 3.1), and hydroxyl radicals are considered the most reactive oxidants known in biochemistry. In this context, the ability to bind and sequester iron has been called the major antioxidant function of

TABLE 46.6. DAILY REQUIREMENTS FOR ESSENTIAL TRACE ELEMENTS		
Trace Element	Enteral Dose	Parenteral Dose
Chromium	200 μg	15 μg
Copper	3 mg	1.5 mg
Iodine	150 μg	150 μg
Iron	10 mg	2.5 mg
Manganese	5 mg	100 μg
Selenium	200 μg	70 μg
Zinc	15 mg	4 mg

Doses represent the maximum daily maintenance doses for each trace element. From Dark DS, Pingleton SK. Nutrition and nutritional support in critically ill patients. Intensive Care Med 1993;8:16–33.

plasma (see Reference 28, Chapter 3). This might explain why hypoferremia is a common occurrence in patients who have conditions associated with hypermetabolism (34) (because this would limit the destructive effects of hypermetabolism.)

In light of this description of iron, **a reduced serum iron level in a critically ill patient should not prompt iron replacement therapy** unless there is evidence of total-body iron deficiency. This latter condition can be detected with a plasma ferritin level; that is, a plasma ferritin below 18 μg/L indicates probable iron deficiency, whereas a plasma ferritin above 100 μg/L means that iron deficiency is unlikely (35).

SELENIUM

Selenium is an endogenous antioxidant by virtue of its role as a cofactor for glutathione peroxidase, one of important endogenous antioxidant enzymes (see Table 3.1). Selenium use is increased in acute illness, and plasma selenium levels can fall to subnormal levels within 1 week after the onset of acute illness (36). Since selenium supplementation is not routinely included in parenteral nutrition support regimens, prolonged parenteral nutrition is accompanied by selenium deficiency (37). The combination of increased selenium use and lack of daily selenium supplementation may make selenium deficiency common in patients in the ICU. Such a condition will promote oxidant cell injury.

The assessment of selenium status is described in Chapter 3. The minimum daily requirement for selenium is 55 μg for women and 70 μg for men (38). This requirement is likely to be much higher in hypermetabolic patients in the ICU. The maximum daily dose of selenium that is considered safe is 200 μg, and this dose is probably more appropriate for ICU patients.

FOOD FOR THOUGHT

Before leaving this chapter, it is important to point out that there is a fundamental problem with the practice of promoting nutrient intake in critically ill patients. This problem relates to the fate of administered nutrients in seriously ill patients.

Abnormal Nutrient Processing

The goal of nutrient intake in the malnourished patient is to correct the malnourished state. However, the malnutrition that accompanies critical illness is different from the malnutrition that accompanies starvation, and this difference has important implications for the value of nutrient intake in each situation. The malnutrition from starvation is due to deficits in the body stores of essential nutrients, and thus nutrient intake will correct this type of malnutrition. However, the malnutrition that accompanies serious illnesses is due to disease-induced abnormal nutrient processing, and thus nutrient intake will not correct this type of malnutrition as long as the underlying disease is active. In other words, the important factor in correcting the malnutrition from critical illness is not the intake of nutrients, but a decrease in the activity of the underlying disease process (39). In fact, in the setting of abnormal nutrient processing, nutrient intake can be used to generate metabolic toxins. This is demonstrated below.

Nutrient Toxicity

In healthy subjects, less than 5% of exogenously administered glucose is metabolized to form lactate. However, in acutely ill patients, up to 85% of an exogenous glucose load can be recovered as lactate (40). The graph in Figure 46.3 demonstrates the ability of exogenous glucose to generate lactic acid in acutely stressed patients undergoing major surgery (41). In this case, patients undergoing abdominal aneurysm surgery were given intraoperative fluid therapy with either Ringer's solutions or 5% dextrose solutions. In the patients who received the 5% dextrose solution (total amount of dextrose infused averaged

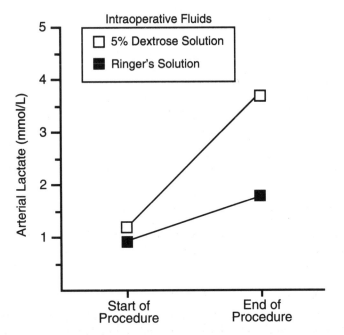

Figure 46.3. Effect of carbohydrate infusion on arterial lactate levels during abdominal aortic surgery. Each point represents a mean lactate level for 10 patients receiving Ringer's solution (closed squares) and 10 patients receiving 5% dextrose solution (open squares) for intraoperative fluid management. Total volume infused is equivalent with both fluids. (Data from Reference 41.)

200 g), the blood lactate increased by 3 mmol/L, whereas in the patients who received an equivalent volume of the glucose-free (Ringer's) solution, the blood lactate level increased only 1 mmol/L. Thus an organic nutrient (carbohydrate) can be used to generate a metabolic toxin (lactic acid) when nutrient processing is abnormal (during the stress of abdominal aneurysm surgery).

The study in Figure 46.3 illustrates that nutrient intake can have very different consequences in different subjects, and that *nutrients can become toxins* in the diseased host. Lucretius realized this more than 2000 years ago when he stated, "What is food to one man may be fierce poison to others." For this reason, one should not immediately jump on the bandwagon for aggressive nutritional support in critically ill patients.

REFERENCES

REVIEWS

1. Mandt JM, Teasley-Strausberg KM, Shronts EP. Nutritional requirements. In: Teasley-Strausberg KM, ed. Nutrition support handbook. Cincinnati, OH: Harvey-Whitney Books, 1992;19–36 (61 references).
2. McClave SA, Snider HL. Use of indirect calorimetry in clinical nutrition. Nutr Clin Pract 1992;7:207–221 (83 references).
3. Dark DS, Pingleton SK. Nutrition and nutritional support in critically ill patients. J Intensive Care Med 1993;8:16–33 (163 references).

DAILY ENERGY EXPENDITURE

4. Harris JA, Benedict FG. A biometric study of basal metabolism in man. Washington, DC: Carnegie Institute of Washington, Publication 279, 1919.
5. Paauw JD, McCamish MA, Dean RE, Ouelette TR. Assessment of caloric needs in stressed patients. J Am Coll Nutr 1984;3:51–59.
6. Mann S, Westenskow DR, Houtchens BA. Measured and predicted caloric expenditure in the acutely ill. Crit Care Med 1985;13:173–177.
7. Weissman C, Kemper M, Askanazi J, et al. Resting metabolic rate of the critically ill patient: measured versus predicted. Anesthesiology 1986;64:673–679.
8. Makk LJK, McClave SA, Creech PW. Clinical application of the metabolic cart to the delivery of total parenteral nutrition. Crit Care Med 1990;18:1320–1327.
9. Burzstein S, Saphar P, Singer P, Elwyn DH. A mathematical analysis of indirect calorimetry measurements in critically ill patients. Am J Clin Nutr 1989;50: 227–230.
10. Weir JB de V. New methods for calculating metabolic rate with special reference to protein metabolism. J Physiol 1949;109:1–9.
11. Westenskow DR, Schipke CA, Raymond JL, et al. Calculation of metabolic expenditure and substrate utilization from gas exchange measurements. J Parent Ent Nutr 1988;12:20–24.
12. Cunningham JJ. Calculation of energy expenditure from indirect calorimetry: assessment of the Weir equation. Nutrition 1990;6:222–223.
13. Koea JB, Wolfe RR, Shaw JHF. Total energy expenditure during total paren-

teral nutrition: ambulatory patients at home versus patients with sepsis in surgical intensive care. Surgery 1995;118:54–62.

NONPROTEIN CALORIES

14. Rodriguez JL, Askanazi J, Weismann C, et al. Ventilatory and metabolic effects of glucose infusions. Chest 1985;88:512–518.
15. Talpers SS, Romberger DJ, Bunce SB, Pingleton SK. Nutritionally associated increased CO_2 production. Chest 1992;102:551–555.
16. Linscheer WG, Vergroesen AJ. Lipids. In: Shils ME, Olson JA, Shike M, eds. Modern nutrition in health and disease. 8th ed. Philadelphia: Lea & Febiger, 1994;47–88.

PROTEIN REQUIREMENTS

17. Crim MC, Munro HN. Proteins and amino acids. In: Shils ME, Olson JA, Shike M, eds. Modern nutrition in health and disease. 8th ed. Philadelphia: Lea & Febiger, 1994;3–35.
18. Blackburn G, Bistrian B, Maini B, et al. Nutritional and metabolic assessment of the hospitalized patient. J Parent Ent Nutr 1977;1:11–22.
19. Velasco N, Long CL, Otto DA, et al. Comparison of three methods for the estimation of total nitrogen losses in hospitalized patients. J Parent Ent Nutr 1990;14:517–522.
20. Konstantinides F, Konstantinides N, Li J, et al. Urinary urea nitrogen: too insensitive for calculating nitrogen balance studies in surgical clinical nutrition. J Parent Ent Nutr 1991;15:189–193.
21. Burge JC, Choban P, McKnight T, et al. Urinary ammonia excretion as an estimate of total urinary nitrogen in patients receiving parenteral nutritional support. J Parent Ent Nutr 1993;17:529–531.

VITAMIN REQUIREMENTS

22. Dempsey DT, Mullen JL, Rombeau JL, et al. Treatment effects of parenteral vitamins in total parenteral nutrition patients. J Parent Ent Nutr 1987;11: 229–237.
23. Beard M, Hatipov C, Hamer J. Acute onset of folate deficiency in patients under intensive care. Crit Care Med 1980;8:500–503.
24. Tanphaichitr V. Thiamine. In: Shils MER, Olson JA, Sike M, eds. Modern nutrition in health and disease. 8th ed. Philadelphia: Lea & Febiger, 1994; 359–365.
25. McConachie I, Haskew A. Thiamine status after major trauma. Intensive Care Med 1988;14:628–631.
26. Seligmann H, Halkin H, Rauchfleisch S, et al. Thiamine deficiency in patients with congestive heart failure receiving long-term furosemide therapy: a pilot study. Am J Med 1991;91:151–155.
27. Dyckner T, Ek B, Nyhlin H, Wester PO. Aggravation of thiamine deficiency by magnesium depletion. Acta Med Scand 1985;218:129–131.
28. Tan GH, Farnell GF, Hemsrud DD, Litin SC. Acute Wernicke's encephalopathy attributable to pure dietary thiamine deficiency. Mayo Clin Proc 1994;69: 849–850.

29. Oriot D, Wood C, Gottesman R, Huault G. Severe lactic acidosis related to acute thiamine deficiency. J Parent Ent Nutr 1991;15:105–109.
30. Skelton WP, Skelton NK. Thiamine deficiency neuropathy: it's still common today. Postgrad Med 1989;85:301–306.
31. Boni L, Kieckens L, Hendrikx A. An evaluation of modified erythrocyte transketolase assay for assessing thiamine nutritional adequacy. J Nutr Sci Vitaminol 1980;26:507–514.

ESSENTIAL TRACE ELEMENTS

32. Fleming CR. Trace element metabolism in adult patients requiring total parenteral nutrition. Am J Clin Nutr 1989;49:573–579.
33. Halliwell B, Gutteridge JMC. Free radicals in biology and medicine. 2nd ed. Oxford: Clarendon Press, 1989;34–38.
34. Shanbogue LKR, Paterson N. Effect of sepsis and surgery on trace minerals. J Parent Ent Nutr 1990;14:287–289.
35. Guyatt GH, Patterson C, Ali M, et al. Diagnosis of iron deficiency anemia in the elderly. Am J Med 1990;88:205–209.
36. Hawker FH, Stewart PM, Switch PJ. Effects of acute illness on selenium homeostasis. Crit Care Med 1990;18:442–446.
37. Sando K, Hoki M, Nezu R, et al. Platelet glutathione peroxidase activity in long-term total parenteral nutrition with and without selenium supplementation. J Parent Ent Nutr 1992;16:54–68.
38. Food and Nutrition Board, National Research Council. Recommended dietary allowances. 10th ed. Washington, DC: National Academy Press, 1989;217–223.

FOOD FOR THOUGHT

39. Marino PL, Finnegan MJ. Nutrition support is not beneficial, and can be harmful, in critically ill patients. Crit Care Clin 1996;12:667–676.
40. Gunther B, Jauch K-W, Hartl W, et al. Low-dose glucose infusion in patients who have undergone surgery. Arch Surg 1987;122:765–771.
41. Degoute C-S, Ray M-J, Manchon M, et al. Intraoperative glucose infusion and blood lactate: endocrine and metabolic relationships during abdominal aortic surgery. Anesthesiology 1989;71:355–361.

SUGGESTED READINGS

Burzstein S, Elwyn DH, Askanazi J, Kinney JM, eds. Energy metabolism, indirect calorimetry, and nutrition. Baltimore: Williams & Wilkins, 1989.
Food and Nutrition Board, National Research Council. Recommended dietary allowances. 10th ed. Washington, DC: National Academy Press, 1989.
Shils ME, Olson JA, Shike M, eds. Modern nutrition in health and disease. 8th ed. Philadelphia: Lea & Febiger, 1994.

47

ENTERAL NUTRITION

One of the important features of the gastrointestinal (GI) tract (as described in Chapters 6 and 33) is the role of the intestinal epithelium as a barrier to invasion by pathogenic microorganisms. As discussed in this chapter, the barrier function of the bowel mucosa is maintained by the intake and processing of bulk nutrients along the digestive tract. Therefore, providing nutrients via the enteral route not only provides nutritional support for the vital organs, but also supports host defenses against invasive infection (1–3).

TROPHIC EFFECT OF ENTERAL NUTRIENTS

Complete bowel rest is accompanied by progressive atrophy and disruption of the intestinal mucosa. This effect becomes evident after just a few days and is not prevented by parenteral (intravenous) nutrition. The influence of luminal nutrients on the morphology of the intestinal mucosa is shown in Figure 47.1 (4). The photomicrograph at the top shows the normal appearance of the small bowel mucosa. Note the fingerlike projections (microvilli), which serve to increase the surface area for nutrient absorption. The photomicrograph at the bottom shows the mucosal changes after 1 week of a protein-deficient diet. Note the shortening of the microvillus on the left of the picture and the generalized disruption of the surface architecture. This demonstrates that **depletion of nutrients in the bowel lumen is accompanied by degenerative changes in the bowel mucosa.**

Observations like those in Figure 47.1 indicate that the bowel mucosa relies on nutrients in the bowel lumen to provide its nutritional needs. One of the nutrients that may play an important role in this process is the amino acid glutamine, which is considered the principal metabolic fuel for intestinal epithelial cells (5). The use of glutamine in enteral feedings is discussed later in this chapter.

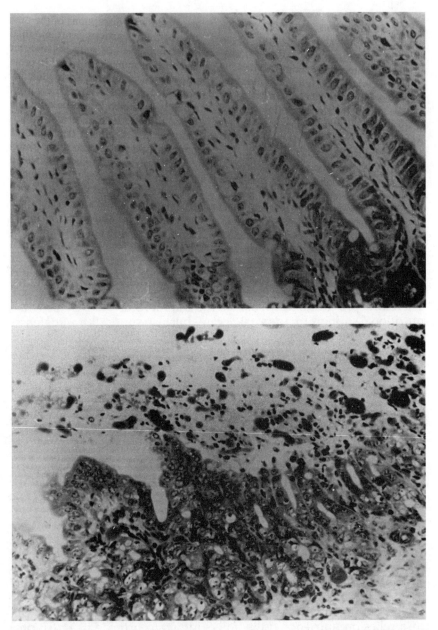

Figure 47.1. Photomicrographs showing the normal appearance of the small bowel mucosa (*upper*), and the mucosal changes after 1 week of a protein-deficient diet (*lower*). (Reprinted with permission from Deitch EA et al. Ann Surg 1987;205:681–690.)

TRANSLOCATION

The process of translocation, where enteric pathogens move across the bowel mucosa and into the systemic circulation, is described in Chapter 6 (see Figure 6.1). Translocation has been documented during periods of bowel rest in critically ill patients (6), and this has been attributed to mucosal disruption from lack of luminal nutrients. This means that enteral nutrition could help prevent translocation and subsequent sepsis by maintaining the functional integrity of the bowel mucosa. The potential for enteral nutrition to prevent sepsis of bowel origin is one of the major reasons why enteral nutrition has become favored over parenteral (intravenous) nutrition in critically ill patients.

PATIENT SELECTION

In the absence of contraindications, enteral tube feedings are indicated when nutrient intake has been inadequate for more than 5 days. In patients who are at risk of bacterial translocation across the bowel (e.g., burn victims), tube feedings should be started as soon as possible after the onset of inadequate nutrient intake (1,2).

CONTRAINDICATIONS

Enteral feedings in any amount are contraindicated in patients with circulatory shock, intestinal ischemia, complete mechanical bowel obstruction, or ileus.

Total enteral nutrition is not advised in patients with the following conditions: partial mechanical bowel obstruction, severe or unrelenting diarrhea, pancreatitis, or high-volume (more than 500 mL daily) enterocutaneous fistulas. Partial (low volume) enteral support is, however, possible in these conditions (1). In the case of pancreatitis, enteral feedings can be delivered into the jejunum (see "Jejunostomy Feedings").

FEEDING TUBES

Standard nasogastric tubes (14 to 16 French) are no longer favored for enteral tube feedings because of patient discomfort. Although there has been concern about gastroesophageal reflux with these tubes, clinical studies do not support this concern (7). The feeding tubes that are currently favored are narrower (8 to 10 French) and more flexible than standard nasogastric tubes (8). Because these tubes are so flexible, a rigid stylet is also provided to facilitate insertion.

INSERTION

Feeding tubes are inserted through the nares and advanced into the stomach or duodenum. The distance that the tube must be advanced

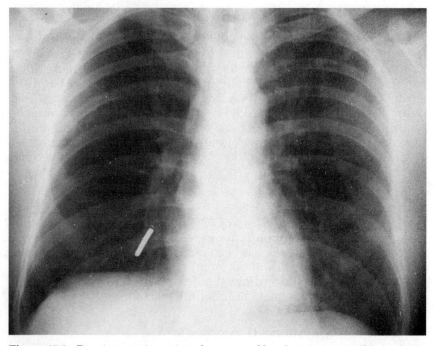

Figure 47.2. Routine postinsertion chest x-ray film showing a small-bore feeding tube in the lower lobe of the right lung.

to reach the stomach can be estimated by measuring the distance from the tip of the nose to the earlobe and then to the xiphoid process (9).

Proper placement in the stomach is sometimes possible to determine by measuring the pH (with litmus paper) of a specimen aspirated from the tip of the feeding tube (10). If the specimen has a pH less than 5, the tip of the tube is likely to be in the stomach. Feeding tubes that are equipped with a pH sensor (GrapHprobe, FT Zinetics Corp., Salt Lake City, Utah) are also available. Remember that pH testing will be unreliable in patients receiving histamine H_2-blockers.

TRACHEAL INTUBATION

The principal complication of feeding tube placement is accidental tracheal intubation (8). Because feeding tubes are narrow, they readily pass through the larynx and around the inflated cuffs on tracheal tubes. Accidental **intubation of the trachea is often asymptomatic** (probably because of sedation, depressed consciousness, or an abnormal cough reflex), and in the absence of symptoms, tubes can be advanced into the distal airways. This is illustrated in Figure 47.2, which shows the tip of a small-bore feeding tube in the lower lobe of the right lung. If feeding tubes are advanced too far into the lungs, the rigid stylet makes it easy to puncture the visceral pleura and produce a pneumothorax (8).

Because of the risk of asymptomatic intubation of the lungs, a postinsertion chest x-ray study is often required to evaluate tube placement (unless pH testing confirms gastric placement). **Auscultation of the upper abdomen** while insufflating air through the tube **is not a reliable method for excluding tube malposition in the lungs** because sounds emanating from a tube in the lower airways can be transmitted into the upper abdomen (8).

DUODENAL PLACEMENT

For those who prefer tube feedings placed in the duodenum instead of the stomach, gastric tubes must be advanced past the pylorus and into the duodenum. This can sometimes be accomplished by specialized maneuvers at the bedside (see Reference 11) or may require fluoroscopic guidance. Tube passage into the duodenum can be confirmed by an increase in the pH of feeding tube aspirates to above 6.0 (7), or by radiographic localization.

Feeding Site

The proposed advantage of duodenal feedings is a reduced risk of reflux of feeding solution into the esophagus and subsequent pulmonary aspiration. However, clinical studies show that **the risk of aspiration in duodenal feedings is the same as that in gastric feedings** (3,12). Therefore, the time and effort devoted to advancing gastric tubes into the duodenum is not justified.

FEEDING FORMULAS

More than 80 liquid feeding formulas are available for enteral nutrition (13). The formulas that are most commonly used are described in Tables 47.1 through 47.5.

TABLE 47.1. CHARACTERISTICS OF SELECTED ENTERAL FEEDING FORMULAS				
Formula	Caloric Density (kcal/mL)	Protein (g/L)	Osmolarity (mOsm/L)	Volume to Meet US RDA*
Isocal	1.1	34	270	1890
Isocal HN	1.1	44	270	1180
Enrich	1.1	40	480	1390
Ensure	1.1	37	470	1890
Osmolite	1.1	37	300	1890
Osmolite HN	1.1	44	300	1320
Travasorb	1.0	35	450	1896
Ultracal	1.1	37	500	1180
Vivonex TEN	1.0	38	630	2000
Vital HN	1.0	42	500	1500
*Indicates the volume needed to provide 100% of the recommended daily allowances (RDAs) for vitamins and essential trace elements.				

TABLE 47.2. ENTERAL FORMULAS WITH A HIGH CALORIC DENSITY

Formula	Caloric Density (kcal/mL)	Osmolarity (mOsm/L)	Volume to Meet US RDA
Ensure Plus	1.5	690	1420
Deliver 2.0	2.0	640	1000
Isocal HCN	2.0	640	1000
Magnacal	2.0	590	1000
TwoCal HN	2.0	950	950

TABLE 47.3. FEEDING FORMULAS WITH AN ALTERED LIPID COMPOSITION

Formula	Feature	Proposed Benefit
Pulmocare (Ross)	High lipid content. Lipids provide 55% of the calories in the formula.	Limits nutrition-induced CO_2 retention in respiratory failure.
Impact (Sandoz)	Contains arginine, RNA, and fatty acids derived from marine oils.	Enhances immune function and limits inflammatory-mediated tissue injury.
Perative (Ross)	Contains beta-carotene and fatty acids derived from marine oils.	Limits inflammatory-mediated tissue injury.

TABLE 47.4. GLUTAMINE-ENRICHED FEEDING FORMULAS

Formula	Manufacturer	Glutamine (g/1000 kcal)
AlitraQ	Ross	12.7
Reabilan HN	O'Brien/KMI	7.0
Reabilan	O'Brien/KMI	5.0
Replete	Clintec	5.0
Vivonex TEN	Norwich Eaton	4.9
Isotein HN	Sandoz	4.5
Isocal HCN	Mead Johnson	3.6
Osmolite HN	Ross	3.2
Peptamen	Clintec	3.0
Ensure	Ross	2.7
Criticare HN	Mead Johnson	1.7

Data on AlitraQ from the manufacturer. Other data from Shronts EP, Havala T. Enteral formulas. In: Teasley-Strausberg KM et al, eds. Nutrition support handbook. Cincinnatti, OH: Harvey Whitney Books, 1992;175.

TABLE 47.5. FIBER-ENRICHED ENTERAL FEEDING FORMULAS			
Formula	Fiber (g/L)	Formula	Fiber (g/L)
Enrich	14.3	Jevity	14.3
Entera with Fiber	14.0	Nutrition Isofiber	14.3
Fibersource	10.0	Nutren 1.0 w/Fiber	14.0
Fibersource HN	6.8	Profiber	12.0
Glucerna	14.3	Ultracal	14.1

The following is a brief description of some of the features of enteral feeding formulas.

CALORIC DENSITY

The caloric density of feeding formulas is determined primarily by the carbohydrate content. Most formulas provide 1 to 2 kilocalories per liter of solution. The formulas that provide 1 to 1.5 kcal/L (standard caloric density) are listed in Table 47.1, and the formulas that provide 1.5 to 2 kcal/L (high caloric density) are listed in Table 47.2. The energy-rich formulas in Table 47.2 are well-suited for patients with excessive daily energy needs and for patients who are volume-restricted.

OSMOLALITY

The osmolality of liquid feeding formulas varies from 280 to 1100 mOsm/kg H_2O. The major determinant of osmolality is the carbohydrate content (because this is the most abundant nutrient in most feeding formulas). Because carbohydrates also determine caloric density, osmolality and caloric density are directly related. Formulas with the lowest caloric density (1 kcal/L) have the lowest osmolalities (approximately 300 mOsm/kg H_2O) and are usually isotonic to the body fluids. Formulas with the highest caloric density (2 kcal/L) have the highest osmolalities (1000 mOsm/kg H_2O) and are markedly hypertonic to the body fluids.

Hypertonic formulas should be infused into the stomach to take advantage of the dilutional effects of the gastric secretions.

PROTEIN

Liquid feeding formulas provide 35 to 40 grams of protein per liter. Although some formulas are designated as being protein-rich (these formulas often have the suffix HN to indicate "high nitrogen"), they provide only 20% more protein than the standard feeding formulas.

Protein Complexity

Most enteral formulas provide intact proteins that are broken down into amino acids in the upper GI tract. Because small peptides are absorbed more rapidly than amino acids, some feeding formulas contain small peptides instead of intact protein to facilitate absorption. Peptide-based formulas such as Peptamen (Clintec) and Vital HN (Ross) can be used in patients with impaired intestinal absorption (e.g., from inflammatory bowel disease). These formulas also promote water reabsorption from the bowel (13), and thus they could prove beneficial in patients with severe or unrelenting diarrhea.

LIPIDS

The lipid emulsions used in feeding formulas are rich in long-chain triglycerides derived from vegetable oils. These lipids represent a concentrated source of calories, with an energy yield (9 kcal/g) that is almost three times that of carbohydrates (3.4 kcal/g). Because excessive fat ingestion is not well tolerated (i.e., it promotes diarrhea), the lipid content of most feeding formulas is limited to 30% of the total calories. Some formulas with an altered lipid composition are described in the following sections. These formulas are summarized in Table 47.3.

Lipid-Rich Formula

One liquid feeding formula with a high fat content is Pulmocare (Ross), which uses lipids to provide 55% of the total calories. This formula is intended for patients with respiratory failure. The proposed benefit is based on the low rate of CO_2 production relative to O_2 consumption associated with lipid metabolism (see Table 46.1). Thus when lipids replace carbohydrates as the principal nutrient substrate, metabolic CO_2 production will decline and there will be less of a tendency for CO_2 retention in patients with compromised lung function (14).

Alternative Lipids

The two feeding formulas described in Table 47.3 contain dietary fat from sources other than vegetable oils. Polyunsaturated fatty acids from vegetable oils can serve as precursors for inflammatory mediators (eicosanoids) that are capable of producing widespread cell injury (15). Fatty acids derived from alternative sources such as marine oils (e.g., fish oil) do not promote the production of harmful inflammatory mediators, and thus they might be preferred to the standard dietary fats to limit the risk of inflammatory-mediated tissue injury.

Two feeding formulas contain fatty acids from marine oils, and both are included in Table 47.3. Impact (Sandoz Nutrition) also contains arginine, which promotes immunocompetence (16), and Perative (Ross

Labs) has beta-carotene, a vitamin A analogue that can have antioxidant activity. Both formulas are intended for patients with systemic inflammation who are at risk for inflammatory-mediated tissue injury. Impact is also supposed to improve immune function.

ADDITIVES

GLUTAMINE

As mentioned earlier, **glutamine is the principal fuel for the bowel mucosa** (5). Therefore, daily supplementation with glutamine seems a reasonable measure for maintaining the functional integrity of the bowel mucosa. Although glutamine is not an essential amino acid (because it is produced in skeletal muscle), tissue glutamine stores decline precipitously in acute, hypercatabolic states. Therefore, glutamine can become an essential nutrient in the hypermetabolic, stressed patient (17).

Glutamine Enriched Formulas

Because glutamine is a natural constituent of proteins, all feeding formulas that contain intact protein will also contain glutamine (18). However, little of this glutamine is in the free or unbound form. The formulas that contain glutamine as a free amino acid are listed in Table 47.4. With the exception of AlitraQ (Ross Laboratories), the glutamine content of enteral feeding formulas is low and may be insufficient to provide a benefit (19,20). In one study of glutamine administration in healthy adults (20), the average glutamine dosage (oral and intravenous) was 0.35 g/kg/day, or 24.5 g/day for a 70-kg subject. Assuming a daily caloric intake of 2000 kcal, the only feeding formula in Table 47.4 that will provide a glutamine dosage of 0.35 g/kg/day is AlitraQ. In the setting of hypercatabolism, the glutamine provided by most enteral formulas will be even more inadequate. Therefore, although the use of glutamine-fortified enteral formulas seems reasonable, the amount of glutamine provided by most formulas may be inadequate.

DIETARY FIBER

The term *fiber* refers to a group of plant products that are not degradable by human digestive enzymes. These products are classified by their fermentative properties.

> **Fermentable fiber** (cellulose, pectin, gums) is degraded by intestinal bacteria to form short-chain fatty acids (e.g., acetate), which are used as an energy substrate by the large bowel mucosa. This type of fiber can slow gastric emptying and bind bile salts, and both of these actions can help alleviate diarrhea.
> **Nonfermentable fiber** (lignins) is not degraded by intestinal bac-

teria, but it can create an osmotic force that adsorbs water from the bowel lumen. This type of fiber can therefore reduce the tendency for watery diarrhea.

Thus fiber has several actions that can reduce the tendency for diarrhea during enteral feedings. Furthermore, fermentable fiber can serve as a source of metabolic support for the mucosa of the large bowel (21). This latter effect could play an important role in limiting the tendency for translocation across a disrupted large bowel mucosa.

Several feeding formulas contain fiber, and they are shown in Table 47.5. The added fiber in all cases is soy polysaccharide, which is a fermentable fiber. Thus there is little difference between the fiber enriched formulas, either in type or in content of fiber. Fiber enhanced feedings can also be achieved by adding Metamucil (nonfermentable fiber) or Kaopectate (fermentable fiber) to the feeding regimen.

Performance

The effects of fiber enriched feedings on the incidence of diarrhea have been inconsistent, with some studies showing a reduced incidence of diarrhea (22), and others showing no effect (23). However, relying on fiber to prevent diarrhea neglects the source of the diarrhea; the focus of prevention should be to eliminate or treat the process responsible for the diarrhea.

MISCELLANEOUS

Branched Chain Amino Acids

The branched chain amino acids (BCAAs) isoleucine, leucine, and valine are available in feeding formulas intended for trauma victims and patients with hepatic encephalopathy. In trauma victims, the BCAAs can be used as a fuel source in skeletal muscle, thereby sparing the degradation of other muscle proteins to provide energy. In hepatic encephalopathy, the BCAAs can antagonize the uptake of aromatic amino acids (e.g., tryptophan) into the central nervous system, and this helps prevent the subsequent breakdown of the aromatic amino acids to form false neurotransmitters, which have been implicated in the pathogenesis of hepatic encephalopathy (24).

Examples of feeding formulas enriched with BCAAs include Traum-Aid (McGaw) and Stresstein (Sandoz) for trauma victims, and Hepatic-Aid II (McGaw) and Travasorb Hepatic (Clintec) for hepatic encephalopathy. The benefits of these formulas are unproven.

Carnitine

Carnitine is necessary for the transport of fatty acids into mitochondria for fatty acid oxidation (25). Deficiency of carnitine can occur in prolonged states of hypercatabolism or when carnitine intake is eliminated. The clinical consequences of carnitine deficiency include cardiomyopathy, skeletal muscle myopathy, and hypoglycemia.

The recommended **daily dose of carnitine is 1 to 3 g in adults** (13). Enteral formulas that are supplemented with carnitine include Glucerna (Ross), Isocal HN (Mead Johnson), Jevity (Ross), and Peptamen (Clintec).

FEEDING REGIMEN

Tube feedings are usually infused for 12 to 16 hours in each 24-hour period. Continuous infusion without a period of bowel rest is an unrelenting stress to the bowel mucosa and promotes malabsorption and diarrhea. Intermittent bolus feedings more closely approximate the normal condition, but the volumes required are often too large to be given safely.

GASTRIC RETENTION

Before gastric feedings are started, it is necessary to determine how much volume will be retained in the stomach over a 1-hour period because this will determine how fast the feedings can be administered. A volume of water that is equivalent to the desired hourly feeding volume should be infused over 1 hour. After the infusion is complete, the feeding tube should be clamped for 30 minutes. The tube should then be unclamped, and any residual volume should be aspirated from the stomach. If the residual volume is less than 50% of the volume infused, gastric feeding can proceed (9). If the residual volume is excessively high, duodenal or jejunal feedings may be more appropriate. When the gastric residual volume is measured, it is important not to administer the volume as a bolus because this will produce acute gastric distension and lead to overestimation of the residual volume.

STARTER REGIMENS

The traditional approach to initiating tube feedings is to begin with dilute formulas and a slow infusion rate and gradually advance the formula concentration and infusion rate over the next few days until the desired nutrient intake is achieved. This presumably allows the atrophic bowel mucosa time to regenerate after a period of bowel rest. The drawback with starter regimens is the fact that nutrient intake is inadequate for the time required to advance to full nutritional support. In the malnourished patient, this added period of inadequate nutrition adds to the malnutrition.

Studies involving intragastric feedings show that full feedings can be delivered immediately without troublesome vomiting or diarrhea (26,27). This is presumably due to the ability of gastric secretions to dilute the feeding formula and reduce the osmotic load associated with the feedings. Therefore, **starter regimens are unnecessary for gastric feedings.** Because of the limited reservoir function of the small bowel, starter regimens are usually required for duodenal and jejunal feedings.

COMPLICATIONS

The complications associated with enteral feedings include occlusion of the feeding tube, reflux of gastric contents into the airways, and diarrhea.

TUBE OCCLUSION

Narrow-bore feeding tubes can become occluded by accumulation of residue from the feeding formulas. One important mechanism is the precipitation of proteins in the feeding solution by acidic gastric juice that refluxes up the feeding tubes (28). Standard preventive measures include flushing the feeding tubes with 30 mL of water every 4 hours, and using a 10-mL water flush after medications are instilled (29).

Relieving the Obstruction

If there is still some flow through the tube, warm water should be injected into the tube and agitated with a syringe. This can relieve the obstruction in 30% of cases (30). If this is ineffective, **pancreatic enzyme** can be used as follows (30):

Dissolve 1 tablet of Viokase and 1 tablet of sodium carbonate (324 mg) in 5 mL of water. Inject this mixture into the feeding tube and clamp for 5 minutes. Follow with a warm water flush.

This should relieve the obstruction in approximately 75% of cases (30). If the tube is completely occluded and it is impossible to introduce warm water or pancreatic enzyme, an attempt should be made to insert a flexible wire or a drum cartridge catheter to clear the obstruction.

ASPIRATION

Retrograde regurgitation of feeding formula is reported in as many as 80% of patients receiving gastric or duodenal feedings (8). As stated earlier, the risk of reflux in gastric feedings is the same as that in duodenal feedings (3,12). Elevating the head of the bed to 45 degrees can reduce—although not eliminate—the risk of reflux (8).

Glucose Reagent Strips

Aspiration of feeding formulas into the airways can be detected by testing tracheal aspirates with glucose oxidase reagent strips. The

TABLE 47.6. SORBITOL-CONTAINING LIQUID DRUG PREPARATIONS

Agent	Preparation	Usual Dosage	Daily Sorbitol Dose (g)
Acetaminophen	Tylenol Elixir	650 mg QID	16
Cimetidine	Tagamet Liquid	300 mg QID	10
Ferrous sulfate	Iberet Liquid	75 mg TID	22
Metaclopramide	Reglan Syrup	10 mg QID	20
Potassium chloride	Kolyum Powder	20 mEq BID	25
Theophylline	Theolar Liquid	200 mg QID	23
Trimethoprim–sulfamethoxazole	Septra Suspension	800/160 mg BID	18

From Cheng EY et al. Unsuspected source of diarrhea in an ICU patient. Clin Intensive Care 1992;3:33–36.

results are measured with an automated glucose meter (AccuCheck, Boehringer Mannheim). A **glucose concentration greater than 20 mg/ dL in tracheal aspirates is evidence of aspiration** (31). Coloring the feeding formulas with food coloring and inspecting the color of the tracheal secretions is an insensitive method for detecting aspiration (31).

DIARRHEA

Diarrhea occurs in approximately 30% of patients receiving enteral tube feedings (32). Although the hypertonicity of enteral feeding formulas can induce an osmotic diarrhea, in most cases of diarrhea associated with enteral feedings, the feeding formula is not responsible for the diarrhea (32,33). **The cause of the diarrhea in many cases is a medicinal elixir that contains sorbitol** (an osmotic agent) to improve palatability (32,34). Some of the sorbitol-containing liquid drug preparations are shown in Table 47.6 (34). Also shown is the daily dosage of sorbitol that would accompany each drug when given in the usual therapeutic dosages (34). In most cases, the daily dosage of sorbitol can be enough to induce an osmotic diarrhea. Therefore, a search for sorbitol-containing medicinal elixirs should be the first concern in the evaluation of diarrhea during enteral tube feedings.

Stool Osmolal Gap

Clostridium difficile enterocolitis is also a possible cause of diarrhea during enteral feedings. One method of differentiating the secretory diarrhea caused by *C. difficile* enterocolitis from the osmotic diarrhea caused by hypertonic feedings or medicinal elixirs is to calculate the stool osmolal gap as follows:

$$\text{Osmolal gap} = \text{Measured stool osmolality} - 2 \times (\text{Stool } [\text{Na}^+] - \text{Stool } [\text{K}^+]) \tag{47.1}$$

A stool osmolal gap greater than 160 mOsm/kg H_2O suggests an osmotic diarrhea secondary to hypertonic tube feedings or medicinal elixirs, whereas a smaller (or negative) osmolal gap suggests a secretory diarrhea caused by *C. difficile* enterocolitis. (For more information on the diagnosis and treatment of *C. difficile* enterocolitis, see Chapter 33.)

JEJUNOSTOMY FEEDINGS

Although abdominal surgery usually is accompanied by 24 to 48 hours of gastric hypomotility, the motility of the small bowel is often unimpaired (35). Infusion of liquid feeding formulas into the jejunum takes advantage of the continued small bowel motility after abdominal surgery and allows immediate postoperative nutrition. Jejunal feedings can also be performed for nutritional support of patients with pancreatitis.

NEEDLE CATHETER JEJUNOSTOMY

A feeding jejunostomy can be performed as a "complimentary" procedure during laparotomy. A needle catheter jejunostomy is shown in Figure 47.3 (36). A loop of jejunum (15 to 20 cm distal to the ligament

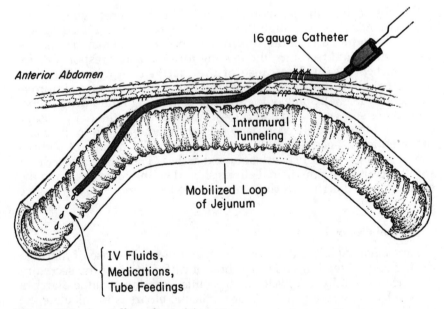

Figure 47.3. A needle catheter jejunostomy.

of Treitz) is mobilized to the anterior abdominal wall, and a 16-gauge catheter is tunneled through the submucosa of the jejunum for a distance of 30 to 45 cm and then advanced into the bowel lumen. The jejunum is then secured to the peritoneum on the underside of the abdominal wall, and the catheter is secured to the skin.

Feeding Method

As mentioned, the small bowel does not have the reservoir capacity of the stomach, so starter regimens are recommended for jejunal feedings. Feedings are usually initiated at a rate of 15 to 25 mL/hour, and the infusion rate is gradually increased over the next few days until full nutritional support is achieved (37). Catheters are flushed with 10 mL of isotonic saline every 6 hours to promote catheter patency.

Complications

The principal complications of needle catheter jejunostomies are diarrhea and occlusion of the narrow feeding catheters (37). Because of the latter complication, needle catheter jejunostomies are used only for temporary nutritional support (approximately 1 week). If more prolonged jejunal feedings are desired, a needle catheter jejunostomy can be converted to a standard jejunostomy (which uses a 12 French feeding tube) using a technique described in Reference 38.

REFERENCES

GUIDELINES

1. A.S.P.E.N. Board of Directors. Guidelines for the use of parenteral and enteral nutrition in adult and pediatric patients. J Parent Ent Nutr 1993;17(Suppl): 1SA–51SA.
2. American Gastroenterological Association Medical Position Statement: Guidelines for the use of enteral nutrition. Gastroenterology 1995;108:1280–1281.

REVIEWS

3. Benya R, Mobarhan S. Enteral alimentation: administration and complications. J Am Coll Nutr 1991;10:209–219 (92 references).

TROPHISM

4. Deitch EA, Wintertron J, Li MA, Berg R. The gut as a portal of entry for bacteremia. Ann Surg 1987;205:681–690.
5. Herskowitz A, Souba WW. Intestinal glutamine metabolism during critical illness: a surgical perspective. Nutrition 1990;6:199–206.
6. Mainous MR, Deitch EA. The gut barrier. In: Zaloga GP, ed. Nutrition in critical care. St. Louis: Mosby, 1994;557–568.

FEEDING TUBES

7. Dotson RG, Robinson RG, Pingleton SK. Gastroesophageal reflux with nasogastric tubes. Am J Respir Crit Care Med 1994;149:1659–1662.
8. Metheny N. Minimizing respiratory complications of nasoenteric tube feedings: state of the science. Heart Lung 1993;22:213–223.
9. Rombeau JL, Caldwell MD, Forlaw L, Guenter PA, eds. Atlas of nutritional support techniques. Boston: Little, Brown, 1989;77–106.
10. Metheny NA, Clouse RE, Clark JM, et al. pH testing of feeding-tube aspirates to determine placement. Nutr Clin Pract 1994;9:185–190.
11. Zaloga GP. Bedside method for placing small bowel feeding tubes in critically ill patients. Chest 1991;100:1643–1646.
12. Strong RM, Condon SC, Solinger MR, et al. Equal aspiration rates from postpylorus and intragastric-placed small-bore nasoenteric feeding tubes: a randomized, prospective study. J Parent Ent Nutr 1992;16:59–63.

FEEDING FORMULAS

13. Shronts EP, Havala T. Enteral formulas. In: Teasley-Strausburg KM, Cerra F, Lehmann S, Shronts EP, eds. Nutrition support handbook. Cincinnati, OH: Harvey Whitney Books, 1992;147–186.
14. Al-Saady NM, Blackmore CM, Bennett ED. High fat, low carbohydrate, enteral feeding lowers $Paco_2$ and reduces the period of ventilation in artificially ventilated patients. Intensive Care Med 1989;15:290–295.
15. Bagley JS, Wan JMF, Georgieff M, et al. Cellular nutrition in support of multiorgan failure. Chest 1991;100(Suppl):182S–188S.
16. Daly JM, Lieberman MD, Goldfine J, et al. Enteral nutrition with supplemental arginine, RNA, and omega-3 fatty acids in patients after operation: immunologic, metabolic, and clinical outcome. Surgery 1992;112:56–67.

ADDITIVES

17. Lacey JM, Wilmore DW. Is glutamine a conditionally essential amino acid? Nutr Rev 1990;48:297–310.
18. Swails WS, Bell SJ, Borlase BC, et al. Glutamine content of whole proteins: implications for enteral formulas. Nutr Clin Pract 1992;7:77–80.
19. AlitraQ. Manufacturer's product description. Ross Laboratories, 1991.
20. Ziegler TR, Benfell K, Smith RJ, et al. Safety and metabolic effects of L-glutamine administration in humans. J Parent Ent Nutr 1990;14(Suppl):137S–146S.
21. Palacio JC, Rombeau JL. Dietary fiber: a brief review and potential application to enteral nutrition. Nutr Clin Pract 1990;5:99–106.
22. Homan H-H, Kemen M, Fuessenich C, et al. Reduction in diarrhea incidence by soluble fiber in patients receiving total or supplemental enteral nutrition. J Parent Ent Nutr 1994;18:486–490.
23. Frankenfield DC, Beyer PL. Soy-polysaccharide fiber: effect on diarrhea in tube-fed, head-injured patients. Am J Clin Nutr 1989;50:533–538.
24. Alexander WF, Spindel E, Harty RF, Cerda JJ. The usefulness of branched chain amino acids in patients with acute or chronic hepatic encephalopathy. Am J Gastroenterol 1989;84:91–96.
25. Vockley J. The changing face of disorders of fatty acid oxidation. Mayo Clin Proc 1994;69:249–257.

FEEDING REGIMEN

26. Rees RGP, Keohane PP, Grimble GK, et al. Elemental diet administered nasogastrically without starter regimens to patients with inflammatory bowel disease. J Parent Ent Nutr 1986;10:258–262.
27. Mizock BA. Avoiding common errors in nutritional management. J Crit Illness 1993;10:1116–1127.

COMPLICATIONS

28. Marcuard SP, Perkins AM. Clogging of feeding tubes. J Parent Ent Nutr 1988; 12:403–405.
29. Benson DW, Griggs BA, Hamilton F, et al. Clogging of feeding tubes: a randomized trial of a newly designed tube. Nutr Clin Pract 1990;5:107–110.
30. Marcuard SP, Stegall KS. Unclogging feeding tubes with pancreatic enzyme. J Parent Ent Nutr 1990;14:198–200.
31. Potts RG, Zaroukian MH, Guerrero PA, Baker CD. Comparison of blue dye visualization and glucose oxidase test strip methods for detecting pulmonary aspiration of enteral feedings in intubated adults. Chest 1993;103:117–121.
32. Edes TE, Walk BE, Austin JL. Diarrhea in tube-fed patients: feeding formula not necessarily the cause. Am J Med 1990;88:91–93.
33. Eisenberg PG. Causes of diarrhea in tube-fed patients: a comprehensive approach to diagnosis and management. Nutr Clin Pract 1993;8:119–123.
34. Cheng EY, Hennen CR, Nimphius N. Unsuspected source of diarrhea in an ICU patient. Clin Intensive Care 1992;3:33–36.

JEJUNOSTOMY FEEDINGS

35. Sagar PM, Kreuger G, Macfie J. Nasogastric intubation and elective abdominal surgery. Br J Surg 1992;79:1127–1131.
36. Nance ML, Gorman RC, Morris JB, Mullen JL. Techniques for long-term jejunal access. Contemp Surg 1995;46:21–25.
37. Collier P, Kudsk KA, Glezer J, Brown RO. Fiber-containing formula and needle catheter jejunostomies: a clinical evaluation. Nutr Clin Pract 1994;9:101–103.
38. Antinori CH, Andrew C, Villanueva DT, et al. A technique for converting a needle catheter jejunostomy into a standard jejunostomy. Am J Surg 1992;164: 68–69.

SUGGESTED READINGS

Lipman TO, ed. A bibliography for specialized nutrition support. 4th ed. Silver Springs, MD: American Society of Parenteral and Enteral Nutrition, 1994.

Rombeau JL, Caldwell MD, eds. Clinical nutrition: enteral and tube feeding. 2nd ed. Philadelphia: WB Saunders, 1990.

Teasley-Strausburg KM, Cerra F, Lehmann S, Shronts EP, eds. Nutrition support handbook. Cincinnati, OH: Harvey Whitney Books, 1992.

Zaloga GP, ed. Nutrition in critical care. St. Louis: Mosby, 1994.

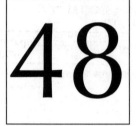

c h a p t e r

PARENTERAL NUTRITION

When full nutritional support is not possible with enteral tube feedings, the intravenous delivery of nutrients can be used to supplement or replace enteral nutrition. This chapter introduces the basic features of intravenous nutritional support (1,2) and explains how to create a total parenteral nutrition (TPN) regimen to meet the needs of individual patients.

INTRAVENOUS NUTRIENT SOLUTIONS

DEXTROSE SOLUTIONS

As mentioned in Chapters 46 and 47, the standard nutritional support regimen uses carbohydrates to supply approximately 70% of the daily (nonprotein) calorie requirement. These are provided by dextrose (glucose) solutions, which are available in the strengths shown in Table 48.1. Because dextrose is not a potent metabolic fuel (see Table 46.1), the dextrose solutions must be concentrated to provide enough calories to satisfy daily requirements. As a result, the dextrose solutions used for TPN are hyperosmolar and should be infused through large central veins.

	TABLE 48.1. INTRAVENOUS DEXTROSE SOLUTIONS		
Strength	Concentration (g/L)	Energy Yield* (kcal/L)	Osmolarity (mOsm/L)
5%	50	170	250
10%	100	340	505
20%	200	680	1010
50%	500	1700	2525
70%	700	2380	3535
* Based on an oxidative energy yield of 3.4 kcal/g for dextrose.			

	TABLE 48.2. STANDARD AND SPECIALTY AMINO ACID SOLUTIONS			
Features	Aminosyn (7%)	Aminosyn-HBC (7%)	Aminosyn RF (5.2%)	HepatAmine (8%)
Indications	Standard TPN	Hypercatabolism	Renal Failure	Hepatic Failure
Nitrogen Content (g/L)	11	Not listed	7.7	12
Essential AAs (% Total)	50%	63%	89%	55%
Branched Chain AAs (% Total)	25%	46%	33%	33%
Osmolarity (mOsm/L)	700	665	475	785

AMINO ACID SOLUTIONS

Amino acid solutions are mixed together with the dextrose solutions to provide the daily protein requirements. A variety of amino acid solutions are available for specific clinical settings, as demonstrated in Table 48.2. The standard amino acid solutions contain approximately 50% essential amino acids (N = 9) and 50% nonessential (N = 10) plus semiessential (N = 4) amino acids (3). The nitrogen in essential amino acids is partially recycled for the production of nonessential amino acids, so the metabolism of essential amino acids produces less of a rise in the blood urea nitrogen concentration than metabolism of nonessential amino acids. For this reason, amino acid solutions designed for use in renal failure are rich in essential amino acids (see Aminosyn RF in Table 48.2). Finally, for reasons stated in Chapter 47, nutritional formulas for hypercatabolic conditions (e.g., trauma) and hepatic failure can be supplemented with branched chain amino acids (isoleucine, leucine, and valine), and two specialty amino acid solutions for each of these conditions are included in Table 48.2. It is important to emphasize that none of these specialized nutrient formulas have improved the outcomes in the disorders for which they are designed (4).

Glutamine

As mentioned in Chapter 47, glutamine is the principal metabolic fuel used by intestinal epithelial cells, and lack of glutamine may be at least partly responsible for the atrophy of the bowel mucosa that accompanies prolonged periods of bowel rest (5). Glutamine-enriched TPN has been shown to reduce the atrophic changes in the bowel mucosa during periods of bowel rest (5). Therefore, glutamine-supplemented TPN may play an important role in maintaining the functional

TABLE 48.3. AMINO ACID SOLUTIONS WITH GLUTAMATE		
Preparation	Manufacturer	Glutamate Content
Aminosyn II, 10%	Abbott	738 mg/dL
Novamine 15%	Clintec	499 mg/dL
Novamine 15% plus BranchAmin 4%	Clintec	250 mg/dL

integrity of the bowel mucosa and preventing bacterial translocation (6).

Although glutamine is not an essential amino acid (because it is produced in skeletal muscle), glutamine levels in blood and tissues drop precipitously in acute, hypercatabolic conditions (e.g., trauma), so glutamine may be a "conditionally essential" amino acid (5). The amino acids that contain glutamic acid are shown in Table 48.3. Glutamine is formed when glutamic acid combines with ammonia in the presence of the enzyme glutamine synthetase, so glutamic acid can be an exogenous source of glutamine. The value of these glutamate-containing amino acid solutions is unknown at present.

LIPID EMULSIONS

Intravenous lipid emulsions are long-chain triglycerides from vegetable oils (safflower or soybean oils) and are rich in linoleic acid, an essential, polyunsaturated fatty acid that is not produced by the human body (7). As shown in Table 48.4, lipid emulsions are available in 10% and 20% strengths (the percentage refers to grams of triglyceride per 100 mL of solution). The 10% emulsions provide approximately 1 kcal/mL, and the 20% emulsions provide 2 kcal/mL. Unlike the hypertonic dextrose solutions, lipid emulsions are roughly isotonic to plasma and can be infused through peripheral veins. The lipid emulsions are available in unit volumes of 50 to 500 mL and can be infused

TABLE 48.4. INTRAVENOUS LIPID EMULSIONS FOR CLINICAL USE						
	Intralipid		Liposyn III		NutriLipid	
Feature	10%	20%	10%	20%	10%	20%
Calories (kcal/mL)	1.1	2.0	1.1	2.0	1.1	2.0
% Calories as EFAs*	41%	45%	45%	49%	45%	49%
Osmolarity (mOsm/L)	280	330	284	292	280	315
Unit volumes (mL)	50	50	100	200	50	250
	100	100	200	500	100	500
	500	250	500		250	
		500			500	

* The essential fatty acid (EFA) in lipid emulsions is linoleic acid. To prevent EFA deficiency, approximately 3% of the total daily calories should be provided by EFAs.

separately (at a maximum rate of 50 mL/hour) or added to the dextrose–amino acid mixtures. The triglycerides introduced into the bloodstream are not cleared for 8 to 10 hours, and lipid infusions often produce a transient, lipemic-appearing (whitish) plasma.

Lipid Restriction

Lipids are used to provide up to 30% of the daily (nonprotein) calorie requirements. However, because dietary lipids are oxidation-prone and can promote oxidant-induced cell injury (8), restricting the use of lipids in critically ill patients (who often have high oxidation rates) seems wise. Although lipid infusion is necessary to prevent essential fatty acid deficiency (cardiomyopathy, skeletal muscle myopathy), this can be accomplished with minimal amounts of lipid (see footnote in Table 48.3).

ADDITIVES

Commercially available mixtures of electrolytes, vitamins, and trace elements are added directly to the dextrose–amino acid mixtures.

ELECTROLYTES

Most electrolyte mixtures contain sodium, chloride, potassium, and magnesium; they also may contain calcium and phosphorous. The daily requirement for potassium or any specific electrolyte can be specified in the TPN orders. If no electrolyte requirements are specified, the electrolytes are added to replace normal daily electrolyte losses.

VITAMINS

Aqueous multivitamin preparations are added to the dextrose–amino acid mixtures. One unit vial of a standard multivitamin preparation will provide the normal daily requirements for most vitamins (see Table 46.4), with the exception of vitamin K (9). Enhanced vitamin requirements in hypermetabolic patients in the ICU may not be satisfied. Furthermore, some vitamins are degraded before they are delivered. Two examples are vitamin A (which is degraded by light) and thiamine (which is degraded by sulfite ions used as preservatives for amino acid solutions) (10).

TRACE ELEMENTS

A variety of trace element additives are available, and two commercial mixtures are shown in Table 48.5. Most trace element mixtures contain chromium, copper, manganese, and zinc, but they do not contain iron and iodine. Some mixtures contain selenium, and others do

TABLE 48.5. TRACE ELEMENT PREPARATIONS AND DAILY REQUIREMENTS			
Trace Element	Daily Parenteral Requirement	Trace Metals Additive (Abbot)	MTE-5 (Lyphomed)
Chromium	15 μg	10 μg	12 μg
Copper	1.5 mg	1 mg	1.2 mg
Iodine	150 μg	—	—
Iron	2.5 mg	—	—
Manganese	100 μg	800 μg	300 μg
Selenium	70 μg	—	60 μg
Zinc	4 mg	4 mg	4 mg

not. Considering the importance of selenium in endogenous antioxidant protection (see Chapter 3), it seems wise to select a trace element additive that contains selenium. Routine administration of iron is not recommended in critically ill patients because of the prooxidant actions of iron (see Chapter 3 and Chapter 46).

CREATING A TPN REGIMEN

The following stepwise approach shows how to create a TPN regimen for an individual patient. The patient in this example is a 70-kg adult who is not nutritionally depleted and has no volume restrictions.

Step 1

The first step is to estimate the daily protein and calorie requirements as described in Chapter 46. For this example, the daily calorie requirement will be 25 kcal/kg, and the daily protein requirement will $≲$ 1.4 g/kg. Therefore, for the 70-kg patient, the protein and calorie requirements are as follows:

$$\text{Calorie requirement} = 25 \text{ (kcal/kg)} \times 70 \text{ (kg)} = 1750 \text{ kcal/day}$$
$$\text{Protein requirement} = 1.4 \text{ (g/day)} \times 70 \text{ (kg)} = 98 \text{ g/day} \quad (48.1)$$

Step 2

The next step is to take a standard mixture of 10% amino acids (500 mL) and 50% dextrose (500 mL) and determine the volume of this mixture that is needed to deliver the estimated daily protein requirement. Although the dextrose–amino acid mixture is referred to as A_{10}–D_{50}, the final mixture actually represents 5% amino acids (50 grams of protein per liter) and 25% dextrose (250 grams dextrose per liter). Therefore, the volume of the A_{10}–D_{50} mixture needed to provide the daily protein requirement is as follows:

$$\text{Volume of } A_{10}\text{–}D_{50} = 98 \text{ (g/day)}/50 \text{ (g/L)} = 1.9 \text{ L/day} \quad (48.2)$$

If this mixture is infused continuously over 24 hours, the infusion rate will be 1900 mL/24 hours = 81 mL/hour (or 81 microdrops/minute).

Step 3

Using the total daily volume of the dextrose–amino acid mixture determined in Step 2, the next step is to determine the total calories that will be provided by the dextrose in the mixture. Using an energy yield of 3.4 kcal/g for dextrose, the total dextrose calories can be determined as follows:

Amount of dextrose = 250 (g/L) × 1.9 (L/day) = 475 g/day
Dextrose calories = 475 (g/day) × 3.4 (kcal/g) = 1615 kcal/day
$$(48.3)$$

Because the estimated requirement for calories is 1750 kcal/day, the dextrose will provide all but 135 kcal/day. These remaining calories can be provided by an intravenous lipid emulsion.

Step 4

If a 10% lipid emulsion (1 kcal/mL) is used to provide 135 kcal/day, the daily volume of the lipid emulsion will be 135 mL/day. Because the lipid emulsion is available in unit volumes of 50 mL, the volume can be adjusted to 150 mL/day to avoid wastage. Thus volume can be infused at half the maximum recommended rate (50 mL/hour) to minimize the tendency to develop lipemic serum during the infusion.

Step 5

The daily TPN orders for the previous example can then be written as follows:

1. Provide standard TPN with A_{10}–D_{50} to run at 80 mL/hour.
2. Add standard electrolytes, multivitamins, and trace elements.
3. Give 10% Intralipid: 150 mL to infuse over 6 hours.

TPN orders are rewritten each day. Specific electrolyte, vitamin, and trace element requirements are added to the daily orders as needed.

The example just presented applies to the separate administration of dextrose–amino acid mixtures and lipid emulsions. Another practice that is gaining popularity is to add the nutrient solutions and additives together to form a total nutrient admixture (TNA). Although this simplifies nutrient administration and reduces cost, there are lingering concerns regarding compatibility (e.g., multivitamin preparations may not be compatible with lipid emulsions).

COMPLICATIONS

A multitude of complications are associated with parenteral nutrition (2,11). Some of the more prominent ones are mentioned in the following paragraphs.

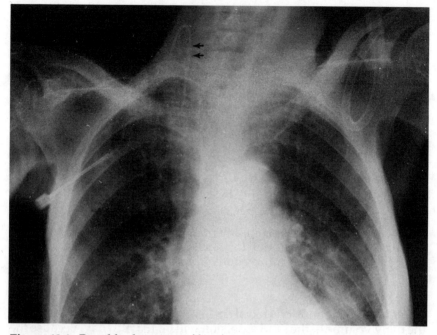

Figure 48.1. Portable chest x-ray film showing a central venous catheter that has been advanced up into the neck.

CATHETER-RELATED COMPLICATIONS

Because the dextrose and amino acid solutions are hyperosmolar (Tables 48.1 and 48.2), TPN is administered through large, central veins. The complications associated with central venous catheters are described in Chapters 5 and 6.

One complication that can be particularly frustrating is the misdirected catheter, like the one shown in Figure 48.1. In this case, a catheter inserted into the right subclavian vein has entered the internal jugular vein and advanced in a retrograde direction up into the neck. When this occurs, the catheter can be repositioned over a guidewire as follows (13).

Catheter Repositioning

When a catheter has been misdirected up into the neck, the patient should be placed in a semirecumbent or upright position if possible and the catheter should be withdrawn until only a few centimeters of the catheter tip remains inserted. A flexible guidewire is then inserted through the catheter and advanced 10 cm. The catheter is removed over the guidewire, and a new catheter is inserted and advanced 15 cm. The guidewire is removed and a Doppler probe (the one used by nurses to detect pedal pulses) is placed over the internal jugular vein in the neck. A bolus of saline is then injected through the catheter. If the catheter has been rethreaded up into the neck, the bolus injection will produce an audible noise from the Doppler probe. If this occurs, a new catheter will need to be inserted into the internal jugular vein on the same side. If no sound is detected, a repeat chest x-ray study should be obtained to determine whether the catheter has been repositioned in the superior vena cava.

CARBOHYDRATE INFUSIONS

Hyperglycemia

Glucose intolerance is one of the most common complications of TPN. Even though this problem can be reduced by providing fewer nonprotein calories as glucose (and more as lipids), persistent hyperglycemia usually requires the addition of insulin to the TPN solutions. It is important to emphasize that **insulin adsorbs to all plastics and glass used in intravenous infusion sets.** The amount lost to adsorption varies with the amount of insulin added, but an average loss of 20 to 30% should be expected (13). Albumin has been used to reduce insulin binding to intravenous infusion sets (13), but this is a costly and unreliable measure. Instead, the insulin dosage is adjusted to achieve the desired glycemic control. When TPN is discontinued, the insulin requirement will be less than that needed during TPN.

Hypophosphatemia

The effects of TPN on the serum phosphate level is shown in Figure 43.2. This effect is due to enhanced uptake of phosphate into cells associated with glucose entry into cells. The phosphate is then used to form thiamine pyrophosphate, an important cofactor in carbohydrate metabolism.

Fatty Liver

When glucose calories exceed the daily calorie requirements, there is lipogenesis in the liver and this can progress to fatty infiltration of the liver and elevated levels of transaminase enzymes in the blood (11,14). It is unclear whether this process has any pathologic consequences or whether it merely serves as a marker of excess carbohydrate calories.

Hypercapnia

Excess carbohydrates promote CO_2 retention in patients with respiratory insufficiency. Although this has been attributed to the high respiratory quotient associated with carbohydrate metabolism (see Table

46.1), this may be a reflection of overfeeding in general and not specific overfeeding with carbohydrates (15).

LIPID INFUSIONS

Oxidant Injury

One of the major (and often overlooked) toxicities associated with lipid infusions is an **increased risk of oxidation-induced cell injury** (8). The damaging effects associated with oxidation of membrane lipids is described in Chapter 3. The same oxidation-prone lipids in cell membranes (i.e., polyunsaturated fatty acids) are also abundant in intravenous lipid emulsions. Because excessive and unprotected biological oxidation is likely to be common in patients in the ICU (see Table 3.2), infusion of oxidation-prone exogenous lipids could promote widespread oxidant damage in these patients. This consideration deserves much more attention that it currently receives.

Impaired Oxygenation

Lipid infusions are associated with impaired oxygenation (16). Free fatty acids are well known for their ability to damage the pulmonary capillaries (e.g., fat embolism syndrome), and infusions of oleic acid (a fatty acid present in lipid emulsions) are used to produce acute respiratory distress syndrome (ARDS) in experimental animals. This effect of lipids may be caused by oxidant-induced injury to the pulmonary capillary endothelium.

GASTROINTESTINAL COMPLICATIONS

Two indirect complications of TPN are related to the absence of bulk nutrients in the bowel.

Mucosal Atrophy

The absence of bulk nutrients in the bowel produces atrophy and disruption of the bowel mucosa. This is described in Chapter 47 and is illustrated in Figure 47.1. These changes can predispose to translocation of enteric pathogens across the bowel mucosa and subsequent septicemia. Because TPN is usually accompanied by bowel rest, one of the indirect complications of TPN is bacterial translocation and sepsis of bowel origin (17). As mentioned earlier, glutamine-supplemented TPN may help reduce the risk of this complication.

Acalculous Cholecystitis

The absence of lipids in the proximal small bowel prevents cholecystokinin-mediated contraction of the gallbladder and the bile stasis that results may promote acalculous cholecystitis (2). This disorder is described in Chapter 33.

PERIPHERAL PARENTERAL NUTRITION

Parenteral nutrition can occasionally be delivered via peripheral veins for short periods. The goal of peripheral parenteral nutrition (PPN) is to provide just enough nonprotein calories to spare the breakdown of proteins to provide energy (i.e., protein-sparing nutritional support). PPN does not create enough of a positive nitrogen balance to build up protein stores, and thus it is not intended for patients who are protein depleted or for patients who are hypercatabolic and at risk of becoming protein depleted.

The osmolarity of peripheral vein infusates should be kept below 900 mOsm/L to prevent osmotic damage to the vessels (18). Therefore, PPN must be delivered with dilute amino acid and dextrose solutions. Because lipid emulsions are isotonic to plasma, lipids can be used to provide a significant proportion of the nonprotein calories in PPN.

METHOD

A common admixture used in PPN is a mixture of 3% amino acids and 20% dextrose. This mixture produces a final concentration of 1.5% amino acids (15 grams of protein per liter) and 10% dextrose (100 grams of dextrose per liter), with an osmolarity of approximately 500 mOsm/L. The dextrose will provide 340 kcal/L, so 2.5 L of the mixture will provide 850 kcal. If 250 mL of 20% Intralipid is added to the regimen (adding 500 kcal), the total nonprotein calories will increase to 1350 kcal/day. This should be close to the nonprotein calorie requirement of an average-size adult at rest (25 kcal/kg/day). In hypermetabolic patients, large volumes of PPN are required to satisfy daily energy requirements.

In summary, peripheral intravenous nutrition can be used as a temporary measure to prevent or limit protein breakdown in patients who are not already protein depleted and are expected to begin oral feedings within a few days. Postoperative patients seem best suited for this form of nutritional support.

REFERENCES

GUIDELINES

1. A.S.P.E.N. Board of Directors. Guidelines for the use of parenteral and enteral nutrition in adult and pediatric patients. J Parent Ent Nutr 1993;17(Suppl): 1SA–52SA.

REVIEWS

2. Phelps SJ, Brown RO, Helms RA, et al. Toxicities of parenteral nutrition in the critically ill patient. Crit Care Clin 1991;7:725–753 (212 references).

INTRAVENOUS NUTRIENT SOLUTIONS

3. Teasley-Stausburg KM. Amino acid solutions. In Teasley-Strausburg KM, Cerra FB, Lehmann S, Shronts EP, eds. Nutrition support handbook. Cincinnati, OH: Harvey Whitney Books, 1992:47–72.
4. Andris DA, Krzywda EA. Nutrition support in specific diseases: back to basics. Nutr Clin Pract 1994;9:28–32.
5. Souba WW, Klimberg VS, Plumley DA, et al. The role of glutamine in maintaining a healthy gut and supporting the metabolic response to injury and infection. J Surg Res 1990;48:383–391.
6. Grant J. Use of L-glutamine in total parenteral nutrition. J Surg Res 1988;44: 506–510.
7. Warshawsky KY. Intravenous fat emulsions in clinical practice. Nutr Clin Pract 1992;7:187–196.
8. Hardin TC. Cytokine mediators of malnutrition: clinical implications. Nutr Clin Pract 1993;8:55–59.
9. Manufacturer's product description for M.V.I.-12. Westborough, MA: Astra USA, 1995.
10. LaFrance RJ, Miyagawa CI. Pharmaceutical considerations in total parenteral nutrition. In: Fischer JE, ed. Total parenteral nutrition. 2nd ed. Boston: Little, Brown, 1991;57–98.

COMPLICATIONS

11. Perry DA, Markin RS, Rose SG, Schenken JR. Changes in laboratory values in patients receiving total parenteral nutrition. Lab Med 1990;21:97–102.
12. Benotti PN, Bistrian BR. Practical aspects and complications of total parenteral nutrition. Crit Care Clin 1987;3:115–131.
13. Trissel LA. Handbook on injectable drugs. 8th ed. Bethesda, MD: American Society of Hospital Pharmacists, 1994;585–590.
14. Freund HR. Abnormalities of liver function and hepatic damage associated with total parenteral nutrition. Nutrition 1991;7:1–6.
15. Talpers SS, Romberger DJ, Bunce SB, Pingleton SK. Nutritionally associated increased carbon dioxide production. Chest 1992;102:551–555.
16. Sleie B, Askanazi J, Rothkopf M, et al. Intravenous fat emulsions and lung function: a review. Crit Care Med 1988;16:183–193.
17. Alverdy JC, Aoys E, Moss GS. Total parenteral nutrition promotes bacterial translocation from the gut. Surgery 1988;104:185–190.

PERIPHERAL PARENTERAL NUTRITION

18. Teasley-Strausburg KM. Indications for parenteral and enteral nutrition. In: Teasley-Strausburg KM, Cerra FB, Lehmann S, Shronts EP, eds. Nutrition support handbook. Cincinnati, OH: Harvey Whitney Books, 1992;37–46.

SUGGESTED READINGS

Fischer JE. Total parenteral nutrition. 2nd ed. Boston: Little, Brown, 1991.
Grant JP. Handbook of total parenteral nutrition. 2nd ed. Philadelphia: WB Saunders, 1992.
Lipman TO, ed. A bibliography for specialized nutrition support. 4th ed. Silver Springs, MD: American Society of Parenteral and Enteral Nutrition, 1994.
Teasley-Strausburg KM, Cerra F, Lehmann S, Shronts EP, eds. Nutrition support handbook. Cincinnati, OH: Harvey Whitney Books, 1992.
Zaloga GP, ed. Nutrition in critical care. St. Louis: Mosby, 1994.

chapter

49

ADRENAL AND THYROID DYSFUNCTION

Endocrine disorders that involve the adrenal and thyroid glands are noted for their ability to act as catalysts for serious, life-threatening conditions while escaping notice themselves. This chapter explains how to unmask an underlying or occult disorder of adrenal or thyroid function and how to treat each disorder appropriately (1–8).

ADRENAL INSUFFICIENCY

The adrenal gland plays a major role in the adaptive response to stress. The adrenal cortex releases glucocorticoids and mineralocorticoids that promote glucose availability and maintain extracellular volume, while the adrenal medulla releases catecholamines that support the circulation. Attenuation or loss of this adrenal response (i.e., adrenal insufficiency) leads to hemodynamic instability, volume depletion, and defective energy metabolism. The important feature of adrenal insufficiency is its ability to remain silent until the adrenal gland is called on to respond to a physiologic stress. When this occurs, adrenal insufficiency becomes an occult catalyst that speeds the progression of acute, life-threatening conditions (1–3).

Adrenal insufficiency can be a primary or secondary disorder (the latter being due to hypothalamic–pituitary dysfunction). The description that follows pertains to primary adrenal insufficiency.

PREDISPOSING CONDITIONS

Several conditions that are common in patients in the ICU can predispose to primary adrenal insufficiency. These include major surgery, circulatory failure, septic shock, severe coagulopathy, and human immunodeficiency virus (HIV) infections (1,2). In some of these conditions, the adrenal insufficiency is caused by pathologic destruction of the adrenal gland (e.g., coagulopathy with adrenal hemorrhage). In others, the problem is diminished adrenal responsiveness (e.g., septic shock).

INCIDENCE

In surveys of random ICU patients, the incidence of adrenal insufficiency has varied from 0 to 30% in different reports (1,2). In patients with septic shock, the incidence is higher at 25 to 40% (9–11). In many of these cases, adrenal insufficiency was not evident clinically but was uncovered by biochemical evidence of abnormal adrenal responsiveness. In patients with laboratory evidence of adrenal insufficiency, the mortality is more than double that of patients with normal adrenal responsiveness (9–11).

CLINICAL MANIFESTATIONS

In critically ill patients, the most prominent manifestation of adrenal insufficiency is **hypotension that is refractory to vasopressors** (1,2,9–11). Other features of adrenal insufficiency, such as electrolyte abnormalities (hyponatremia, hyperkalemia), weakness, and hyperpigmentation, are either uncommon or not specific enough to suggest the diagnosis in ICU patients.

Hemodynamics

In mild or chronic cases of adrenal insufficiency, the hemodynamic changes are often a reflection of hypovolemia (low filling pressures, low cardiac output, high systemic vascular resistance). In acute adrenal failure, the hemodynamic changes are similar to those of hyperdynamic shock (high cardiac output, low systemic vascular resistance) (10,12). Because many cases of adrenal insufficiency are uncovered in patients with septic shock, where the hemodynamic changes are similar to those of acute adrenal failure (i.e., hyperdynamic shock), it is often impossible to identify adrenal failure based on hemodynamic profiles in critically ill patients.

ACTH STIMULATION TEST

Adrenal insufficiency should be suspected in any patient in the ICU who develops sudden hypotension of unclear etiology or has hypotension that is refractory to vasopressors. In critically ill patients, the diagnostic test of choice for primary adrenal insufficiency is the rapid adrenocorticotropic hormone (ACTH) stimulation test (1–3). This test evaluates the acute adrenal response to a bolus injection of synthetic ACTH (Cortrosyn).

METHOD

The rapid ACTH stimulation test can be performed at any time and is not influenced by diurnal variations in cortisol secretion (which are often absent in critically ill patients anyway). An initial blood sample is obtained for a plasma cortisol level, and synthetic ACTH (0.25 mg) is injected intravenously. A post-ACTH plasma cortisol level is then obtained 1 hour after the ACTH injection.

Results

The graph in Figure 49.1 shows the plasma cortisol level before and after ACTH injection in three different situations. Under normal conditions, there is more than a twofold increase in the plasma cortisol level 1 hour after the ACTH injection. In the presence of a physiological stress (which pertains to most ICU patients), the baseline plasma cortisol level is higher than normal, but the response to ACTH is blunted. In the setting of adrenal insufficiency, the baseline cortisol is below normal, and the response to ACTH is markedly diminished.

Interpretation

The interpretation of the ACTH stimulation test is outlined in Table 49.1. In the presence of a physiologic stress, a baseline plasma cortisol level that is above 15 μg/dL (414 nmol/L) indicates normal adrenal function. An increment in plasma cortisol (at 1 hour after ACTH injection) of less than 7 μg/dL (193 nmol/L) is evidence of a limited adrenal reserve (as would be seen when the adrenal gland is maximally stimulated). A baseline plasma cortisol of less than 15 μg/dL and a poststimulation increment in plasma cortisol of less than 7 μg/dL is evidence of primary adrenal insufficiency.

STEROID THERAPY

In patients with suspected adrenal insufficiency who have severe or refractory hypotension, **steroids can be started immediately, before the ACTH stimulation test is performed.** Steroid administration can proceed as follows:

1. Dexamethasone (Decadron) will not interfere with plasma cortisol assay (13) and thus can be given before or during the ACTH stimulation test. The initial dose should be 10 mg (as an intravenous bolus), which is equivalent to 270 mg of hydrocortisone (cortisol).
2. Methylprednisolone (Solu-Medrol) will not interfere with the cortisol assay if a radioimmunoassay (RIA) is performed (13). The initial dose of methylprednisolone is 60 mg (as an intravenous bolus), which is equivalent to 300 mg of hydrocortisone.
3. After the ACTH stimulation test is completed, empiric therapy

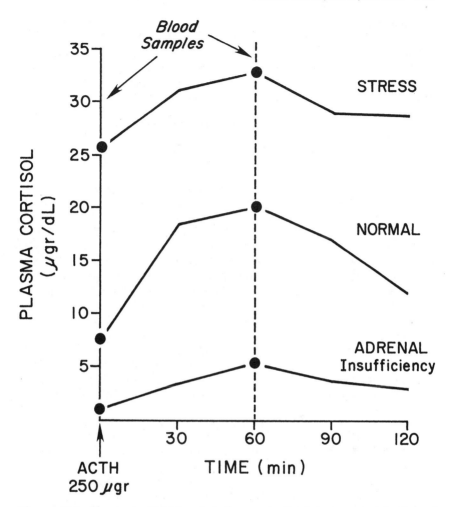

Figure 49.1. Plasma cortisol levels before and after intravenous injection of synthetic *ACTH* (Cortrosyn). (Redrawn from Chernow B. Hormonal and metabolic considerations in critical care medicine. In: Thompson WL, Shoemaker W, eds. Critical care: state of the art. Volume 3. Fullerton, CA: Society of Critical Care Medicine, 1982.)

TABLE 49.1. INTERPRETATION OF THE ACTH STIMULATION TEST		
Plasma Cortisol (μg/dl)		
Baseline	**Increment**	**Interpretation**
>15	>7	Normal adrenal function
>15	<7	Limited adrenal reserve
<15	<7	Adrenal insufficiency

TABLE 49.2. THE LABORATORY EVALUATION OF THYROID FUNCTION	
Serum Assay	**Comments**
Thyroxine (T$_4$)	Measures protein-bound and free T$_4$. Is unreliable for the evaluation of thyroid function in patients in the ICU.
Free thyroxine index (FTI)	An indirect method of determining free T$_4$ levels. The FTI is the product of the serum T$_4$ and the T$_3$ resin uptake test.
Free thyroxine (free T$_4$)	The most reliable test of thyroid function, but may not be routinely available.
Thyroid-stimulating hormone (TSH)	Can differentiate a primary thyroidal disorder from pituitary–hypothalamic dysfunction. Useful only in hypothyroidism.

can begin with hydrocortisone (Solu-Cortef). The initial dose is 250 mg (intravenous bolus), followed by 100 mg given intravenously (IV) every 6 hours until the test results are available.

4. If the ACTH stimulation test is normal, the hydrocortisone can be abruptly discontinued, without a taper. If the test reveals primary adrenal insufficiency, the hydrocortisone should be continued at the dosage of 100 mg IV every 6 hours until the patient is no longer in a stressed condition. When this occurs, the daily dose of hydrocortisone should be reduced to 20 mg (which is equivalent to the amount of cortisol secreted daily by the adrenal glands).

EVALUATION OF THYROID FUNCTION

Laboratory tests of thyroid function can be abnormal in 75% of hospitalized patients (14) and 90% of critically ill patients (15). In most cases, the abnormality represents an adaptive response to nonthyroidal illness and is not a sign of pathologic thyroid disease (14–16). This section describes the laboratory evaluation of thyroid function (17) and explains how to determine whether a laboratory abnormality represents a disorder of thyroid function or a condition known as *euthyroid sick*. A summary of the pertinent thyroid function tests is shown in Table 49.2.

SERUM THYROXINE

Thyroxine (T$_4$) is the principal hormone secreted by the thyroid gland, but the active form of the hormone is triiodothyronine (T$_3$), which is formed by the deiodination of thyroxine in extrathyroidal tissues. Despite being the active form of thyroid hormone, T$_3$ levels in plasma are not a reliable index of thyroid function. Serum T$_3$ levels can be normal in 30% of patients with hypothyroidism, and subnormal in 70% of patients who are euthyroid sick (17). Therefore, measurements of T_3 levels in the blood are not advised for the evaluation of thyroid function (17).

T_4 in plasma is partly bound to carrier proteins such as thyroid binding globulin. However, the free (unbound) T_4 is the active form of the hormone. The assay for T_4 in plasma is an RIA that measures both the protein-bound (inactive) and free (active) hormone levels. Thus, an abnormal "total" T_4 assay can represent an abnormality in protein binding and not an abnormality in thyroid function. The total serum T_4 is subnormal in 50% of patients in the ICU (17), even though most of these patients do not have abnormal thyroid function. Therefore, **the routine assay for (total) T_4 levels in plasma is not recommended for the evaluation of thyroid function in patients in the ICU (17).**

FREE THYROXINE INDEX

The free thyroxine index (FTI) is an indirect assessment of free (unbound) T_4 levels in plasma. The FTI is the product of the total serum T_4 level and the T_3 resin uptake (T_3RU). The latter test measures the binding capacity of carrier proteins for T_3. An increase in the T_3RU indicates a decrease in the binding capacity of plasma proteins (which could occur when the amount of protein-bound T_4 has increased or when protein concentration has decreased). A decrease in the T_3RU indicates an increase in protein binding capacity (which could occur when there is a decrease in the amount of protein-bound T_4 or when there is an increase in the protein concentration).

When the total T_4 and T_3RU change in opposite directions (FTI unchanged), the change in the total T_4 is due to altered binding by carrier proteins (euthyroid state). When the total T_4 and T_3RU change in the same direction (FTI changed), the change in total T_4 is due to abnormal thyroid function. The FTI is increased in hyperthyroidism and decreased in hypothyroidism.

FREE THYROXINE

The amount of free T_4 in plasma can be measured by allowing the plasma to pass through a semipermeable membrane that allows only the free (unbound) T_4 to pass. This test is the most reliable laboratory measure of thyroid function, but it is a complex assay and is not performed routinely in many clinical laboratories.

THYROID-STIMULATING HORMONE

When abnormal thyroid function is detected by the FTI or free T_4 assay, the level of thyroid-stimulating hormone (TSH) in plasma can help determine whether the problem is a primary thyroid disorder or the result of hypothalamic–pituitary dysfunction. For example, in

TABLE 49.3. MANIFESTATIONS OF THYROID DYSFUNCTION	
Hyperthyroidism	**Hypothyroidism**
Cardiovascular:	Effusions:
Sinus tachycardia	Pericardial effusion
Atrial fibrillation	Pleural effusion
Neurologic:	Miscellaneous:
Agitation	Hyponatremia
Lethargy (elderly)	Skeletal muscle myopathy
Fine tremors	Elevated creatinine
Thyroid Storm:	Myxedema Coma:
Fever	Hypothermia
Hyperdynamic shock	Dermal infiltration
Obtundation	Depressed consciousness

hypothyroidism caused by pathologic injury of the thyroid gland (primary hypothyroidism), the negative feedback effect of T_4 on TSH secretion will be lost and the plasma level of TSH will be elevated. On the other hand, in hypothyroidism caused by hypothalamic–pituitary dysfunction, the level of TSH in plasma will be subnormal.

The normal concentration of TSH in plasma is 0.5 to 3.5 4 mU/L (6). Because TSH is normally present in a low concentration, only an elevated TSH level is interpretable. In primary hypothyroidism, TSH levels usually rise above 20 mU/L. Both dopamine and high-dosage glucocorticoids can suppress the increase in TSH in primary hypothyroidism, so a normal TSH in patients receiving dopamine infusions or high-dosage steroids does not rule out the possibility of primary hypothyroidism.

HYPERTHYROIDISM

Most cases of hyperthyroidism are due to primary thyroidal disorders (e.g., Grave's disease, autoimmune thyroiditis). Chronic therapy with amiodarone, an iodine-containing antiarrhythmic agent, can also cause hyperthyroidism (18).

CLINICAL MANIFESTATIONS

Some of the common or characteristic manifestations of hyperthyroidism are listed in Table 49.3. It is important to note that **elderly patients with hyperthyroidism may be lethargic** rather than agitated (apathetic thyrotoxicosis). The combination of lethargy and unexplained atrial fibrillation is characteristic of apathetic thyrotoxicosis in the elderly (7,19).

Thyroid Storm

An uncommon but severe form of hyperthyroidism known as thyroid storm can be precipitated by acute illness or surgery. This condition, characterized by fever, severe agitation, and high-output heart failure, can progress to hypotension and coma (20) and is uniformly fatal if overlooked and left untreated.

DIAGNOSIS

As mentioned in the previous section, hyperthyroidism will be accompanied by an elevated FTI and an increased free T_4 level in plasma. Because hyperthyroidism is usually caused by primary thyroidal disorders, the TSH is not a valuable test in hyperthyroidism.

MANAGEMENT

β-Receptor Antagonists

Immediate management of troublesome tachyarrhythmias can be achieved by administering intravenous propanolol (1 mg every 5 minutes until the desired effect is achieved). Oral maintenance therapy (20 to 120 mg every 6 hours) can be used until antithyroid drug therapy is effective.

Antithyroid Drugs

The two drugs used to suppress thyroxine production are methimazole and propylthiouracil (PTU). **Methimazole** is usually preferred to PTU because it causes a more rapid decline in serum thyroxine levels and has a lower incidence of serious side effects (agranulocytosis) (8). Both antithyroid drugs are given orally. The initial dose of methimazole is **10 to 20 mg once a day,** and the initial dose of PTU is 75 to 100 mg TID (8). The dose of both drugs is reduced by 50% after 4 to 6 weeks of therapy.

Iodide

In severe cases of hyperthyroidism, iodide (which blocks thyroxine release from the thyroid gland) can be added to therapy with PTU. Iodide can be given orally as Lugol's solution (4 drops every 12 hours) or intravenously as sodium iodide (500 to 1000 mg every 12 hours). If the patient has an iodide allergy, lithium (300 mg orally every 8 hours) can be used as a substitute.

Thyroid Storm

In addition to the above measures, the treatment of thyroid storm often requires aggressive volume infusion (to replace fluid losses as a result of vomiting, diarrhea, and heightened insensible fluid loss). Thyroid storm can accelerate glucocorticoid metabolism and create a relative adrenal insufficiency. Thus in cases of thyroid storm associated with severe or refractory hypotension, hydrocortisone (300 mg IV as a loading dose, followed by 100 mg IV every 8 hours) may help correct the hypotension. Successful management of thyroid storm also requires treatment of the precipitating event (20).

HYPOTHYROIDISM

Hypothyroidism is uncommon in hospitalized patients. When present, most cases represent primary hypothyroidism (16).

CLINICAL MANIFESTATIONS

Some of the more common or characteristic manifestations of hypothyroidism are listed in Table 49.3. The most common cardiovascular manifestation is **pericardial effusion** (21), which develops in approximately 30% of cases, and is the most common cause of an enlarged cardiac silhouette in patients with hypothyroidism (21). These effusions usually accumulate slowly and do not cause cardiac compromise. Pleural effusions are also common in hypothyroidism. The pleural and pericardial effusions are due to an increase in capillary permeability and are exudative in quality.

Hypothyroidism can also be associated with hyponatremia and a skeletal muscle myopathy, with elevations in muscle enzymes (creatine phosphokinase, aldolase, lactate dehydrogenase). Enhanced release of creatinine from skeletal muscles can also raise the serum creatinine in the absence of renal dysfunction (22).

Myxedema Coma

Advanced cases of hypothyroidism are accompanied by hypothermia and depressed consciousness. Although this condition is called myxedema coma, frank coma is uncommon (5). The edematous appearance in myxedema is due to intradermal accumulation of proteins (5) and does not represent accumulation of interstitial edema fluid.

DIAGNOSIS

As mentioned earlier, hypothyroidism should be accompanied by a decrease in the FTI and a decrease in the free T_4 levels in plasma. Furthermore, primary hypothyroidism will be accompanied by an elevated serum TSH level (usually greater than 20 mU/L). A normal total serum T_4 level will virtually exclude the diagnosis of hypothyroidism.

THRYROID REPLACEMENT THERAPY

The treatment for mild to moderate hypothyroidism is levothyroxine, which is given orally in a single daily dose of 50 to 200 μg(6).

The initial dose is usually 50 μg/day, and this is increased in 50 μg/day increments every 3 to 4 weeks. The optimal replacement dose of levothyroxine is determined by monitoring the serum TSH level. The optimal dose is the lowest dose of levothyroxine that returns the TSH to within the normal range (0.5 to 3.5 mU/L). In 90% of cases, this occurs with a levothyroxine dose of 100 to 200 μg/day (6).

Oral thyroxine therapy can also be effective in severe hypothyroidism, but intravenous therapy is often recommended (at least initially) because of the risk of impaired gastrointestinal motility in severe hypothyroidism. One recommended regimen includes an initial intravenous thyroxine dose of 250 μg, followed on the next day by a dose of 100 μg, and followed thereafter by a daily dose of 50 μg (5).

T_3 Replacement Therapy

Because the conversion of T_4 to T_3 (the active form of thyroid hormone) can be depressed in critically ill patients (5), oral therapy with T_3 can be used to supplement thyroxine replacement therapy. In patients with depressed consciousness, oral T_3 can be given in a dose of 25 μg every 12 hours until the patient awakens (23). However, the benefits of T_3 supplementation are unproven.

REFERENCES

REVIEWS: ADRENAL DYSFUNCTION

1. Knowlton AI. Adrenal insufficiency in the intensive care setting. J Intensive Care Med 1988;4:35–45 (111 references).
2. Chin R. Adrenal crisis. Crit Care Clin 1991;7:23–42 (58 references).
3. Oelkers W. Adrenal insufficiency. N Engl J Med 1996;335:1206–1212 (43 references).

REVIEWS: THYROID DYSFUNCTION

4. Brent GA. The molecular basis of thyroid hormone action. N Engl J Med 1994; 331:847–853 (59 references).
5. Myers L, Hays J. Myxedema coma. Crit Care Clin 1991;7:43–56 (48 references).
6. Toft AD. Thyroxine therapy. N Engl J Med 1994;331:174–180 (74 references).
7. Reasner CA 2nd, Isley WL. Thyrotoxicosis in the critically ill. Crit Care Clin 1991;7:57–74 (117 references).
8. Franklyn JA. The management of hyperthyroidism. N Engl J Med 1994;330: 1731–1738 (89 references).

ADRENAL INSUFFICIENCY

9. Rothwell PM, Udwadia ZF, Lawler PG. Cortisol response to corticotrophin and survival in septic shock. Lancet 1991;337:582–583.
10. Moran JL, Chapman MJ, O'Fathartaigh MS, et al. Hypocortisolemia and adre-

nocortical responsiveness at onset of septic shock. Intensive Care Med 1994; 20:489–495.
11. Soni A, Pepper GM, Wyrwinski PM, et al. Adrenal insufficiency occurring during septic shock: incidence, outcome, and relationship to peripheral cytokine levels. Am J Med 1995;98:266–271.
12. Dorin RI, Kearns PJ. High output circulatory failure in acute adrenal insufficiency. Crit Care Med 1988;16:296–297.
13. Passmore JM Jr. Adrenal cortex. In: Geelhoed SW, Chernow B, eds. Endocrine aspects of acute illness. Clinics in critical care medicine. Volume 5. New York: Churchill Livingstone, 1985;97–134.

EVALUATION OF THYROID FUNCTION

14. Simons RJ, Simon JM, Demers LM, Santen RJ. Thyroid dysfunction in elderly hospitalized patients. Arch Intern Med 1990;150:1249–1253.
15. Sumita S, Ujike Y, Namika A, et al. Suppression of the thyrotropin response to thyrotropin-releasing hormone and its association with severity of critical illness. Crit Care Med 1994;22:1603–1609.
16. Isley WL. Thyroid dysfunction in the severely ill and elderly. Postgrad Med 1993;94:111–128.
17. Surks MI, Chopra IJ, Mariash CN, et al. American Thyroid Association guidelines for use of laboratory tests in thyroid disorders. JAMA 1990;263: 1529–1532.

HYPERTHYROIDISM

18. Trip MD, Wiersinga W, Plomp TA. Incidence, predictability, and pathogenesis of amiodarone-induced thyrotoxicosis and hypothyroidism. Am J Med 1991; 91:507–511.
19. Klein I. Thyroid hormone and the cardiovascular system. Am J Med 1990;88: 631–637.
20. Ehrmann DA, Sarne DH. Early identification of thyroid storm and myxedema coma. Crit Illness 1988;3:111–118.

HYPOTHYROIDISM

21. Ladenson PW. Recognition and management of cardiovascular disease related to thyroid dysfunction. Am J Med 1990;88:638–641.
22. Lafayette RA, Costa ME, King AJ. Increased serum creatinine in the absence of renal failure in profound hypothyroidism. Am J Med 1994;96:298–299.
23. McCulloch W, Price P, Hinds CJ, Wass JAH. Effects of low dose triiodothyronine in myxedema coma. Intensive Care Med 1985;11:259–262.

section XIII
NEUROLOGIC DISORDERS

There is no delusion more damaging than to get the idea in your head that you understand the functioning of your own brain.

Lewis Thomas

c h a p t e r

50

DISORDERS OF MENTATION

Abnormal mental function is one of the most recognizable signs of serious illness. In patients in the ICU, abnormal mental function is associated with a higher mortality rate, a prolongation of mechanical ventilation, and a longer stay in the ICU (1,2). This chapter focuses on two disorders of mental function that are common in critically ill patients: depressed consciousness and delirium. The final section of this chapter describes the most severe disorder of mental function that will ever be encountered: brain death.

MENTAL FUNCTION

The "mental" aspects of nervous system function are responsible for the manner in which individuals interact with their environment. Mental function can be considered normal when all the following mental processes are intact:

1. Awareness of self and surroundings
2. Accurate perception of what is experienced (orientation)
3. Ability to process input data to generate more meaningful information (judgment and reasoning)
4. Ability to store and retrieve information (memory)

The first mental process is known as consciousness, and the latter three mental processes make up what is known as cognition. The disorders of mental function can therefore be classified as disorders of consciousness and disorders of cognition.

DEPRESSED CONSCIOUSNESS

Consciousness has two components: arousal (or wakefulness) and awareness (or responsiveness). Because awareness is not possible without arousal, the tendency for arousal is the most important determinant of the level or degree of consciousness. The following are some definitions of level of consciousness based on the tendency for arousal.

LEVELS OF CONSCIOUSNESS

Awake—aroused and aware
Somnolent—easily aroused and aware
Stuporous—aroused with difficulty, impaired awareness
Comatose—unarousable and unaware
Vegetative state—aroused but unaware

Because coma is characterized by the absence of arousal, it must also be characterized by the absence of awareness (responsiveness). Therefore, coma can be defined as a state of unarousable unresponsiveness.

Vegetative State

A vegetative state is produced by diffuse cerebral injury without involvement of the brainstem reticular activating system (which determines arousal). In this condition, the patient is awake (eyes open) but is unresponsive to verbal or noxious stimuli. A condition that can mimic the vegetative state is called the **locked-in syndrome.** The patient with this condition is awake and aware but unable to generate a motor response to verbal and noxious stimuli. Locked-in syndrome can be produced by destruction of the motor pathways in the ventral portion of the lower brainstem or by the induction of neuromuscular paralysis without adequate sedation.

ETIOLOGIES

The common causes of a depressed level of consciousness in patients who have not sustained a head injury are listed in Figure 50.1. Most of the conditions listed in this figure can be classified as types of encephalopathies (i.e., infectious, ischemic, drug-related, or metabolic encephalopathies). These conditions are included in the simplified pneumonic **SMASHED** (3):

S—Substrate deficiencies (e.g., glucose, thiamine)
M—Meningoencephalitis or Mental illness (e.g., malingering, psychogenic coma)
A—Alcohol or Accident (i.e., cerebrovascular accident)
S—Seizures
H—Hypers (e.g., hypercapnia, hyperglycemia, hyperthyroid, hyperthermia) or Hypos (e.g., hypoxia, hypotension, hypothyroid, hypothermia)
E—Electrolyte abnormalities (e.g., hypernatremia, hyponatremia, hypercalcemia) and Encephalopathies (e.g., hepatic, septic, uremic)

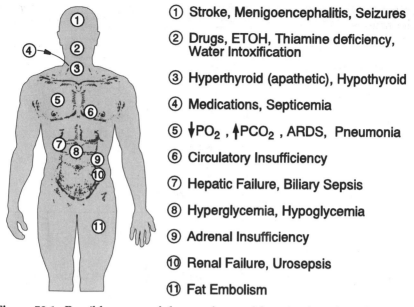

① Stroke, Menigoencephalitis, Seizures

② Drugs, ETOH, Thiamine deficiency, Water Intoxification

③ Hyperthyroid (apathetic), Hypothyroid

④ Medications, Septicemia

⑤ $\downarrow PO_2$, $\uparrow PCO_2$, ARDS, Pneumonia

⑥ Circulatory Insufficiency

⑦ Hepatic Failure, Biliary Sepsis

⑧ Hyperglycemia, Hypoglycemia

⑨ Adrenal Insufficiency

⑩ Renal Failure, Urosepsis

⑪ Fat Embolism

Figure 50.1. Possible causes of abnormal mental function (i.e., depressed consciousness and delirium) in patients who have not sustained a head injury.

D—Drugs (e.g., opioid analgesics, sedative–hypnotic agents).

In one survey of neurologic complications in a medical ICU (1), **ischemic stroke** was the most common cause of depressed consciousness in patients admitted to the ICU and **septic encephalopathy** was the most common cause of depressed consciousness that developed after admission to the ICU.

Septic Encephalopathy

The condition known as septic encephalopathy applies to all infections other than primary infections of the central nervous system (4). Encephalopathy is reported in 70% of patients in the ICU with sepsis and can appear as an early sign of sepsis (4). The underlying mechanism is unclear. Multiple, small microabscesses in both cerebral hemispheres is the most consistent finding in fatal cases of septic encephalopathy (4), but the incidence of these lesions in less advanced cases is unknown. The amino acid alterations that are characteristic of hepatic encephalopathy (i.e., increased aromatic amino acids and decreased branched chain amino acids in plasma) are also found in septic encephalopathy (5), but the significance of this abnormality is unclear. Septic encephalopathy may be one feature of a more widespread multiorgan injury associated with the systemic inflammatory response (see Chapter 33). If this is the case, oxidant-induced cell injury may play a role in the pathogenesis of septic encephalopathy.

TABLE 50.1. CONDITIONS THAT AFFECT PUPILLARY SIZE AND REACTIVITY		
Dilated Pupils	**Midposition Pupils**	**Constricted Pupils**

Reactive:
  Atropine (usual
  doses)
  Sympathomimetics
	Reactive:
	  Metabolic
	  encephalopathy
	  Sedative-hypnotic
	  overdose
		Reactive:
		  Pontine destruction
		  Opiates

Unreactive:
  Supratentorial
  damage
  Ocular trauma
  Atropine (high-dose)
  Dopamine (high-dose)
	Unreactive:
	  Barbiturates
	  (high-dose)
	  Glutethimide
		Unreactive:
		  Opiates
		  (high-dose)
		  Pilocarpine eye
		  drops

BEDSIDE EVALUATION

The following features of the bedside evaluation of depressed consciousness deserve mention.

Pupils

The conditions that affect pupillary size and light reactivity are shown in Table 50.1 (6–9). Dilated and unreactive pupils are usually signs of supratentorial (cerebral) injury. If the injury is due to diffuse cerebral ischemia, the pupillary abnormality is bilateral. If the injury is due to a mass lesion or cerebral edema with herniation, the pupillary abnormality will be unilateral (9). When atropine is given in the usual doses during cardiopulmonary resuscitation, the pupils will dilate but they usually remain reactive (6). If the pupils remain unreactive for longer than 6 hours after resuscitation from cardiac arrest, the prognosis for neurologic recovery is very poor (8).

Ocular Motility

Spontaneous eye movements (conjugate or dysconjugate) are a nonspecific sign in comatose patients. However, a fixed gaze preference involving one or both eyes is highly suggestive of a mass lesion or seizures (9).

Ocular Reflexes

The ocular reflexes can be used to evaluate the functional integrity of the lower brainstem (9). These reflexes are illustrated in Figure 50.2.

The **oculocephalic reflex** is elicited by rotating the patient's head from side to side (slowly at first, then briskly). When the cerebral hemispheres are impaired but the lower brainstem is intact, the eyes will deviate away from the direction of rotation (see the upper left panel in Figure 50.2). Because this eye movement resembles the fixed

Brainstem Intact

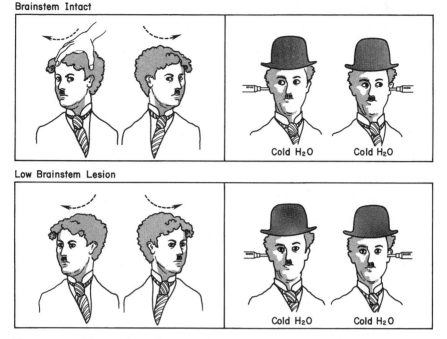

Low Brainstem Lesion

Figure 50.2. The ocular reflexes in the evaluation of coma. The oculocephalic reflex is demonstrated in the panels on the left, and the oculovestibular reflex is demonstrated in the panels on the right.

forward gaze of a doll's eyes, it is popularly known as the *doll's-eyes* movement (9). When the lower brainstem is damaged (or when the patient is awake), the eyes will follow the direction of head rotation (see the lower left panel in Figure 50.2). The oculocephalic reflex should not be attempted in patients with cervical arthritis or a suspected injury involving the cervical spine.

The **oculovestibular reflex** is elicited by injecting 30 mL of cold saline or tap water in the external auditory canal (using a 50-mL syringe and a 2-inch plastic catheter). When the brainstem is functionally intact, both eyes will deviate toward the irrigated ear. This conjugate eye movement is lost when the lower brainstem is damaged.

The Extremities

Clonic movements elicited by flexing the patient's hands or feet (asterixis) is a sign of a diffuse metabolic encephalopathy (4). A focal motor or sensory defect in the extremities (e.g., hemiparesis or asymmetric reflexes) can also be associated with a diffuse metabolic encephalopathy. However, the presence of focal neurologic defects should always prompt further investigation (with computed tomography) for a structural brain lesion.

THE GLASGOW COMA SCALE

The severity of a depressed level of consciousness is often evaluated with the Glasgow Coma Scale, which is shown in Table 50.2. Although this scale was originally proposed for patients with head injuries (10), it has gained widespread acceptance for use in the evaluation of non-traumatic coma as well (11–15). In the initial evaluation of nontraumatic coma, patients with a Glasgow Coma score of 6 or higher (out of a maximum score of 15) are seven times more likely to awaken than patients with a score of 5 or lower (11).

Limitations

The Glasgow Coma Scale is based on three indicators of cerebral function: eye opening, verbal communication, and motor responses to verbal and noxious stimuli. The verbal communication component is a problem in patients in the ICU who are intubated because these patients are unable to communicate verbally (13,14). The predictive value of the other components of the Glasgow Coma Scale are shown in Table 50.3. In this case, the predictive value refers to the chances of a satisfactory neurologic recovery in patients who remain comatose after resuscitation from cardiac arrest (15). In patients who show no response to verbal or noxious stimuli 1 hour after the cardiac arrest, 70 to 80 % will not have a satisfactory neurologic recovery. If these deficits persist for more than 3 days after the cardiac arrest, the chances of a satisfactory neurologic recovery are practically nil. Therefore, the

TABLE 50.2. THE GLASGOW COMA SCALE		
Eye Opening:	Points	
Spontaneous	4	
To speech	3	
To pain	2	
None	1	☐ Points
Verbal Communication:		
Oriented	5	
Confused conversation	4	
Inappropriate words	3	
Incomprehensible sounds	2	
None	1	☐ Points
Motor Response:		
Obeys commands	6	
Localizes to pain	5	
Withdraws to pain	4	
Abnormal flexion	3	
Abnormal extension	2	
None	1	☐ Points
	Total Points*	☐

* Best score is 15 points; worst score is 3 points.

TABLE 50.3. PREDICTIVE VALUE OF THE GLASGOW COMA SCALE			
	Negative Predictive Value Postarrest		
Parameter	1 hour (%)	24 hours (%)	3 days (%)
No eye opening to pain	69	92	100
No motor response to pain	75	91	100
No response to verbal stimuli	67	75	94
Glasgow Coma Score ≤5	69	—	100

Data from Edgren E et al. Assessment of neurologic prognosis in comatose survivors of cardiac arrest. Lancet 1994;343:1055–1059.

Glasgow Coma Scale can still provide prognostic information in patients who are intubated and unable to verbalize.

The data in Table 50.3 also demonstrates that the Glasgow Coma Scale does not reach its full predictive power in the first few hours after cardiac arrest. Therefore, **the Glasgow Coma Scale should not be used** to predict the chances for neurologic recovery **in the first few hours after cardiac arrest.**

DELIRIUM

Delirium is the most common mental disorder in hospitalized elderly patients (16–19), and it is the most common postoperative complication in the elderly (20). Surveys of hospitalized patients have found delirium in up to 50% of the elderly patients (19). Unfortunately, as many as three-fourths of the cases of delirium will be missed by physicians and nurses caring for the patients (16).

CLINICAL FEATURES

The clinical features of delirium are summarized in Table 50.4 (20). Delirium is a cognitive disorder that is characterized by attention deficits, disordered thinking, and a fluctuating symptomatology. The hallmark of delirium (and the features that distinguish delirium from dementia) is its acute onset and fluctuating clinical course.

Hypoactive Delirium

There is a tendency to consider delirium as a state of agitation (as in the delirium tremens syndrome). However, as shown in Table 50.4, there is also a hypoactive form of delirium that is characterized by lethargy rather than agitation. In fact, **hypoactive delirium (with lethargy) is the most common form of delirium in the elderly** (20), and this is certainly a source of many missed diagnoses of delirium in elderly patients.

TABLE 50.4. THE CLINICAL FEATURES OF DELIRIUM	
Feature	Description
1 Attention deficit	Inability to maintain or shift attention
2 Acute onset	Onset in hours to a few days
3 Fluctuating course	Day–night fluctuations; symptoms usually worse at night
4 Disorganized thinking	Illogical or irrelvant thoughts; incoherent or rambling speech
5 Altered consciousness	Hyperactive and hyperalert (agitated) or hypoactive and hypoalert (lethargic)
Delirium = 1 + 2 + 3 plus 4 or 5	

Adapted from Inouye SK et al. Clarifying confusion: the Confusion Assessment Method; a new method for detection of delirium. Ann Intern Med 1990;113: 941–948.

Delirium versus Dementia

Delirium and dementia are distinct mental disorders that are easily confused because they have overlapping clinical features (e.g., attention deficits and disordered thinking) (21). As mentioned earlier, the principal features of delirium that distinguish it from dementia are its acute onset and fluctuating course. However, as many as three-fourths of cases of delirium are superimposed on an underlying dementia (20), so the diagnosis of delirium in any individual patient does not exclude the presence of dementia.

ETIOLOGIES

The possible causes of delirium are listed in Figure 50.1. Any type encephalopathy (i.e., infectious, ischemic, drug-related, or metabolic) can cause a state of delirium. **Drugs** are implicated as causative or contributory factors in up to 40% of cases of delirium in the elderly (17–19). The drugs that are most likely to be responsible for delirium in patients in the ICU are listed in Table 50.5. The principal offenders in this list are alcohol (withdrawal), long-acting benzodiazepines (diazepam and flurazepam), and opiates (particularly meperidine) (17–19).

MANAGEMENT

The management of delirium should focus on identifying and treating the underlying cause of the problem. If agitation and disruptive behavior become a problem, the administration of sedatives is advised.

TABLE 50.5. DRUGS THAT CAN CAUSE DELIRIUM*	
Alcohol	Isoniazid
Amphotericin	Lidocaine
Aminoglycosides	Metaclopramide
Benzodiazepines	Metronidazole
β-Blockers	Opiates
Cephalosporins	Penicillin (high-dose)
Cimetidine	Phenytoin
Cocaine	Ranitidine
Corticosteroids (high-dose)	Theophylline
Digitalis	Trimethoprim–Sulfamethoxazole
Ibuprofen	

* List is limited to drugs that are likely to be encountered in patients in the ICU. From Med Lett 1986;28:81–86.

The choice of sedative is determined by the cause of the delirium (22–25), as indicated in the following.

ICU and Postoperative Delirium

For delirium that is ICU-related or develops postoperatively, the sedative of choice is haloperidol (22). (See Table 8.6 for haloperidol dosing recommendations.) The only drawback with intravenous haloperidol is its delayed onset of action (approximately 10 minutes). If rapid sedation is desired, a benzodiazepine (e.g., midazolam) can be used in the initial stages of management. However, **benzodiazepines should be avoided** for continued management because they can aggravate ICU-related and postoperative delirium (22).

Delirium Tremens

The management of delirium that accompanies alcohol withdrawal is the opposite of the management for ICU-related delirium. In this situation, the preferred sedatives are benzodiazepines, whereas haloperidol can aggravate the delirium and lower the seizure threshold (24,25). (See Table 8.3 for benzodiazepine dosing recommendations.)

If troublesome hypertension is a feature of delirium tremens, adjunctive therapy with clonidine (a centrally-acting α_2-agonist) can help both decrease the blood pressure and add to the sedation produced by benzodiazepines (24,25). The dose of clonidine is 0.1 mg orally every 2 hours until the pressure is controlled or a cumulative dose of 0.5 mg has been given (26). Clonidine is also available in a transdermal patch, but this is not recommended because of the delayed onset of action.

Cocaine-Induced Delirium

The management of cocaine-induced delirium is essentially the same as has been described for delirium tremens: benzodiazepines are the preferred sedatives, and haloperidol is not advised (23).

BRAIN DEATH

Brain death is a condition characterized by irreversible cessation of life-supporting function in the central nervous system (27,28). This condition is most often the result of severe intracranial injury or massive intracerebral hemorrhage or infarction. It is not a common consequence of the conditions listed in Figure 50.1.

DIAGNOSIS

A checklist for the diagnosis of brain death is shown in Table 50.6. Each of the criteria on this checklist should be satisfied on two separate occasions. The principal feature of brain death is the irreversible cessation of all purposeful electrical activity in the brain, including activity in the lower brainstem respiratory centers. This cessation of activity should have no contribution from sedating drugs or hypothermia.

Apnea Testing

The hallmark of the brain death determination is the demonstration of persistent apnea despite the presence of a hypercapnic stimulus to ventilation. To perform this apnea test, the patient is separated from the ventilator to allow the arterial Pco_2 to rise at least 10 mm Hg above the normal or baseline levels (the baseline arterial Pco_2 should not be below normal before this test). To prevent life-threatening hypoxemia during the apnea test, the test is preceded by a 10 to 15 minute period of ventilation with 100% oxygen (29,30). In addition, 100% oxygen can be insufflated into the trachea at a rate of 15 L/minute during the period of apnea (30). After the patient has been separated from the ventilator for a predetermined period (usually 10 minutes), an arterial blood gas measurement is obtained to document the desired increase in arterial Pco_2. If apnea persists despite the desired increase in arterial Pco_2, the test is confirmatory for the diagnosis of brain death.

ORGAN DONATION

If a patient with suspected or documented brain death is a candidate for organ donation, the following measure can be used to preserve organ viability during and after the brain death determination (31).

TABLE 50.6. CHECKLIST FOR THE DIAGNOSIS OF BRAIN DEATH

Brain death has occurred if the following criteria are met on two consecutive occasions, at least two hours apart.

1. Does not localize in response to noxious stimuli* ☐

2. Body temperature above 34° C ☐

3. Serum levels of the following are negligible or subtherapeutic:
   a. Ethanol
   b. CNS depressant drugs ☐

4. The following movements are absent:
   a. Decorticate posturing
   b. Decerebrate posturing
   c. Shivering
   d. Spontaneous movements ☐

5. The following reflexes are absent bilaterally†:
   a. Pupillary light reflex
   b. Corneal reflex
   c. Oculovestibular reflex
   d. Oculocephalic reflex (doll's eyes) ☐

6. EEG is isoelectric at maximal gain‡ ☐

7. Apnea test confirmatory§
   a. Pao_2 at end of test _____
   b. $Paco_2$ at end of test _____ ☐

* Painful stimuli should be localized to cranial nerve areas because of the risk of spinal cord reflexes with peripheral stimuli. The favored test is supraorbital pressure.

† Pupillary light reflexes can be absent after eye injury, neuromuscular blocking agents, atropine, mydriatics, scopolamine, and opiates.

‡ Isoelectric EEG does not exclude brainstem activity and is not to be used in isolation to make the diagnosis of brain death.

§ The apnea test is confirmatory if there is no evidence of spontaneous ventilatory efforts for at least 3 minutes and the $Paco_2$ is above 60 mm Hg at the end of the test. If there is a history of chronic CO_2 retention, the Pao_2 should be below 55 mm Hg at the end of the test.

Modified from the University of Pittsburgh criteria for brain death, with permission of B. C. Decker, Inc., Philadelphia.

A Safer Apnea Test

To prevent damaging hypoxemia during apnea testing, an alternative method is available in which the arterial Pco_2 is allowed to rise while the patient continues to receive assisted ventilation (32). This alternative method involves mechanical ventilation with 100% oxygen using intermittent mandatory ventilation (IMV). Hypoventilation is then induced by decreasing the number of machine breaths delivered by the ventilator, which allows the arterial Pco_2 to rise. This method is demonstrated in Figure 50.3. The total ventilation delivered by the ventilator is abruptly decreased from 11 to 1 L/minute, and the rise in arterial Pco_2 is monitored noninvasively with an end-tidal Pco_2 monitor. Note that the arterial oxygen saturation (Sao_2), which

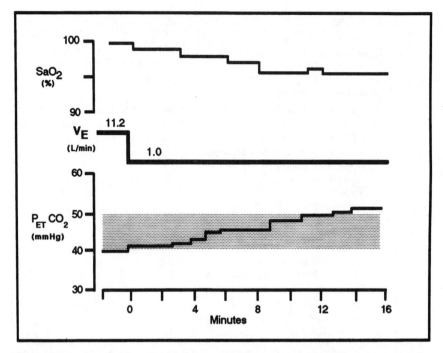

Figure 50.3. A safer apnea test that produces progressive hypercapnia while the patient continues to receive assisted ventilation. The step decrease in minute ventilation (from 11 to 1 L/minute) is produced by reducing the number of machine breaths delivered during intermittent mandatory ventilation (IMV). The rise in arterial P_{CO_2} is monitored noninvasively using an end-tidal CO_2 monitor ($P_{ET}CO_2$), and arterial oxygenation (SaO_2) is monitored continuously using a pulse oximeter. (From Gutmann DH, Marino PL. An alternative apnea test for the evaluation of brain death. Ann Neurol 1991; 30:852–853.)

is monitored continuously with a pulse oximeter, is maintained above 90% during the entire period of progressive hypercapnia (because the patient continues to receive some assisted ventilation). When the arterial P_{CO_2} rises to the desired level, the patient can then be separated from the ventilator to observe for persistent apnea.

Hemodynamics

Hypotension or an impaired cardiac output in potential organ donors should be corrected by infusing dobutamine (for positive inotropic effects) or dopamine (for positive inotropic and vasoconstrictor effects) as described in Chapter 18. If a pulmonary artery catheter is in place, the goal of hemodynamic management should be a systemic oxygen uptake above 100 mL/min/m^2 and a serum lactate concentration below 4 mmol/L (see Chapter 13).

Pituitary Failure

More than half of patients with brain death will develop pituitary failure with diabetes insipidus and secondary adrenal insufficiency (31). Both conditions can lead to profound hypovolemia (and reduced organ perfusion) and hypertonic hypernatremia (and cell dehydration). If there is evidence of a central diabetes insipidus (i.e., spontaneous diuresis with a urine osmolality below 200 mOsm/L), treatment with **desmopressin** (a form of vasopressin that does not cause vasoconstriction) is advised (31). If there is evidence of adrenal insufficiency (i.e., hypotension refractory to vasopressors), treatment with **hydrocortisone** (see dosages in Chapter 49) is advised.

REFERENCES

INTRODUCTION

1. Bleck TP, Smith MC, Pierre-Louis J-C, et al. Neurologic complications of critical medical illnesses. Crit Care Med 1993;21:98–103.
2. Kelly BJ, Matthay MA. Prevalence and severity of neurologic dysfunction in critically ill patients. Chest 1993;104:1818–1824.

DEPRESSED CONSCIOUSNESS

3. Roberts JR, Wason S, Soegel E. Pneumonic for diagnosis of acute mental status changes. Ann Emerg Med 1990;19:221–222.
4. Mahler J, Young GB. Septic encephalopathy. Intensive Care Med 1993;38:177–187.
5. Sprung CL, Cerra FB, Freund HR, et al. Amino acid alterations and encephalopathy in the sepsis syndrome. Crit Care Med 1991;19:753–757.
6. Goetting MG, Contreras E. Systemic atropine administration during cardiac arrest does not cause fixed and dilated pupils. Ann Emerg Med 1991;20:55–57.
7. Ong GL, Bruning HA. Dilated fixed pupils due to administration of high doses of dopamine hydrochloride. Crit Care Med 1981;9:658–660.
8. Steen-Hansen JE, Hansen NN, Vaagenes P, Schreiner B. Pupil size and light reactivity during cardiopulmonary resuscitation: a clinical study. Crit Care Med 1988;16:69–70.
9. Weisberg LA. Differential diagnosis of coma: a step-by-step strategy. J Crit Illness 1989;4:97–108.

GLASGOW COMA SCALE

10. Teasdale G, Jennett B. Assessment of coma and impaired consciousness. Lancet 1974;2:81–84.
11. Sacco RL, VanGool R, Mohr JP, Hauser WA. Nontraumatic coma: Glasgow Coma Score and coma etiology as predictors of 2-week outcome. Arch Neurol 1990;47:1181–1184.
12. Hamel MB, Goldman L, Teno J, et al. Identification of comatose patients at high risk for death or severe disability. JAMA 1995;273:1842–1848.

13. Segatore M, Way C. The Glasgow Coma Scale: time for change. Heart Lung 1992;21:548–557.
14. Marion D. The Glasgow Coma Scale score: contemporary application. Intensive Care World 1994;11:101–102.
15. Edgren E, Hedstrand U, Kelsey S, et al. Assessment of neurologic prognosis in comatose survivors of cardiac arrest. Lancet 1994;343:1055–1059.

DELIRIUM

16. Inouye SK. The dilemma of delirium: clinical and research controversies regarding diagnosis and evaluation of delirium in hospitalized elderly medical patients. Ann Intern Med 1994;97:278–288.
17. Rummans TA, Evans JM, Krahn LE, Fleming KC. Delirium in elderly patients: evaluation and management. Mayo Clin Proc 1995;70:989–998.
18. Francis J, Martin D, Kapoor WN. A prospective study of delirium in the hospitalized elderly. JAMA 1990;263:1097–1101.
19. Marcantonio ER, Juarez G, Goldman L, et al. The relationship of postoperative delirium with psychoactive medications. JAMA 1994;272:1518–1522.
20. Inouye SK, van Dyck CH, Alessi CA, et al. Clarifying confusion: the confusion assessment method: a new method for detection of delirium. Ann Intern Med 1990;113:941–948.
21. Fleming KC, Adams AC, Petersen RC. Dementia: diagnosis and evaluation. Mayo Clin Proc 1995;70:1093–1107.
22. Weissman C. Strategies for managing delirium in critically ill patients. J Crit Illness 1996;11:295–307.
23. Hoffman RS. An effective strategy for managing cocaine-induced agitated delirium. J Crit Illness 1994;9:139–149.

DELIRIUM TREMENS

24. Lohr RH. Treatment of alcohol withdrawal in hospitalized patients. Mayo Clin Proc 1995;70:777–782.
25. Crippen DW. Strategies for managing delirium tremens in the ICU. J Crit Illness 1997;12:140–149.
26. Gales MA. Oral antihypertensives for hypertensive urgencies. Ann Pharmacother 1994;28:352–357.

BRAIN DEATH

27. Curry PD, Bion JF. The diagnosis and management of brain death. Curr Anaesth Crit Care 1994;5:36–40.
28. Wijdicks EFM. Diagnosis and management of brain death in the intensive care unit. In: Neurology of critical illness. Philadelphia: FA Davis, 1995;323–337.
29. Benzel EC, Gross CD, Hadden TA, et al. The apnea test for the determination of brain death. J Neurosurg 1989;71:191–194.
30. Marks SJ, Zisfein J. Apneic oxygenation in apnea tests for brain death. Arch Neurol 1990;47:1066–1068.
31. Detterbeck FC, Mill MR, Williams W, Egan TM. Organ donation and the management of the multiple organ donor. Contemp Surg 1993;42:281–285.
32. Gutmann D, Marino PL. An alternative apnea test for the evaluation of brain death. Ann Neurol 1991;30:852–853.

SUGGESTED READINGS

Grotta JC, ed. Management of the acutely ill neurologic patient. New York: Churchill Livingstone, 1993.

Plum F, Posner JB. The diagnosis of stupor and coma. 3d ed. Philadelphia: FA Davis, 1982.

Wijdicks EFM. Neurology of critical illness. Philadelphia: FA Davis, 1995.

51

DISORDERS OF MOVEMENT

This chapter focuses on three general types of movement disorders encountered in critically ill patients: involuntary movements (seizures), weak or ineffective movements (neuromuscular weakness), and no movements (neuromuscular blockade).

SEIZURES

Seizures are second only to metabolic encephalopathies as the most common neurologic complication encountered in patients in the ICU (1).

DEFINITIONS

The following definitions will prove helpful in the description, evaluation, and treatment of seizures (2,3).

Types of Movement

Seizures can be accompanied by any of the following patterns of muscle contraction: tonic contractions (sustained muscle contraction), atonic contractions (absence of muscle contraction), clonic contractions (periodic muscle contractions with a regular amplitude and frequency), or myoclonus (periodic muscle contractions with an irregular amplitude and frequency). Seizures may also be accompanied by familiar movements called automatisms (e.g., lip smacking or chewing).

Generalized Seizures

Generalized seizures arise from symmetric and synchronous electrical discharges involving the entire cerebral cortex. These seizures may or may not be accompanied by muscle contractions. Generalized seizures that are not accompanied by prominent muscle contractions are called *absence* seizures (formerly known as petit-mal seizures).

Partial Seizures

Partial seizures arise from electrical discharges that are confined to a focal or restricted part of the cerebral cortex. They are subdivided into simple partial seizures (do not impair consciousness) and complex partial seizures (cause impaired consciousness). Two types of partial complex seizures that deserve mention are temporal lobe seizures (characterized by a motionless stare and automatisms) and *epilepsia partialis continua* (characterized by persistent tonic-clonic movements of the facial muscles and limb muscles on one side of the body).

Status Epilepticus

Status epilepticus is defined as more than 30 minutes of continuous seizure activity or two or more sequential seizures without an intervening period of consciousness.

ETIOLOGIES

New-onset seizures can be the result of a drug intoxication (e.g., theophylline), drug withdrawal (e.g., ethanol), infections (e.g., meningoencephalitis, abscess), ischemic injury (e.g., focal or diffuse), space-occupying lesions (e.g., tumor or hemorrhage), or metabolic derangements (e.g., hepatic or uremic encephalopathy, hypoglycemia, hyponatremia, hypocalcemia). In one survey of new-onset seizures in patients in the ICU, the most common causes were drug intoxications and drug withdrawal (4). The drugs most likely to be implicated as a cause of seizures in patients in the ICU are listed in Table 51.1 (5).

TABLE 51.1. DRUG-RELATED SEIZURES IN THE ICU	
Drug withdrawal:	Barbiturates
	Benzodiazepines
	Ethanol
	Opiates
Drug intoxication:	
Drugs of Abuse:	Amphetamines
	Cocaine
	Phencyclidine
Pharmaceuticals:	Ciprofloxacin
	Imipenem
	Lidocaine
	Penicillin
	Theophylline
	Tricyclics

Status Epilepticus

Approximately 50% of cases of status epilepticus occur as new-onset seizures. The most common cause is acute cerebrovascular injury (ischemia, hemorrhage). Hypoglycemia and central nervous system infections are uncommon offenders.

Evaluation

The evaluation of new-onset seizures should focus on the etiologies previously mentioned. In the absence of an obvious metabolic or drug-related cause or when the physical examination reveals a focal abnormality, further evaluation (with neuroimaging studies and lumbar puncture) is advised.

MANAGEMENT

Most seizures encountered in the ICU are generalized or partial seizures associated with tonic-clonic movements (i.e., convulsive seizures). The acute management of convulsive seizures is summarized in Table 51.2, which uses the recommendations for status epilepticus (6).

Benzodazepines

Intravenous benzodiazepines are the initial drugs of choice for suppression of convulsive seizures. Intravenous diazepam (Valium) in a dose of 0.2 mg/kg will terminate seizure activity within 5 minutes in approximately 80% of cases, but the effect lasts only 30 minutes (6).

TABLE 51.2. DRUG TREATMENT OF CONVULSIVE STATUS EPILEPTICUS		
Drug	**Indication**	**Parenteral Dose**
Diazepam	Initial treatment	0.2 mg/kg at 5 mg/min. Can be repeated in 5 minutes if necessary. Can be infused at 0.1 to 0.2 mg/kg/hr (if history of hypersensitivity to phenytoin).
Lorazepam	Initial treatment	0.1 mg/kg at 2 mg/min.
Phenytoin	Following treatment with diazepam	15 to 20 mg/kg at a maximum rate of 50 mg/min. (Use lower dose in the elderly.)
Phenobarbital	Persistent seizures after above treatment	20 mg/kg at a maximum rate of 100 mg/min.
From the Epilepsy Foundation of America Working Group on Status Epilepticus. Treatment of convulsive status epilepticus. JAMA 1993;270:854–859.		

Intravenous lorazepam (Ativan) in a dose of 0.1 mg/kg is as effective as diazepam and has a longer duration of action (12 to 24 hours).

Phenytoin

Because of its short duration of action, intravenous diazepam should always be followed by phenytoin to prevent recurrence of seizures. The standard intravenous dose of phenytoin is 20 mg/kg in adults, but a smaller dose of 15 mg/kg is recommended for elderly patients (6). A maximum infusion rate of 50 mg/minute is advised to reduce the risk of cardiovascular depression from phenytoin (which may be related to the propylene glycol solvent used in intravenous phenytoin preparations) (7). If the initial dose of phenytoin is unsuccessful, additional doses of 5 mg/kg can be given to a total cumulative dose of 30 mg/kg (6). The therapeutic serum level for phenytoin is 10 to 20 mg/L.

In patients with a history of anticonvulsant hypersensitivity syndrome (fever, rash, and lymphadenopathy in response to phenytoin administration), status epilepticus can be managed with a continuous intravenous infusion of diazepam using the infusion rate shown in Table 51.2 (8).

Phenobarbital

The combination of benzodiazepines and phenytoin will control seizures in 90% of cases of status epilepticus. In the remaining 10% of cases, intravenous phenobarbital will achieve control in approximately half the cases (6). Phenobarbital is given in a dose of 100 mg/minute until the seizures are controlled or a maximum dose of 20 mg/kg is achieved. The therapeutic serum level for phenobarbital is 10 to 40 mg/L. The higher dosage range will produce profound and prolonged sedation, so the patient may not awaken for several hours after the seizures are suppressed.

Approximately 5% of patients with status epilepticus will be refractory to benzodiazepines, phenytoin, and phenobarbital. These refractory cases may require inhalational anesthesia and neuromuscular paralysis (9). At this stage, a neurologic consultation should be obtained immediately.

NEUROMUSCULAR WEAKNESS

The following is a brief description of three neuromuscular disorders that can produce severe and life-threatening neuromuscular weakness. Some of the comparative features of these disorders are included in Table 51.3.

MYASTHENIA GRAVIS

Myasthenia gravis is an autoimmune disease characterized by antibody-mediated destruction of postsynaptic acetylcholine receptors at

TABLE 51.3. COMPARATIVE FEATURES OF THREE NEUROMUSCULAR DISORDERS			
Features	Myasthenia Gravis	Guillain-Barré Syndrome	Critical Illness Polyneuropathy
Ocular findings	Yes	No	No
Fluctuating weakness	Yes	No	No
Bulbar weakness	Yes	Yes	No
Deep tendon reflexes	Intact	Depressed	Depressed
Autonomic instability	No	Yes	No
Nerve conduction	Normal	Abnormal	Abnormal

neuromuscular junctions. The illness is uncommon and affects approximately 1 in every 100,000 adults (10).

Clinical Features

The weakness in myasthenia gravis characteristically becomes worse with repeated activity. Signs of weakness are usually first evident in the eyelids and extraocular muscles, and generalized weakness follows in 85% of cases (10). The proximal limb muscles are often affected, and weakness can involve the diaphragm and thoracic musculature. Rapid progression to respiratory failure and ventilator dependence, called *myasthenic crisis,* can occur. The deficit in myasthenia is purely motor, with no sensory involvement. Deep tendon reflexes are usually preserved.

In addition to concurrent illness and surgery, several drugs can precipitate or aggravate the myasthenic syndrome. The principal offenders are antibiotics (e.g., aminoglycosides), cardiac drugs (e.g., lidocaine, procainamide, quinidine), and magnesium (11). Aminoglycosides can precipitate a myasthenic syndrome that resolves when the drugs are discontinued. Magnesium blocks the presynaptic release of acetylcholine and can be particularly detrimental in myasthenic patients.

Diagnosis

The diagnosis of myasthenia gravis is based on the characteristic pattern of muscle weakness (e.g., eyelid or extraocular muscle weakness, worse with activity) and the finding of enhanced muscle strength after the administration of an anticholinesterase inhibitor such as edrophonium (Tensilon). A radioimmunoassay for acetylcholine receptor antibodies in the blood is positive in 85% of cases (10) and confirms the diagnosis. Once the diagnosis is confirmed, a search for associated conditions such as thymic tumors (10% of cases) and hyperthyroidism (5% of cases) is advised.

Treatment

Anticholinesterase agents are the first line of therapy in myasthenia gravis. Pyridostigmine (Mestinon) is started at a dosage of 60 mg orally (or 2 mg intramuscularly) every 8 hours and can be increased if necessary to a maximum dosage of 120 mg orally (or 4 mg intramuscularly) every 8 hours. Immunotherapy is added if needed with prednisone (20 to 60 mg/day), azathioprine (2 to 3 mg/kg/day), or cyclosporine (5 mg/kg/day) (10). In advanced cases requiring mechanical ventilation, plasmapheresis (to remove acetylcholine antibodies) is often effective in producing short-term improvement. Surgical thymectomy is often advised in patients under 60 years of age to reduce the need for immunosuppressive therapy (10).

GUILLAIN-BARRÉ SYNDROME

Guillain-Barré syndrome is an acute inflammatory demyelinating polyneuropathy that is preceded by an acute infectious illness in two-thirds of cases (12,13). The disorder is considered to be immune in origin, but the precise mechanism remains unclear.

Clinical Features

This condition presents with paresthesias and symmetric limb weakness that evolves over a period of a few days to a few weeks. Symptoms of a preceding infection usually subside before the weakness becomes apparent. Approximately 20% of patients progress to respiratory failure that requires mechanical ventilation (12,13). Advanced cases can also be characterized by autonomic instability and bulbar paralysis. The condition resolves spontaneously in approximately 85% of cases, but residual neurologic deficits are common (12).

Diagnosis

The diagnosis is based on the clinical picture (i.e., progressive, symmetric limb weakness following an acute infectious illness). Axonal degeneration can be documented by nerve conduction studies if necessary.

Treatment

The treatment of Guillain-Barré syndrome mostly involves supportive care. In severe cases requiring mechanical ventilation, both plasmapheresis and intravenous immune globulin (0.4 g/kg/day) can produce transient improvement (14), but the treatment effects are much less marked than in myasthenia gravis. Because this disorder resolves spontaneously in most cases, careful attention to complications (e.g., respiratory failure, thromboembolism) is mandatory for a satisfactory outcome. The respiratory management of this disorder is described later in the chapter.

CRITICAL ILLNESS POLYNEUROPATHY

In patients with systemic sepsis and multiorgan dysfunction (see Chapter 31), one of the organs that can be affected is the peripheral nervous system. The result is a diffuse peripheral neuropathy called critical illness polyneuropathy (15).

Clinical Features

As many as 70% of patients with systemic sepsis and multiorgan dysfunction will have evidence of a combined motor and sensory polyneuropathy on nerve conduction studies (16). This disorder is clinically silent in most cases, but it can produce severe limb and truncal weakness on occasion. Most cases occur in patients who have been ventilator-dependent for at least 1 week (17). The weakness usually becomes evident when the sepsis begins to resolve, and it can delay weaning from mechanical ventilation (17). Many of the patients have received neuromuscular blocking agents, and the condition presents as persistent weakness after neuromuscular paralysis is discontinued. Autonomic dysfunction and bulbar weakness are uncommon, which helps distinguish this condition from Guillain-Barré syndrome (17).

The diagnosis of critical illness polyneuropathy is suggested by the clinical setting (i.e., limb and truncal weakness associated with severe sepsis and multiorgan dysfunction) and by the exclusion of other neuromuscular disorders. Nerve conduction studies or electromyography can performed to document axonal degeneration (17), but these studies should not be necessary in most cases. No specific treatment exists, but spontaneous recovery occurs in many cases.

PULMONARY COMPLICATIONS

The pulmonary consequences of progressive neuromuscular weakness are summarized in Table 51.4. Respiratory muscle strength must

TABLE 51.4. Respiratory Consequences of Neuromuscular Weakness		
Vital Capacity (mL/kg)	Consequences	Management
70	Normal respiratory muscle strength	Observe
30	Impaired cough, with difficulty clearing secretions	Chest physiotherapy
25	Accumulation of secretions, with risk of infection and airways obstruction	Tracheal intubation
20	Atelectasis and progressive hypoxemia	Supplemental oxygen
10	Alveolar hypoventilation and hypercapnia	Mechanical ventilation

decrease considerably before pulmonary complications appear. The earliest complication is a depressed cough with difficulty clearing secretions. This can lead to retained secretions with infection and airways obstruction. When patients are unable to clear secretions adequately, tracheal intubation is indicated to help clear secretions. As the neuromuscular weakness progresses, atelectasis and hypoxemia become prominent, followed by alveolar hypoventilation and progressive CO_2 retention.

One of the important features to note in Table 51.4 is the fact that tracheal intubation is often necessary before the appearance of progressive hypoxemia and hypercapnia. In other words, in neuromuscular disorders that involve the respiratory muscles, **early intubation before the onset of respiratory failure is often necessary** (13,18) The most sensitive measure of respiratory muscle strength is the maximum inspiratory pressure (P_{Imax}) (19), which is described in Chapter 29. A P_{Imax} that falls below 30 cm H_2O is evidence of severe respiratory muscle weakness and is an indication for tracheal intubation and assisted ventilation.

NEUROMUSCULAR BLOCKADE

Drug-induced neuromuscular blockade is a common practice in ICUs for managing ventilator-dependent patients who are agitated and difficult to ventilate. However, this practice has serious drawbacks (20), as described later.

MECHANISMS

Neuromuscular blocking agents act by binding to acetylcholine receptors on the postsynaptic side of the neuromuscular junction. Once bound, there are two different modes of action. The *depolarizing agents* act like acetylcholine and depolarize the postsynaptic membrane. However, they produce a sustained depolarization, which blocks the propagation of electrical impulses along the muscle. The *nondepolarizing agents* act by blocking acetylcholine-induced activation of the postsynaptic membrane.

NEUROMUSCULAR BLOCKERS

The neuromuscular blocking drugs that are used most commonly in the ICU are shown in Table 51.5 (21). All three agents in this table are nondepolarizing blockers.

Pancuronium (Pavulon) is a relatively long-acting neuromuscular blocker (duration of action is 1 to 2 hours) that was introduced for clinical use in 1972. The initial popularity of this agent has dwindled because of its long duration of action (can accumulate with repeated use) and vagolytic effects (which can produce tachycardia and hyper-

TABLE 51.5. COMPARATIVE FEATURES OF NEUROMUSCULAR BLOCKERS			
	Pancuronium (Pavulon)	Vecuronium (Norcuron)	Atracurium (Tracrium)
Initial dose	0.10 mg/kg	0.10 mg/kg	0.50 mg/kg
Usual dose	0.02 mg/kg	0.02 mg/kg	0.1 mg/kg
Duration of action	60–90 min	25–30 min	20–35 min
Infusion rate	1 μg/kg/min	1 μg/kg/min	7 μg/kg/min
Approximate cost of equipotent dose*	$2.00	$5.80	$6.30

* Cost represents 1 hour of neuromuscular blockade in a 70-kg adult. Drug costs (per mg) from Reference 22. Drug doses from Reference 21.

tension). Although pancuronium can be given by continuous infusion, it is usually given as intermittent bolus doses because of the risk of drug accumulation. Pancuronium is excreted by the kidneys, and dosage reductions are often necessary in renal failure.

Vecuronium (Norcuron) is a chemical analog of pancuronium but is shorter acting and has no vagolytic effects. The dosing of vecuronium is similar to that for pancuronium. Because of its short duration of action (30 minutes), it is often given by continuous infusion.

Atracurium (Tracrium) is also shorter acting than pancuronium and can be given by continuous infusion. This agent can release histamine from mast cells and produce hypotension when given too rapidly. For this reason, bolus injections should be given over 2 to 4 minutes.

Succinylcholine (Anectine) is a depolarizing agent that is not included in Table 51.5 because it is used relatively infrequently. This agent is ultra-short acting and is most often used to facilitate tracheal intubation. An intravenous dose of 1 to 2 mg/kg produces paralysis within 2 minutes, and the effect disappears within 10 minutes. The prolonged depolarization produced by this agent is accompanied by a large efflux of potassium out of muscle cells, and this results in a transient rise in serum potassium of 0.5 to 1.0 mEq/L (21). Life-threatening increases in serum potassium have been recorded in patients with acute neurologic injury and burns.

MONITORING

The standard method of monitoring the adequacy of neuromuscular blockade involves stimulating the ulnar nerve at the wrist to produce adduction of the thumb. The stimulating electrical current is small (50 to 80 milliamps) and it is imperceptible to the patient. Because nondepolarizing neuromuscular blockade is exaggerated by repeated nerve stimulation, a series of repetitive stimuli can be applied to the ulnar nerve and the movement of the thumb can be observed for evidence of a progressive decrement in response. The standard method is to apply a series of 4 stimuli in succession and compare the thumb movement in response to the first and fourth stimuli. This method is called the *train-of-four* stimulation technique (23). Total absence of thumb movement is evidence for excessive neuromuscular blockade, whereas absence of a decrement in thumb contractions with repetitive nerve stimulation is evidence of inadequate blockade.

DISADVANTAGES

Inadequate Sedation

Neuromuscular blocking drugs do not produce sedation, and because paralysis is an extremely frightening and even painful experience, heavy sedation is *mandatory* during neuromuscular blockade. Unfortunately, it is impossible to determine whether sedation is adequate in a patient who is paralyzed, so generous doses of sedative agents is advised. Because immobilization is often a painful experience, opiates may be preferred for sedation.

Prolonged Paralysis

A number of reports have documented prolonged neuromuscular paralysis after discontinuing therapy with neuromuscular blocking agents (24). This phenomenon often occurs after prolonged neuromuscular blockade (longer than 1 week), but it can also occur after just a few doses of neuromuscular blockers. There is no evidence that this problem is related to the drug that is used. Shorter periods and intermittent cessation of neuromuscular blockade have been recommended to limit the risk of prolonged paralysis (24). However, the best preventive measure is to eliminate the use of neuromuscular blockade whenever possible.

Hypostatic Pneumonia

Clearance of respiratory secretions is inadequate during neuromuscular paralysis. Endotracheal suction catheters are unable to reach the distal airways, and in the absence of cough to help clear secretions, there will be pooling of secretions in dependent lung regions. This can lead to hypostatic pneumonia.

Venous Thromboembolism

Loss of the milking action of muscle contraction on the venous return from the legs predisposes to venous thrombosis during neuromuscular paralysis. Therefore, prophylaxis for venous thrombosis (as described in Chapter 7) is mandatory during neuromuscular paralysis.

In summary, the risks of neuromuscular paralysis are considerable enough to consider avoiding the use of neuromuscular blocking agents whenever possible. With the aggressive use of sedation, avoiding these agents will be easier than anticipated.

REFERENCES

SEIZURES

1. Bleck TP, Smith MC, Pierre-Louis SJ-C, et al. Neurologic complications of critical medical illnesses. Crit Care Med 1993;21:98–103.
2. Mosewich RK, So EL. A clinical approach to the classification of seizures and epileptic syndromes. Mayo Clin Proc 1996;71:405–414.
3. Seamens CM, Slovis CM, Kramer D, Gavin LJ. Seizures: current clinical guidelines for evaluation and emergency management. Emerg Med Rep 1995;16: 23–30.
4. Wijdicks EFM, Sharbrough FW. New-onset seizures in critically ill patients. Neurology 1993;43:1042–1044.
5. Wijdicks EFM. Seizures in the intensive care unit. In: Neurology of critical illness. Philadelphia: FA Davis, 1995;18–33.
6. Epilepsy Foundation of America's Working Group on Status Epilepticus. Treatment of Convulsive Status Epilepticus. JAMA 1993;270:854–859.
7. Louis S, Kott H, McDonell F. The cardiocirculatory changes caused by intravenous Dilantin and its solvent. Am Heart J 1967;74:523–529.
8. Bertz RJ, Howrie DL. Diazepam by continuous intravenous infusion for status epilepticus in anticonvulsant hypersensitivity syndrome. Ann Pharmacother 1993;27:298–301.
9. Jagoda A, Riggio S. Refractory status epilepticus in adults. Ann Emerg Med 1993;22:1337–1348.

MYASTHENIA GRAVIS

10. Drachman DB. Myasthenia gravis. N Engl J Med 1994;330:1797–1810.
11. London SF, Ringel SP. Neuromuscular emergencies. In: Weiner WJ, ed. Emergent and urgent neurology. Philadelphia: JB Lippincott, 1992;59–78.

GUILLAIN-BARRÉ SYNDROME

12. Ropper AH. Guillain-Barré syndrome. N Engl J Med 1992;326:1130–1136.
13. Hund EF, Borel CO, Cornblath DR, et al. Intensive management and treatment of Guillain-Barré syndrome. Crit Care Med 1993;21:433–446.
14. van der Meche FGA, Schmitz PIM, the Dutch Guillain-Barré Study Group. A randomized trial comparing intravenous immune globulin and plasma exchange in Guillain-Barré syndrome. N Engl J Med 1992;326:1123–1129.

CRITICAL ILLNESS POLYNEUROPATHY

15. Bolton CF. Polyneuropathy in critically ill patients. J Neurol Neurosurg Psychiatry 1984;47:1223–1231.
16. Witt NJ, Zochodne DW, Bolton CF, et al. Peripheral nerve function in sepsis and multiple organ failure. Chest 1991;99:176–184.
17. Leijten FSS, Harinck-de Weerd JE, Poortvliet DCJ, de Weerd AW. The role of

polyneuropathy in motor convalescence after prolonged mechanical ventilation. JAMA 1995;274:1221–1225.

PULMONARY COMPLICATIONS

18. Newton-John H. Prevention of pulmonary complications in severe Guillain-Barré syndrome by early assisted ventilation. Med J Aust 1985;142:444.
19. Mier-Jedrzejowicz AK, Brophy C, Green M. Respiratory muscle function in myasthenia gravis. Am Rev Respir Dis 1988;138:867–873.

NEUROMUSCULAR BLOCKADE

20. Hansen-Flaschen J, Cowen J, Raps E. Neuromuscular blockade in the intensive care unit. More than we bargained for. Am Rev Respir Dis 1993;147:234–236.
21. Prielipp RC, Coursin DB. Applied pharmacology of common neuromuscular blocking agents in critical care. New Horiz 1994;2:34–47.
22. Armstrong DK, Crisp CB. Pharmacoeconomic issues of sedation, analgesia, and neuromuscular blockade in critical care. New Horiz 1994;2:85–93.
23. Davidson JE. Neuromuscular blockade: indications, peripheral nerve stimulation, and other concurrent interventions. New Horiz 1994;2:75–84.
24. Watling SM, Dasta JF. Prolonged paralysis in intensive care unit patients after the use of neuromuscular blocking agents: a review of the literature. Crit Care Med 1994;22:884–893.

SUGGESTED READINGS

Grotta JC, ed. Management of the acutely ill neurologic patient. New York: Churchill Livingstone, 1993.
Wijdicks EFM. Neurology of critical illness. Philadelphia: FA Davis, 1995.

chapter

52

STROKE AND RELATED DISORDERS

Stroke (a poorly descriptive term for acute brain injury of vascular origin) is the third leading cause of death in the United States and is responsible for approximately one-fourth of all deaths in the adult population. Considering these credentials, stroke should occupy a top position in the hierarchy of life-threatening conditions. However, stroke has traditionally received little attention from critical care specialists. This has changed in recent years. The current view of acute cerebral infarction emphasizes the similarities to acute myocardial infarction and stresses the value of approaching a *brain attack* with the same aggressive measures used in the approach to a heart attack (1,2).

DEFINITIONS

The clinical disorders described in this chapter are cerebrovascular disorders. The following are some definitions and classifications for these disorders proposed by the National Institute of Neurologic Disorders and Stroke (3).

STROKE

Stroke is a clinical condition with all the following features (3,4):

1. An **acute** neurologic disorder
2. Produced by **nontraumatic** injury in the central nervous system that is vascular in origin
3. Accompanied by **focal** rather than global neurologic dysfunction
4. Persists for **longer than 24 hours** or results in death within the first 24 hours

Classifications

Stroke can be classified as ischemic or hemorrhagic based on the type of pathologic injury. Approximately 80% of strokes are ischemic and 15% are hemorrhagic (10% caused by intracerebral hemorrhage, and 5% caused by subarachnoid hemorrhage) (5). Ischemic strokes can be further classified as thrombotic or embolic in origin. Thrombotic strokes originate in the same fashion as described for acute myocardial infarction (MI) (see Chapter 19). Embolic strokes account for 20% of ischemic strokes (6). Most emboli originate from thrombi in the left atrium (from atrial fibrillation) and left ventricle (from acute MI), but occasionally they can arise from deep vein thrombosis in the legs that embolized through a patent foramen ovale (7).

Stroke can also be classified according to the rapidity of neurologic recovery. A minor stroke, also called a *reversible ischemic neurologic deficit* (RIND), is characterized by complete recovery of neurologic function within 3 weeks after the acute event (3). A major stroke is characterized by neurologic deficits that persist for longer than 3 weeks after the event.

TRANSIENT ISCHEMIC ATTACK

A transient ischemic attack (TIA) is an episode of focal loss of brain function (as a result of ischemia) that lasts less than 24 hours (3). The major distinction between TIA and stroke is the underlying pathology; i.e., ischemia in TIA versus infarction or hemorrhage in stroke. This, in turn, determines the duration of the neurologic deficits: less than 24 hours in TIA and longer than 24 hours in stroke.

BEDSIDE EVALUATION

The patient with a suspected stroke will have new-onset focal neurologic deficits that are not traumatic in origin. If the deficits have been present for less than 24 hours, it is often impossible to distinguish TIA from stroke. The following features of the clinical presentation can be useful in the evaluation of suspected stroke (8). These features are included in Table 52.1.

Seizures

Generalized convulsive seizures and convulsive status epilepticus are uncommon in TIA and stroke. Seizures develop in approximately 10% of cases of stroke (4). They usually appear in the first 24 hours and are focal rather than generalized in most cases.

Fever

Fever is uncommon in TIA but can be present in approximately 50% of patients with stroke (9). In most cases of fever associated with stroke,

TABLE 52.1. THE BEDSIDE EVALUATION OF SUSPECTED STROKE	
Manifestation	Comment
Fever	Fever can be present in 50% of patients with stroke, but it is usually the result of conditions other than the stroke.
Seizures	Generalized convulsive seizures and convulsive status epilepticus are uncommon in ischemic stroke.
Coma	Coma is not expected in cerebral infarction and suggests possible intracerebral hemorrhage, massive infarction with cerebral edema, or seizures.
Aphasia	The presence of aphasia indicates probable ischemia or infarction involving the left middle cerebral artery.
Limb weakness	Demonstrated by inability to hold arm in a raised position for 10 seconds or inability to hold leg 30° above the horizontal plane for 5 seconds.

the fever is due to a process other than the stroke (e.g., infection or thromboembolism).

Consciousness

The reticular activating system in the brainstem is responsible for arousal or wakefulness (consciousness). Because most cases of stroke are the result of *cerebral* infarction, loss of consciousness is not a common finding in uncomplicated stroke (1,4). When focal neurologic deficits are accompanied by coma, the most likely diagnoses are intracerebral hemorrhage, massive cerebral infarction with cerebral edema, brainstem infarction, or seizures (nonconvulsive seizures or postictal state).

Aphasia

The left cerebral hemisphere is the dominant hemisphere for speech in 90% of subjects. Damage involving the left cerebral hemisphere produces a condition known as aphasia, which is defined as a disturbance in the comprehension and formulation of language (10). Patients with aphasia can have difficulty understanding verbal remarks (receptive aphasia), difficulty in verbal expression (expressive aphasia), or both (global aphasia). Most patients with aphasia will have a cerebral infarction in the distribution of the left middle cerebral artery (10). Other causes of aphasia are tumors, head injury, and Alzheimer's dementia.

Weakness

The hallmark of ischemia or hemorrhagic injury involving the cerebral hemispheres is weakness in the contralateral limbs. Limb weakness is present if the patient is unable to hold the arm in 90 degrees of abduction for 10 seconds or unable to hold the leg 30 degrees above the horizontal plane for 5 seconds (11). The presence of a hemiparesis supports the diagnosis of TIA or stroke. However, hemiparesis has also been described in metabolic encephalopathy caused by renal failure (12) and sepsis (13).

DIAGNOSTIC EVALUATION

The diagnostic evaluation of suspected stroke has traditionally proceeded at a slow pace. However, as mentioned in the introduction to this chapter, the current view of ischemic stroke stresses the similarities with acute MI, and the need to approach acute stroke with the same alacrity used in the approach to acute MI. According to the U.S. National Stroke Association, the evaluation of suspected stroke should be completed within 6 hours after the onset of symptoms (14). Or stated more succinctly, *time is brain* (15).

ROUTINE STUDIES

The evaluation of suspected stroke should include blood chemistries to search for hypoglycemia, hyponatremia, hypernatremia, and renal failure. Additional routine studies should include an INR if the patient is being treated with coumadin, an electrocardiogram if atrial fibrillation is suspected, and a chest x-ray if the patient has fever.

COMPUTED TOMOGRAPHY

Computed tomography (CT) of the brain can identify ischemic infarction and hemorrhage and can distinguish between the two (16). The sensitivity of CT scans is 70% for cerebral infarction (17) and over 90% for intracerebral hemorrhage (1). However, the sensitivity of CT scans is influenced by the time passed from the onset of stroke to the time the scans are performed.

Timing

The influence of timing on the diagnostic yield from CT scans is illustrated in Figure 52.1. **For cerebral infarctions, the diagnostic yield from CT scans is 50% lower if the scans are performed within 24 hours after the infarction** (16). Therefore, an unrevealing CT scan performed within 24 hours after the onset of suspected stroke does not rule out the possibility of cerebral infarction.

Indications

Two major benefits are derived from CT scans in suspected stroke. First, CT scans can distinguish infarction from hemorrhage, which is

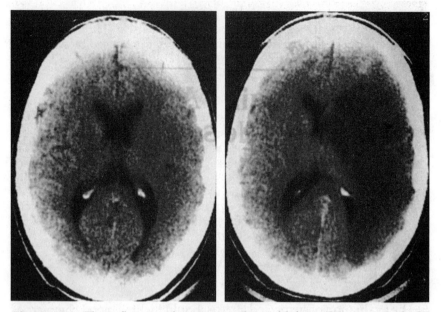

Figure 52.1. The influence of timing on the yield from CT scans. Both CT scans are from the same patient with suspected stroke. The scan on the left was obtained within 24 hours after the onset of symptoms and is unrevealing. The scan on the right was obtained 3 days later and shows a large hypodense area (infarction) with mass effect in the left cerebral hemisphere. (Reproduced with permission from Reference 16.)

important for selecting the appropriate therapy. Second, CT scans will identify the occasional case of suspected stroke caused by a space-occupying lesion (tumor or abscess). For these reasons, CT scans are recommended as a routine diagnostic procedure in patients with suspected stroke (1).

Cost

As may be expected, CT scans are costly. At Presbyterian Medical Center (University of Pennsylvania), the charge to the patient for an unenhanced CT scan of the head is **$1342** (charge for the fiscal year 1996).

MAGNETIC RESONANCE IMAGING

Magnetic resonance imaging (MRI) has a higher diagnostic yield than CT scans for bland infarctions (particularly those involving the cerebellum and brainstem) (18). The value of MRI in suspected stroke

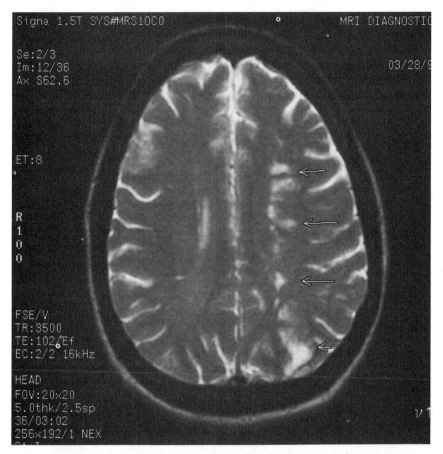

Figure 52.2. A T_2-weighted MRI scan from a 39-year-old woman with acute onset of right-sided weakness and a normal CT scan. The arrows point to hyperdense areas of infarction along the distribution of the left middle cerebral artery. (Case history and MRI scan courtesy of Dr. Sami Khella, M.D.)

is illustrated by the case in Figure 52.2. The MRI scan in this figure is from a previously healthy 39-year-old woman who experienced acute onset of right arm and leg weakness. The initial CT scan was unrevealing, but the MRI scan reveals multiple (hyperdense) infarctions along the course of the left middle cerebral artery (whereas infarctions are hypodense on CT scans, they are hyperdense on MRI scans). This prompted a cerebral angiogram, which revealed probable vasculitis as a cause of the cerebral infarction.

Indications

MRI is reserved for the occasional case of suspected stroke in which CT scans are unrevealing. However, because of the expense of MRI (see below), it should be reserved for cases in which the results of MRI will lead to improved therapy and a better chance for recovery.

Contraindications

Because MRI uses magnetic pulses, it is contraindicated in patients with implanted pacemakers, cerebral aneurysm clips, intraocular metal, and cochlear implants (18). Other metal implants and vena cava filters are relative contraindications to MRI (18).

Cost

At Presbyterian Medical Center (University of Pennsylvania), the patient charge for an MRI of the brain is **$1761** (for fiscal year 1996).

OTHER DIAGNOSTIC TESTS

The following tests are appropriate for the indications cited.

1. **Lumbar puncture** is not indicated in most patients with suspected stroke. It can be useful in the occasional case when a CT scan reveals equivocal evidence of subarachnoid hemorrhage or when an abscess is in close proximity to the subarachnoid space.
2. **Echocardiography** is indicated when stroke is associated with atrial fibrillation, acute MI, or left-sided endocarditis. It may also be indicated in stroke of undetermined etiology to identify a patent foramen ovale (and possible paradoxical cerebral embolism).
3. **Electroencephalography** is indicated in cases in which seizures are suspected as the cause of the neurologic deficits.

EARLY MANAGEMENT

The following discussion refers to the management in the first 24 hours after acute stroke.

HYPERTENSION

Hypertension is common in the early period after acute stroke, but antihypertensive therapy is not advised as a routine practice for two reasons. First, cerebral autoregulation may be lost in the region of the brain that is damaged, and thus acute lowering of the blood pressure could enhance the extent of injury. This is verified by a clinical study showing that acute lowering of blood pressure in hypertensive stroke victims is often accompanied by worsening of the neurologic deficits (19). This is applied to patients with severe hypertension (diastolic blood pressure above 120 mm Hg) as well. The second reason to avoid antihypertensive therapy is the tendency for the hypertension to re-solve spontaneously in the days following an acute stroke (20).

The Stroke Council of the American Heart Association recommends antihypertensive treatment when the systolic pressure is above 220 mm Hg or when the mean blood pressure is above 130 mm Hg (1). However, this recommendation lacks experimental validation. If anti-hypertensive therapy is used, the goal must be *gradual* rather than prompt reduction of blood pressure. Both **nitroglycerin and nitro-prusside should be avoided** because these cerebral vasodilators can increase intracranial pressure (1). Nicardipine (a calcium channel blocker that preserves cerebral blood flow) or angiotensin-converting enzyme inhibitors (which have little effect on cerebral vessels) may be the most appropriate agents for lowering blood pressure in acute stroke.

ANTICOAGULATION

Approximately 20% of patients with acute ischemic stroke develop progressive neurologic deficits over the ensuing 4 days (21,22). Thera-peutic anticoagulation with heparin has been the traditional practice for patients with progressive ischemic stroke (22). Although early studies showed a possible benefit from this practice, these studies were not well designed. More recent studies reveal **little or no benefit from full anticoagulation in progressive ischemic stroke** (22).

THROMBOLYTIC THERAPY

Considering the similarities between acute thrombotic infarction of the brain and acute (thrombotic) MI and the success with thrombolytic therapy in acute MI (see Chapter 19), it follows that thrombolytic ther-apy should be evaluated in acute ischemic stroke. The studies of thrombolytic therapy in ischemic stroke have not been encouraging. However, in the most recent study, which was sponsored by the Na-tional Institute of Neurologic Disorders and Stroke (NINDS) (23), pa-tients given tissue plasminogen activator (0.9 mg/kg over 1 hour) within 3 hours after the onset of ischemic stroke showed significantly fewer neurologic deficits 3 months later. (The clinical course in the early period after acute ischemic stroke was not favorably influenced by thrombolytic therapy in this study.)

Based on the NINDS study just described, **the Food and Drug Ad-ministration has approved the use of tissue plasminogen activator in the first 3 hours after the onset of acute ischemic stroke** (24). How-ever, because a CT scan must be obtained to rule out hemorrhage before thrombolytic therapy is started, this means that patients with ischemic stroke must seek treatment in the emergency department *and* have a CT scan completed within 3 hours to be candidates for thrombolytic therapy. In light of these strict requirements, it is unlikely that thrombolytic therapy will become a common treatment modality in acute ischemic stroke.

INCREASED INTRACRANIAL PRESSURE

Increased intracranial pressure can be the result of intracerebral hemorrhage or massive infarction with cerebral edema. In either case, it carries a poor prognosis. Several measures are used to lower intracranial pressure following head injury (25). However, many of these are aimed at reducing cerebral blood flow, which can aggravate an ischemic stroke. The use of selected methods to lower intracranial pressure in acute ischemic stroke can be summarized as follows:

1. Intracranial pressure monitoring is of unproven value for managing intracranial hypertension in ischemic stroke (1) and is not recommended as a routine measure.
2. Elevating the head of the bed to 30 degrees will reduce intracranial pressure by promoting venous return from the head (25), and this measure is recommended for all patients with intracranial hypertension (1).
3. Endotracheal suctioning can increase intracranial pressure, even when hypoxemia is prevented by a preceding period of 100% oxygen inhalation (26). Therefore, endotracheal suctioning should be reduced in frequency and duration (if possible) in patients with intracranial hypertension (26).
4. Hyperventilation to induce hypocapnia and reduce cerebral blood flow does not improve outcome in patients with a head injury (25). This lack of documented benefit, together with the risk of exaggerated ischemia during hyperventilation, makes hyperventilation an undesirable intervention is ischemic stroke.
5. High-dosage corticosteroids do not improve outcome in ischemic stroke with cerebral edema and can increase the risk of infection (1). Therefore, steroids should be avoided in all cases of intracranial hypertension.
6. Mannitol lowers intracranial pressure by drawing water out of cerebral tissues (27). Although of unproven value, mannitol can be given in cases of severe or progressive cerebral edema from acute stroke. The dose is 0.25 to 0.5 g/kg IV over 20 minutes. Hypertonic fluids like mannitol can increase the permeability of the blood-brain barrier (25), which favors the entry of mannitol into cerebral tissues. Because of this risk, mannitol should not be given in repeated doses to control intracranial pressure (25).

SUBARACHNOID HEMORRHAGE

Subarachnoid hemorrhage (SAH) is usually the result of aneurysmal rupture or bleeding from an arteriovenous malformation. Predisposing factors for SAH include cocaine abuse and bleeding disorders (28).

Although classified as a type of stroke (5), SAH can differ from the other types of stroke in both presentation and management.

CLINICAL PRESENTATION

The hallmark of the clinical presentation of SAH is headache. The full-blown syndrome may be preceded by a severe but self-limited headache called a sentinel headache (29), which is presumably the result of aneurysmal dilation or a small hemorrhagic leak. The headache of SAH is usually abrupt in onset, persistent and progressive, and worse with exertion. Severe headache that is worse with exertion is more characteristic of SAH than the myriad other causes of headache (29). Although the headache of SAH tends to be centered at the base of the skull or in the cervical region, this feature is not specific for SAH. Other manifestations, such as nausea and vomiting, mental status changes, and stiff neck, may or may not be present.

DIAGNOSTIC EVALUATION

As mentioned earlier, CT scans of the head (unenhanced) have a 90% sensitivity for the detection of hemorrhage, including subarachnoid hemorrhage, and thus are the initial diagnostic test of choice for suspected SAH. However, CT scans can miss SAH in the posterior fossa (where the brainstem and cerebellum are located). The image in Figure 52.3 is an MRI scan from a 30-year-old woman with severe and persistent headache who had a normal CT scan of the head. The MRI scan shows a hyperdense area (indicated by the arrows) just ventral to the pons, which represents a SAH. Thus, even though CT scans have a high sensitivity for SAH, a negative CT scan does not eliminate the possibility for SAH.

MANAGEMENT

The morbidity and mortality in SAH is related to two processes: recurrence of the hemorrhage and cerebral vasospasm.

Recurrent SAH

In most cases of SAH, the bleeding has subsided at the time of diagnosis. To prevent a recurrence of the SAH, cerebral angiography is performed to identify the responsible vascular abnormality for surgical correction. However, angiography is usually delayed until the patient is awake and clinically recovered.

Cerebral Vasospasm

The neurologic deficits in SAH are caused by vasospasm of cerebral vessels with resultant cerebral ischemia. The vasospasm is produced

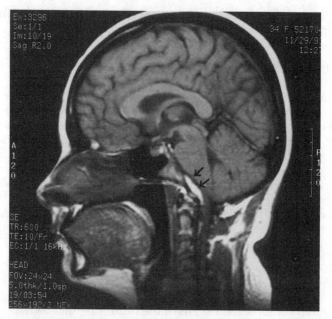

Figure 52.3. An MRI scan from a 30-year-old woman with severe, persistent headache and a normal CT scan of the head. Note the arrows pointing to a hyperdense area ventral to the brainstem. This represents a prepontine subarachnoid hemorrhage. Lumbar puncture confirmed the presence of blood in the subarachnoid space. (Case history and MRI scan courtesy of Dr. Sami Khella, M.D.)

by blood in the subarachnoid space, although the exact mechanism is unclear. This vascular response is attenuated by nimodipine, a calcium channel blocker that has a preferential vasodilating effect on cerebral vessels. Nimodipine in a dosage of 0.35 mg/kg orally every 4 hours has proven effective in reducing vasospasm (30) and improving neurologic function (31) in patients with SAH. As a result, this agent is used routinely in SAH.

REFERENCES

REVIEWS

1. Stroke Council of the American Heart Association. Guidelines for the management of patients with acute ischemic stroke. Circulation 1994;90:1588–1601 (179 references).
2. Naradzay JFX, Gaasch WR. Acute stroke. Emerg Med Clin North Am 1996; 14:197–216 (123 references).

DEFINITIONS

3. Special Report from the National Institute of Neurologic Disorders and Stroke. Classification of cerebrovascular diseases III. Stroke 1990;21:637–676.

4. Bamford J. Clinical examination in diagnosis and subclassification of stroke. Lancet 1992;339:400–405.
5. D'Costa DF. Subclassification of strokes. Lancet 1992;339:1541.
6. Hart RG. Cardioembolic stroke. Am J Med 1996;100:465–474.
7. Di Tullio M, Sacco RL, Gopal A, et al. Patent foramen ovale as a risk factor for cryptogenic stroke. Ann Intern Med 1992;117:461–465.

BEDSIDE EVALUATION

8. Goldstein LB, Matchar DB. Clinical assessment of stroke. JAMA 1994;271: 1114–1120.
9. Oppenheimer S, Hachinski V. Complications of acute stroke. Lancet 1992;339: 721–724.
10. Damasio A. Aphasia. N Engl J Med 1992;326:531–559.
11. Brott T, Adams HP, Olinger CP, et al. Measurements of acute cerebral infarctions: a clinical examination scale. Stroke 1989;20:864–870.
12. Bolton CF, Young GB. Neurologic complications of renal failure. Toronto: Butterworths, 1990.
13. Maher J, Young GB. Septic encephalopathy. Intensive Care Med 1993;8: 177–187.

DIAGNOSTIC EVALUATION

14. National Stroke Association Consensus Statement. Stroke: the first 6 hours. Stroke, Clinical Updates. Vol. IV. Englewood, CO: National Stroke Association, 1993.
15. McCarthy M. Time is brain. Lancet 1993;341:1339–1340.
16. Graves VB, Partington VB. Imaging evaluation of acute neurologic disease. In: Goodman LR, Putman CE, eds. Critical care imaging. 3rd ed. Philadelphia: WB Saunders, 1992;391–409.
17. Bryan RN, Levy LM, Whitlow WD, et al. Diagnosis of acute cerebral infarction: comparison of CT and MR imaging. Am J Neuroradiol 1991;12:611–620.
18. Kent DL, Haynor DR, Longstreth WT, Larson EB. The clinical efficacy of magnetic resonance imaging in neuroimaging. Ann Intern Med 1994;120:856–874.

MANAGEMENT

19. Phillips SJ. Pathophysiology and management of hypertension in acute, ischemic stroke. Hypertension 1994;23:131–136.
20. O'Connell JE, Gray CS. Treating hypertension after stroke. BMJ 1994;308: 1523–1524.
21. Britton M, Roden A. Progression of stroke after arrival at hospital. Stroke 1985; 16:629–633.
22. Rothrock JF, Hart RG. Antithrombotic therapy in cerebrovascular disease. Ann Intern Med 1991;115:885–895.
23. The National Institute of Neurologic Disorders and Stroke rt-PA Stroke Study Group. Tissue plasminogen activator for acute ischemic stroke. N Engl J Med 1995;333:1581–1587.
24. Bleck TP. Thrombolysis for acute ischemic stroke: how, when, and why. J Crit Illness 1996;11:645–657.
25. Cold GE, Holdgaard HO. Treatment of intracranial hypertension in acute head

injury with social reference to the role of hyperventilation and sedation with barbiturates: a review. Intensive Care World 1992;9:172–178.
26. Rudy EB, Turner BS, Baun M, et al. Endotracheal suctioning in adults with head injury. Heart Lung 1991;20:667–674.
27. Nath F, Galbraith S. The effect of mannitol on cerebral white matter water content. J Neurosurg 1986;65:41–43.

SUBARACHNOID HEMORRHAGE

28. Ozer MN, Materson RS, Caplan LR. Management of persons with stroke. St. Louis: Mosby, 1994;83–84.
29. Saper JR. Headache: urgent considerations in diagnosis and treatment. In: Weiner WJ. Emergent and urgent neurology. Philadelphia: JB Lippincott, 1992; 509–531.
30. Allen GS, Ahn HS, Preziosi TJ, et al. Cerebral arterial spasm—a controlled trial of nimodipine in patients with subarachnoid hemorrhage. N Engl J Med 1983;308:619–624.
31. Petruk KC, West M, Mohr G, et al. Nimodipine treatment in poor-grade aneurysm patients: results of a multicenter double-blind placebo-controlled trial. J Neurosurg 1988;68:505–517.

SUGGESTED READINGS

Ozer MN, Materson RS, Caplan LR. Management of persons with stroke. St. Louis: Mosby, 1994.
Wijdicks EFM. Neurology of critical illness. Philadelphia: FA Davis, 1995.

section XIV
PHARMACEUTICAL CONSIDERATIONS

The desire to take medicine is, perhaps, the great feature that distinguishes man from other animals.

Sir William Osler

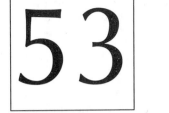

c h a p t e r

53

PHARMACEUTICAL TOXINS AND ANTIDOTES

Poisons and medicine are oftentimes the same substance given with different intents.
Peter Latham (1865)

There is little doubt that pharmaceutical mishaps are a source of considerable morbidity and even mortality. Adverse drug reactions are responsible for at least 10% of hospital admissions and as many as 20% of ICU admissions (1,2). Once in the hospital, as many as 30% of patients experience an adverse drug reaction before discharge (3). The average patient in the ICU receives 6 to 9 different medications daily and 8 to 12 different medications during the ICU stay (1). Therefore, the ICU is a fertile environment for pharmaceutical misadventures.

This chapter describes the clinical toxicity associated with the pharmaceutical agents listed below, and the treatment of each with specific antidotes (shown in parentheses). Included are toxic drug ingestions that prompt admission to the ICU and toxic drug reactions that surface after admission to the ICU. (For a list of the most common toxic ingestions in the United States, see the Appendix.)

Acetaminophen (acetylcysteine)
Benzodiazepines (flumazenil)
β-Blockers (glucagon)
Calcium antagonists (calcium, glucagon)
Digitalis (antibody fragments)
Nitroprusside (nitrites, thiosulfate)
Opioids (naloxone)
Tricyclic antidepressants (bicarbonate)

ACETAMINOPHEN

Acetaminophen gained widespread popularity in the 1960s as a less toxic analgesic–antipyretic agent than aspirin. Ironically, acetaminophen is now the **second leading cause of toxic drug ingestions in the United States** (4). Although it is safe when administered in the usual therapeutic dosages (less than 4 g daily), acetaminophen can be a lethal hepatotoxin when ingested in large doses.

TOXIC MECHANISM

The toxicity of acetaminophen is related to its metabolism, which is shown in Figure 53.1. The bulk of acetaminophen metabolism involves the formation of sulfate and glucuronide conjugates in the liver, which are then excreted in the urine. Approximately 5% of the metabolism involves oxidation by cytochrome P-450–dependent enzymes to form a highly reactive intermediate that can promote oxidant injury in hepatic parenchymal cells. This toxic metabolite is normally removed by conjugation with glutathione (an intracellular antioxidant described in Chapter 3). Large doses of acetaminophen prompt increased use of the glutathione pathway, and this can lead to glutathione depletion. When hepatic glutathione stores fall to 30% of normal levels, the toxic metabolite can accumulate and promote widespread hepatocellular damage (5).

Predisposing Conditions

According to the metabolic sequence in Figure 53.1, the following conditions predispose to acetaminophen hepatotoxicity (5–8):

Therapy with drugs that enhance hepatic microsomal oxidation, such as barbiturates, phenytoin, and rifampin
Conditions associated with glutathione depletion, such as chronic

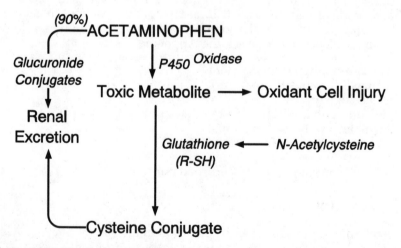

Figure 53.1. The hepatic metabolism of acetaminophen and the mechanism of action of N-acetylcysteine.

ethanol ingestion, malnutrition, and infections with the human immunodeficiency virus (HIV)

These conditions are important to consider when interpreting serum acetaminophen levels, as discussed later in this chapter.

CLINICAL PRESENTATION

The period following acetaminophen overdose is divided into three stages (5). In the initial stage (the first 24 hours), symptoms are either absent or nonspecific (e.g., nausea) and no laboratory evidence of hepatic injury exists. In patients who develop hepatotoxicity, a second stage (24 to 72 hours after drug ingestion) occurs, during which clinical manifestations continue to be minimal or absent, but laboratory evidence of hepatic injury (i.e., elevated serum transaminases) begins to appear. In advanced cases of hepatic injury, a third stage follows (after 72 hours after ingestion) that is characterized by clinical and laboratory evidence of progressive hepatic injury and hepatic insufficiency (e.g., encephalopathy and coagulopathy), occasionally combined with renal insufficiency.

DIAGNOSIS

In most cases of acetaminophen overdose, the initial presentation occurs within 24 hours after drug ingestion, when no manifestations of hepatic injury are present. The principal task at this time is to identify the patients who are likely to develop hepatotoxicity in later stages. Two variables can have prognostic value in this regard.

Ingested Dose

The toxic dose of acetaminophen can vary in individual patients. However, when the ingested dose of acetaminophen is known, the following criteria can be used to predict the likelihood of hepatotoxicity.

Ingested Dose	Hepatotoxicity
250 mg/kg	Probable
>140 mg/kg	Possible
> 70 mg/kg	Possible (high-risk conditions)

Serum Drug Levels

The serum acetaminophen level is the most reliable predictor of toxic risk in the early period after drug ingestion (5,6). Figure 53.2 shows a widely used nomogram that relates toxic risk to the serum acetaminophen level (in micrograms/milliliter) in the first 24 hours after drug ingestion. The first 4 hours after drug ingestion is not included in the nomogram because serum drug levels may not reach

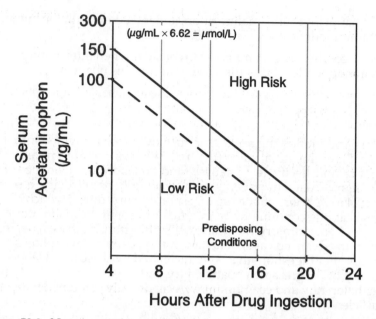

Figure 53.2. Nomogram for predicting the risk of hepatotoxicity from the serum acetaminophen level in the first 24 hours after drug ingestion. Any serum level that falls on or above the threshold lines is an indication to begin therapy with N-acetylcysteine. The normal threshold (*solid line*) is from Reference 5, and the threshold for predisposing conditions (*dashed line*) is from Reference 6.

steady-state levels during this time. The dotted line (lower threshold) is used for patients with a condition that predisposes to acetaminophen hepatotoxicity (9); the solid line is used for all other patients. If a serum acetaminophen level falls in the high-risk region of the nomogram, the risk of developing hepatotoxicity is 60% or higher (5), and this is sufficient to warrant the treatment described here.

N-ACETYLCYSTEINE

The goal of therapy in acetaminophen overdose is to limit or prevent accumulation of the toxic metabolite. Because glutathione does not readily cross cell membranes, the administration of exogenous glutathione is not well suited for this task. N-acetylcysteine (NAC) is a glutathione analog that can cross cell membranes and act as an intracellular glutathione surrogate (10). As shown in Figure 53.1, NAC contains a sulfhydryl group that allows it to act as a reducing agent and inactivate the toxic acetaminophen metabolite. This ability to act as a reducing agent also allows N-acetylcysteine to function as an antioxidant agent, as described in Chapter 3. In fact, the toxic effect of the acetaminophen metabolite is an oxidant-induced injury, similar to the cell injury produced by oxygen metabolites, and N-acetylcystein protects against acetaminophen toxicity because of its antioxidant actions.

Timing

Therapy with NAC provides protection against acetaminophen hepatotoxicity when treatment is initiated within 24 hours after drug ingestion (5,6,11). Although some evidence exists that NAC can be protective when given 24 to 36 hours after drug ingestion (12), the consensus is that **N-acetylcysteine is indicated only when therapy can be started within 24 hours after acetaminophen overdose.** Protection is greatest when therapy starts within 8 hours after drug ingestion (11), and thereafter the protective effects of NAC decline steadily with time. Therefore, avoiding treatment delays is the single most important measure for ensuring optimal therapy with N-acetylcysteine.

Therapeutic Regimens

NAC can be given orally or intravenously using the dosing regimens shown in Table 53.1. The intravenous route is preferred in most countries except the United States, where orally administered NAC is the only regimen approved for clinical use. Despite the preference for oral therapy in the United States, both routes of therapy are considered equally effective.

Adverse Reactions

The sulfur content of NAC gives the liquid drug preparation a very disagreeable taste (often described as rotten eggs). As a result, oral administration of NAC often incites vomiting. NAC can be diluted in grapefruit juice to improve tolerance, but in many instances, a nasogastric tube must be inserted to administer therapy. The oral regimen of

---

TABLE 53.1 TREATMENT OF ACETAMINOPHEN OVERDOSE WITH N-ACETYLCYSTEINE (NAC)

Preparations: 10% NAC (100 mg/mL) and 20% NAC (200 mg/mL)
Oral Regimen
Dilute 10% NAC (1:2) in water or juice to make a 5% solution (50 mg/mL).
  Initial dose: 140 mg/kg
  Maintenance dosage: 70 mg/kg q 4 h for 17 doses
  Total dose: 1330 mg/kg over 72 h
Intravenous Regimen
Use 20% NAC for each of the doses below, and infuse in sequence.
  1. 150 mg/kg in 200 mL D_5W over 15 min
  2. 50 mg/kg in 500 mL D_5W over 4 h
  3. 100 mg/kg in 1000 mL D_5W over 16 h
  Total dose: 300 mg/kg over 20 h

NAC is also associated with a dose-dependent diarrhea that appears in approximately half the patients who complete the 72-hour regimen (13). Fortunately, this diarrhea resolves with continued therapy in over 90% of cases. Intravenous NAC can cause troublesome anaphylactoid reactions (14), but these reactions are uncommon.

ACTIVATED CHARCOAL

Acetaminophen is completely absorbed from the gastrointestinal tract in the first few hours after drug ingestion (5). Therefore, activated charcoal (1 g/kg body weight) is recommended only in the first 4 hours after acetaminophen overdose (5,15). Although charcoal can also adsorb N-acetylcysteine, this interaction is probably not significant (5).

BENZODIAZEPINES

Benzodiazepines are the most commonly overdosed prescription drugs in the United States (4). However, admissions for drug overdose are not the only source of benzodiazepine toxicity in the ICU. Surveys reveal that roughly 50% of patients in the ICU receive benzodiazepines for sedation (16,17), and adverse reactions to benzodiazepine sedation are likely to be a significant source of clinical toxicity. The use of benzodiazepines for sedation in the ICU is described in Chapter 8.

CLINICAL TOXICITY

Benzodiazepines produce a dose-dependent depression in the level of consciousness, but this effect usually is not accompanied by respiratory depression or cardiovascular depression. The lack of significant respiratory or cardiovascular depression explains why benzodiazepine overdose is rarely fatal (18). However, several factors in the ICU can promote respiratory and cardiovascular depression with benzodiazepines. These include advanced age, combined therapy with opioid analgesics, and prolonged drug therapy.

Drug Accumulation

As mentioned in Chapter 8, the benzodiazepines are lipophilic agents, and thus have a tendency to accumulate in lipid-rich tissues such as the central nervous system. This can result in oversedation when benzodiazepines are given for prolonged periods (19–22). This tendency for drug accumulation is underappreciated, particularly with midazolam, which is considered a rapidly acting agent. There is a general misconception that the short elimination half-life of midazolam (90 minutes) indicates that the drug is rapidly cleared from the body. However, the elimination of midazolam from the circulation is caused largely by uptake into the central nervous system and other lipid-laden tissues. Therefore, **the short elimination half-life of mida-zolam does not represent rapid elimination from the body.** As a result, prolonged infusions of midazolam can be associated with significant drug accumulation in the central nervous system, leading to oversedation and delays in weaning from mechanical ventilation (21,22).

FLUMAZENIL

Flumazenil is a benzodiazepine antagonist that binds to benzodiazepine receptors in the central nervous system but does not exert any agonist actions (23). It is most effective in reversing the sedative effects of the benzodiazepines but is inconsistent in reversing benzodiazepine-induced respiratory depression (24). Flumazenil can also improve the sensorium in ethanol intoxication (25), but the doses required are large (5 mg) and potentially hazardous.

Drug Administration

Flumazenil is given as an intravenous bolus. The initial dose is 0.2 mg, and this can be repeated at 1-minute intervals if necessary to a cumulative dose of 1.0 mg. The response is rapid in onset (1 to 2 minutes), and lasts for approximately 1 hour (19,21,23). Because flumazenil has a shorter duration of action than the benzodiazepines, resedation is common after 30 to 60 minutes. Because of the risk of resedation, the initial bolus dose of flumazenil is often followed by a continuous infusion at 0.3 to 0.4 mg/hour (19).

Adverse Reactions

Flumazenil produces few undesirable side effects (23,26,27). It can precipitate a benzodiazepine withdrawal syndrome in patients with a long-standing history of benzodiazepine use (26). Flumazenil can also precipitate seizures in patients receiving benzodiazepines for seizure control and in mixed overdoses involving tricyclic antidepressants (28).

Clinical Uses

Because of the benign nature of benzodiazepine toxicity, flumazenil is a treatment in search of an illness. The principal use of flumazenil is in patients with known or suspected benzodiazepine overdose, but only when a mixed overdose involving tricyclic antidepressants is not suspected, and only in patients who are not taking benzodiazepines for seizure control. Flumazenil has even fewer uses in the ICU. Although flumazenil can reverse oversedation with benzodiazepines in ventilator-dependent patients (19–22), the hazards of oversedation are minimal in patients receiving ventilatory support. Flumazenil has been reported to hasten weaning from mechanical ventilation (21–23), but

TABLE 53.2. COMPARISON OF INTRAVENOUS
β-RECEPTOR ANTAGONISTS

Antagonist	Target Receptors	Relative Potency	Intravenous Dosage	Lipid Solubility	Metabolism
Propranolol	All β	1	1–10 mg	+ + +	Hepatic
Metoprolol	β-1	1	5–15 mg	+	Hepatic
Atenolol	β-1	1	5–10 mg	0	Renal
Timolol	All β	6	0.3–1 mg	+	Hepatic and renal
Labetalol	α, all β	0.3	2 mg/kg	+ +	Renal
Esmolol	All β	0.06	0.5–1 mg/kg 0.1–0.3 mg/ kg/min	0	Plasma

this application seems limited by the lack of respiratory depression in benzodiazepine sedation.

β-RECEPTOR ANTAGONISTS

Toxic ingestion of β-receptor antagonists is increasing yearly, and more than 5000 cases of β-blocker overdose were reported in 1992 (4). Intentional overdose is not the only source of β-blocker toxicity in the ICU. β Blockers are used to manage several conditions in the ICU, including hypertension, narrow-complex tachycardias, unstable angina, and acute myocardial infarction, and these uses create an additional source of β-blocker toxicity. The β-receptor antagonists used most often in the ICU are shown in Table 53.2.

CLINICAL TOXICITY

The manifestations of β-receptor blockade arise primarily from the cardiovascular system and the central nervous system (29,30).

Cardiovascular Toxicity

The most common manifestations of β-blocker toxicity are **bradycardia** and **hypotension** (29,30). The bradycardia is usually sinus in origin and is well tolerated. The hypotension can be caused by peripheral vasodilation (renin blockade) or a decrease in cardiac output (β-1 receptor blockade). Hypotension that is sudden in onset is usually a reflection of a decrease in cardiac output and is an ominous sign.

The more lipophilic β-blockers (e.g., propranolol) have a membrane-stabilizing or quinidine-like action that can prolong atrioventricular (AV) conduction. This effect, which is not the result of β-blockade, can produce various degrees of **heart block.**

Neurotoxicity

Most β-blockers are lipid soluble to some degree and thus have a tendency to accumulate in lipid-rich organs such as the central nervous system. As a result, β-blocker overdose is often accompanied by lethargy, **depressed consciousness,** and **generalized seizures.** The latter manifestation is more prevalent than suspected and has been reported in 60% of overdoses with highly lipophilic agents such as propranolol (30). Like prolonged AV conduction, the neurologic manifestations are not the result of β-receptor blockade.

GLUCAGON

The cardiovascular depression from β-receptor blockade is resistant to conventional therapy with atropine (1 mg intravenously), isoproterenol (0.1 to 0.2 mg/minute), and transvenous pacing (29). The regulatory hormone glucagon is the agent of choice for reversing the cardiovascular depression in β-receptor blockade.

Mechanism of Action

The diagram in Figure 53.3 shows the chain of events responsible for the positive inotropic actions of β-1 receptor activation in the heart. The β-receptor is functionally linked (via specialized G proteins) to the adenyl cyclase enzyme on the inner surface of the cell membrane. Activation of the receptor–enzyme complex results in the hydrolysis

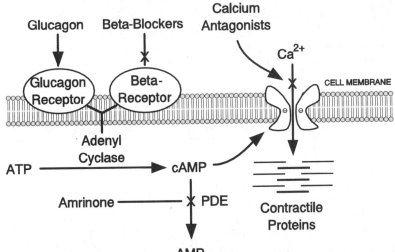

Figure 53.3. The mechanism of action of drugs that affect the strength of cardiac contraction. ATP = adenosine triphosphate, $cAMP$ = cyclic adenosine monophosphate, PDE = phosphodiesterase, AMP = adenosine monophosphate.

of adenosine triphosphate (ATP) to form cyclic adenosine monophosphate (cAMP). The cAMP then activates a protein kinase that promotes the inward movement of calcium through the cell membrane. The influx of calcium promotes interactions between contractile proteins and thereby augments the strength of cardiac contraction.

The diagram in Figure 53.3 shows that glucagon can activate adenyl cyclase through a membrane receptor that is distinct from the β-receptor. This allows glucagon to mimic the positive inotropic effects of β-receptor activation when the β-receptors are quiescent.

Indications

Glucagon is indicated for the treatment of hypotension and *symptomatic* bradycardia associated with toxic exposure to β-blockers (Table 53.3). When used at the appropriate dosages, glucagon elicits a favorable response in 90% of patients (29). Glucagon is *not* indicated for reversing the prolonged AV conduction or neurologic abnormalities in β-blocker overdose because these effects are not mediated by β-receptor blockade.

Preparation

Glucagon is provided as a powder that must be reconstituted. The diluent provided by the manufacturer usually includes phenol (carbolic acid) as a preservative. Phenol can cause a variety of toxic side effects, including agitation, seizures, and hypotension. The threshold tolerance for phenol in adults is 50 mg (31), and this threshold will be reached after 5 hours with a glucagon infusion at the standard dosage (i.e., glucagon at 5 mg/hour delivers phenol at 10 mg/hour). Therefore, **the commercial phenol-containing diluent should be avoided** and glucagon should be reconstituted in saline or sterile water.

TABLE 53.3. ANTIDOTE THERAPY WITH GLUCAGON

Indications:
For toxic exposure to β-blockers or calcium channel blockers accompanied by
  • Symptomatic bradycardia or
  • Hypotension
Preparation:
Supplied as a powder (1 mg or 10 mg). *Do not* use commercial diluent (contains phenol). Reconstitute with saline or sterile water to a concentration of 1 mg/mL.
Administration:
Initial bolus dose: 0.05 mg/kg (or 3 mg) intravenously over 1 min. Then 0.07 mg/kg (or 5 mg) if necessary.
Continuous infusion: 0.07 mg/kg/h (or 5 mg/h)

Dosing Recommendations

The effective dose of glucagon can vary in individual patients, but **a bolus dose of 3 to 5 mg intravenously should be effective in most adults** (29,30). The initial dose is 3 mg (or 0.05 mg/kg), and this can be followed by a second dose of 5 mg (or 0.07 mg/kg) when necessary. The response to glucagon is most pronounced when the plasma ionized calcium is normal (32). The effects of glucagon can be short-lived (5 minutes), so a favorable response should be followed by a continuous infusion (5 mg/hour).

Adverse Effects

Nausea and vomiting are common at glucagon doses above 5 mg/hour. Mild hyperglycemia is common, and it is caused by glucagon-induced glycogenolysis and gluconeogenesis. The insulin response to the hyperglycemia can drive potassium into cells and promote hypokalemia. Finally, glucagon stimulates catecholamine release from the adrenal medulla, and this can raise blood pressure in hypertensive patients. This hypertensive response is exaggerated in pheochromocytoma, so glucagon is contraindicated in patients with pheochromocytoma.

CALCIUM ANTAGONISTS

The calcium antagonists are responsible for more than 6000 cases of drug overdose each year and are the fourth leading cause of death from toxic drug ingestions in the United States (4). The three original calcium antagonists (verapamil, nifedipine, and diltiazem) are responsible for most of the clinical experience with calcium antagonist toxicity.

MECHANISMS

Calcium has a profound influence on the electrical and mechanical performance of smooth muscle. Its role in the contraction of cardiac smooth muscle is shown in Figure 53.3. The inward movement of calcium across the cell membrane (triggered by depolarization of the cell membrane or by activation of the cAMP pathway) promotes the interaction between contractile proteins that ultimately determines the strength of muscle contraction. Although not shown in the figure, calcium influx also triggers calcium release from the sarcoplasmic reticulum, which is another source of calcium for muscle contraction. This process from membrane depolarization to muscle contraction is called excitation–contraction coupling (33).

Calcium also participates in the propagation of electrical impulses in smooth muscle. The depolarization-triggered inward movement of calcium facilitates the propagation of electrical impulses in cardiac muscle, and speeds conduction through the AV node.

The calcium antagonists block the inward movement of calcium across smooth muscle membranes, but not across the sarcoplasmic reticulum. This blockade can result in negative inotropic and chronotropic effects, prolonged atrioventricular conduction (negative dromotropic effect), decreased arrhythmogenicity, vascular dilation, and bronchial dilation. The individual calcium antagonists differ in their ability to elicit these responses.

CLINICAL TOXICITY

The toxic manifestations of the three most popular calcium antagonists (verapamil, nifedipine, and diltiazem) are shown in Table 53.4 (34). Verapamil is most likely to produce hypotension and prolonged AV conduction. Verapamil is only a weak vasodilator, and the hypotension is caused by a decrease in cardiac output (negative inotropic effect) without compensatory vasoconstriction. Nifedipine is predominantly a vasodilator (hence the high incidence of sinus tachycardia) and has little influence on AV conduction. Diltiazem is similar to verapamil in its ability to prolong AV conduction, but it causes less cardiac depression than verapamil and less vasodilation than nifedipine.

Noncardiovascular manifestations of calcium blocker toxicity include lethargy and depressed consciousness (most common), generalized seizures, and hyperglycemia (caused by inhibition of insulin release, which is calcium-dependent) (34,35).

TREATMENT

There are two approaches to calcium channel blockade (29). The first involves the administration of calcium to antagonize the blockade on the outer surface of the cell membrane. The second involves the use of drugs that activate the cAMP pathway, which antagonizes the blockade from the inner surface of the cell membrane.

TABLE 53.4. CLINICAL FEATURES OF OVERDOSES WITH DIFFERENT CALCIUM ANTAGONISTS

Clinical Manifestation	Incidence		
	Verapamil	Nifedipine	Diltiazem
Hypotension	53%	32%	38%
Sinus tachycardia	23	57	26
Sinus bradycardia	29	14	29
Prolonged AV conduction	55	18	29
Data from Ramoska EA et al. (34).			

TABLE 53.5 ANTIDOTE THERAPY WITH INTRAVENOUS CALCIUM		
Characteristics	10% Calcium Chloride	10% Calcium Gluconate
Unit volume	10 mL per ampule	10 mL per ampule
Calcium content	13.6 mEq per ampule	4.6 mEq per ampule
Dose to prevent calcium channel blockage	⅓ ampule	1 ampule
Dose to reverse calcium channel blockage	1 ampule	3 ampules

Intravenous Calcium

Intravenous calcium is the traditional first-line therapy for reversing calcium channel blockade and elicits favorable responses in 35 to 75% of cases (34–36). As described in Chapter 43, there are two calcium salts for intravenous use (calcium chloride and calcium gluconate), and equivalent amounts of each salt do not contain equivalent amounts of elemental calcium. This is shown in Table 53.5; 1 g (1 ampule) of 10% calcium chloride contains roughly three times as much elemental calcium as 1 g (1 ampule) of 10% calcium gluconate. Therefore, the common practice of ordering calcium by ampules, without identifying the calcium salt, is inappropriate.

Although the calcium dosage varies widely in clinical reports, calcium is most effective when given in dosages that increase the serum calcium level (35). The dosage of calcium for reversing calcium channel blockade shown in Table 53.5 should be sufficient to raise the serum calcium level. The response to calcium may last only 10 to 15 minutes, so the initial response to calcium should be followed by a continuous infusion at 0.3 to 0.7 mEq/kg/hour (29). Calcium infusions are *not* recommended for patients being treated with digitalis.

Glucagon

Glucagon is emerging as a promising antidote for calcium channel blockade (37). However, the experience with glucagon is limited to individual case reports (38–40). There is some evidence that the effective dosage of glucagon may be higher for calcium channel blockade than for β-receptor blockade (38). However, until further studies are available, the recommended dosage of glucagon for β-blockade (Table 53.3) is a reasonable estimate of the effective dosage for calcium channel blockade.

Catecholamines

A variety of catecholamines have been used to antagonize calcium channel blockade, but **dopamine** (starting at 5 μg/kg/minute) seems to produce the most favorable responses (29). Cases that are refractory to dopamine can be treated with high-dose epinephrine (starting at 1 μg/kg/minute) (29).

Phophodiesterase Inhibitors

The phosphodiesterase inhibitor amrinone can add to the effects of glucagon and catecholamines in reversing the cardiovascular toxicity of calcium antagonists (40,41). However, the experience with amrinone is limited to case reports at present.

PREVENTIVE THERAPY

Hypotension is a common complication of therapy with intravenous verapamil for supraventricular tachyarrhythmias. The initial recommendation for eliminating this risk was to pretreat with 1 ampule of 10% calcium chloride (13.6 mEq calcium). However, this dose of calcium can produce transient sinus bradycardia and atrioventricular blockade (42). More recent experience indicates that pretreatment with one-third of an ampule of calcium chloride or 1 ampule of 10% calcium gluconate (4.6 mEq calcium) is effective in preventing verapamil-induced hypotension in most cases (Table 53.5) (36).

DIGITALIS

Digoxin is the fifth most commonly prescribed medication in the United States (43), and toxic reactions are reported in up to 25% of patients receiving the drug (44). It is the second leading cause of adverse drug reactions in hospitalized patients (45) and the seventh leading cause of death from pharmaceutical exposures (4).

TOXIC MANIFESTATIONS

Neurotoxicity

The neurologic manifestations of digitalis toxicity include lethargy and depressed consciousness, delirium, psychosis with hallucinations, and seizures (46). Visual disturbances, including decreased acuity, scotomata, and the appearance of colored halos around lights, are reported in over 90% of cases (44). Anorexia, nausea, and vomiting, which originate from chemoreceptor trigger zones in the lower brainstem, are each reported in over 40% of cases of digitalis toxicity (44).

Cardiotoxicity

Digitalis toxicity can produce a variety of cardiac rhythm disturbances. The spectrum includes sinus arrest, sinoatrial block, Mobitz type I AV block, ectopic atrial tachycardia with AV block, atrial fibrillation with AV junctional escape, AV junctional tachycardia (more than 80 beats/minute), AV junctional exit block, AV dissociation, ventricular ectopic depolarizations, ventricular tachycardia, and ventricular fibrillation (47). None of these rhythm disturbances are specific for digitalis toxicity. The one that is most predictive of digitalis toxicity is atrial fibrillation with a junctional rhythm (i.e., atrial fibrillation with a regular R–R interval).

Others

Abdominal pain and diarrhea are reported in 65% and 40% of cases of digitalis toxicity, respectively (44). Severe hyperkalemia is an uncommon but life-threatening manifestation of digitalis toxicity, and can be resistant to conventional therapy (48).

CONVENTIONAL MANAGEMENT

Activated Charcoal

As much as 30% of a digoxin dose (oral or intravenous) is excreted in the bile, and repeated doses of activated charcoal (1 g/kg every 4 hours) enhances clearance of digoxin from the bloodstream (49), and may be particularly valuable in aiding digoxin clearance in patients with renal insufficiency. However, digoxin has a large volume of distribution (6 to 7 L/kg in adults) and attempts to enhance drug elimination by any means (e.g., hemodialysis and gastrointestinal dialysis) have limited success (44).

Magnesium

Digitalis cardiotoxicity is believed to be the result of inhibition of the magnesium-dependent membrane pump for sodium and potassium. Therefore, depletion of magnesium, which is common in patients receiving digitalis, can promote digitalis cardiotoxicity. Magnesium deficiency also promotes potassium depletion, which is another predisposing factor for digitalis cardiotoxicity. For these reasons, intravenous magnesium is recommended for digitalis cardiotoxicity (except bradycardia and prolonged AV conduction), particularly when accompanied by hypokalemia.

Dosing Regimen. Give 2 g magnesium intravenously over 20 minutes and follow with a continuous infusion of 1 to 2 g/hour to maintain a serum magnesium of 4 to 5 mEq/L.

Magnesium infusion is not recommended for patients with renal insufficiency (for more on magnesium, see Chapter 42).

Antiarrhythmic Agents

Dilantin and lidocaine are favored for suppressing digitalis-induced ventricular ectopic rhythms because they do not prolong AV conduction. Dilantin can actually enhance AV conduction, but lidocaine is often preferred because it is given by continuous infusion and is easily titrated.

Lidocaine. Load with 1 to 2 mg/kg intravenously and follow with a continuous infusion at 1 to 4 mg/minute.

Dilantin. Infuse at 25 to 50 mg/minute until arrhythmia is suppressed or the total dose is 15 mg/kg. Follow with oral therapy at 400 to 600 mg/day.

Quinidine and procainamide are contraindicated because they depress AV conduction (quinidine also elevates serum digoxin levels), and bretylium is contraindicated because it can be proarrhythmic (44).

Atropine (0.5 to 1 mg as an intravenous bolus, repeated every 5 to 10 minutes as needed) can be used to reverse mild forms of digitalis-induced bradyarrhythmias (e.g., sinus bradycardia and low-grade AV block). Cardiac pacing is indicated for complete heart block. Temporary external pacing (pending immunotherapy) may be preferred to transvenous pacing because of the myocardial irritability that accompanies digitalis toxicity (44).

IMMUNOTHERAPY

Digoxin-specific antibody fragments (Digibind, Burroughs Wellcome) were introduced for clinical use in 1986 and have proven effective in life-threatening cases of digoxin toxicity (48,49).

Indications

The indications for digoxin-specific antibody fragments (Fab) are listed in Table 53.6. All of the conditions in this table are life-threatening, and many are resistant to therapy with conventional modalities. The largest clinical experience with antibody therapy has been in cases of hyperkalemia, high-grade AV block, and malignant ventricular arrhythmias. In these conditions, immunotherapy has elicited favorable responses in 90% of cases (50).

TABLE 53.6. INDICATIONS FOR IMMUNOTHERAPY OF DIGITALIS TOXICITY

Any one of the following:
- Digoxin dose > 10 mg
- Serum digoxin level > 6 ng/mL
- Serum potassium > 5.5 mEq/L*
- High-grade atrioventricular block*
- Malignant ventricular ectopic rhythms*
  - Multifocal ventricular ectopias
  - Bigeminy/trigeminy
  - Ventricular tachycardia/fibrillation

*When the condition is (or likely to be) refractory to conventional treatment modalities.

> **TABLE 53.7. DOSING RECOMMENDATIONS FOR DIGOXIN-SPECIFIC ANTIBODY FRAGMENTS (FAB)**
>
> **Total Body Load (TBL)**
>
> TBL = Oral digoxin dose (mg) × 0.8*
>
> $$TBL = \frac{Serum\ digoxin\ level\ (ng/mL) \times 5.6\ (L/g) \times Weight\ (kg)}{1000}$$
>
> | **Fab Dose** | **Cost†** |
> |---|---|
> | Fab (mg) = TBL (mg) × 66.6 | 1 mg Fab = $9.65 |
> | Fab (vials) = $\frac{TBL\ (mg)}{0.6\ (mg/vial)}$ | 1 vial Fab = $386 |
> | Empiric dose = 800 mg or 20 vials | Empiric Fab = $7720 |
>
> * Adjust oral dosage by 0.8 (bioavailability factor) only for digoxin tablets, not for digoxin capsules or elixir.
> † Based on the average wholesale price listed in the 1994 Red Book. Montvale, NJ: Medical Economics, 1994:169.

Dosage Recommendations

The dosage of antibody fragments is determined according to the relationships shown in Table 53.7. Each vial of Digibind contains 40 mg of antibody fragments, and binds 0.6 mg of digoxin. The total body content of digoxin (estimated using the digoxin dose or the serum digoxin level) is used to determine the appropriate dose of antibody fragments. If neither the dose nor the serum digoxin level is known, antibody fragments can be given in the empiric dose shown in Table 53.7.

The dose of antibody fragments is usually infused over 30 minutes but can be given by rapid intravenous injection (48). Because the response is not immediate, bolus injection may be preferred when a rapid response is desirable. Most responses are evident within 1 hour after drug administration, and peak responses require another 3 hours to develop (50).

Plasma Digoxin Levels

An increase in plasma digoxin levels occurs in all patients who receive digoxin-specific antibody fragments. The antibody fragments have such a high affinity for digoxin that they displace digoxin from tissue binding sites, and this raises the amount of Fab-bound digoxin in extracellular fluid. Within minutes after antibody administration, plasma levels of digoxin (most bound to Fab) can be 20 times higher than pretreatment levels (51). These levels gradually decline over the next few days, as Fab fragments are cleared by the kidneys. The clinical laboratory uses a radioimmunoassay that measures both free and bound forms of digoxin, so monitoring plasma digoxin levels is misleading in the first few days following antibody therapy.

Financial Burden

Therapy with antibody fragments is extremely costly, as indicated in Table 53.7. As a result, immunotherapy should be limited to cases in which it is clearly indicated.

NITROPRUSSIDE

Nitroprusside is a rapidly acting vasodilator whose therapeutic uses and potential for toxicity are described in Chapter 18. The toxic potential of nitroprusside is a reflection of its **cyanide** content, which **accounts for 44% of the molecular weight of nitroprusside** (52–54). Nitroprusside-induced cyanide intoxication may be responsible for over 1000 deaths each year (52), and this has led to the recommendation that nitroprusside be abandoned for clinical use (52).

CYANIDE METABOLISM

The nitroprusside molecule is a ferricyanide complex that contains five cyanide atoms and a nitrosyl group bound to iron in the oxidized (Fe-III) state. The molecule is disrupted in circulating blood, releasing the nitrosyl group as nitric oxide, which mediates the vasodilator actions of nitroprusside. The fate of the free cyanide that is released is shown in Figure 53.4 (53–55). When cyanide combines with the oxidized iron in cytochrome oxidase, it blocks the use of oxygen and inhibits the production of high-energy phosphate compounds. Two chemical reactions prevent cyanide from reacting with cytochrome oxidase. One involves the binding of cyanide to the oxidized iron in methemoglobin. The other reaction involves the transfer of sulfur from a donor molecule (thiosulfate) to cyanide to form a thiocyanate compound, which is then cleared by the kidneys. The latter transulfuration reaction is the principal mechanism for removing cyanide from the human body.

Capacity for Cyanide Removal

Healthy adults of average size have enough methemoglobin to bind the cyanide in 18 mg of nitroprusside, and enough thiosulfate to bind the cyanide in 50 mg of nitroprusside (53). When taken together, the human body has the capacity to detoxify 68 mg of nitroprusside. At a nitroprusside infusion of 2 µg/kg/minute (therapeutic range) in an 80-kg adult, this 68 mg capacity is reached 500 minutes (8.3 hours) after the onset of infusion. This illustrates the limited capacity of the human body to detoxify nitroprusside, even under ideal conditions. The removal of cyanide is further limited by thiosulfate depletion, which is common in smokers and postoperative patients (53,54).

CYANIDE INTOXICATION

The limited capacity of the human body to remove cyanide was not appreciated when nitroprusside was introduced for clinical use in 1976 (53). As a result, **cyanide accumulation is common during nitroprus-**

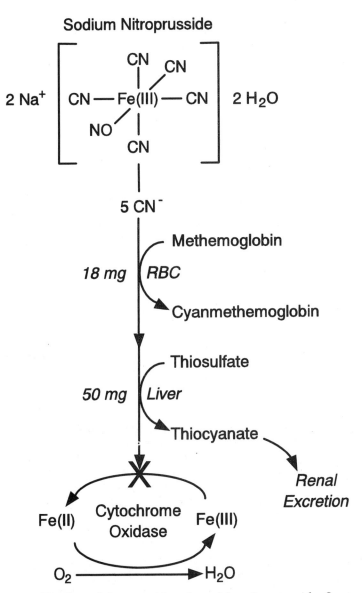

Figure 53.4. The fate of free cyanide released by nitroprusside. See text for explanation.

side infusions, even in low therapeutic doses (e.g., 1 μg/kg/minute) (53,54). The clinical manifestations of cyanide intoxication are listed in Table 53.8. One of the early signs of cyanide accumulation is nitroprusside tachyphylaxis (53). Signs of impaired oxygen use (i.e., a decrease in oxygen extraction ratio and lactic acidosis) often do not appear until the late stages of cyanide intoxication (55). Lactic acidosis

TABLE 53.8. CYANIDE INTOXICATION: DIAGNOSIS AND THERAPY

Clinical Features

Early: Behavioral changes   Late: Coma, convulsions
        Narrowed (Sao_2–Svo_2) $Svo_2 > 85\%$
        Nitroprusside tachyphylaxis   Lactic acidosis

Blood Cyanide Level*

Toxicity	Micrograms/mL	Micromoles/L
None	<0.5	<20
Mild	0.5–2.5	20–95
Severe	>2.5	>95
Fatal	>3.0	>114

Cyanide Antidote Kit[†]

Amyl nitrate inhaler, inhale for 1 min, or 3% sodium nitrite, 10 mL (300 mg) intravenously over 15 min and 25% sodium thiosulfate, 50 mL (12.5 g) intravenously over 15 min

* From Hall AH, Rumack BH. Clinical toxicology of cyanide. Ann Emerg Med 1986;15:1067.
[†] Eli Lilly & Co.

is not a sensitive marker of cyanide intoxication (53,54), and **the absence of lactic acidosis during nitroprusside infusion does not exclude the possibility of cyanide accumulation.**

Diagnosis

Whole blood cyanide levels can be used to document cyanide intoxication, as shown in Table 53.8. However, the results of cyanide assays are not immediately available (a STAT specimen usually requires 3 to 4 hours to be processed) (54), so immediate decisions regarding cyanide intoxication are often based on the clinical presentation. **Nitroprusside tachyphylaxis is an important early marker of cyanide accumulation.**

Prevention

Because cyanide intoxication is common and often overlooked, measures aimed at preventing cyanide accumulation during nitroprusside therapy are particularly valuable. The most effective preventive measure is to avoid the use of nitroprusside. Another effective measure is **adding thiosulfate to the nitroprusside infusate,** using the doses presented in Chapter 18 (54). This latter measure **should be a mandatory practice for nitroprusside infusions.**

Therapy

Treatment of cyanide intoxication should begin with the inhalation of 100% oxygen. The **Cyanide Antidote Kit** (Eli Lilly & Co.) can be used as described in Table 53.8 (56). Nitrites promote the oxidation of hemoglobin to methemoglobin and promote cyanide binding to methemoglobin. The cyanide bound to methemoglobin must eventually be eliminated from the body by transulfuration, so thiosulfate should always be given with nitrites.

Because nitrite therapy creates methemoglobinemia, alternative methods of cyanide binding have been explored. The affinity of cyanide for cobalt has led to the use of hydroxocobalamin (100 mL of a 5% solution infused over 15 minutes) (57), which combines with cyanide to form cyanocobalamin (vitamin B_{12}), which is then excreted in the urine. This strategy is popular in Europe, but the lack of a suitable hydroxocobalamin preparation has hampered its use in the United States.

THIOCYANATE INTOXICATION

The most important mechanism for cyanide removal involves the formation of thiocyanate, which is slowly excreted in the urine. When renal function is impaired, thiocyanate can accumulate and produce a toxic syndrome that is distinct from cyanide intoxication (53,54). The clinical features include anxiety, confusion, pupillary constriction, tinnitus, hallucinations, and generalized seizures (53,54). Thiocyanate can also produce hypothyroidism by blocking the thyroid uptake of iodine (54).

The diagnosis of thiocyanate toxicity is established by the serum thiocyanate level. Normal levels are below 10 mg/L, and clinical toxicity is usually accompanied by levels above 100 mg/L (54). Thiocyanate intoxication can be treated by hemodialysis or peritoneal dialysis.

OPIOIDS

The opioids are common offenders in overdoses involving illicit street drugs, and the opioid analgesic morphine is the most common cause of toxic drug reactions involving hospitalized patients (45). The adverse side effects of the opioid analgesics are described in Chapter 8. The following description focuses on the treatment of opioid intoxication with the opioid antagonist naloxone.

NALOXONE

Naloxone is a pure opioid antagonist that binds to endogenous opioid receptors but does not elicit any agonist responses. It is most effective in blocking μ-receptors (analgesia, respiratory depression) and κ-receptors (sedation, pupillary constriction), and least effective in blocking σ-receptors (delirium, hallucinations).

Routes of Administration

Naloxone (0.4 mg/mL or 1 mg/mL) is usually given intravenously (58), but it can also be given endotracheally (59), by intralingual injection, or by submental injection (60,61). The **submental injection** of naloxone is easily performed with a 23-gauge, 1.5-in. needle inserted in the midline about halfway between the mandible and thyroid cartilage. The needle is directed superiorly and advanced approximately 1 in. to make the injection. The drug is introduced into the muscles at the base of the tongue and is absorbed into the sublingual circulation. This approach is safe and can elicit a response in less than 2 minutes (61).

Dosing Recommendations

In opioid overdose, reversal of the sedation usually requires smaller doses of naloxone than reversal of the respiratory depression.

Depressed mental state. For patients with a depressed sensorium but no respiratory depression, the initial dose of naloxone should be 0.4 mg intravenous push. This can be repeated in 2 minutes, if necessary. A total dose of 0.8 mg should be effective if the mental status changes are caused by an opioid derivative (62). In patients with known opioid dependency, the bolus dose of naloxone should be reduced to 0.1 or 0.2 mg (62).

Respiratory depression. For patients who have evidence of respiratory depression the initial dose of naloxone should be 2 mg intravenous push. This dose is repeated every 2 minutes if necessary, to a total dose of 10 mg (58,62).

The effects of naloxone last approximately 60 to 90 minutes, which is less than the duration of action of most opioids. Therefore, a favorable response to naloxone should be followed by repeat doses at 1-hour intervals or by a continuous infusion. For a **continuous naloxone infusion,** the hourly dose of naloxone should be two-thirds of the effective bolus dose (a 6-hour dose can be added to 250 or 500 mL of saline and the solution infused over 6 hours) (63). To achieve steady-state drug levels in the early infusion period, a second bolus of naloxone (at one-half the original bolus dose) is given 30 minutes after the infusion is started. The duration of the infusion varies (according to the drug and the dose ingested), but the average duration is 10 hours (62).

Empiric Therapy

Patients with a depressed mental state of undetermined etiology are often given naloxone (0.8 to 2 mg intravenous push) as empiric therapy. This practice has been questioned because it elicits a favorable response in fewer than 5% of cases (64). An alternative approach has been proposed where **empiric naloxone is indicated only for patients with pinpoint pupils who have circumstantial evidence of opioid abuse** (e.g., needle tracks) (62,64). When naloxone is used in this manner, a favorable response is expected in approximately 90% of patients (64).

Adverse Reactions

Naloxone has few side effects. The most common adverse reaction is the opioid withdrawal syndrome (anxiety, abdominal cramps, vomiting, and piloerection). There are case reports of acute pulmonary edema (most in the early postoperative period) and generalized seizures following naloxone administration (62), but these complications are rare.

TRICYCLIC ANTIDEPRESSANTS

Overdose of tricyclic antidepressants (e.g., amitriptyline, desipramine, doxepin, and imipramine) is the leading cause of death from pharmaceutical drug overdose in the United States (4).

TOXIC MANIFESTATIONS

The toxic effects of the tricyclic antidepressants result primarily from their anticholinergic actions and their ability to block the reuptake of neurotransmitters such as norepinephrine (65). Serious toxicity usually emanates from the central nervous system or cardiovascular system.

Central Nervous System

Early manifestations include fever, agitation, and pupillary dilatation. Advanced cases are characterized by delirium, coma, and generalized seizures. The neurotoxic manifestations are attributed to anticholinergic effects.

Cardiovascular

Early signs include tachycardia and hypertension, which are attributed to blockade of norepinephrine reuptake. Depletion of norepinephrine in nerve terminals leads to postural and supine hypotension. Cardiac conduction abnormalities (prolonged QRS interval), arrhythmias (ventricular ectopics, wide-complex tachycardias), and a decreased cardiac output are seen in advanced cases.

CLINCAL EVALUATION

Admission to the ICU is warranted for patients with life-threatening complications, such as delirium, coma, seizures, cardiac arrhythmias, or hypotension. Toxic manifestations often require 6 to 12 hours to become apparent, and in the early period after drug ingestion, the principal task is to identify patients who are likely to develop serious toxicity. Plasma drug levels can be useful in confirming the diagnosis of tricyclic overdose but not in predicting progression to serious toxicity (65). The electrocardiogram has the greatest predictive value in asymptomatic patients.

Prolongation of the QRS interval can be a prognostic sign for progression to seizures (QRS above 0.10 second) and serious arrhythmias (QRS above 0.16 second) (66). Therefore, asymptomatic patients with a prolonged QRS interval usually are admitted for observation (admission to a telemetry area is appropriate).

MANAGEMENT

Management of tricyclic overdose in the ICU usually involves seizures, cardiac arrhythmias, or hypotension.

Seizures

Benzodiazepines usually are effective in treating generalized seizures in tricyclic overdose. Diazepam (5 to 10 mg) and lorazepam (1 to 2 mg) are equally effective. Seizures refractory to these agents have responded to midazolam (10 mg intravenously, then 6 mg/hour) (67). Barbiturates can also be used for refractory seizures, but phenytoin has limited efficacy (65).

Arrhythmias

The treatment of choice for serious arrhythmias in tricyclic overdose is alkalinization of the blood with **sodium bicarbonate** (68). Alkalinization reverses the cardiotoxic actions of the tricyclics by an unknown mechanism. The goal of alkalinization is a serum pH of 7.50 to 7.55, which can be achieved by intermittent bolus doses of sodium bicarbonate at a dosage of 1 to 2 mEq/kg. Alkalinization has also been accompanied by an improved mental status and resolution of hypotension in tricyclic overdoses (68).

Hypotension

Hypotension in tricyclic overdose can be the result of cardiac dysfunction, peripheral vasodilation, or both. Therefore, hypotension that does not respond to volume infusion should prompt insertion of a pulmonary artery catheter to guide management. If the problem is a cardiac dysfunction, dobutamine should be used; if the problem is a low systemic vascular resistance, norepinephrine should be used. Dopamine can promote arrhythmias in tricyclic overdose and should be avoided (65).

REFERENCES

INTRODUCTION

1. Dasta JF. Drug prescribing issues in the intensive care unit: finding answers to common questions. Crit Care Med 1994;22:909–912.
2. Trunet P, Borda IT, Rouget AV, et al. The role of drug-induced illness in admissions to an intensive care unit. Intensive Care Med 1986;12:43–46.
3. Jankel CA, Speedie SM. Detecting drug interactions: a review of the literature. DICP Ann Pharmacother 1990;24:982–989.

ACETAMINOPHEN

4. Litovitz TL, Holm KC, Clancy C, et al. 1992 Annual Report of the American Association of Poison Control Centers Toxic Exposure Surveillance System. Am J Emerg Med 1993;11:494–555.
5. Anker AL, Smilkstein MJ. Acetaminophen: concepts and controversies. Emerg Med Clin North Am 1994;12:335–350.
6. Janes J, Routledge PA. Recent developments in the management of paracetamol (acetaminophen) poisoning. Drug Safety 1992;7:170–177
7. Whitcomb DC, Block GD. Association of acetaminophen hepatotoxicity with fasting and ethanol use. JAMA 1994;272:1845–1850.

8. Dequay B, Malinverni R, Lauterburg BH. Glutathione depletion in HIV-infected patients: role of cysteine deficiency and effect of oral N-acetylcysteine. AIDS 1992;6:815–820.
9. British National Formulary No. 27. London: British Medical Association, 1994; 20–21.
10. Holdiness MR. Clinical pharmacokinetics of N-acetylcysteine. Clin Pharmacokinet 1991;20:123–134.
11. Smilkstein MJ, Knapp GL, Kulig KW, Rumack BH. Efficacy of oral N-acetylcysteine in the treatment of acetaminophen overdose. Analysis of the National Multicenter Study. N Engl J Med 1988;319:1557–1562.
12. Harrison PM, Keays R, Bray GP, et al. Improved outcome of paracetamol-induced fulminant hepatic failure by late administration of N-acetylcysteine. Lancet 1990;335:1572–1573.
13. Miller LF, Rumack BH. Clinical safety of high doses of acetylcysteine. Semin Oncol 1983;10(Suppl 1):76–85.
14. Sunman W, Hughes A, Sever P. Anaphylactoid response to intravenous acetylcysteine. Lancet 1992;339:1231–1232.
15. Spiller HA, Krenzelok EP, Grande GA, et al. A prospective evaluation of the effect of activated charcoal before oral N-acetylcysteine in acetaminophen overdose. Ann Emerg Med 1994;23:519–523.

BENZODIAZEPINES

16. Dasta JF, Fuhrman TM, McCandles C. Patterns of prescribing and administering drugs for agitation and pain in a surgical intensive care unit. Crit Care Med 1994;22:974–980.
17. Hansen-Flaschen JH, Brazinsky S, Basile C, Lanken PN. Use of sedating drugs and neuromuscular blocking agents in patients requiring mechanical ventilation for respiratory failure. JAMA 1991;266:2870–2875.
18. Gaudreault P, Guay J, Thivierge RL, Verdy I. Benzodiazepine poisoning. Drug Safety 1991;6:247–265.
19. Bodenham A. Reversal of prolonged sedation using flumazenil in critically ill patients. Anesthesia 1989;44:603–605.
20. Ritz R, Elsasser S, Schwander J. Controlled sedation in ventilated intensive care patients. Resuscitation 1988;16(Suppl):S83–S89.
21. Pepperman ML. Double-blind study of the reversal of midazolam-induced sedation in the intensive care unit with flumazenil (RO 15-1788): effect on weaning from ventilator. Anesth Intensive Care 1990;18:38–44.
22. Breheny FX. Reversal of midazolam sedation with flumazenil. Crit Care Med 1992;20:736–739.
23. Howland MA. Flumazenil. In: Goldfrank LR, Flomenbaum NE, Lewin NA, et al., eds. Goldfrank's toxicologic emergencies. Norwalk, CT: Appleton & Lange, 1994;805–810.
24. Shalansky SJ, Naumann TL, Englander FA. Therapy update: effect of flumazenil on benzodiazepine-induced respiratory depression. Clin Pharmacol 1993;12:483–487.
25. Martens F, Koppel C, Ibe K, et al. Clinical experience with the benzodiazepine antagonist flumazenil in suspected benzodiazepine or ethanol poisoning. J Toxicol Clin Toxicol 1990;28:341–356.
26. Doyon S, Roberts JR. Reappraisal of the "coma cocktail." Emerg Med Clin North Am 1994;12:301–316.
27. Chern TL, Hu SC, Lee CH, Deng JF. Diagnostic and therapeutic utility of flumazenil in comatose patients with drug overdose. Am J Emerg Med 1993; 11:122–124.
28. Haverkos GP, DiSalvo RP, Imhoff TE. Fatal seizures after flumazenil administration in a patient with mixed overdose. Ann Pharmacother 1994;28:1347–1349.

BETA RECEPTOR ANTAGONISTS

29. Kerns W II, Kline J, Ford MD. Beta blocker and calcium channel blocker toxicity. Emerg Med Clin North Am 1994;12:365–390.
30. Weinstein RS. Recognition and management of poisoning with beta-adrenergic blocking drugs. Ann Emerg Med 1984;13:1123–1131.
31. Brancato DJ. Recognizing potential toxicity of phenol. Vet Hum Toxicol 1982; 24:29–30.
32. Chernow B, Zaloga G, Malcolm D, et al. Glucagon's chronotropic action is calcium-dependent. J Pharmacol Exp Ther 1987;241:833–837.
33. Lucchesi BR. The role of calcium in excitation–contraction coupling in cardiac and vascular smooth muscle. Circulation 1989;80:IV1–IV10.

CALCIUM ANTAGONISTS

34. Ramoska EA, Spiller HA, Winter M, Borys D. A one-year evaluation of calcium channel blocker overdoses: toxicity and treatment. Ann Emerg Med 1993;22: 196–200.
35. Ramoska EA, Spiller HA, Myers A. Calcium channel blocker toxicity. Ann Emerg Med 1990;19:649–653.
36. Jameson SJ, Hargarten SW. Calcium pretreatment to prevent verapamil-induced hypotension in patients with SVT. Ann Emerg Med 1992;21:84 (editorial).
37. Zaritsky A, Morowicz M, Chernow B. Glucagon antagonism of calcium blocker-induced myocardial dysfunction. Crit Care Med 1988;16:246–251.
38. Doyon S, Roberts J. The use of glucagon in a case of calcium channel blocker overdose. Ann Emerg Med 1993;22:1229–1233.
39. Walter FG, Frye G, Mullen JT, et al. Amelioration of nifedipine poisoning associated with glucagon therapy. Ann Emerg Med 1993;22:1234–1237.
40. Wolf LR, Spadafora MP, Otten EJ. Use of amrinone and glucagon in a case of calcium channel blocker overdose. Ann Emerg Med 1993;22:1225–1228.
41. Goenen M, Col J, Compere A, et al. Treatment of severe verapamil poisoning with combined amrinone-isoproterenol therapy. Am J Cardiol 1986;58: 1142–1143.
42. Kuhn M. Severe bradyarrhythmias following calcium pretreatment. Am Heart J 1991;121:1813–1814.

DIGITALIS

43. Red Book. 100th ed. Montvale, NJ: Medical Economics, 1996;98.
44. Krisanda TJ. Digitalis toxicity. Postgrad Med 1992;91:273–284.
45. Evans PS, Pestotnik SL, Classen DC, et al. Preventing adverse drug events in hospitalized patients. Ann Pharmacother 1994;28:523–527.
46. McDonnell Cooke D. The use of central nervous system manifestations in the early detection of digitalis toxicity. Heart Lung 1993;22:477–481.
47. Moorman JR, Pritchett ELC. The arrhythmias of digitalis intoxication. Arch Intern Med 1986;145:1289–1292.
48. Martiny SS, Phelps SJ, Massey KL. Treatment of digitalis intoxication with digoxin-specific antibody fragments: a clinical review. Crit Care Med 1988; 16:629–635.
49. Lalonde RL, Deshpande R, Hamilton PP, et al. Acceleration of digoxin clearance by activated charcoal. Clin Pharmacol Ther 1985;37:367–371.
50. Antmann EM, Wenger TL, Butler VP, et al. Treatment of 150 cases of life-threatening digitalis intoxication with digoxin-specific Fab antibody fragments. Circulation 1990;81:1744–1752.
51. Ujhelyi MR, Robert S, Cummings DM, et al. Influence of digoxin immune Fab

therapy and renal dysfunction on the disposition of total and free digoxin. Ann Intern Med 1993;119:273–277.

NITROPRUSSIDE

52. Robin ED, McCauley R. Nitroprusside-related cyanide poisoning. Time (long past due) for urgent, effective interventions. Chest 1992;102:1842–1845.
53. Curry SC, Arnold-Capell P. Nitroprusside, nitroglycerin, and angiotensin-converting enzyme inhibitors. In: Blumer JL, Bond GR, eds. Toxic effects of drugs used in the ICU. Critical care clinics. Philadelphia:WB Saunders, 1991;555–582.
54. Hall VA, Guest JM. Sodium nitroprusside-induced cyanide intoxication and prevention with sodium thiosulfate prophylaxis. Am J Crit Care 1992;2:19–27.
55. Arieff AI. Is measurement of venous oxygen saturation useful in the diagnosis of cyanide poisoning? Am J Med 1992;93:582–583.
56. Kirk MA, Gerace R, Kulig KW. Cyanide and methemoglobin kinetics in smoke inhalation victims treated with the Cyanide Antidote Kit. Ann Emerg Med 1993;22:1413–1418.
57. Curry SC, Connor DA, Raschke RA. Effect of the cyanide antidote hydroxocobalamin on commonly ordered serum chemistry studies. Ann Emerg Med 1994;24:65–67.

OPIOIDS

58. Naloxone hydrochloride. AHFS Drug Information 95. Bethesda, MD: American Society of Hospital Systems Pharmacists, 1995;1418–1420.
59. Tandleberg D, Abercrombie D. Treatment of heroin overdose with endotracheal naloxone. Ann Emerg Med 1982;11:443–445.
60. Maio RF, Gaukel B, Freeman B. Intralingual naloxone injection for narcotic-induced respiratory depression. Ann Emerg Med 1987;16:572–573.
61. Salvucci AA Jr, Eckstein M, Iscovich AI. Submental injection of naloxone. Ann Emerg Med 1995;25:719–720.
62. Doyon S, Roberts J. Reappraisal of the "coma cocktail." Emerg Med Clin 1994; 12:301–316.
63. Goldfrank L, Weisman RS, Errick JK, et al. A dosing nomogram for continuous infusion intravenous naloxone. Ann Emerg Med 1986;15:566–569.
64. Hoffman JR, Schriger DL, Luo JS. The empiric use of naloxone in patients with altered mental status: a reappraisal. Ann Emerg Med 1991;20:246–252.

TRICYCLIC ANTIDEPRESSANTS

65. Weisman R, Howland MA, Hoffman RS, Cohen H. et al. Cyclic antidepressants. In: Goldfrank LR, Flomenbaum NE, Lewin NA, et al., eds. Goldfrank's toxicologic emergencies. 5th ed. Norwalk, CT: Appleton & Lange, 1994; 725–734.
66. Boehnert M, Lovejoy FH Jr. Value of the QRS duration versus the serum drug level in predicting seizures and ventricular arrhythmias after acute overdose of tricyclic antidepressants. N Engl J Med 1985;313:474–479.
67. Kumar A, Bleck TP. Intravenous midazolam for the treatment of refractory status epilepticus. Crit Care Med 1992;20:483–488.
68. Hoffman JR, Votey SR, Bayer M, Silver L. Effect of hypertonic sodium bicarbonate in the treatment of moderate to severe cyclic antidepressant overdose. Am J Emerg Med 1993;11:336–341.

SUGGESTED READING

Goldfrank LR, Flomenbaum NE, Lewin NA, et al., eds. Goldfrank's toxicologic emergencies. 5th ed. Norwalk, CT: Appleton & Lange, 1994.

chapter

54

DRUG DOSING ADJUSTMENTS IN THE ICU

This final chapter is a compilation of some of the important drug dosing adjustments mentioned throughout the book. The information is presented in tabular form, with each drug or group of drugs listed in alphabetical order. Included for each drug is the normal or usual dosage, along with pertinent dosage adjustments for drug interactions, renal insufficiency, hepatic insufficiency, and advanced age. The sources for the recommended dosage alterations are listed in the bibliography at the end of this chapter. The information in this chapter is by no means exhaustive (as this would require a separate text of its own), but it does provide a quick reference of dosage adjustments for drugs that are commonly used in the ICU. Most of the recommendations in this chapter are for parenteral drug therapy.

GLOMERULAR FILTRATION RATE

Many of the dose alterations in this chapter are based on the glomerular filtration rate (GFR). This can be estimated in adults using the equation shown below (see Cockroft and Gault, 1976).

$$\text{GFR (mL/min)} = \frac{(140 - \text{Age}) \times \text{wt (kg)} \times (0.85 \text{ for women})}{72 \times \text{Serum creatinine (mg/dL)}}$$

(54.1)

Note the additional factor of 0.85 for women, indicating that the GFR in women is 85% of the GFR in men. The body weight in this calculation should be the *ideal* or lean body weight (see the Reference Tables in the Appendix for a list of ideal body weights in adult men and women). However, if a patient has a body weight that is below the ideal weight, the *actual* body weight should be used in the calculation (see Robert et al, 1993). Estimates of GFR based on the Cockcroft–Gault equation shown here are reported to be more accurate than estimates of GFR based on urinary creatinine clearances in critically ill patients (see Robert et al, 1993).

The Elderly

Note that the Cockroft–Gault equation predicts that the GFR in adults will decline with advancing age. After the age of 40, the GFR decreases approximately 1 mL/minute each year (see Zawada and Boice, 1993). This means that a 70-year-old patient will have a GFR that is 30 mL/minute less than that of a 40-year-old patient. This age-related decline in GFR can influence the dosing guidelines for drugs that are eliminated by the kidneys. Therefore, **the GFR is an important consideration for dosing adjustments in elderly patients** as well as in patients with renal disease.

Drug	Normal Dose	Conditions	Recommendation
Acetaminophen	650 mg q6hr	Hepatic insufficiency Patients with: HIV infection Malnutrition Chronic ETOH	Avoid acetaminophen. Increased risk of hepatotoxicity from acetaminophen. Avoid acetaminophen if possible, or use with extreme caution.
Acetazolamide	250 mg q6hr	GFR <30 mL/min	Avoid acetazolamide.
Adenosine	6–12 mg IV	Administration through central venous catheter	Reduce dosage by 50%.
		Combined treatment with: β Blockers Calcium blockers Dipyridamole	Reduce dosage by 50%.
		Theophylline (blocks adenosine receptors)	Avoid combined treatment.
Aminoglycosides Amikacin Gentamicin Tobramycin	2–3 mg/kg q8hr 1–1.5 mg/kg q8hr 1–1.5 mg/kg q8hr	GRF 10–50 mL/min GFR <10 mL/min	Reduce single doses by 30 to 70% and give q12–18hr. Reduce single doses by 70% and give q24–48hr.
Amphotericin	0.5–1 mg/kg/day	GFR <10 mL/min TPN solutions	Extend dosage interval to 48 or 72 hr. Do not add to TPN solutions (incompatible).
Ampicillin	1–3 g q6hr	GFR <15 mL/min	Extend dosage interval to 24 hr.
Amrinone	5–10 µg/kg/min	GFRI <10 mL/min	Reduce dosage rate 25 to 50%.

Drug	Normal Dose	Conditions	Recommendation
Aztreonam	1–2 g q8–12 hr	GFR <10 mL/min	Reduce dosage by 70%.
		Hepatic insufficiency	Reduce dosage by 25%.
Benzodiazepines Diazepam Midazolam	See Tables 8.3 and 8.4.	Combined treatment with: Cimetidine Erythromycin Isoniazid Ketoconazole Metoprolol Propranolol Valproic acid	Impaired metabolism of diazepam and midazolam may lead to increased dose requirements. Avoid erythromycin–midazolam combination. Otherwise, adjust benzodiazepine dosage only as needed.
		Combined treatment with theophylline	Avoid theophylline (antagonizes benzodiazepine sedation) if sedation an important goal.
		Combined treatment with rifampin	Enhanced metabolism of midazolam and diazepam may lead to increased dosage requirements.
		Obesity	Use ideal body weight for midazolam dosing.
Calcium	200 mg IV over 10 minutes	Digitalis treatment	Avoid if possible, or reduce dosage by 50% and infuse over 30 minutes.
		Digitalis toxicity	Avoid calcium infusions.
Cephalosporins Cefazolin	1 g q8hr	GFR <10 mL/min	Extend dosage interval to 24–48 hr.
Cefotaxime	2 g q8hr	GFR <10 mL/min	Extend dosage interval to 24 hr.
Ceftazidime	2 g q8hr	GFR 10–50 mL/min	Extend dosage interval to 24 hr.
		GFR <10 mL/min	Extend dosage interval to 48 hr.
Cimetidine	Continuous infusion: Start at 37.5 mg/hr. Increase in 12.5 mg/hr increments if needed to a maximum of 100 mg/hr.	GFR 20–50 mL/min	Reduce dosage rate by 25% and do not exceed rate of 67 mg/hr.
		GFR <20 m/min	Reduce dosage rate by 75% and do not exceed rate of 33 mg/hr.

Note: Cimetidine blocks renal creatinine secretion and can increase serum creatinine without a change in GFR. This can cause a falsely low estimate of GFR.

Drug	Normal Dose	Conditions	Recommendation
Ciprofloxacin	400 mg IV q12hr	GFR <10 mg/min	Reduce dosage by 50%.
		Combined treatment with: Coumadin Theophylline	See recommendations for coumadin and theophylline.
Coumadin	5–10 mg PO daily	Combined treatment with: Amiodarone Ciprofloxacin Cimetidine Erythromycin Fluconazole Isoniazid Metronidazole Quinidine Salicylates Trimothoprim–sulfamethoxazole	Possible enhanced anticoagulant effect. Avoid combined treatment with amiodarone, metronidazole, and salicylates. Otherwise, monitor INR.
		Combined treatment with: Corticosteroids Estrogen Nafcillin Phenobarbital Rifampin Sucralfate	Possible reduced anticoagulant effect. Monitor INR.
Digoxin	0.125–0.5 mg qd	Combined treatment with: Amiodarone Quinidine Verapamil Captopril Diltiazem	Possible enhanced digoxin effect. Reduce digoxin dosage by 50% for combined treatment with amiodarone, quinidine, and verapamil. Otherwise, monitor serum digoxin levels.
		GFR <10 mL/min	Decrease single dose by 75% and administer every 48 hr.

Note: In renal failure, there may be a spuriously high serum digoxin level by radioimmunoassay.

Drug	Normal Dose	Conditions	Recommendation
Fluconazole	200 to 400 mg/day	GFR 20–50 mL/min	Reduce dosage by 50%.
		GFR <20 mL/min	Reduce dosage by 75%.
		Combined treatment with: Phenytoin Warfarin	See recommendations for phenytoin and warfarin.
Haloperidol	See Table 8.6.	Prolonged QT Interval	Avoid haloperidol.

Drug	Normal Dose	Conditions	Recommendation
Heparin	See Table 7.4.	Morbid obesity (body weight >130 kg)	Heparin dose may be much smaller than recommended in the standard weight-based dosing nomogram.
		High–dosage nitroglycerin (>350 μg/min)	May be increased heparin requirement. Monitor PTT.
Imipenem	0.5–1 g q6hr	GFR 20–50 mL/min	Extend dosage interval to 8 hr.
		GFR <20 mL/min	Extend dosage interval to 12 hr.
		Seizure disorder	Do not exceed a daily dose of 2 g or 25 mg/kg.
Insulin	Variable	Treatment with ACE Inhibitors	Possible decrease in insulin requirement. Monitor blood glucose.
		IV fluid containers and infusion sets	Expect 20 to 30% loss of insulin dose as a result of adsorption to plastic and glass in IV infusion sets.
Ketorolac	15 to 30 mg q6hr	GFR <50 mL/min	Reduce dosage by 50%.
Lidocaine	1–4 mg/min	Hepatic insufficiency Low cardiac output Combined treatment with: Cimetidine β-Blockers	Reduce dosage by 50% because of impaired lidocaine metabolism.
		Elderly patients	Limit lidocaine infusion to less than 12 hr.
Metronidazole	7.5 mg/kg q6hr	GFR <10 mL/min	Reduce dosage by 50%.
		Combined treatment with phenytoin	See recommendations for phenytoin.
Nitroglycerin	10–200 μg/min	Polyvinychloride tubing	Nitroglycerin absorbs to PVC. Use Nitrostat infusion sets (nonadsorbent material).
		Increased intracranial pressure	Avoid nitroglycerin.

Drug	Normal Dose	Conditions	Recommendation
Nitroprusside	0.2–10 μg/kg/min	GFR <10 mL/min	Avoid nitroprusside.
Opioids			
Meperidine	50–100 mg q4hr	GFR <50 mL/min	Avoid (neurotoxic metabolite accumulates when renal function is impaired).
Morphine	1–6 mg/hr	GFR <10 mL/min	Reduce dosage by 50%.
		Hepatic insufficiency	Avoid if possible.
Fentanyl	30–100 μg/hr	GFR <10 mL/min	Reduce dosage by 50%.
Pentamidine	4 mg/kg/day	GFR <10 mL/min	Extend dosage interval to 48 hr
Phenytoin	300–400 mg/day	Combined treatment with: Amiodarone Fluconazole Isoniazid Metronidazole	Possible enhanced phenytoin toxicity. Monitor serum levels.
		Hypoalbuminemia	Same as above.
		Combined treatment with: Coumadin Diazepam Glucocorticoids Phenobarbital Theophylline Valproic acid	Possible reduction in phenytoin efficacy. Monitor serum levels.
		Glucose-containing intravenous fluids	Do not add phenytoin to glucose-containing fluids (incompatible).
Procainamide	2–6 mg/min	Mild heart failure	Reduce dosage by 25%.
		Elderly patients with renal dysfunction	Reduce dosage by 50%.
		Cimetidine treatment	Possible increase in serum procainamide levels. Monitor serum levels.
		GFR <10 mL/min	Avoid if possible.
Propofol	See Table 8.4.	Obesity	Dose is determined by ideal body weight.
Ranitidine	50 mg IV q8–10hr	GFR <50 mL/min	Extend dosage interval to 24 hr.

Drug	Normal Dose	Conditions	Recommendation
Theophylline	See Table 25.4.	Low cardiac output Hepatic insufficiency	Reduce dosage by 50% and follow serum drug levels.
		Combined treatment with: Cimetidine Ciprofloxacin Erythromycin Enoxacin Propranolol Verapamil	Reduce dosge by 30 to 50% and follow serum theophylline levels.
		Combined treatment with: Phenytoin Phenobarbital Obesity	Normal dosing may be subtherapeutic. Follow serum theophylline levels. Dosing by ideal body weight may be subtherapeutic. Follow serum drug levels.
Thiamine	3–100 mg/day	Hypomagnesemia	Thiamine will be ineffective until magnesium depletion is corrected.
		Parenteral nutrition	Do not add thiamine to amino acid solutions (may be degraded by sulfites in the solutions).
Trimethoprim–sulfamethoxazole (TMP–SMX)	For *Pneumocystis carinii* pneumonia (PCP): 20 mg TMP/kg/day and 100 mg SMX/kg/day in 3 to 4 divided doses	GFR 15 to 30 mL/min	Normal dose for 48 hr, then reduce daily dose by 50% and extend dose interval to 12 hr.
		GFR <15 mL/min	Reduce daily dose by 50%, and extend dosage interval to 12 hr.
Vancomycin	500 mg IV q6hr	GFR 10–30 mL/min	Extend dosage interval to 48 hr.
		GFR <10 mL/min	Extend dosage interval to 4 days.
		Heparin infusion	Heparin degrades vancomycin. Use a separate IV line.
Verapamil	5–10 mg IV	Combined treatment with: ACE inhibitors β-blockers Quinidine	Possible enhanced negative inotropic and vasodilator effects of verapamil. Avoid combined treatment if possible.
		Digoxin treatment	See recommendations for digoxin.

REFERENCES

GENERAL DRUG INFORMATION SOURCES

1. Young DS. Effects of drugs on clinical laboratory tests. 3d ed. Washington, DC: American Association for Clinical Chemistry, 1990.
2. Rizock MA, Hillman CDM, eds. The Medical Letter handbook of adverse drug interactions. New Rochelle, NY: The Medical Letter, 1991.
3. Schrier RW, Gambertoglio JG, eds. Handbook of drug therapy in liver and kidney disease. Boston: Little, Brown, 1991.
4. Trissel LA. Handbook on injectable drugs. 8th ed. Bethesda, MD: American Society of Hospital Pharmacists, 1994.
5. Bennett WM, Aronoff GR, Golper TA, et al. Drug prescribing in renal failure: dosing guidelines for adults. 3d ed. Philadelphia: American College of Physicians, 1994.
6. Chernow B, ed. The pharmacologic approach to the critically ill patient. 3d ed. Baltimore: Williams & Wilkins, 1994.
7. McEvoy GK, ed. AHFS Drug Information, 1995. 38th ed. Bethesda, MD: American Society of Health-System Pharmacists, 1995.
8. Semla TP, Beizer JL, Higbee MD. Geriatric dosage handbook. 2nd ed. Hudson, OH: Lexi-Comp Inc., 1995.

REVIEWS

1. Bass NM, Williams RL. Guide to drug dosage in hepatic disease. Clin Pharmacokinet 1988;15:396–420.
2. Zawada ET, Boice JL. Clinical pharmacology in aged intensive care unit patients. J Intensive Care Med 1993;8:289–297 (38 references).
3. Kubisty CA, Arns PA, Wedlund PJ, Branch RA. Adjustment of medications in liver failure. In: Chernow B, ed. The pharmacologic approach to the critically ill patient. 3d ed. Baltimore: Williams & Wilkins, 1994;95–113 (186 references).
4. Kroh UF. Drug administration in critically ill patients with acute renal failure. New Horiz 1995;3:748–759 (42 references).
5. Preston L, Briceland LL, Lomaestro BM, et al. Dosing adjustment of 10 antimicrobials for patients with renal impairment. Ann Pharmacother 1995;29:1202–1207.

GLOMERULAR FILTRATION RATE

1. Cockroft DW, Gault MN. Prediction of creatinine clearance from serum creatinine. Nephron 1976;16:31–41.
2. Robert S, Zarowitz BJ, Peterson EL, et al. Predictability of creatinine clearance estimates in critically ill patients. Crit Care Med 1993;21:1487–1495.

ADENOSINE

1. McCollam PL, Uber W, Van Bakel AB. Adenosine-related ventricular asystole. Ann Intern Med 1993;118:315–316.
2. Rankin AC, Brooks R, Ruskin JM, McGovern BA. Adenosine and the treatment of supraventricular tachycardia. Am J Med 1992;92:655–664.

3. Chronister C. Clinical management of supraventricular tachycardia with adenosine. Am J Crit Care 1993;2:41–47.

AMINOGLYCOSIDES

1. See Bennett WM et al, pp. 18-19.

AMPHOTERICIN

1. See Bennett WM et al, p. 31.

AMRINONE

1. Bottorff MB, Rutledge DR, Pieper JA. Evaluation of intravenous amrinone: the first of a new class of positive inotropic agents with vasodilator properties. Pharmacotherapy 1984;5:227–236.

AZTREONAM

1. See Bennett WM et al, p. 25.
2. McLeod CM, Bartley EA, Payne JA, et al. Effects of cirrhosis on kinetics of aztreonam. Antimicrob Agents Chemother 1984;26:493–497.

BENZODIAZEPINES

1. Levine RL. Pharmacology of intravenous sedatives and opioids in critically ill patients. Crit Care Clin 1994;10:709–731.
2. Hoegholm A, Steptoe P, Fogh B, et al. Benzodiazepine antagonism by aminophylline. Acta Anesth Scand 1989;33:164–166.
3. Olkkola KT, Aranko K, Luurila H, et al. A potentially hazardous interaction between erythromycin and midazolam. Clin Pharmacol Ther 1993;53:298–305.

CEPHALOSPORINS

1. Gustaffero CA, Steckelberg JM. Cephalosporin antimicrobial agents and related compounds. Mayo Clin Proc 1991;66:1064–1073.

CIMETIDINE

1. Ben-Menachem T, Fogel R, Patel RV, et al. Prophylaxis for stress-related gastric hemorrhage in the medical intensive care unit. Ann Intern Med 1994;121:568–575.

COUMADIN

1. Crussel-Porter LL, Rindone JP, Ford MA, Jaskar DW. Low-dose fluconazole therapy potentiates the hypoprothrombinemic response to warfarin. Arch Intern Med 1993;153:102–104.
2. See McEvoy GK, ed., p. 928.

DIGOXIN

1. Marcus MI. Pharmacokinetic interactions between digoxin and other drugs. J Am Coll Cardiol 1985;5:82A–90A.

FLUCONAZOLE

1. Terrell CL, Hughes CE. Antifungal agents used for deep-seated mycotic infections. Mayo Clin Proc 1992;67:69–91.

HEPARIN

1. Holliday DM, Watling SM, Yanos J. Heparin dosing in a morbidly obese patient. Ann Pharmacother 1994;28:1110–1111.
2. Jaffrani NA, Ehrenpreis S, Laddu A, Somburg J. Therapeutic approach to unstable angina: nitroglycerin, heparin, and combined therapy. Am Heart J 1993; 126:1239–1242.

IMIPENEM

1. Hellinger WC, Brewer NS. Imipenem. Mayo Clin Proc 1991;66:1074–1081.
2. Vos MC, Vincent HH, Yzerman EPF. Clearance of imipenem/cilastatin in acute renal failure patients treated by continuous hemodiafiltration (CAVHD). Intensive Care Med 1992;18:282–285.

INSULIN

1. See Trissel LA, pp. 585–590.

LIDOCAINE

1. Marcus FI, Opie LH. Antiarrhythmic drugs. In: Opie LH, ed. Drugs for the heart. 4th ed. Philadelphia: WB Saunders, 1995;221–222.

NITROGLYCERIN

1. See Trissell LA, pp. 777–780.

NITROPRUSSIDE

1. Curry SC, Arnold-Cappell P. Nitroprusside, nitroglycerin, and angiotensin-converting enzyme inhibitors. Crit Care Clin 1991;7:555–582.

2. FDA Medical Bulletin 21:3–4, March, 1991.

OPIATES

1. Shochet RB, Murray GB. Neuropsychiatric toxicity of meperidine. J Intensive Care Med 1988;3:246–252.
2. Chauvin M, Sandouk P, Scherrmann JM, et al. Morphine pharmacokinetics in renal failure. Anesthesiology 1987;66:327–331.

PHENYTOIN

1. Cadle RM, Zenon GJ, Rodriguez-Barradas MC, Hamill RJ. Fluconazole-induced symptomatic phenytoin toxicity. Ann Pharmacother 1994;28:191–195.
2. Smart HL, Somerville KW, Williams J, et al. The effects of sucralfate upon phenytoin absorption in man. Br J Pharmacol 1985;20:238–240.
3. Lindow J, Wijdicks EFM. Phenytoin toxicity associated with hypoalbuminemia in critically ill patients. Chest 1994;105:602–604.
4. Wijdicks EFM. Seizures in the intensive care unit. In Neurology of critical illness. Philadelphia: FA Davis, 1995;19–33.
5. Epilepsy Foundation of America's Working Group on Status Epilepticus. Treatment of convulsive status epilepticus. JAMA 1993;270:854–859.

PROCAINAMIDE

1. Marcus FI, Opie LH. Antiarrhythmic drugs. In: Opie LH, ed. Drugs for the heart. Philadelphia: WB Saunders, 1995;216–217.

PROPOFOL

1. Barr J. Propofol: A new drug for sedation in the intensive care unit. Int Anesthesiol Clin 1993;31:131–154.

RANITIDINE

1. McEvoy GK. AHFS Drug Information 1995. Bethesda, MD: American Society of Health System Pharmacists, 1995;2057–2062.

THEOPHYLLINE

1. Sessler CN, Brady W. Theophylline toxicity: How to minimize the potential risk. J Crit Illness 1991;6:1045–1054.
2. Joeng CS, Huang SC, Jones DW. Theophylline disposition in Korean patients with congestive heart failure. Ann Pharmacother 1994;28:396–401.
3. Spivey JM, Laughlin PH, Goss TF. Theophylline toxicity secondary to ciprofloxacin administration. Ann Emerg Med 1991;20:1131–1134.
4. Rizzo A, Mirabella A, Bonanno A. Effect of body weight on the volume of distribution of theophylline. Lung 1988;166:269–276.

THIAMINE

1. Dyckner T, Nyhlin H, Wester PO. Aggravation of thiamine deficiency by magnesium depletion. Acta Med Scand 1985;218:129–131.
2. LaFrance RJ, Miyagawa CI. Pharmaceutical considerations in total parenteral nutrition. In: Fischer JE, ed. Total parenteral nutrition. 2nd ed. Boston: Little, Brown, 1991;57–98.

TRIMETHOPRIM–SULFAMETHOXAZOLE

1. Paap CM, Nahata MC. Trimethoprim/sulfamethoxazole dosing during renal dysfunction. Ann Pharmacother 1995;29:1300.

VANCOMYCIN

1. Brown DL, Manro LS. Vancomycin dosing chart for use in patients with renal impairment. Am J Kidney Dis 1988;11:15–19.

VERAPAMIL

1. Piepho RW, Culbertson VL, Rhodes RS. Drug interactions with the calcium entry blockers. Circulation 1987;75:V181–V194.
2. See McEvoy GK, ed., pp. 1153–1154.

section XV
APPENDICES

Thus in dealing with any subject matter, find out what entities are undeniably involved, and state everything in terms of these entities.

Bertrand Russell

Section XV

APPENDICES

appendix

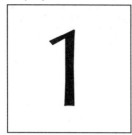

UNITS AND CONVERSIONS

The units of measurement in the medical sciences are taken from the metric system (centimeter, gram, second) and the Anglo-Saxon system (foot, pound, second). The metric units were introduced during the French Revolution and were revised in 1960. The revised units are called Système International (SI) units and are currently the worldwide standard. The United States initially refrained from adopting the SI units, but this position has softened in recent years.

UNITS OF MEASUREMENT IN THE SYSTÈME INTERNATIONAL (SI)

Parameter	Dimensions	Basic SI Unit (Symbol)	Equivalences
Length	L	Meter (m)	1 inch = 2.54 cm
Area	L^2	Square meter (m^2)	1 square centimeter (cm^2) = 10^4 m^2
Volume	L^3	Cubic meter (m^3)	1 liter (L) = 0.001 m^3
			1 milliliter (ml) = 1 cubic
			centimeter (cm^3)
Mass	M	Kilogram (kg)	1 pound (lb) = 453.5 g
			1 kg = 2.2 lbs
Density	M/L^3	Kilogram per cubic meter	1 kg/m^3 = 0.001 kg/dm^3
		(kg/m^3)	Density of water = 1.0 kg/dm^3
			Density of mercury = 13.6 kg/dm^3
Velocity	L/T	Meters per second (m/sec)	1 mile per hour (mph) = 0.4 m/sec
Acceleration	L/T^2	Meters per second squared	1 ft/sec^2 = 0.03 m/sec^2
		(m/sec^2)	
Force	$M \times (L/T^2)$	Newton (N)	1 dyne = 10^{-5} N
		= kg × (m/sec^2)	
Pressure	$\dfrac{M \times (L/T^2)}{L^2}$	Pascal (Pa) = N/m^2	1 kPa = 7.5 mm Hg
			= 10.2 cm H_2O
			1 mm Hg = 1.00000014 torr
			(See conversion table for kPa and
			mmHg)
Heat	$M \times (L/T^2)$ $\times$ L	Joule (J) = N × m	1 kilocalorie (kcal) = 4184 J
Temperature	None	Kelvin (K)	0° C = −273 K
			(See conversion table for °C and °F)
Viscosity	M, 1/L, 1/T	Newton × second per	Centipoise (cP) = 10^{-3}N · sec/m^2
		square meter	
		(N · sec/m^2)	
Amount of a	N	Mole (mol) = molecular	Equivalent (Eq) = mol × valence
substance		weight in grams	
Concentration	N/L^3	mol/m^3 = Molarity	Ionic strength = mol/kg
	N/M	mol/kg = Molality	

TEMPERATURE CONVERSIONS

(°C)	(°F)
100	212
41	105.8
40	104
39	102.2
38	100.4
37	98.6
36	96.8
35	95
34	93.2
33	91.4
32	89.6
31	87.8
30	86
0	32

°F = (9/5 °C) + 32
°C = 5/9 (°F − 32)

APOTHECARY AND HOUSEHOLD CONVERSIONS	
Apothecary	**Household**
1 grain = 60 mg	1 teaspoonful = 15 mL
1 ounce = 30 g	1 dessertspoonful = 10 mL
1 fluid ounce = 30 mL	1 tablespoonful = 15 mL
1 pint = 500 mL	1 wineglassful = 60 mL
1 quart = 1000 mL	1 teacupful = 120 mL
	1 tumblerful = 240 mL
	1 petroleum barrel = 42 gal

PRESSURE CONVERSIONS					
mmHg	**kPa**	**mmHg**	**kPa**	**mmHg**	**kPa**
41	5.45	61	8.11	81	10.77
42	5.59	62	8.25	82	10.91
43	5.72	63	8.38	83	11.04
44	5.85	64	8.51	84	11.17
45	5.99	65	8.65	85	11.31
46	6.12	66	8.78	86	11.44
47	6.25	67	8.91	87	11.57
48	6.38	68	9.04	88	11.70
49	6.52	69	9.18	89	11.84
50	6.65	70	9.31	90	11.97
51	6.78	71	9.44	91	12.10
52	6.92	72	9.58	92	12.24
53	7.05	73	9.71	93	12.37
54	7.18	74	9.84	94	12.50
55	7.32	75	9.98	95	12.64
56	7.45	76	10.11	96	12.77
57	7.58	77	10.24	97	12.90
58	7.71	78	10.37	98	13.03
59	7.85	79	10.51	79	13.17
60	7.98	80	10.64	100	13.90

Kilopascal (kPa) = 0.133 × mmHg
mmHg = 7.50 × kPa

pH AND HYDROGEN ION CONCENTRATION	
pH	[H$^+$] (nEq/L)
6.8	160
6.9	125
7.0	100
7.1	80
7.2	63
7.3	50
7.4	40
7.5	32
7.6	26
7.7	20
7.8	16

SIZES OF PLASTIC TUBE DEVICES			
French Size	Outside Diameter*		Device
	inches	mm	
1	0.01	0.3	Vascular catheters
4	0.05	1.3	
8	0.10	2.6	Small-bore
10	0.13	3.3	feeding tubes
12	0.16	4.0	
14	0.18	4.6	Nasogastric tubes
16	0.21	5.3	
18	0.23	6.0	
20	0.26	6.6	Chest tubes
22	0.28	7.3	
24	0.31	8.0	
26	0.34	8.6	
28	0.36	9.3	
30	0.39	10.0	
32	0.41	10.6	
34	0.44	11.3	
36	0.47	12.0	
38	0.50	12.6	

* Diameters can vary with manufacturers. However, a useful rule of thumb is OD (mm) × 3 = French size.

SIZES OF INTRAVASCULAR CATHETERS			
	Outside Diameter*		
Gauge	inches	mm	Type of Catheter
26	0.018	0.45	Butterfly devices
25	0.020	0.50	
24	0.022	0.56	
23	0.024	0.61	
22	0.028	0.71	Peripheral vascular catheters
21	0.032	0.81	
20	0.036	0.91	
19	0.040	1.02	
18	0.048	1.22	Central venous catheters
16	0.064	1.62	
14	0.080	2.03	Introducer catheters
12	0.104	2.64	
10	0.128	3.25	
* Diameters can vary with manufacturers.			

appendix

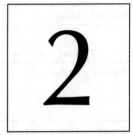

SELECTED REFERENCE RANGES

REFERENCE RANGES FOR SELECTED CLINICAL LABORATORY TESTS

Substance	Fluid*	Traditional Units	× k =	SI Units
Acetoacetate	P, S	0.3–3.0 mg/dL	97.95	3–30 μmol/L
Alanine aminotransferase (SGPT)	S	0–35 U/L	0.016	0–0.58 μkat/L
Albumin	S	4–6 g/dL	10	40–60 g/L
	CSF	11–48 mg/dL	0.01	0.11–0.48 g/L
Aldolase	S	0–6 U/L	16.6	0–100 nkat/L
Alkaline phosphatase	S	(F)30–100 U/L	0.016	0.5–1.67 μkat/L
		(M)45–115 U/L		0.75–1.92 μkat/L
Ammonia	P	10–80 μg/dL	0.587	5–50 μmol/L
Amylase	S	0–130 U/L	0.016	0–2.17 μkat/L
Aspartate aminotransferase (SGOT)	S	0–35 U/L	0.016	0–0.58 μkat/L
β-Hydroxybutyrate	S	<1.0 mg/dL	96.05	<100 μmol/L
Bicarbonate	S	22–26 mEq/L	1	22–26 mmol/L
Bilirubin: Total	S	0.1–1.0 mg/dL	17.1	2–18 μmol/L
Conjugated	S	≤0.2 mg/dL		≤4 μmol/L
Blood urea nitrogen (BUN)	P, S	8–18 mg/dL	0.367	3.0–6.5 mmol/L
Calcium: Total	S	8.5–10.5 mg/dL	1	2.2–2.6 mmol/L
Ionized	P	2.2–2.3 mEq/L		1.10–1.15 mmol/L
Chloride	P, S	95–105 mEq/L	1	95–105 mmol/L
	CSF	120–130 mEq/L		120–130 mmol/L
	U	10–200 mEq/L		10–200 mmol/L
Creatinine	S	0.6–1.5 mg/dL	0.09	0.05–0.13 mmol/L
	U	15–25 mg/kg/24 hr	0.009	0.13–0.22 mmol/kg/24 h
Cyanide: Nontoxic	WB	<5 μg/dL	3.8	<19 μmol/L
Lethal		>30 μg/dL		>144 μmol/L
Fibrinogen	P	150–350 mg/dL	0.01	1.5–3.5 g/L
Fibrin split products	S	<10 μg/mL	1	<10 mg/L
Glucose (fasting)	P	70–100 mg/dL	0.06	3.9–6.1 mmol/L
	CSF	50–80 mg/dL		2.8–4.4 mmol/L
Lactate: Resting	P	<2.0 mEq/L	1	<2 mmol/L
Exercise		<4.0 mEq/L		<4 mmol/L
Lactate dehydrogenase (LDH)	S	50–150 U/L	0.017	0.82–2.66 μkat/L
Lipase	S	0–160 U/L	0.017	0–2.66 μkat/L
Magnesium	P, S	1.8–3.0 mg/dL	0.41	0.8–1.2 mmol/L
		1.5–2.4 mEq/L	0.5	0.8–1.2 mmol/L
Osmolality	S	280–296 mOsm/kg	1	280–296 mmol/kg
Phosphate	S	2.5–5.0 mg/dL	0.32	0.80–1.60 mmol/L
Potassium	P, S	3.5–5.0 mEq/L	1	3.5–5.0 mmol/L
Total protein	P, S	6.0–8.0 g/dL	10	60–80 g/L
	CSF	<40 mg/dL	0.01	<0.40 g/L
	U	<150 mg/24 hr	0.01	<1.5 g/24 hr
Sodium	P, S	135–147 mEq/L	1	135–147 mmol/L
Thyroxine: Total	S	4–11 μg/dL	12.9	51–142 nmol/L
Free		0.8–2.8 ng/dL		10–36 pmol/L
Triiodothyronine (T₃)	S	75–220 ng/dL	0.015	1.2–3.4 nmol/L

* *P* = Plasma, *S* = serum, *U* = urine, *WB* = whole blood, *CSF* = cerebrospinal fluid, *RBC* = red blood cell.

Adapted from the New England Journal of Medicine SI Unit Conversion Guide. Waltham, MA: Massachusetts Medical Society, 1992.

REFERENCE RANGES FOR VITAMINS AND TRACE ELEMENTS

Substance	Fluid*	Traditional Units	× k =	SI Units
Chromium	S	0.14–0.15 ng/mL	17.85	2.5–2.7 nmol/L
Copper	S	70–140 µg/dL	0.16	11–22 µmol/L
Folate	RBC	140–960 ng/mL	2.26	317–2169 nmol/L
Iron	S	(M)80–180 µg/dL	0.18	(M)14–32 µmol/L
		(F)60–160 µg/dL		(F)11–29 µmol/L
Ferritin	P, S	(M)20–250 ng/mL	1	(M)20–250 µg/L
		(F)10–120 ng/mL		(F)10–120 µg/L
Manganese	WB	0.4–2.0 µg/dL	0.018	0.7–3.6 µmol/L
Pyridoxine	P	20–90 ng/mL	5.98	120–540 nmol/L
Riboflavin	S	2.6–3.7 µg/dL	26.57	70–100 nmol/L
Selenium	WB	58–234 µg/dL	0.012	0.7–2.5 µmol/L
Thiamine (total)	P	3.4–4.8 µg/dL	0.003	98.6–139 µmol/L
Vitamin A	P, S	10–50 µg/dL	0.349	0.35–1.75 µmol/L
Vitamin B$_{12}$	S	200–1000 pg/mL	0.737	150–750 pmol/L
Vitamin C	S	0.6–2 mg/dL	56.78	30–100 µmol/L
Vitamin D	S	24–40 ng/mL	2.599	60–105 nmol/L
Vitamin E	P, S	0.78–1.25 mg/dL	23.22	18–29 µmol/L
Zinc	S	70–120 µg/dL	0.153	11.5–18.5 µmol/L

*P = plasma, S = serum, WB = whole blood, RBC = red blood cell.
Adapted from the New England Journal of Medicine SI Unit Conversion Guide, Waltham, MA: Massachusetts Medical Society, 1992.

LABORATORY MEASUREMENTS THAT ARE INFLUENCED BY BODY POSITION

	% Decrease When Upright	
Measurement	Average	Range
Hemoglobin	5	3–7
Hematocrit	6	4–9
Serum calcium	4	2–6
Total protein	9	7–10
Serum albumin	9	6–14
Cholesterol	9	5–15
Alkaline phosphatase	9	5–11
Alanine aminotransferase	7	4–14

From Ravel R. Clinical laboratory medicine, Chicago: Yearbook Medical Publishing, 1989;4.

VOLUME USED BY AUTOMATED ANALYZERS IN THE CLINICAL LABORATORY

Laboratory Test	Instrument Volume (mL)
Arterial blood gases	1.0
Electrolyte panel	0.15
Complete blood cell count	0.125
Glucose	0.04

For serum assays, the volume of whole blood to be withdrawn is:

$$\text{Whole blood volume} = \frac{\text{Serum volume}}{1 - \text{Hematocrit}}$$

From Mayo Clin Proc 1993;68:255.

DESIRABLE WEIGHTS FOR ADULTS*				
Height		**Males**		
Feet	**Inches**	**Small Frame**	**Medium Frame**	**Large Frame**
5	2	128–134	131–141	138–150
5	3	130–136	133–143	140–153
5	4	132–138	135–145	142–156
5	5	134–140	137–148	144–160
5	6	136–142	139–151	146–164
5	7	138–145	142–154	149–168
5	8	140–148	145–157	152–172
5	9	142–151	148–160	155–176
5	10	144–154	151–163	158–180
5	11	146–157	154–166	161–184
6	0	149–160	157–170	164–188
6	1	152–164	160–174	168–192
6	2	155–168	164–178	172–197
6	3	158–172	167–182	172–202
6	4	162–176	171–187	181–207
		Females		
4	10	102–111	109–121	112–131
4	11	103–113	111–123	120–134
5	0	104–115	113–126	122–137
5	1	106–118	115–129	125–140
5	2	108–121	118–132	128–143
5	3	111–124	121–135	131–147
5	4	114–127	124–138	134–151
5	5	117–130	127–141	137–155
5	6	120–133	130–144	140–159
5	7	123–136	133–147	143–163
5	8	126–139	136–150	146–167
5	9	129–142	139–153	149–170
5	10	132–145	142–156	152–173
5	11	135–148	145–159	155–176
6	0	138–151	148–162	158–179

* Unclothed weights associated with the longest life expectancies. From the statistics bureau of the Metropolitan Life Insurance Company, 1983.

BASAL METABOLIC RATES		
Body Weight (kg)	kcal/24 hours	
	Male	**Female**
40	1340	1241
50	1485	1399
52	1505	1429
54	1555	1458
56	1580	1487
58	1600	1516
60	1630	1544
62	1660	1572
64	1690	1599
66	1725	1626
68	1765	1653
70	1785	1679
72	1815	1705
74	1845	1731
76	1870	1756
78	1900	1781
80	—	1805

From Talbot FB. Am J Dis Child 1938;5:455–459.

DETERMINATIONS OF BODY SIZE

Ideal Body Weight*

$$\text{Males: IBW (kg)} = 50 + 2.3 \text{ (Ht in inches} - 60)$$
$$\text{Females: IBW (kg)} = 45.5 + 2.3 \text{ (Ht in inches} - 60)$$

Body Mass Index†

$$BMI = \frac{\text{Wt (in lbs)}}{\text{Ht (in inches)}^2 \times 703}$$

Body Surface Area

Dubois Formula‡

$$BSA \text{ (m}^2) = \text{Ht (in cm)}^{0.725} \times \text{Wt (in kg)}^{0.425} \times 0.007184$$

Jacobson Formula§

$$BSA \text{ (m}^2) = \frac{\text{Ht (in cm)} + \text{Wt (in kg)} - 60}{100}$$

* Devine BJ. Drug Intell Clin Pharm 1974;8:650.
† Matz R. Ann Intern Med 1993;118:232.
‡ Dubois EF. Basal metabolism in health and disease. Philadelphia: Lea & Febiger, 1936.
§ Jacobson B. Medicine and clinical engineering. Englewood Cliffs, NJ: Prentice-Hall, 1977.

BODY BUILD AND BLOOD VOLUME IN ADULTS		
	Average Blood Volume (mL/kg)	
Body Build	**Males**	**Females**
Thin	65	60
Normal	70	65
Muscular	75	70
Obese	60	55
From Documenta Geigy Scientific Tables. 7th ed. Basel, Switzerland: JR Geigy, SA, 1970;528.		

BLOOD VOLUMES IN THE ELDERLY		
Volume	**Elderly Men**	**Elderly Women**
Whole blood	$(3809 \times BSA) - 2362$	$(1591 \times BSA) + 889$
Plasma	$(1{,}9995 \times BSA) - 667$	$(925 \times BSA) + 802$
Erythrocytes	$(1761 \times BSA) - 1609$	$(716 \times BSA) + 14$
From Cordtes PR et al. Surg Gynecol Obstet 1992;175:243–248.		

BODY FLUID DISTRIBUTION IN HEALTHY ADULTS			
Parameter	**Derivation**	**Male**	**Female**
Total body water	$0.55 \times$ body wt (kg)	600 mL/kg	500 mL/kg
Interstitial fluid	$0.16 \times$ body wt (kg)	160 mL/kg	160 mL/kg
Blood volume (BV)	$0.065 \times$ body wt (kg)	70 mL/kg	65 mL/kg
Erythrocyte volume (EV)	$EV = BV \times Hct$	33 mL/kg	27 mL/kg
Plasma volume (PV)	$PV = BV - EV$	37 mL/kg	38 mL/kg
Hematocrit (Hct)	$EV/BV \times 100$	47% (mean)	42% (mean)
		40–54%	37–47%
		(range)	(range)
From Documenta Geigy Scientific Tables. 7th ed. Basel, Switzerland: JR Geigy SA, 1970.			

PEAK EXPIRATORY FLOW RATES FOR HEALTHY MALES					
		Average Peak Flow (L/min)			
Age (yr)	Ht:	60"	65"	70"	75"
20		602	649	693	740
25		590	636	679	725
30		577	622	664	710
35		565	609	651	695
40		552	596	636	680
45		540	583	622	665
50		527	569	607	649
55		515	556	593	634
60		502	542	578	618
65		490	529	564	603
70		477	515	550	587

Peak Flow (L/min) = [3.95 − (0.0151 × Age)] × Ht (cm)

Regression equation from Leiner GC et al. Am Rev Respir Dis 1963;88:646.

PEAK EXPIRATORY FLOW RATES FOR HEALTHY FEMALES					
		Average Peak Flow (L/min)			
Age (yr)	Ht:	55"	60"	65"	70"
20		309	423	460	496
25		385	418	454	490
30		380	413	448	483
35		375	408	442	476
40		370	402	436	470
45		365	397	430	464
50		360	391	424	457
55		355	386	418	451
60		350	380	412	445
65		345	375	406	439
70		340	369	400	432

Peak Flow (L/min) = [2.93 − (0.0072 × Age)] × Ht (cm)

Regression equation from Leiner GC et al. Am Rev Respir Dis 1963;88:647.

appendix

3

CLINICAL SCORING SYSTEMS

The APACHE (Acute Physiology and Chronic Health Evaluation) scoring system was developed to provide an objective assessment of severity of illness in patients in the ICU. The scoring system is not meant for burn patients or post–cardiopulmonary bypass patients. Although there are limitations in predicting mortality in individual patients in the ICU, the APACHE scoring system is widely used in clinical studies to provide some measure of disease severity in the study patients. The following pages demonstrate how to generate an APACHE II score (1). Although there is an APACHE III scoring system (2), the APACHE II score is more widely used.
The APACHE II score is made up of three components:

1. **Acute Physiology Score (APS).** The largest component of the APACHE II score is derived from 12 clinical measurements that are obtained within 24 hours after admission to the ICU. The *most abnormal measurement* is selected to generate the APS component of the APACHE II score. If a variable has not been measured, it is assigned zero points.
2. **Age Adjustment.** From one to six points is added for patients older than 44 years of age.
3. **Chronic Health Evaluation.** An additional adjustment is made for patients with severe and chronic organ failure involving the heart, lungs, kidneys, liver, and immune system.

ACUTE PHYSIOLOGY SCORE

Points:	+4	+3	+2	+1	0	+1	+2	+3	+4
Temperature (°C)	≥41	39–40.9		38.5–38.9	36–38.4	34–35.9	32–33.9	30–31.9	≤29.9
Mean arterial pressure	≥160	130–159	110–129		70–109		50–69		≤49
Heart rate	≥180	140–179	110–139		70–109		55–69	40–54	≤39
Respiratory rate	≥50	35–49		25–34	12–24	10–11	6–9		≤5
[1]A-aPO$_2$	≥500	350–499	200–349		<200				
[2]PAO$_2$					>70	61–70		55–60	<55
Arterial pH	≥7.7	7.6–7.69		7.5–7.59	7.33–7.49		7.25–7.32	7.15–7.24	<7.15
[3]Serum bicarbonate (mEq/L)	≥52	41–51.9		32–40.9	23–31.9		18–21.9	15–17.9	<15
Serum sodium (mEq/L)	≥180		160–179	155–159	150–154	130–149	120–129	111–119	≤110
Serum potassium (mEq/L)	≥7	6–6.9		5.5–5.9	3.5–5.4	3–3.4	2.5–2.9		<2.5
Serum creatinine (mg/dL)	≥3.5	2–3.4	1.5–1.9		0.6–1.4		<0.6		
Hematocrit	≥60		50–59.9	46–49.9	30–45.9		20–29.9		<20
WBC count	≥40		20–39.9	15–19.9	3–14.9		1–2.9		<1
[4]15 − (Glasgow Coma Score) =									

1. If Fio$_2$ >50. 2. If Fio$_2$ <50%. 3. Use only if no ABGs.
Scoring Method
    1. Select the *most abnormal measurement* for each parameter in the first 24 hours after ICU admission.
    2. If a parameter has not been measured, assign it zero points.
    3. Add the corresponding points for all 12 parameters to obtain the Acute Physiology Score.
    4. Glasgow Coma Scale follows.

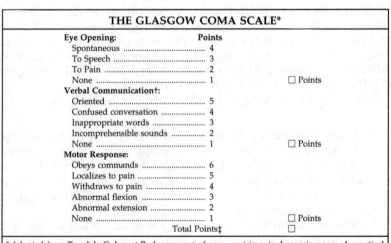

THE GLASGOW COMA SCALE*

Eye Opening: Points
    Spontaneous 4
    To Speech 3
    To Pain 2
    None 1   ☐ Points

Verbal Communication†:
    Oriented 5
    Confused conversation 4
    Inappropriate words 3
    Incomprehensible sounds 2
    None 1   ☐ Points

Motor Response:
    Obeys commands 6
    Localizes to pain 5
    Withdraws to pain 4
    Abnormal flexion 3
    Abnormal extension 2
    None 1   ☐ Points
                Total Points‡   ☐

* Adapted from Teasdale G, Jennet B. Assessment of coma and impaired consciousness. A practical approach. Lancet 1974;2:81–86.
† For intubated patients, assign a score of 1 for verbal communication
‡ Best score is 15 points; worst score is 3 points.

AGE ADJUSTMENT	
Age (yr)	**Points**
<44	0
45–54	2
55–64	3
65–74	5
>75	6

CHRONIC HEALTH ADJUSTMENT

For any of the following:
1. Biopsy proven cirrhosis.
2. Heart failure: NYHA Class IV
3. Severe COPD (hypercapnia, home oxygen)
4. Chronic dialysis
5. Immunocompromised

Add 2 points for elective surgery or neurosurgery, 5 points for emergency surgery.

TOTAL APACHE II SCORE

APS score _____

Age adjustment _____

Chronic health adjustment _____

Total APACHE II score _____

APACHE II SCORE AND MORTALITY IN 5815 ICU PATIENTS		
	Hospital Mortality (%)	
APACHE II Score	**Nonoperative**	**Postoperative**
0–4	4	1
5–9	6	3
10–14	12	6
15–19	22	11
20–24	40	29
25–29	51	37
30–34	71	71
≥35	82	87

Data from Knaus WA et al. Crit Care Med 1985;13:818–829.

Limitations

The following limitations of the APACHE II score deserve mention.

1. The APS score has no adjustments for measurements obtained in the presence of interventions such as hemodynamic support drugs, mechanical ventilation, or antipyretic therapy.

2. There is an exaggerated penalty for old age. For example, age greater than 65 years adds more points than an A-a P_{O_2} gradient above 500 mm Hg (6 points versus 4 points, respectively).
3. There is no consideration for malnutrition or cachexia in the chronic health evaluation.

MULTIPLE ORGAN DYSFUNCTION SCORE

The multiple organ dysfunction score was developed because of the direct relationship between the number of major organ systems failed and mortality in ICU patients. Unlike the APACHE II scoring system, which can only be used on admission to the ICU, the multiple organ dysfunction score can be determined daily. This allows identification of changing mortality risks in individual patients during the ICU stay.

THE MULTIPLE ORGAN DYSFUNCTION SCORE					
	Points				
Parameter	0	1	2	3	4
P_{AO_2}/F_{IO_2}	>300	226–300	151–225	76–150	≤75
Serum creatinine (μmol/L)	≤100	101–200	201–350	351–500	≥500
Serum bilirubin (μmol/L)	≤20	21–60	61–120	121–240	>240
Pulse-adjusted heart rate*	≤10	10.1–15	15.1–20	20.1–30	>30
Platelet count (per μL)	>120	81–120	51–80	21–50	≤20
Glasgow Coma Score[†]	15	13–14	10–12	7–9	≤6

* PAR = HR × (RAP/MAP); HR = heart rate, RAP = right atrial pressure, MAP = mean arterial pressure.
[†] The best estimate in the absence of sedation.
Scoring Method
  1. Select the *most abnormal result* for each parameter over a 24-hour period.
  2. If a parameter has not been measured, assign it zero points.
  3. Add the corresponding points for all 6 parameters to obtain the final score.
  4. A new score can be obtained for any subsequent 24-hour period.
From Marshall JC et al. Multiple organ dysfunction score: a reliable predictor of a complex clinical outcome. Crit Care Med 1995;23:1638–1652.

MULTIPLE ORGAN DYSFUNCTION SCORE AND ICU MORTALITY*			
Score	Mortality (%)	Score	Mortality (%)
0	0	13–16	50
1–4	1	17–20	75
5–8	3	>20	100
9–12	25		

* Mortality recorded in 692 patients in a Surgical ICU.
From Marshall JC et al. Crit Care Med 1995;23:1638–1652.

REFERENCES

1. Knaus WA, Draper EA, Wagner DP, Zimmerman JE. APACHE II: A severity of disease classification system. Crit Care Med 1985;13:818–828.
2. Knaus WA, Wagner DP, Draper EA, et al. The APACHE III Prognostic system. Chest 1991;100:1619–1636.

HEALTH CARE AND VITAL STATISTICS

CHARGES TO THE PATIENT FOR SELECTED HOSPITAL CARE SERVICES IN 1996*

Inpatient Laboratory Tests

Sodium	$52.75
Chloride	$51.75
Glucose	$24.50
BUN	$40.50
Creatinine	$129.00
Na, K, Cl, Creat	$170.75
Calcium	$29.75
Phosphate	$29.75
Magnesium	$70.00
Heme Panel	$35.25
WBC differential	$44.00
Arterial blood gas	$173.00
Urinalysis	$20.50
CPK	$258.25
Stat charge per test	$25.00

Average Daily Room Charge

Regular room	$993.00
Intermediate care unit	$1253.00
Intensive care unit	$1759.00

Radiographic Imaging

Chest, single view	$126.00
Chest, two views	$167.00
Abdomen, one view	$158.00
Abdomen, complete	$215.00
Portable charge	$100.00
Ultrasound, abdomen	$800.00
CT, abdomen (enhanced)	$1201.00
MRI, abdomen	$1761.00
CT, head (unenhanced)	$1342.00
CT, head (enhanced)	$1437.00
MRI, head	$1761.00

Miscellaneous

Echo, 2D	$1149.00
ECG	$222.00
Chest physical therapy	$149.00
Oxygen, hourly	$16.00

* Patient charges are those of the University of Pennsylvania Health System, Presbyterian Medical Center, for the 1996 fiscal year.

ANNUAL COST OF HEALTH CARE IN THE UNITED STATES

(Billions of dollars)

	1960	1970	1980	1990	1994
All health-related services	$26.9	$73.2	$247.2	$697.5	$949.4
Hospital care	$9.3	$28.0	$102.7	$256.5	$338.5
Physician services	$5.3	$13.6	$45.2	$140.5	$189.4
Medications	$4.2	$8.8	$21.6	$61.2	$78.6
Health-related research	$0.7	$2.0	$5.6	$8.5	$15.9

From Office of National Health Statistics, Health Care Financing Administration.

LIFE EXPECTANCY IN THE UNITED STATES

Years Expected At Birth

	White		Black	
Year	Female	Male	Female	Male
1950	72.2	60.8	62.9	59.1
1960	74.1	67.4	66.3	61.1
1970	75.6	68.0	69.4	61.3
1980	78.1	70.7	73.6	65.3
1990	79.4	72.9	75.2	67.0
1995	79.6	73.4	74.0	65.4

From National Center for Health Statistics, U.S. Department of Health and Human Services.

ANNUAL MORTALITY IN THE UNITED STATES

Year	Total Deaths*	Deaths per 1000 Population
1960	1,711,982	9.5
1970	1,921,031	9.5
1980	1,986,000	8.7
1990	2,162,000	8.6
1991	2,169,518	8.6
1992	2,175,613	8.5
1993	2,268,000	8.8
1994	2,286,000	8.8

* Excludes fetal deaths and deaths outside the United States.
From National Center for Health Statistics, US Department of Health and Human Services.

THE ELDERLY POPULATION IN THE UNITED STATES			
Year	Total U.S. Population (in millions)	Elderly Population (in millions)	
		>65 yr	>85 yr
1960	179.3	16.0 (8.9%)	0.9 (<0.01%)
1990	248.7	31.2 (12.6%)	3.1 (1.2%)
1995	262.8	33.5 (12.8%)	3.6 (1.4%)
2010	297.7	39.4 (13.2%)	5.6 (1.9%)
2050	393.9	78.8 (20.0%)	18.2 (4.6%)
From Bureau of the Census, U.S. Department of Commerce.			

WORLD POPULATION GROWTH RATE	
World Population (in billions)	Time for Each Growth Increment (yr)
1	2,000,000
2	100
3	30
4	15
5	7
From Rifkin J. Entropy and the greenhouse world. New York: Bantam Books, 1989;118.	

RELATIVE SIZE OF THE MEDICAL SPECIALTIES IN 1995			
Most Popular		Least Popular	
Specialty	Physicians	Specialty	Physicians
Internal medicine	88,241	Forensic pathology	466
Family practice	59,110	Aerospace medicine	575
Pediatrics	43,609	Colorectal surgery	990
Psychiatry	38,089	Preventive medicine	1269
General surgery	37,570	Nuclear medicine	1435
Ob–Gyn	33,519	Public health	1760
Anesthesiology	32,853	Thoracic surgery	2310
Orthopedics	22,037	Occupational medicine	3031
Radiology	19,808	Radiation oncology	3360
Emergency medicine	19,112	Allergy/immunology	4040
From 1997 World Almanac and Book of Facts. Mahwah NJ: World Almanac Books, 1997;969.			

MOST COMMONLY DISPENSED PRESCRIPTION DRUGS IN THE UNITED STATES IN 1995	
1. Premarin (estrogen)	11. Cardizem (diltiazem)
2. Synthroid (levothyroxine)	12. Coumadin (warfarin)
3. Zantac (ranitidine)	13. Zoloft (sertraline HCL)
4. Trimox (amox/TMP/SMX)	14. Zestril (lisonopril)
5. Lanoxin (digoxin)	15. Augmentin (amox/clav)
6. Amoxil (amoxicillin)	16. Biaxin (clarithromycin)
7. Procardia (nifedipine)	17. Triamterene/HCTZ
8. Vasotec (enalapril)	18. Ventolin (albuterol)
9. Proventil (albuterol)	19. Cipro (ciprofloxacin)
10. Prozac (fluoxetine)	20. Hydrocodone w/APAP

From 1996 Red Book. Montvale NJ: Medical Economics Co., 1996.

MOST COMMONLY REPORTED TOXIC INGESTIONS

Drugs	Cases Reported No.	Cases Reported Rank	Deaths No.	Deaths Rank
Acetaminophen (adult)	25,742	#2	18	#8
Aspirin (adult)	5,411	#6	8	#10
Benzodiazepines	33,516	#1	54	#2
β-Blockers	5,308	#7	16	#9
Calcium antagonists	6,683	#4	38	#4
Digitalis	2,310	#10	19	#7
Cocaine	3,713	#9	52	#3
Opiates	4,474	#8	33	#6
Theophylline	5,735	#5	35	#5
Tricyclic antidepressants	20,619	#3	146	#1

From Annual Report of the American Association of Poison Control Centers Toxic Exposure Surveillance System. Am J Emerg Med 1993;11:494.

Index

Note: Page numbers in *italics* indicate illustrations; those followed by t indicate tables.

in oxygen therapy, 389–390
shunt fraction and, 341–342, 343
variability in, 346t, 346–347
ventilation-perfusion ratio and, 339
wedged, 172–173, 173t
venous
in acid-base disorders, 590, 590–591
in cardiopulmonary resuscitation, 272
Blood lactate (See Lactate)
Blood loss (See also Bleeding; Hemorrhage; Hypovolemia)
classification of, 209t, 209–210
evaluation of, 210–214
fatal, 207
mild, response to, 208–209
pneumatic compression in, 218–219
Trendelenburg position in, 217–218
volume replacement for, 219–225 (See also Fluid resuscitation)
Blood pressure, 143–152
arterial pressure waveforms and, 148–149, 149
distortion of, 149–151, 150
direct measurement of, 147–152
flush test for, 150, 150–151
limitations of, 148
recording artifacts in, 149–152
resonant systems and, 149, 150
waveform distortion on, 149–151, 150
estimated mean, 151
in hypovolemia, 209t, 210
indirect measurement of, 143–147
accuracy of, 143, 144, 146, 146t
auscultatory method for, 145–146
bedside method of, 144–145
cuff bladder in
application of, 144–145
dimensions of, 144, 144–145
in low flow states, 145–146, 146t
oscillometric method for, 146–147, 147
mean arterial pressure and, 148–149, 151–152
pharmacologic maintenance of, 278–296
(See also Hemodynamic drugs)
pressure vs. flow waves in, 148
radial artery pressure and, 152
Blood products (See also Transfusion[s])
allergic reaction to, 701t, 703
resuscitative efficacy of, 219, 220
Blood salvage
intraoperative, 705
postoperative, 705–706
Blood sampling, pseudohyperkalemia and, 653–654
Blood transfusion (See Transfusion[s])
Blood volume
estimation of, 208
fluid volume and, 20, 208t
reference ranges for, 207–208, 873t
Blood warmers, in erythrocyte transfusion, 700

Body fluids (See under Fluid)
Body mass index, determination of, 872t
Body position (See Positioning)
Body size, determination of, 872t
Body surface area
calculation of, 872t
hemodynamic parameters and, 159
Body temperature
elevated (See Fever)
normal, 485–486
scales for, 485, 486t
Body weight
ideal, determination of, 872t
reference ranges for, 871t
Bohr equation, 343
Bowel, as occult source of catheter-related sepsis, 91, 91t
Bowel infarction, 497, 497–498
Bowel mucosa, changes in, nutritional deficits and, 737, 738, 762
Bowel rest
microbial translocation and, 95, 96, 534, 739
mucosal atrophy in, 737, 738, 755, 762
Brachiocephalic vein, length of, 64t
Bradycardia (See also Arrhythmias)
benzodiazepines and, 828, 830
opioids and, 127
Brain death, 788–791, 789t, 790
hemodynamic management in, 790–791
pituitary failure in, 791
Brain injury, postresuscitation, 224
Brainstem depression, alveolar hypoventilation in, 352t, 352–353
Branched-chain amino acids, in enteral formulas, 746
Breathing, rapid, in ventilator weaning, 476–477
Bretylium, for ventricular tachycardia, 331t, 332
Bronchoalveolar lavage, 526, 526t
in acute respiratory distress syndrome, 379–380
Bronchodilators, 404–411
aerosol administration of, 405, 405–407, 406
for anaphylaxis, 512, 513t
β-blockers as, 404t, 404–409
administration of, 405, 405–407, 406
for asthma, 407
side effects of, 407–409
response to
auto-PEEP and, 404
in mechanical ventilation, 429–430
peak expiratory flow and, 402, 403t
peak inspiratory pressure and, 403–404
theophylline as, 409t, 409–411, 410t
Bronchoscopy
fever and, 491
in HIV-related pneumonia, 550